APPLIED STATISTICAL DESIGNS FOR THE RESEARCHER

Biostatistics: A Series of References and Textbooks

Series Editor

Shein-Chung Chow

Vice President, Clinical Biostatistics and Data Management
Millennium Pharmaceuticals, Inc.
Cambridge, Massachusetts

Adjunct Professor
Temple University
Philadelphia, Pennsylvania

1. *Design and Analysis of Animal Studies in Pharmaceutical Development*, edited by Shein-Chung Chow and Jen-pei Liu
2. *Basic Statistics and Pharmaceutical Statistical Applications*, James E. De Muth
3. *Design and Analysis of Bioavailability and Bioequivalence Studies, Second Edition, Revised and Expanded*, Shein-Chung Chow and Jen-pei Liu
4. *Meta-Analysis in Medicine and Health Policy*, edited by Dalene K. Stangl and Donald A. Berry
5. *Generalized Linear Models: A Bayesian Perspective*, edited by Dipak K. Dey, Sujit K. Ghosh, and Bani K. Mallick
6. *Difference Equations with Public Health Applications*, Lemuel A. Moyé and Asha Seth Kapadia
7. *Medical Biostatistics*, Abhaya Indrayan and Sanjeev B. Sarmukaddam
8. *Statistical Methods for Clinical Trials*, Mark X. Norleans
9. *Causal Analysis in Biomedicine and Epidemiology: Based on Minimal Sufficient Causation*, Mikel Aickin
10. *Statistics in Drug Research: Methodologies and Recent Developments*, Shein-Chung Chow and Jun Shao
11. *Sample Size Calculations in Clinical Research*, Shein-Chung Chow, Jun Shao, and Hansheng Wang
12. *Applied Statistical Designs for the Researcher*, Daryl S. Paulson

ADDITIONAL VOLUMES IN PREPARATION

Advances in Clinical Trials Biostatistics, Nancy L. Geller

APPLIED STATISTICAL DESIGNS FOR THE RESEARCHER

DARYL S. PAULSON

BioScience Laboratories, Inc.
Bozeman, Montana, U.S.A.

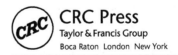

CRC Press
Taylor & Francis Group
Boca Raton London New York

CRC Press is an imprint of the
Taylor & Francis Group, an **informa** business

CRC Press
Taylor & Francis Group
6000 Broken Sound Parkway NW, Suite 300
Boca Raton, FL 33487-2742

First issued in paperback 2019

© 2003 by Taylor & Francis Group, LLC
CRC Press is an imprint of Taylor & Francis Group, an Informa business

No claim to original U.S. Government works

ISBN-13: 978-0-8247-4085-6 (hbk)
ISBN-13: 978-0-367-39506-3 (pbk)

Library of Congress Cataloging-in-Publication Data
A catalog record for this book is available from the Library of Congress.

Visit the Taylor & Francis Web site at
http://www.taylorandfrancis.com

and the CRC Press Web site at
http://www.crcpress.com

Series Introduction

The primary objectives of the *Biostatistics* series are to provide useful reference books for researchers and scientists in academia, industry, and government, and also to offer textbooks for undergraduate and/or graduate courses in the area of biostatistics. This book series will provide comprehensive and unified presentations of statistical designs and analyses of important applications in biostatistics, such as those in biopharmaceuticals. A well-balanced summary will be given of current and recently developed statistical methods and interpretations for both statisticians and researchers/scientists with minimal statistical knowledge who are engaged in the field of applied biostatistics. The series is committed to providing easy-to-understand, state-of-the-art references and textbooks. In each volume, statistical concepts and methodologies will be illustrated through real world examples.

Medical and pharmaceutical research are lengthy and costly processes, which involves discovery, formulation, laboratory development, animal studies, clinical development, and regulatory submission. These lengthy processes are necessary not only for understanding of the target disease but also for providing substantial evidence regarding efficacy and safety of the pharmaceutical entity under investigation prior to regulatory approval. In addition, it provides assurance that the pharmaceutical entity will possess good characteristics such as identity, strength, quality, purity, and stability after regulatory approval. Statistics plays an important role in medical and pharmaceutical research not only to provide a valid and fair assessment of the pharmaceutical entity under investigation prior to regulatory approval, but also to assure that the pharmaceutical entity possesses good characteristics with a desired accuracy and reliability. *Applied Statistical Designs for the Researcher* is a condensation of various useful experimental designs that are commonly employed in the medical and pharmaceutical industries. It covers important topics in medical and pharmaceutical research and development such as complete randomized two-factor factorial designs, small scale pilot designs, and nested designs. This volume provides useful approaches to medical and pharmaceutical research. It would be beneficial to biostatisticians, medical researchers, and pharmaceutical scientists who are engaged in the areas of medical and pharmaceutical research.

Shein-Chung Chow

Preface

This book is a condensation of the most useful experimental designs I have employed over the past twenty years. Initially, I was trained in medical microbiology with a strong background in applied statistics. Once I finished graduate school, I began work in the medical–pharmaceutical industry. Then, I worked on solid dosage form process validations, from which I learned the problems of using very complex statistical designs requiring many theoretical assumptions that were assumed to be true, but could not be assured. Reproducibility was the major problem. I began to use practical, robust, and easily understood designs whenever possible from that moment forward.

It was not long before I began working in clinical trials of both parenteral and topical drugs. Most of my experience in this area was in bioequivalency using regression analysis. From this I learned the value of small-scale pilot studies, determining which product of several was the most effective, as well as determining use or label instructions. When I launched my own biotechnology company, BioScience Laboratories, Inc., in 1991, the opportunity arose for greatly expanding statistically based studies in microbial death-rate kinetics, skin biotechnology, and clinical trials of topical antimicrobials.

This book represents the most useful approaches to research based on what I have learned over these years. The first chapter, "Research and Statistics," is a broad discussion of experimental process. Chapter 2, "Basic Review of Parametric Statistics," is a review of basic statistics. It is assumed that the reader knows how to perform basic statistical operations, such as deriving values of the mean and the standard deviation. However, no other knowledge is required. Chapter 3, "Exploratory Data Analysis," provides methods that enable the researcher to evaluate quickly the form of the data prior to computing a statistic. It involves the researcher intimately with the data so as to see the general data distribution, skewness, and outliers. Chapter 4, "Two-Sample Tests," is an in-depth view of the statistical workhorse, the Student's *t*-test. Three varieties are covered: comparisons of two different groups with different variances, two groups with the same variance, and matched, paired groups. The power, the detectable differences, and sample size calculations are also provided.

Chapter 5, "Completely Randomized One-Factor Analysis of Variance," introduces the analysis of variance (ANOVA) design; Chapter 6, "One and Two Restrictions on Randomization," further expands ANOVA designs and introduces Latin square designs; and Chapters 7, "Completely Randomized Two-Factor Factorial Designs," and 8, "Two-Factor Factorial Completely Randomized Blocked Designs," present more complex ANOVA designs.

Chapter 9, "Useful Small-Scale Pilot Designs: 2^k Designs" presents very useful screening approaches to comparing two factors and their interactions. Chapter 10, "Nested Statistical Designs," provides the reader with a background on common hierarchical ANOVA designs. Chapter 11, "Linear Regression," is a complete introduction to regression analysis, as well as to many ways of comparing the various confidence levels within the analysis.

Chapter 12, "Nonparametric Statistics," presents nonparametric analysis analogs to the parameteric ones previously presented. Unique to this book, the nonparametric analogs of their parametric counterparts are classified according to the strength of the collected data: nominal (qualitative non-rankable), ordinal (qualitative rankable), and interval continuous quantitative data. Finally, Chapter 13, "Introduction to Research Synthesis and Meta-Analysis and Concluding Remarks," provides a brief introduction to meta-analysis.

I wish to dedicate this book to my first statistics professor and the person who stimulated my love of statistics, the late Edward Perrasini of Great Falls, Montana. He was a teacher's teacher.

I want to thank John A. Mitchell, Ph.D., for his excellent and persistent editing of this book, Tammy Anderson for managing the process, and the wonderful personnel at Marcel Dekker, Inc., specifically Maria Allegra and Brian Black.

Daryl S. Paulson

Contents

1

Research and Statistics

The vast majority of researchers are familiar with, if not *experts* in, a specialized field outside statistics, such as chemistry, biology, microbiology, medicine, pharmacy, animal science, sports medicine, botany, or zoology. This book is written for them.

Researchers do not need to be statisticians in order to perform quality research as long as they understand the basic principles of experimental design and apply them. In this way, the statistical method can usually be kept relatively simple and can provide straightforward answers. Underlying all research is the need to present the findings in a clear, concise manner. This is particularly important if one is defending those findings before a regulatory agency, explaining them to management, or looking for funding from a particular group.

Research validity can be assured by understanding how to use statistics properly. Compromised research validity can occur when conducting an experiment prior to designing the study and, afterward, determining *what the numbers mean* [1]. In this situation, researchers generally need to consult a professional statistician to extract any useful information because there is no easy repair. An even more serious situation can occur when a researcher evaluates the data using several statistical methods and selects the one that provides the results most favorable to a preconceived conclusion. It is important, then, that the statistical method to be used is chosen prior to conducting the study.

I. EMPIRICAL RESEARCH

Valid statistical methods, as described in this text, require objective observation and measurement, consisting of observing an event or phenomenon under controlled conditions where as many extraneous influences as possible are eliminated [2]. Valid statistical methods employed in experimentation require at least four characteristics [3]:

1. Collection of sample data, performed in a unbiased manner
2. Accurate, objective observation and measurement
3. Interpretation of data-based results
4. Reproducibility of the observations and measurements

The controlled experiment is a fundamental tool for the researcher. In controlled experiments, a researcher selects samples at random from the population or populations of interest. One sample set is usually designated the control group and is the standard, or reference, for comparison. The other group (or groups) is the test group, the one to be subjected to the specific test condition one wishes to observe and measure. Other than the test condition(s), the control and test groups are treated in the same way. For example, if an experiment is designed to evaluate the effectiveness of a surgical scrub solution in removing normal microflora from the hands, individuals from a population of healthy volunteers are assigned randomly to either the control group (no scrub) or the test group (scrub). Randomization ensures that each person is as likely to be assigned to the test group as to the control group.

II. BIASES

Measurement error has two components, a random one and a systematic one. Random error is unexplainable fluctuation in the data that remains beyond the researcher's ability to attribute a specific cause. We discuss random error in Sec. IV of this chapter. Systematic error, or bias, is error that is not the consequence of chance alone. And systematic error, unlike random fluctuation, has a direction and magnitude.

Researchers cannot will themselves to take a purely objective perspective on research, even if they think they can [4]. The researcher has personal desires, needs, wants, and fears that *unconsciously* come into play by filtering, to some degree, the research, particularly when interpreting the data's meaning [5]. Also, shared, *cultural* values of the scientific research community bias the researcher's interpretations with preset expectations. This makes it very difficult to *get outside the box* to perform new and creative research. Particularly dangerous is the belief of a researcher that he or she is without bias.

Knowing the human predisposition to bias, it is important to collect data by methods of randomization and *blinding*. It is also helpful to the researcher to hone his or her mind continually by developing several important characteristics:

Openness
Discernment
Understanding

A. Openness

It is important that the research problem, the research implementation, and the interpretation of the data receive the full, *open* attention of the researcher. Open attention can be likened to the Taiost term *wu wei*, or noninterfering awareness. That is, the researcher does not try to interpret initially but, instead, is aware. In this respect, even though unconscious bias remains, the researcher does not consciously overlay data with theoretical constructs concerning how the results should appear. One should strive to avoid consciously bringing to the research process any preconceived values. This is difficult because those of us who perform research have conscious and unconscious biases. Probably the best way to remain consciously open for *what is* is to avoid becoming overly invested in specific theories and explanations.

B. Discernment

Accompanying openness is discernment—the ability not only to be passively aware but also to go a step further, to see into the heart or root of the experiment and uncover information not immediately evident while not adding information that is not present. Discernment can be thought of as one's internal nonsense detector. Unlike openness, discernment enables the researcher to draw upon experience to differentiate fact from supposition, association from causation, and intuition from fantasy. Discernment is accurate discrimination with respect to sources, relevance, pattern, and motives by grounding interpretation in the data and one's direct experience.

C. Understanding (Verstehen)

Interwoven with openness and discernment is understanding. Researchers must understand—that is, correctly interpret—the data, not merely observe an experiment. Understanding what is, then, is knowing accurately and precisely what the phenomena mean. This type of understanding is attained when intimacy with the data and their meaning is achieved *and* integrated.

In research, it is not possible to gain understanding by merely observing phenomena and analyzing them statistically. One must interpret the data correctly, a process enhanced by at least three conditions:

1. *Familiarity* with the mental processes by which understanding, and hence meaning, is obtained must exist. And much of this meaning is shared. Researchers do not live in isolation but live within a culture—albeit scientific—that, nevertheless, operates through shared meaning, shared values, shared beliefs, and shared goals. In addition, one's language—both technical and conversant—is held together by both shared meaning and concepts. Because each researcher tries to communicate meaning to others, understanding the semiotics of communication is important [6]. For example, the letters—marks—on this page are *signifiers*. They are symbols that refer to collectively defined (by language) objects, or concepts, known as *referents*. However, each individual has a slightly unique concept of each referent stored in memory, termed the *signified*. For instance, when one says or writes *tree*, the utterance or letter markings of t-r-e-e, this signifier represents a culturally shared referent, the symbol of a wooden object with branches and leaves. Yet, unavoidably, you and I have slightly different concepts of the referent tree. My mental signified may be an oak tree; yours may be a pine tree.

2. *Realization* that an event and the conception of an event are not the same. Suppose a researcher observes event A_1 at time t_1 (Fig. 1). The researcher describes what she or he witnessed at time t_1, which is now a description, A_2, of event A_1 at time t_2. Later, the researcher distances himself or herself even farther from event A_1 by reviewing the laboratory notes on A_2, a process that produces A_3. Notice that this process hardly represents a direct, unbiased view of A_1. The researcher generally interprets data (A_3) that, themselves, are interpretations of data to some degree (A_2) based on the actual occurrence of the event, A_1 [7].

3. *Understanding* that a scientific system itself (e.g., biology, geology) provides a *definition* of most observed events that transfers interpretation, which is again reinterpreted by researchers. This, in itself, is biasing, particularly in that it provides a preconception of what is.

III. THE EXPERIMENTAL PROCESS

In practice, the experimental process is usually iterative. The results of experiment *A* become the starting point for experiment *B*, the next experiment

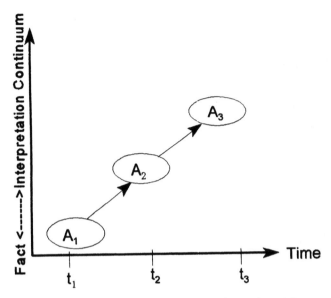

FIGURE 1   Fact–interpretation gradient of experimental processes.

(Fig. 2). The results of experiment *B* become the starting point for experiment *C*. Let us look more closely at the iterative process in an example.

Suppose one desires to evaluate a newly developed antimicrobial at five incremental concentration levels (0.25, 0.50, 0.75, 1.00, and 1.25%) for its antimicrobial effects against two representative pathogenic bacterial species: *Staphylococcus aureus*, a gram-positive bacterium, and *Escherichia coli*, a gram-negative one. The researcher designs a simple, straightforward test to observe the antimicrobial action of the five concentration levels upon challenge for 1 minute with specific inoculum levels of *S. aureus* and *E. coli*. Exposure of the two bacterial species to the five levels of the drug demonstrates that the 0.75 and 1.00% concentrations are equivalent in their antimicrobial effects and 0.25, 0.50, and 1.25% are much less antimicrobially effective.

Encouraged by these results, the researcher designs another study, focusing on the 0.75 and 1.00% drug formulations, to compare their antimicrobial properties, now against 13 different microbial species, and to select the better formulation (more antimicrobially active). However, the two formulations perform equally well against the 13 different species of microorganisms. The researcher then expands the scope of the next study to use the same 13 microorganisms but at reduced exposure times, 15 seconds and 30 seconds, and adds a competitive product to use as a reference.

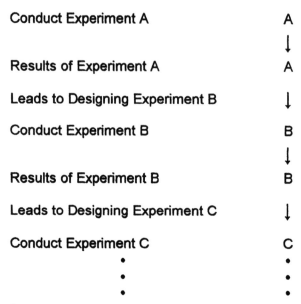

Conduct Experiment A

Results of Experiment A

Leads to Designing Experiment B

Conduct Experiment B

Results of Experiment B

Leads to Designing Experiment C

Conduct Experiment C

FIGURE 2   Iterative approach to research.

The two formulations again perform equally well and significantly better than the competitor. The researcher now believes that one of the formulations may truly be a candidate to market, but which active concentration? Product cost studies, product stability studies, etc. are conducted, and still the two formulations are equivalent.

Finally, the researcher performs a human clinical trial to compare the two products' antibacterial efficacy as well as their skin irritation potential. Although the antimicrobial portion of the study reveals activity equivalence, the skin irritation evaluation demonstrates that the 1.00% product is significantly more irritating to users' hands. Hence, the formulation candidate is the 0.75% product.

This is the type of process commonly employed in new product development projects. Because research and development efforts are generally subject to tight budgets, small pilot studies are preferred to larger, more costly ones. Usually, this is fine because the experimenter has intimate, first-hand knowledge of the research area as well as an understanding of its theoretical aspects. With this knowledge and understanding, the researcher can usually ground the meaning of the data in the observations, even when the number of observations is small.

Yet, researchers must be aware that there is a downside to this step-by-step approach. When experiments are conducted one factor at a time,

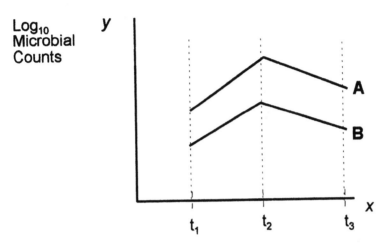

FIGURE 3   No interaction present.

if interaction between factors is present, it will not be discovered. Statistical interaction occurs when two or more products do not produce the same proportional response at different levels of measurement. Figure 3 depicts $\log_{10}$ microbial counts after three time exposures with product A (50% strength) and product B (full strength). No interaction is apparent because, over the three time intervals, the difference between the product responses is constant.

Figure 4 portrays statistical interaction between factors. At time t_1, product A provides more microbial reduction (lower counts) than product B. At time t_2, product A demonstrates less reduction in microorganisms than product B. At time t_3, products A and B are equivalent. When statistical interaction is present, it makes no sense to discuss general effects of products A and B. Instead, one must discuss product performance relative to a specific exposure time frame, that is, at times t_1, t_2, and t_3.

In addition, researchers must realize that reality cannot be broken into small compartments to know it in toto. Although this book is devoted mainly to small study designs and much practical information can be gained by using small studies, by themselves, they rarely provide a clear perspective on the whole situation.

We humans tend to think and describe reality in simple cause-and-effect relationships (e.g., A causes B). But, in reality, phenomena seldom share merely linear relationships, nor do they have a simple, one-factor cause [8]. For example, in medical practice, when a physician examines a patient infected with *S. aureus*, the physician is likely to conclude that *S. aureus* caused the disease and proceed to eliminate the offending microorganism

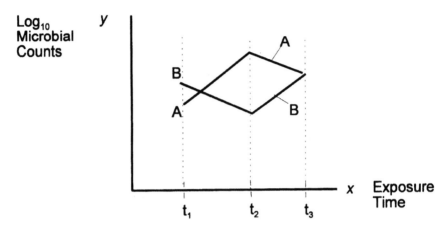

FIGURE 4   Interaction present.

from the body. Yet, this is not the complete story. The person's immune system—composed of the reticuloendothelial system, immunocytes, phagocytes, etc.—acts to prevent infectious diseases from occurring and to fight them once the infectious process begins. The immune system is directly dependent upon genetic predisposition, modified through one's nutritional state, psychological state (e.g., sense of life's meaning and purpose), and stress level. In a simple case like this, in which oral administration of an antibiotic *cures* the disease, knowledge of these other influences usually does not matter. But in more complicated chronic diseases such as cancer, these other factors may play an important part in treatment efficacy and the survival of the patient.

IV.   OTHER DIFFICULTIES IN RESEARCH

There are three other phenomena that may pose difficulties for the experimenter:

    Experimental (random) error
    Confusing correlation with causation
    Employing too complex a study design when a simpler one would be
        as good

A.   Experimental Error

Random variability—experimental error—is produced by a multitude of uncontrolled factors that tend to obscure the conclusions that can be drawn from an experiment with a small sample size. This is a very critical consideration in research in which small sample sizes are the rule because it is often difficult to detect significant treatment effects when they truly exist, a type II error.

One or two *wild* data points (outliers) in a small sample can distort the mean and hugely inflate the variance, making it nearly impossible to make inferences—at least meaningful ones. Therefore, before becoming heavily invested in a research project, the experimenter should have an approximation of what the variability of the data is and establish the tolerable limits for both the alpha (α) and beta (β) errors so that the appropriate sample size is tested. Recall that α error (type I error) occurs when rejecting a true null hypothesis, and β error (type II error) is committed by failing to reject a false null hypothesis. In other words, α error occurs when one states that there is a difference between treatments when there actually is not, and β error occurs when one concludes that there is no difference between treatments when there is.

Traditionally, type I error—α error—is considered the more serious and can be controlled by setting the α level. But in research and development (R&D) studies, type II error is also serious. For example, if one is evaluating several products, particularly when using a small sample size per treatment group, there is a *real* problem of concluding statistically that the products are not different from each other when they are. It should be pointed out that, as one tightens α error, that is, reduces its probability of occurrence, the probability of committing a β error increases. The reverse is also true.

The simplest way to control both α and β errors is to use more experimental replicates, but the increases in cost may prohibit this. Another viable method is to use larger α values to reduce β error. That is, use an α of 0.10 or 0.15 instead of 0.05 or 0.01. Also, using more powerful statistical procedures can immensely reduce the probability of committing β error.

B. Confusing Correlation with Causation

Correlation is a measure of the degree to which two variables vary linearly in relationship to each other. For example, in comparing the number of lightning storms in Kansas with the number of births in New York City, you discover a strong positive correlation: the more lightning storms in Kansas, the more children born in New York City (Fig. 5). Although the two variables appear to be correlated *sufficiently* to claim that the increased incidence of lightning storms in Kansas caused increased childbirth in New York, correlation is not causation. Correlation between two variables, X and Y, often occurs because they are both associated with a third factor, Z, that is unknown. There are a number of empirical ways to verify causation,

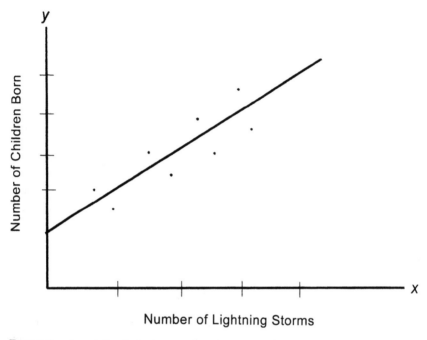

FIGURE 5 Correlation between unrelated variables.

and generally these do not rely on statistical inference. So, until causation is truly demonstrated, it is preferable to state that correlated data are *associated* rather than causally related.

C. Complex Study Design

In many research situations, especially those involving human subjects in medical research clinical trials, the study design must be complex in order to better evaluate the dependent variable(s). But whenever possible, it is wise to use the rule of parsimony. That is, use the simplest and most straightforward study design available. Even simple experiments can quickly become complex. Adding other questions, although interesting, will quickly make them that way. I often find it useful to state formally the study objectives, the choice of experimental factors and levels (that is, independent variables), the dependent variable one intends to measure to fulfill the study objectives, and the study design selection. For example, suppose a biochemist is evaluating the $\log_{10}$ reduction in *S. aureus* bacteria after a 15-second exposure to a new antimicrobial compound produced in several pilot batches. The biochemist wants to determine the 95% confidence interval for the true $\log_{10}$ microbial average reduction. This is simple enough, but then the chemist asks:

1. Is there significant lot-to-lot variation in the pilot batches? If there is, perhaps one is significantly more antimicrobial than the other.
2. What about subculture-to-subculture variability in antimicrobial resistance of the strain of *S. aureus* used in testing? If one is interested in knowing whether the product is effective against *S. aureus*, what number of strains must be evaluated?
3. What about lot-to-lot variability in the culture medium used to grow the bacteria? The chemist remembers supplier A's medium supporting significantly higher microbial populations than that of supplier B. Should both be tested? Does the medium have significant effects on $\log_{10}$ microbial reduction variability?
4. What about procedural error by technicians and variability between technicians? Evaluation of the training records shows technician A to be more accurate than technicians B and C. How should this be handled?

As one can see, even a very simple study can—and often does—become complex.

V. BASIC TOOLS IN EXPERIMENTAL DESIGN

There are three basic tools in statistical experimental design:

Replication
Randomization
Blocking

Replication means that the basic experimental measurement is repeated. For example, if one was measuring the CO_2 concentration of blood, the measurements would be repeated several times under controlled circumstances. Replication serves several important functions. First, it allows the investigator to estimate the experimental or random error through the sample standard deviation (S) or sample variance (S^2). This estimate becomes a basic unit of measurement for determining whether observed differences in the data are statistically significant. Second, if the sample mean ($\bar{X}$) is used to estimate a true population mean (μ), replication enables the investigator to obtain a more precise estimate of the mean. If S^2 is the sample variance of the data for n replicates, then the variance of the sample mean is $S_{\bar{x}}^2 = S^2/n$.

The practical aspect of this is that, if no or few replicates are made, the investigator may be unable to make a useful inference about the value of the population mean, μ. However, if the sample mean computation is based on replicated data, one can estimate the population mean, μ, more accurately and precisely. This will become more evident as we discuss further the mean, the standard deviation, and the $1-\alpha$ confidence intervals.

Randomization of a sampling process is a mainstay of statistical analysis. No matter how careful an investigator is in eliminating bias, it still creeps into the study. In addition, when a variable cannot be controlled, randomized sampling can negate any biasing effect. Randomization schemes can be achieved by using a table of random numbers or a computer-generated randomization subroutine. Through randomization, each experimental unit is as likely to be selected for a particular treatment or measurement as any of the others.

Blocking is another common statistical technique used to increase the precision of an experimental design. It is used to reduce or even eliminate nuisance factors that influence the measured responses but are not of interest to the study. Blocks consist of groups of the experimental unit chosen so that each group is more homogeneous with respect to some variable than the collection of experimental units as a whole. Blocking involves subjecting the block to all the experimental treatments and comparing the treatment effects within each block. For example, in a drug absorption study, an investigator may have four different drugs to compare. The investigator may block according to similar weights of test subjects. The four individuals between 120 and 125 pounds may be in block 1, and each randomly receives one of the four test drugs. Block 2 may contain the four individuals between 130 and 135 pounds. The rationale is that the closer the subjects are to the same weight, the closer the baseline liver functions will be.

The statistical method selected depends, in part, on the data distribution (normal, skewed, bimodal, exponential, binomial, or other). As will be explained (Chap. 3), the use of exploratory data analysis (EDA) procedures can help the investigator select the appropriate statistical method and develop an intuitive *feel* for the data before the actual statistical analysis occurs.

VI. STATISTICAL METHOD SELECTION: OVERVIEW

The statistical method, to be appropriate, must measure and reflect the data accurately and precisely [8, 9, 10, 11]. The test hypothesis should be formulated clearly and concisely. If, for example, the study is designed to test whether products A and B are different, statistical analysis should provide an answer.

Roger H. Green, in his book *Sampling Designs and Statistical Methods for Environmental Biologists,* describes 10 steps for effective statistical analysis [12]. These steps are applicable to any analysis:

1. State the test hypothesis concisely to be sure that what you are testing is what you want to test.
2. Always replicate the treatments. Without replication, measurements of variability may not be reliable.
3. Insofar as possible, keep the number of replicates equal throughout the study. This practice makes it much easier to analyze the data in order to produce more reliable results.
4. When determining whether a particular treatment has a significant effect, it is important to take measurements both where the test condition is present and where it is absent.
5. Perform a small-scale study to assess the effectiveness of the design and statistical method selection before going to the effort and expense of a larger study.
6. Verify that the sampling scheme one devises actually results in a representative sample of the target population. Guard against systematic bias by using techniques of random sampling.
7. Break a large-scale sampling process into smaller components.
8. Verify that the collected data meet the statistical distribution assumptions. In the days before computers were commonly used and programs were readily available, some assumptions had to be made about distributions. Now it is easy to test these assumptions to verify their validity.
9. Test the method thoroughly to make sure that it is valid and useful for the process under study. And, even if the method is satisfactory for one set of data, be certain that it is adequate for other sets of data derived from the same process.
10. Once these nine steps have been carried out, one can accept the results of analysis with confidence. Much time, money, and effort can be saved by following these steps to statistical analysis.

Once an investigator has a general understanding of the products' attributes, she or he must choose a statistical method to analyze the data. At times, the data are such that nonparametric methods are more appropriate than parametric methods. For example, if budgetary or time constraints force the investigator to use only a few replicates per test group or if some requirements of the parametric method, such as a normal distribution of the data, cannot be achieved or determined, then the nonparametric method is the method of choice. There is also another reason. That is, under many conditions, quantitative data cannot be collected. This is particularly true when data are subjective and, hence, qualitative on the basis of arbitrary scales of measure. An applied researcher can face this situation many times. We will address some potential sources of qualitative data in Sec. X of this chapter.

Prior to assembling the large-scale study, the investigator should re-examine (1) the test hypothesis, (2) the choice of variables, (3) the number of replicates required to protect against type I and type II errors, (4) the order of the experimentation process, (5) the randomization process, (6) the appropriateness of the design used to describe the data, and (7) the data collection and data-processing procedures to ensure that they continue to be relevant to the study.

Let us now briefly address the types of parametric and nonparametric statistical methods available.

VII. PARAMETRIC TESTS

The parametric tests addressed in this book require that the data distributions be normal, an often unsubstantiated assumption. Specifically, parametric tests require that certain conditions be met and, generally, these include the following:

1. The data must be collected randomly, which is also a requirement for nonparametric tests. That is, the selection of any one sample item from a population must not be more probable than the selection of any of the others; each sample is then as likely to be selected as any other one.
2. The observations must be normally distributed (fit a bell-shaped curve) or nearly so.
3. When multiple populations are sampled, they must have similar variances (σ^2).
4. The sample data involved must have been measured, at least, on an interval scale or one that approximates it (e.g., some discrete distributions, such as microbial counts, numbers of animals, numbers of cells, can be used).

Interval data can be ranked, as well as be subdivided, into an infinite number of intervals that are objectively meaningful (102.915, 1×10^{-5}, 1.3000, 7.23914,...). Usually, interval data relate to some standard physical measurement (e.g., height, weight, blood pressure, the number of deaths). Subjective perception of degrees of pregnancy, prestige, or social status, for instance, cannot be translated into interval data, despite a number of research studies erroneously categorizing them as such. Extreme caution must be used when using quantitative methods to analyze what are actually qualitative data, or nonsensical analyses result (e.g., variance of subjective preferences).

Common parametric statistical methods include the following:

1. *Student's t-test*. This is probably the most common parametric statistical test used in research. It is often used to compare two groups of data (a test and a control group or two test groups). It can also be used to compare a test group with a specific value, as a *one-tail* test to determine whether one group is significantly *better* or *worse* than other, or as a *two-tail* test to determine whether they simply differ.
2. *Analysis of variance (ANOVA)*: Analysis of variance is a common parametric technique usually used to compare more than two groups. There are a number of variants of ANOVA used to analyze one-factor, two-factor, and three-factor designs as well as cross-over and nested designs.
3. *Regression analysis*: Regression analysis is a common parametric statistical procedure used where rates of change and trending are evaluated.

VIII. NONPARAMETRIC TESTS

Most nonparametric methods do not require the data to fit a normal distribution or to have the same variances, when multiple populations are compared, nor do they require the sample data to be of interval scale. Random sampling, however, is a requirement. Nonparametric tests do not use the usual parameters (mean, standard deviation, or variance), and they can be used to evaluate nominal or ordinal data.

Nominal data can be grouped but not ranked. Data such as right/left, male/female, yes/no, and 0/1 are examples of nominal data, and such data consist of numbers used only to classify an object, person, or characteristic.

Ordinal data can be both grouped and ranked. Examples include good/bad, poor/average/excellent, and lower class/middle class/upper class. Nonparametric methods are also often used for interval data when the sample size is very small or the data distribution cannot be assumed to be *normal*, a requisite for use of parametric tests.

Common nonparametric tests include the following:

1. *Wilcoxon–Mann–Whitney Test*: This test is the nonparametric analog of the two independent sample Student's *t*-test. Unlike the parametric Student's *t*-test that assumes normal distributions, the Wilcoxon–Mann–Whitney test requires only that the sample data are randomly selected and that the population of data is of at least ordinal scale.

2. *Kruskal–Wallis Test*: This is the nonparametric analog of a one-way ANOVA *F*-test, and it is used to compare multiple groups. For example, suppose one wants to evaluate the relative antimicrobial effects of five different hand soaps; the Kruskal–Wallis test can be used for this evaluation.

In many evaluations where the number of human subjects required to perform the study is low and, thus, cost feasible, the best choice may well be a nonparametric test. Many investigators simply will not have the funding necessary to perform larger scale studies. However, there is a price to pay when using nonparametric statistics. They are not as powerful as parametric statistics and tend to err on the conservative side. If a parametric test can barely detect a significant difference between two treatments, the comparable nonparametric test more than likely would not be able to detect a difference.

IX. RESEARCHER'S PLACE IN THE LARGER PICTURE

Most researchers who read this book will recognize that they are parts in a larger whole, a corporate entity, for example. In industrial research, much of a researcher's work will be in new product development and in comparative product studies in industries where intense levels of competition are present. There will also be the pressure from the ever-tightening control of regulating agencies expecting valid scientific and statistical studies. In the medical topical antimicrobial market, for example, product requirements include high, broad-spectrum antimicrobial effectiveness, low skin irritation potential upon repeated and prolonged use, ease of use, and aesthetic appeal. If these aspects have been addressed successfully, the product has a good chance of being a success. But too often, these important factors are ignored, and the product is never really accepted in the market. Because the goal is to introduce products into a market that has multiple determinants of a product's success, it is best to develop the product from a multidimensional perspective. At least four different domains exist and should be addressed in R&D projects: (1) social, (2) cultural, (3) personal objective, and (4) personal subjective. Let me flesh out this type of model so that it is more accessible to readers.

X. FOUR-DOMAIN MODEL

Let us look at the situation of bringing a new antimicrobial product to market.

A. Social Requirements

Social requirements in new antimicrobial product development include conforming to standards set by regulating agencies, such as the Food and Drug Administration (FDA), the Federal Trade Commission (FTC), and the Environmental Protection Agency (EPA), as well as the rules, laws, and regulations they enforce. Before developing a product, it is critical to understand the current legal regulations governing the product and the product's components and their levels as well as product stability and toxicological concerns. Although probably not a great deal of statistical analysis will be used in this domain, it is a critical component in the statistical work. For example, a New Drug Application (NDA) is required in order to market a regulated drug product. For over-the-counter (OTC) products, the active drug and its dosage must be both legal and within allowable limits.

B. Cultural Requirements

Cultural requirements are very important but are often ignored by researchers. Cultural and subcultural requirements include shared interpersonal values, beliefs, goals, and the world views of a society or subgroup of society. Shared values such as perceived *antimicrobial effectiveness* have much influence on consumers, professional and domestic. These values are generally of two types: manifest and latent. A consumer is conscious of manifest (surface) values. For example, consumers buy an antimicrobial soap to be *cleaner* than they can be using a non-antimicrobial soap. But deeper and more fundamental values are also present [13,14]. These are referred to as latent values and are unconscious in that the consumer is not aware of them. In this case, *cleaner* may mean to the consumer such things as being accepted, valued, loved, and worthwhile as a person, spouse, and/or parent.

Most manifest and latent values that we share as a culture are magnified by manufacturers' advertising campaigns. The consumer will be motivated by both the manifest and latent values. For example, if homemakers perceive that they are taking better care of the children by having them use antimicrobial soaps (a manifest value), and if they feel more valuable, more lovable, and/or more needed by their family, etc. (latent values), they will be motivated to purchase the product. Or, in the hospital setting, there are practices considered *better* than others. For example, when chlorhexidine gluconate was first used as a preoperative skin preparation, many surgical staff members refused to use it. The data demonstrated that the product was antimicrobially effective, but it still was not used. It was not until subjective data were collected that nonparametric statistical analysis showed that it was not used because, once it dried on the skin, it could not be seen as readily as the standard povidone iodine. Staff members derived shared meaning and value by being able to see the iodine covering the proposed operative site. To solve this problem, chlorhexidine gluconate manufacturers added a reddish dye to stain the skin.

Finally, much of what consumers believe to be true is not grounded in objective reality. Most of these beliefs are formed from consumers' interpretation of mass media reports, opinions of others, and explanations of phenomena from various notorious sources.

C. Personal Objective Attributes

Physical components of a product include its application, its antimicrobial actions, and its irritating effects on skin and environment (e.g., staining clothing, gowns, and bedding). It is important that products be designed with the individual in mind. Hence, products must be easy to use, easy to open (if in a container), and effective for their intended use (e.g., food service, in-home, or medical and surgical personnel applications). This region is generally subject to both parametric and nonparametric methods.

D. Personal Subjective Attributes

This category includes one's personal interpretation of cultural and subcultural *world views*. In relation to antimicrobials, these include, for example,

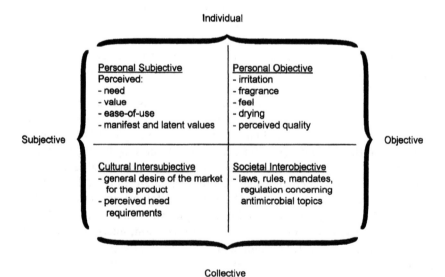

FIGURE 6   Quadrant model of attribute categories.

subjective likes and dislikes of characteristics such as the fragrance and feel of the product, the perceived *quality* of the product, and other aesthetic considerations. As with cultural attributes, there are manifest and latent values in this category. Hence, if one likes the springtime fragrance of a consumer body wash (manifest), the latent or deeper value may be that it makes one feel younger and, therefore, more physically attractive and desirable as a person. This region is usually better approached with nonparametric methods.

These four attribute categories are presented in quadrant form (Fig. 6). Each quadrant interacts with the other three quadrants. For example, cultural values influence personal values and vice versa. Cultural and personal values influence behavior, and behavior influences values.

XI. CONCLUSION

With this said, it certainly cannot be the sole responsibility of a single researcher to evaluate products in all four dimensions. Yet, it is critical from a business perspective that, as a group effort, this be done if a product is to achieve and sustain a competitive advantage.

2

Basic Review of Parametric Statistics

In this chapter, we discuss fundamental statistical procedures. It is assumed that the reader has had an introductory statistical course and this chapter will serve merely as a review.

I. THE NORMAL DISTRIBUTION

For most of the statistical models developed and described in this text, the data are assumed to be from a normal (bell-shaped or Gaussian) distribution. The normal distribution is perhaps the most important distribution encountered in statistical applications. A good reason for this is that many measurements have observed frequency distributions that closely resemble the normal distribution—for example, intelligence quotients, weights and heights of individuals, speeds of runners, and chemical reaction times.

There is another reason why the normal distribution is so important in statistics. A theoretical property of the sample mean, the central limit theorem, allows one to use the normal distribution to find probabilities for various test results, even when the data are not normal, as long as the sample size is large. Hence, the normal distribution has a basic role to play in many situations, particularly in research experiments, when only the sample mean can be known.

Normally distributed data describe a curve (Fig. 1) that is bell-shaped, with a single central peak, termed "unimodal." A normal distribution is symmetric about its center, with the mean, the mode, and the median at that

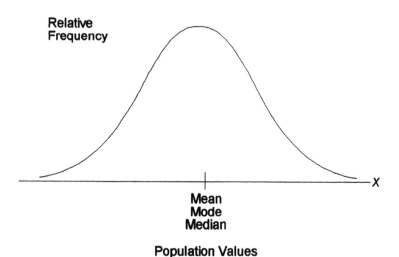

Population Values

FIGURE 1   Frequency distribution for the normal.

center, all with the same value.* Theoretically, the tails of the normal distribution extend to infinity, never quite touching the horizontal (*x*) axis.†

   We say that a population having a shape approximating the normal distribution is approximately "normally distributed." The normal curve is dependent upon two values, μ and σ, the population mean and the standard deviation, respectively. Note also that the area under the curve is always 1.

   Figure 2 provides examples of distributions that are not normal. Distributions A and B are examples of skewed distributions. Curve A is said to be skewed to the left and curve B to the right. Distribution C is a bimodal distribution, and distribution D is a uniform distribution.

   Figure 3 illustrates three different populations, each with a mean equal to 80. Yet, note that the data distributions are different in spread, meaning that their standard deviation values differ. Distributions with small standard deviations have narrow, peaked bells, and those with larger standard deviations have wide, flattened bells. The normal curve is symmetric about the mean and the area under the curve from *a* to *b* depends only on the distance,

---

* Note that the *mode* is the value that occurs most frequently. The *median* is the central value in an ordered array of values.

† If *y* is a "normal" random variable, then the probability distribution function of *y* is

$$f(Y) = \frac{1}{\sigma\sqrt{2\pi}} e^{(\frac{1}{2})(\frac{Y-\mu}{\sigma})^2}$$

where $-\infty < \mu < \infty$ is the mean of the distribution and $\sigma^2 > 0$ is the variance.

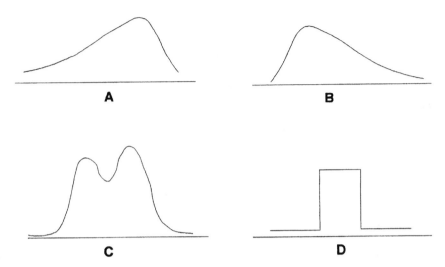

FIGURE 2   Nonnormal distributions.

measured in standard deviations, that separates the end points *a* and *b* from the mean.

For example, about 68% of the values in a normal population lie within one standard deviation (plus and minus) from the mean, from $\mu - \sigma$ to $\mu + \sigma$. That is, the area under the curve between $\mu - \sigma$ and μ and the area under the curve from μ to $\mu + \sigma$, taken together, equal 0.68, or 68% of the data (Fig. 4, curve A). It is also true that about 95% of the normal population lies within 2σ of the mean, from $\mu - 2\sigma$ to $\mu + 2\sigma$, as depicted in curve B, and about

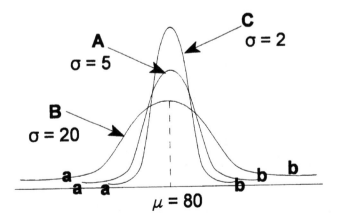

FIGURE 3   Examples of normal distributions.

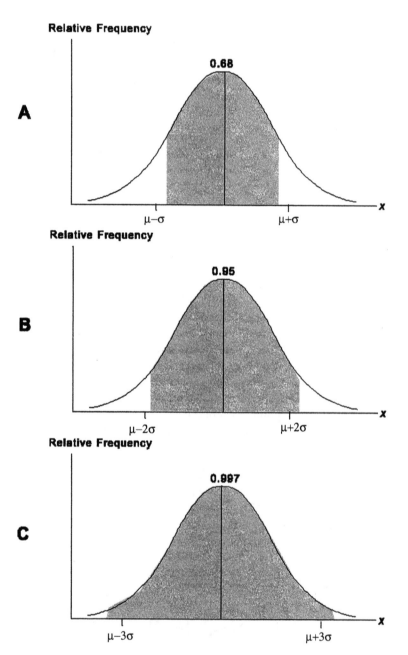

FIGURE 4   Relationship between area under the normal curve and the distance from the mean in standard deviations.

99.7% within three standard deviations of the mean, from $\mu - 3\sigma$ to $\mu + 3\sigma$, as depicted in curve C.

We will occasionally use the notation $X \sim N(\mu, \sigma^2)$ to denote that X is normally distributed with a mean of μ and a variance of σ^2. An important, special case of the normal distribution is the *standard normal distribution*, where $\mu = 0$ and $\sigma^2 = 1$. The statistic is converted to this scale for use of the normal distribution tables A and B. In this case, the random variable, $Z = (X - \mu)/\sigma$, follows the standard normal distribution, $Z \sim N(0, 1)$. This equation transforms any normal random variable, X, into a standard normal random variable, Z, that can then be used in a table of the cumulative standard normal distribution.

A statistical population is the set of all elements under observation. This "population" exists whether all, some, or no observations have been made. It may be real, such as the heights of all 30-year-old males in New York State on January 15, 2005, or it may be hypothetical, such as the longevity of laboratory mice fed a special diet. It is synonymous with "universe" because it consists of all possible elements.

Generally, the true population mean (μ) is not known and must be estimated by the sample mean ($\bar{X}$). The mean is a measure of central tendency, the value around which the other values are distributed. The population variance, designated by σ^2, is the degree to which these values cluster around the arithmetic mean (μ). Generally, like the population mean, the population variance is unknown and is estimated by S^2, the sample variance. Under random sampling (technically, when sampled with replacement), S^2 (the sample variance) is an unbiased estimate of σ^2 (the population variance) [9]. However, the sample standard deviation, S, is not an unbiased estimate of the population standard deviation, σ.

In applied research, one is often interested in comparing two treatments to determine whether the measured response from one treatment group is significantly different from that of the other (two-tail test) or is significantly larger (upper tail) or smaller (lower tail). The basic test for this is Student's t-test, which is covered in detail in Chap. 4. For example, it may be used to compare two chemical purification methods, two skin-moisturizing products, or a new and an old (control) method of active ingredient extractions. The comparison of data from the two groups is usually made in terms of their sample mean values (e.g., $\bar{X}_1$ and $\bar{X}_2$). Let us begin with an example of calculating the mean, variance, and standard deviation, which estimate their population counterparts [10].

Suppose a researcher wants to test two types of paint for their average time before cracking. Paint 1 is an oil-based paint, and paint 2 is a water-based paint. The scores are the numbers of days the paints remain on the test substance in an environmental chamber at 140°F before cracking is

TABLE 1   Data Results

n	Paint 1 score	Paint 2 score
1	85	89
2	87	89
3	92	90
4	80	84
5	84	88

noticed. Five replicate wood carriers are used. The data are presented in Table 1.

II. CALCULATION OF THE ARITHMETIC MEAN AVERAGE

The arithmetic mean, or average, is probably the most commonly encountered statistic. Technically, the mean is computed as:

$$\frac{\sum_{i=1}^{n} X_i}{n}$$

where X_i = value of the ith observation in the sample

n = sample size = total number of values

In applied statistics, one can rarely know the population mean value (μ), so it is estimated by the sample mean ($\bar{X}$). The unbiased, expected value of the sample mean is μ. That is, the sample mean is an unbiased estimate of the population mean.

$$\text{Paint 1} \quad \bar{x}_1 = \frac{\sum x_i}{n} = \frac{85 + 87 + 92 + 80 + 84}{5} = \frac{428}{5} = 85.6 \qquad (1)$$

$$\text{Paint 2} \quad \bar{x}_2 = \frac{\sum x_i}{n} = \frac{89 + 89 + 90 + 84 + 88}{5} = \frac{440}{5} = 88.0 \qquad (2)$$

III. VARIANCE

The dispersion of the data, the scatter of the data about the population mean, is measured by the variance, σ^2. The population variance σ^2 is, again in practice, estimated by the sample variance, S^2. The expression for calculating the population variance is:

$$\sigma^2 = \frac{\sum (X_i - \mu)^2}{N} \tag{3}$$

where N is the population size, and which is estimated by the sample variance:

$$S^2 = \frac{\sum (X_i - \bar{X})^2}{n-1} \tag{4}$$

Notice that the sample variance formula denominator is $n - 1$, not n, as one might expect by analogy with the population variance. This is because one degree of freedom is lost when μ is estimated by $\bar{X}$ in the variance formula.

IV. CALCULATION OF SAMPLE VARIANCE

In practice, the formula:

$$S^2 = \frac{\sum X_i^2 - n\bar{X}^2}{n-1} = \frac{\sum X_i^2 - (\sum X_i)^2/n}{n-1} \tag{5}$$

is much easier to use, particularly with a calculator.

Paint 1

$$s_1^2 = \sum \frac{(x_{1i} - \bar{x}_1)^2}{n-1}$$

$$= \frac{(85 - 85.60)^2 + (87 - 85.60)^2 + (92 - 85.60)^2}{5-1}$$

$$\frac{+(80 - 85.60)^2 + (84 - 85.60)^2}{5-1}$$

$$= \frac{77.20}{4} = 19.30$$

Paint 2

$$s_2^2 = \sum \frac{(x_{2i} - \bar{x}_2)^2}{n-1}$$

$$= \frac{(89 - 88)^2 + (89 - 88)^2 + (90 - 88)^2 + (84 - 88)^2 + (88 - 88)^2}{5-1}$$

$$= \frac{22}{4} = 5.50$$

V. STANDARD DEVIATION

The population standard deviation, σ, has unique properties in that, for a population of size N from a bell-shaped distribution, the mean plus or minus ($\pm$) one standard deviation encompasses approximately 68% of the data. Plus or minus ($\pm$) two standard deviations encompasses approximately 95% of the data, and $\pm$ three standard deviations encompasses approximately 99.7% of the data. More about this later.

The population standard deviation,

$$\sigma = \sqrt{\frac{\sum(X - \mu)^2}{N}} = \sqrt{\sigma^2} \tag{6}$$

is estimated by sample standard deviation,

$$S = \sqrt{\frac{\sum(X_i - \bar{X})^2}{n - 1}} = \sqrt{S^2} \tag{7}$$

This is merely the square root of the variance.

VI. CALCULATIONS OF SAMPLE STANDARD DEVIATION

Paint 1:

$$s_1 = \sqrt{s_1^2} = \sqrt{19.30} = 4.39$$

Paint 2:

$$s_2 = \sqrt{s_2^2} = \sqrt{5.50} = 2.35$$

VII. QUALITATIVE AND QUANTITATIVE VARIABLES

There are two basic kinds of variables in statistics, distinguished by the form of the characteristic of interest. When the characteristic can be expressed numerically, in a meaningful way, such as weight, height, speed, cost, stability, or number, the variable is termed *quantitative.* When the characteristic is nonnumerically operational, such as sex, category, lot, batch, or occupation, the variable is said to be *qualitative.* Different methods will be introduced for describing and summarizing each type of variable. The difference in procedure stems from the fact that arithmetic operations can be performed only on numbers. For example, one can calculate the average weight of a collection of individual laboratory rats, but other procedures must be employed to summarize qualitative data. Qualitative data with a particular characteristic are called *attributes*.

VIII. THE CENTRAL LIMIT THEOREM

The central limit theorem states that, as the value of n increases (i.e., as the sample size increases), no matter what the underlying distribution, the distribution of $\bar{X}$ tends to become normal [2, 3]. The central limit theorem is applicable to any frequency distribution—skewed, bimodal, uniform, or exponential—and its utility lies in enabling the researcher to make an inference about a population without knowing anything more about its frequency distribution than can be found in a sample.

IX. STATISTICAL ESTIMATES

Sample data are what we will use to draw our statistical inferences. A descriptive statistic (mean, median, standard deviation, variance) is generated from a sample and performs the function of an *estimator*. Much statistical theory over the years has been concerned with finding and then using statistics that are appropriate estimators. For example, the sample mean is a good estimator of the population mean, as is the sample variance for the population variance [8]. That is, the expected value of the sample mean is the population mean, and the expected value of the sample variance is the population variance.

$$E(\bar{X}) = \mu$$

$$E(S^2) = \sigma^2$$

Because of chance, the value actually calculated (the "estimate") may not be identical to the population parameter value. That is, the values of the sample mean, $\bar{X}$, and sample variance, S^2, usually differ from the population mean, μ, and the population variance, σ^2. For this reason, we will use estimates in two forms: *point* and *interval*.

A point estimate is a single numerical value used as the best estimate of the unknown population parameter value. The value of a sample mean ($\bar{X}$) is a point estimate of the population mean (μ). The value of the sample variance (S^2) is a point estimate of the population variance (σ^2). Point estimates, although very useful, tend to be interpreted as an *exact* representation of their population counterparts. So, if the average height of a laboratory wheat specimen group is 23 inches, based on a sample, it may be interpreted to mean that the population mean is 23 inches. This is usually not so.

In addition, there is no way to measure the degree of confidence the researcher has with respect to the accuracy of the point estimate. In this example, how confident can the researcher be that 23 inches is close to the true population mean? What does "close" mean?

In cases where the researcher needs an objective measure of the reliability of an estimate, she uses an interval estimate. Interval estimates provide a range of values in which, with a specific confidence, a particular parameter is contained. What does "a $P\%$ confidence interval estimate for μ is (a, b)" mean? It means that, if all possible samples of size n had been drawn from the population and the data from each sample had been used to create a separate confidence interval (CI) estimate of, say, μ, then if somehow later the value of μ became known, $P\%$ of the confidence intervals would include the value μ and the rest would not. In Fig. 5, each horizontal line ($\longleftrightarrow$) represents the CI estimate of μ calculated from a particular sample. The vertical line shows the true value of μ. Note that some intervals capture μ and some do not. For, say, 95% CI, 95% of these intervals would include μ and 5% would not.

Obviously, the researcher draws only one sample of size n, not all possible samples of size n. "A $P\%$ CI for μ is (a, b)" means that the researcher drew a sample, ran the data through the CI formula, and got the numbers a and b. Her best estimate of μ is that $a \le \mu \le b$; i.e., μ is somewhere between a and b. (This is a mathematical translation of a statement such as "the average

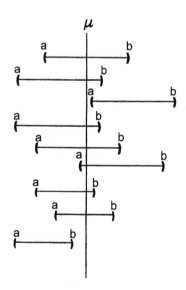

FIGURE 5   Confidence intervals about the true mean.

height of the wheat specimen group is 23 inches, give or take 3 inches," i.e., the mean is estimated to be between $23 - 3 = 20$ inches and $23 + 3 = 26$ inches.)

The researcher does not know and probably will never know whether μ is between a and b,* i.e., whether her interval was one of the $P\%$ of the CI that captures μ or one of the intervals that does not capture μ. She only knows that she used a method of estimation (the CI process) that works $P\%$ of the time. The researcher is "confident" in the procedure and "confident" in the estimate (a, b) of μ that resulted from the procedure.

The word "probability" is not used in this situation; it is incorrect to say, for example, "the probability that μ is between 20 inches and 26 inches is 95%."

A 95% confidence interval about the mean is an interval range of values that, 95% of the time, will include the true mean (μ) within the upper and lower bounds [12]. The true population mean is rarely known; only the probability that it is contained within the interval range of values 95% of the time is known.

In practice, both point and interval estimates are important. They are like a hammer and nail, a saw and board; they complement each other [9].

One of the most common and useful estimators is used to determine the interval estimate of a population mean, μ. It has the form

$$\bar{X} - Z_{\alpha/2}\left(\frac{\sigma}{\sqrt{n}}\right) \leq \mu \leq \bar{X} + Z_{\alpha/2}\left(\frac{\sigma}{\sqrt{n}}\right) \qquad (8)$$

or

$$\bar{X} \pm Z_{\alpha/2}\left(\frac{\sigma}{\sqrt{n}}\right) \qquad (9)$$

where μ = the true population mean

$\bar{X}$ = the sample mean

n = sample size

σ = the population standard deviation

Z = value from a table of the standard normal values used for two-tail α-level tests.

---

*One case where the CI can be checked is in political election polling. Before an election, pollsters estimate the percentage of voters who probably will vote for a particular candidate. After the election, the true percentage of votes the candidate received is known. Statements such as "candidate Jones is projected to receive 52% of the votes ... the poll has a margin of error of 3 percentage points" mean that the pollster's interval estimate is 49 to 55%. If Jones gets only 48% of the votes, his is one of those unlucky intervals that did not capture the parameter value, 48%.

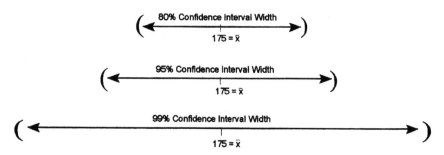

FIGURE 6 Various confidence levels.

The interval is symmetrically centered at $\bar{X}$, and its width is determined by the confidence level percent used (e.g., for $\alpha = 0.20$, $1 - \alpha = 0.80$ or 80%; for $\alpha = 0.05$, $1 - \alpha = 0.95$ or 95%; for $\alpha = 0.01$, $1 - \alpha = 0.99$ or 99%). Recall that the confidence level is set, not calculated by the experimenter. The most commonly used confidence level in science is 95%. If the experimenter desires a greater degree of confidence, the CI width increases (Fig. 6).

For example, if one wants to estimate the true average weight of the population of U.S. males 25 years of age, the point estimate may be 175 pounds and the interval estimate 175 ± 5, or (170, 180), pounds at 80% confidence. At 95% confidence, the point estimate remains 175 pounds, and the interval estimate may be 175 ± 20, or (155, 195), pounds, and at 99% confidence, the interval estimate may be 175 ± 50, or (125, 225), pounds. The more confidence one requires, the wider the confidence interval becomes. But the more confidence one has, the less precise one is. In practice, a trade-off is necessary between confidence and precision.

X. NORMAL TABLES

The standard normal distribution is found in Table A.1. It requires one to transform a value into a *normal* deviate, where it is converted to a Z score. If $X \sim N(\mu, \sigma^2)$, then

$$Z = \frac{X - \mu}{\sigma} \tag{10}$$

is distributed as a standard normal.

Instead of the normal table (Z table in Table A.1), we will generally use Student's t-distribution for work in this book. Student's t-distribution is identical to the normal standard distribution for large sample sizes, $n \geq 120$, and has the added advantage of compensating for sample sizes that are much

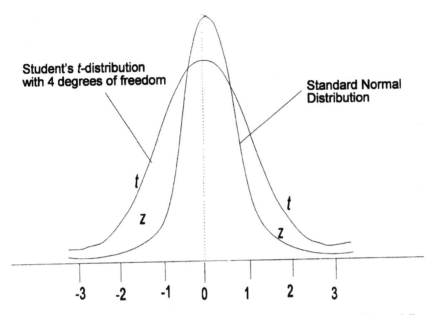

FIGURE 7   Comparison of the relative frequency curves of the standard normal distribution (Z table) and Student's *t*-distribution.

smaller [1,3]. It does this by extending the tails of the sample distribution (see Fig. 7), making it more conservative, lowering the probability of α error.

XI. INTRODUCTION TO STATISTICAL INFERENCE

In 1954, the largest medically related statistical investigation ever performed up to that time was conducted. It dealt with the question, "Does the Salk polio vaccine provide protection against the polio disease?" To answer this question, more than a million children were randomly assigned to two groups—one to be inoculated with the Salk polio vaccine, the other to be inoculated with a salt solution placebo. The data collected from this study would lead to one of two conclusions: (1) If the percentage of children developing polio among those given the vaccine was less than the percentage developing polio among those receiving the placebo, then the vaccine provided a degree of immunity to polio, or (2) if the percentages of children developing polio in both groups were about the same, then the Salk vaccine was not effective against polio.

Such decision problems are called statistical hypothesis tests. The researcher decides between two possible hypotheses. A hypothesis is a statement (or claim) about a parameter of a population, and it is the researcher's purpose to decide, on the basis of experimental or sample evidence, which statement is most probably true. The null hypothesis (H_0) is a mathematical statement that the treatment *is not* effective. The alternative or test hypothesis (H_A) is a statement that the treatment *is* effective. Both hypotheses cannot be true, and both cannot be false. In this example, the null hypothesis, that the vaccine provided no immunity, was to be weighed against the test hypothesis, that the vaccine was effective. Fortunately for posterity, the data failed to support H_0, and H_0 was rejected. The researchers were able to conclude that the Salk polio vaccine worked.

Decision problems such as this are common. Other examples include such issues as the following:

1. A researcher is interested in testing whether a specific presurgical preparation product will show greater antimicrobial efficacy than a control product.
2. A sociologist suggests that certain environmental changes will reduce the crime rate in a community.
3. An agronomist predicts greater yield per acre if farmers use a new hybrid seed.
4. A new packaging process is claimed to reduce damage to goods shipped by mail order businesses.

Collecting valid data to provide evidence for or against the null hypothesis is crucial in statistical inference. When the evidence one collects comes from a representative sample of a larger (often much larger) group called the "population," one can conclude that results seen in the sample-based study would hold true for the entire population. In the polio example, the researchers concluded that the Salk vaccine was effective in reducing the incidence of polio among the children who were vaccinated. Because the sample of children studied was representative of children nationwide, they were also able to conclude that, if children nationwide were given the Salk vaccine, the incidence of polio in the United States would drop significantly. And it did; because of routine vaccination, polio is now a very rare disease in industrialized countries.

Statistical inference is the process of making inductive generalizations from part (the sample) to whole (the population). The process of inference is inherently incorporated in hypothesis testing; only the *sample* data go into the test statistic (which determines whether the null hypothesis is to be rejected), but both hypotheses, H_0 and H_A, are stated in terms of a population parameter. Thus, the conclusion is related to the population, even though the evidence came from only a sample.

XII. STATISTICAL HYPOTHESIS TESTING

The objective of a statistical hypothesis test is to evaluate an assumption or claim made about a specific parameter of a given population. The statistic used in the hypothesis testing is termed the test statistic. We know that the evidence one collects to help make the decision comes from sample data that are, in turn, used in statistical inference procedures.

Many individuals complain of having trouble with hypothesis testing because they get lost in the process—there is so much going on. It is confusing to try to keep track of upper tail, lower tail, and two-tail tests. However, there is a straightforward way to conduct hypothesis tests, which can greatly help the researcher. It was taught to me by my first statistics professor and mentor, Edward Peresini [13], who called it the "six-step procedure." The six steps are as follows:

Step 1. Formulate the test hypothesis (H_A) first, and then the null hypothesis (H_0), which will be the opposite of the test hypothesis (H_A). These serve as the two mutually exclusive alternatives being considered.

Step 2. Select the sample size, n, and set the α level (the probability of a type I [α] error).

Step 3. Select the appropriate test statistic to be used. This selection process is, to a great degree, what this book covers.

Step 4. Formulate the decision rule; that is, decide what the test statistic must show in order to support or reject the null hypothesis (H_0).

Step 5. Collect the sample data, conduct the experiment, and perform the statistical test calculations.

Step 6. Apply the decision rule to the null hypothesis H_0 in terms of accepting or rejecting it at the specified α value.*

---

*In academic writing, as well as in many scientific journals, net; fixed (α) level hypothesis testing is not often done. Instead, a p value is provided for each test. This allows the reader to draw her own conclusions, based on the p value. For some investigators, a smaller p value may be required for a study's results to be significant than would be required by another researcher. Let us look at what the p value means specifically. The p value is the observed significance level. A p value of .047 ($p \leq .047$), say, for a t-test, means the following: the probability of computing a test statistic value as extreme as or more extreme than the one calculated, given that the null hypothesis is true, is less than or equal to .047, the p value. The statement just written can be expressed as:

$$P[(t \geq t_c)|H_0 \text{ is true}] \leq .047$$

assuming this is an upper tail hypothesis test. However, in industrial-type experiments, where decisions must be made, we will use fixed-level hypothesis testing. The reader can easily adapt p values to fixed level tests by calculating the p value and rejecting (H_0) if $p < \alpha$, the level of the test.

Let us look at the first two steps in greater detail.

> *Step 1.* Step 1 requires the formulation of two hypotheses. The first to
> be formulated is the alternative or test statistic (H_A), which is con-
> trasted with the null hypothesis (H_0) or a statement of the status quo.
> For example, one may want to test the hypotheses:
>
>> A new presurgical skin preparation provides faster antimicro-
>> bial effects than the standard one; or
>>
>> A new leave-on antimicrobial soap for food handlers leaves
>> substantially less soap residue on the skin than a rival pro-
>> duct; or
>>
>> A new sanitation program can reduce food contamination
>> levels significantly more than the standard one.

The current position, H_0, or the "no change" position, is the null hypothesis claim. The researcher demands convincing evidence before rejecting the null hypothesis. Statistical tests are predisposed to err on the
conservative side, for it is considered a worse problem to commit a type I,
or α error, than to commit a type II, or β error (i.e., β error is committed when
accepting the null hypothesis as true when it is not). The null hypothesis is
denoted by H_0, and the test or alternative hypothesis is denoted by H_A, H_1,
or k. We use the first notation, H_A, in this book.

The null hypothesis and the alternative hypothesis take on one of the
following formats*: the H_0 statement about a parameter's value will include
one of three possibilities: equal to ($=$), greater than or equal to ($\geq$), or less
than or equal to ($\leq$). The H_A will never include equality. The H_A statement
will use not equal to ($\neq$), less than ($<$), or greater than ($>$) in making a statement about a parameter's value.

1. A two-tail test [tests whether a significant difference exists
   between two population parameters or if a parameter is different
   from a stated value] has the form:

   H_0: Population A's parameter $=$ population B's parameter
   H_A: Population A's parameter $\neq$ population B's parameter

2. An upper tail test has the form:

   H_0: Population A's parameter $\leq$ population B's parameter
   H_A: Population A's parameter $>$ population B's parameter

   (Again, be sure to state H_A first. The H_0 is "less than or equal to.").

---

*In more advanced statistical tests, the same basic hypothesis structure remains.

3. A lower tail test has the form:

H_0: Population A's parameter $\geq$ population B's parameter
H_A: Population A's parameter $<$ population B's parameter

Note that:

1. One sets up the test based on the alternative, or test hypothesis, H_A.
2. The equality symbol is always included with H_0.
3. H_A is a statement that indicates the *test challenge of the researcher* to the status quo (H_0).
4. H_0 is a statement of the commonly accepted belief or standard.

Step 2. Select α (the probability of a type I error) and the sample size, n.

1. The object of testing hypotheses is to make correct decisions. When making a decision in the presence of uncertainty (from a sample that is, by definition, incomplete information about some larger population), one runs the risk of making an error. The probability of making a type I error is denoted by α, where $\alpha = P(\text{type I error}) = P(\text{rejecting } H_0 \text{ when } H_0 \text{ is true})$. The *significance level* of a test is the probability value of α *selected beforehand* for that test.

Condition	Accept H_0	Reject H_0
H_0 true	Correct	Type I error
H_0 false	Type II error	Correct

2. In many parametric hypotheses, the test statistic will have a bell-shaped probability distribution, such as Z or t, as its basis. If we consider the total area beneath a curve to be equal to 1.00, then the chosen value of α, together with whether that particular test is one tail or two tail, enables us to divide the area into two parts called the *region of rejection* and the *region of nonrejection* (or the region of acceptance). Hence, $\alpha =$ probability of observing a test statistic in the rejection region when H_0 is true.
3. Let us look at the test regions for a general, bell-shaped distribution, beginning with a lower tail test.

Lower tail test: The letter L (Fig. 8) defines the *critical value* of the test statistic's distribution (e.g., Z or t) and represents the region of rejection for H_0. If the calculated value of the test statistic falls in the rejection region, H_0

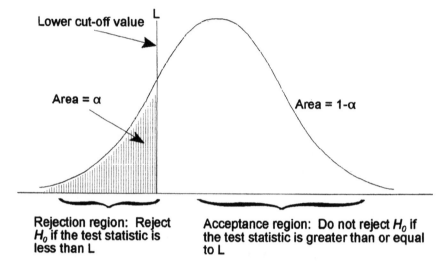

FIGURE 8   Regions of rejection and nonrejection (lower tail).

will be rejected at the α level. For example, H_0: $\mu_1 \geq \mu_2$, and H_A: $\mu_1 < \mu_2$, at $\alpha = 0.05$.

Upper tail test: The letter U (Fig. 9) is called the *critical value* of the test statistic's distribution and represents the region of rejection for H_0. If the calculated value of the test statistic is greater than U, i.e., falls in the rejection

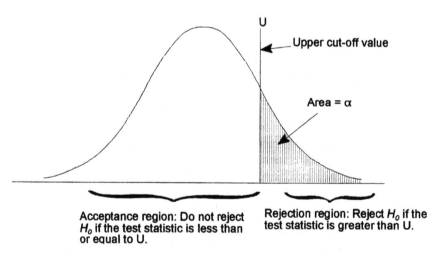

FIGURE 9   Regions of rejection and nonrejection (upper tail).

region, H_0 will be rejected at that α level. For example, H_0: $\mu_1 \le \mu_2$, and H_A: $\mu_1 > \mu_2$, at $\alpha = 0.01$, 0.05.

Two-tail test: The letters L (lower critical value) and U (upper critical value) (Fig. 10) both appear in this diagram because a two-tail test has *two* critical areas, each with area $\alpha/2$, which together equal α. If the value of the test statistic calculated from the sample data is less than L or greater than U, reject H_0. If the value of the test statistic is greater than or equal to L *and* less than or equal to U, do not reject H_0. For example, H_0: $\mu_1 = \mu_2$, and H_A: $\mu_1 \ne \mu_2$, $\alpha = 0.10$.

Note, we *choose* the value of α before conducting the experiment. The value of β can also be estimated, as explained later in this book.

Let us now get an overview of testing using the six-step procedure.

XIII. TEST FOR ONE MEAN WITH σ KNOWN

Step 1. Formulate hypotheses (μ_0 is a specific value of μ which is often also represented by K). There are three possible tests.

1. H_0: $\mu \le \mu_0$ versus H_A: $\mu > \mu_0$ (upper tail, directional test)
2. H_0: $\mu \ge \mu_0$ versus H_A: $\mu < \mu_0$ (lower tail, directional test)
3. H_0: $\mu = \mu_0$ versus H_A: $\mu \ne \mu_0$ (two tail, nondirectional test)

Step 2. State sample size, n, and select α.

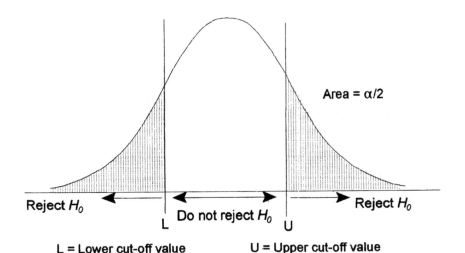

Area = $\alpha/2$

Reject H_0 Do not reject H_0 Reject H_0

L   U

L = Lower cut-off value   U = Upper cut-off value

FIGURE 10   Region of rejection and nonrejection for two-tail test.

Step 3. Write the formula for the test statistic, such as

$$Z_c = \frac{\bar{X} - \mu_0}{\sigma/\sqrt{n}}$$

This test statistic assumes that the data are *normally* distributed or that n is sufficiently large for the central limit theorem to apply.

Step 4. Formulate a decision rule via drawing a normal curve and shading the critical region(s). Call the test statistic's value calculated from the sample data Z_c. Let Z_α be the tabled value of the standard normal that cuts off an area of size α in the upper tail of the distribution. Also, $-Z_\alpha$ is the tabled value that cuts off an area the size of α in the lower-tail region. A two-tail test at α cuts off areas in both the lower and upper regions the size of $\alpha/2$.

Null hypothesis	Test hypothesis	Reject region	Nonreject region
$H_0 = \mu \le \mu_0$	$H_A = \mu > \mu_0$	$z_c > z_\alpha$	$z_c \le z_\alpha$
$H_0 = \mu \ge \mu_0$	$H_A = \mu < \mu_0$	$z_c < -z_\alpha$	$z_c \ge -z_\alpha$
$H_0 = \mu = \mu_0$	$H_A = \mu \ne \mu_0$	$z_c < -z_{\alpha/2}$	$-z_{\alpha/2} \le z_c \le z_{\alpha/2}$
		or $z_c > z_{\alpha/2}$	

Step 5. Collect sample data and perform statistical calculations.

Step 6. Apply decision rule and make decision.

Example 1. The following data represent the number of days a disinfectant (consisting of parts A and B mixed together to form a solution) will remain antimicrobially effective. In 21 independent tests of the product, the following "mixed solution" shelf-life data are provided in days: 27, 28, 30, 31, 29, 30, 26, 26, 30, 21, 34, 31, 33, 35, 24, 25, 28, 32, 34, 30, 34.* The population standard deviation is known to be $\sigma = 11$ days. The firm that manufactures the antimicrobial product wants to state that the mean number of days that the product is stable, when parts A and B are mixed, is greater than 34 days. Based on sample information, can the manufacturer do so?

Step 1. Formulate the hypothesis. (I find it easier to determine the test hypothesis first.)

H_0: $\mu \le 34$

H_A: $\mu > 34$

---

*In order to use this test, we should check that the lifetimes, X_c, are normally distributed (lifetimes often are), or we need to claim $n = 21$ is sufficiently large for the central limit theorem to apply. These distributional considerations are discussed in a later chapter.

Step 2. Set α and n. For the preceding data, $n = 21$. Let's pick $\alpha = 0.05$.
Step 3. Write out the test statistic. Because σ is known, we will use the standard normal distribution as the basis for our test.

We will use $Z_c = (\bar{X} - \mu_0)/(\sigma/\sqrt{n})$ as the test statistic, where the subscript c is used to indicate that this is the Z-score calculated from the data and μ_0 represents a specified value of the mean (here $\mu_0 = 34$).

Step 4. This is a one-tail (upper tail) test at $\alpha = 0.05$ because the average value needed is greater than 34. One can now turn to Table A.1 in the Appendix and find that the Z tabled value (normal deviate), which cuts off an upper tail area of $\alpha = 0.05$, is $Z_t = 1.64$. The decision rule is: if $Z_{\text{calculated}} > Z_{\text{tabled}}$, reject H_0 at $\alpha = 0.05$ (Fig. 11).
Step 5. Perform the calculations.

$$\bar{X} = \frac{\sum x_i}{n} = \frac{27 + 28 + 30 + \cdots + 30 + 34}{21} = \frac{618}{21} = 29.43$$

$$Z_c = \frac{\bar{x} - \mu_0}{\sigma/\sqrt{n}} = \frac{29.43 - 34.0}{11/\sqrt{21}} = -1.90$$

Step 6. Because the calculated value of Z $(Z_c = -1.90)$ is *less than* the tabled value of Z $(Z_t = 1.64)$, one cannot reject H_0 at $\alpha = 0.05$. Conclude that the mean number of days the product is stable is 34, or less. The firm must reformulate.

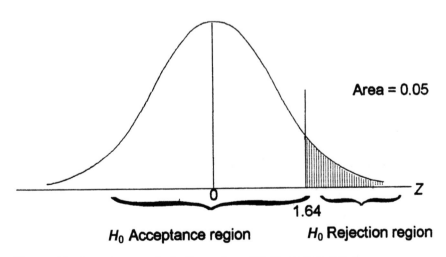

Area = 0.05

Z

1.64

H_0 Acceptance region H_0 Rejection region

FIGURE 11   Acceptance and rejection regions of H_0 (Example 1, step 4).

XIV. TEST FOR ONE MEAN WITH σ UNKNOWN

Recall that for a large sample size, n, the Z and t distributions are virtually identical. For this reason, many authors recommend using the preceding Z-test if $n \geq 30$ and σ is unknown. However, for a sample size $n < 30$, it is better to use Student's t-test, using Student's t-distribution. Steps 1, 2, 5, and 6 are exactly as described in the problem with one mean, σ known. The formula in step 3 changes because σ is not known and is, therefore, estimated by S, the sample standard deviation. And, in step 4, each z_c is replaced by the t_c because z_c is used to signify a normal distribution, whereas t_c indicates Student's t-distribution.

The test statistic is distributed as Student's t, with $n - 1$ degrees of freedom (df). Hence, $t_c = (\bar{X} - \mu_0)/(S/\sqrt{n})$, with $n - 1$ df.

Example 2. Suppose we work the previous example,* ignoring the fact that the value of σ was given.

Step 1.   State hypothesis.

$$H_0 : \mu \leq 34$$

$$H_A : \mu > 34$$

Step 2.   Specify α and n.

$$\alpha = 0.05$$

$$n = 21$$

Step 3.   Write out the test statistic

$$t_c = \frac{\bar{X} - 34}{S/\sqrt{n}} \quad \text{with } n - 1 \text{ df}$$

where

$$S = \sqrt{\frac{\sum (x_i - \bar{x})^2}{n - 1}}$$

A simplified calculation for S is:

$$S = \sqrt{\frac{\sum x_i^2 - n\bar{x}^2}{n - 1}}$$

---

*As before, the data need to be tested for normality; this will be discussed in Chapter 3.

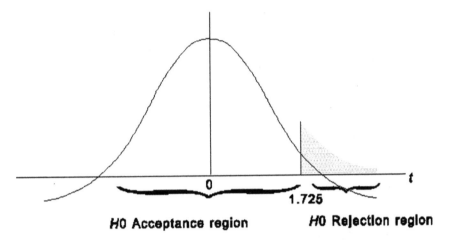

FIGURE 12   Acceptance and rejection regions of H_0 (Example 2, step 4).

Step 4.   Formulate the decision rule.
Student's *t*-table (Appendix Table B) shows that, with $21-1=20$ df,
the value of *t* that cuts off an upper tail area of $\alpha = 0.05$ is $t_t = 1.725$
(Fig. 12). The tabled *t* value, t_t, is also known as the critical value.
Decision rule: If $t_c > t_t$, reject H_0 at $\alpha = 0.05$.

Step 5.   Calculate the test statistic.

$$\bar{x} = \frac{618}{21} = 29.43$$

$$S^2 = \frac{\sum x_i^2 - n(\bar{X})^2}{n-1}$$

$$S^2 = \frac{18{,}460 - 21(29.43)^2}{21-1}$$

$$S^2 = \frac{18{,}460 - 18{,}189}{20} = 13.55$$

$$S = \sqrt{13.55} = 3.68$$

$$\sum x_i^2 = 27^2 + 28^2 + 30^2 + 31^2 + 29^2$$
$$+ 30^2 + 26^2 + 26^2 + 30^2 + 21^2$$
$$+ 34^2 + 31^2 + 33^2 + 35^2 + 24^2$$
$$+ 25^2 + 28^2 + 32^2 + 34^2$$
$$+ 30^2 + 34^2$$
$$= 18{,}460$$

Thus,

$$t_c = \frac{29.43 - 34}{3.68/\sqrt{21}} = \frac{-4.57}{0.80} = -5.71$$

Step 6.   Draw conclusion.
Because $-5.71 < 1.725$, one cannot reject H_0 at $\alpha = 0.05$.

Example 3. Consider the following set of $\log_{10}$ measurements*:0.91, 1.32, 1.72, 1.43, 1.66, 1.95, 1.61, 2.07, 2.02, 1.65, 1.52, 1.21, 1.30, 1.59, 1.82, 2.02, 1.69, 2.33, 1.75, 1.46. Could one conclude that the mean of the population is less than 1.70 (in the $\log_{10}$ scale)? In order to answer this question, apply the six-step process.

Step 1. Formulate hypotheses. The test question, $\mu < 1.70$, is the alternative or test hypothesis. The null hypothesis is simply $\mu \geq 1.70$. The hypotheses are:

$H_0: \mu \geq 1.70$

$H_A: \mu < 1.70.$

Step 2. Set n and α.
Let $n = 20$ and $\alpha = 0.025$.

Step 3. Specify the test statistic. It is

$$t_c = \frac{\bar{X} - \mu_0}{S/\sqrt{n}}$$

Step 4. Formulate the decision rule. Because this is a lower tail test, we need the tabled t value with $n - 1 = 20 - 1 = 19$ df, which cuts off an area of $\alpha = 0.025$ in the *lower* (left) tail. The critical value t_t is, therefore, -2.093 (Fig. 13).

Decision rule: If $t_t < -2.093$, reject H_0 at $\alpha = 0.025$.

Step 5. Perform calculations.

$$\bar{x} = \frac{\sum x_i}{n} = \frac{33.03}{20} = 1.6515$$

$$s = \sqrt{\frac{\sum x_i^2 - n(\bar{x})^2}{n - 1}} = 0.3346$$

$$t_c = \frac{1.6515 - 1.70}{0.3346/\sqrt{20}} = -0.6482$$

Step 6. Determine conclusion.
Because $t_c(-0.6482) > t_t(-2.093)$, one cannot reject H_0 at $\alpha = 0.025$.

---

*The $\log_{10}$ measurements need to be checked for normality; this will be discussed later.

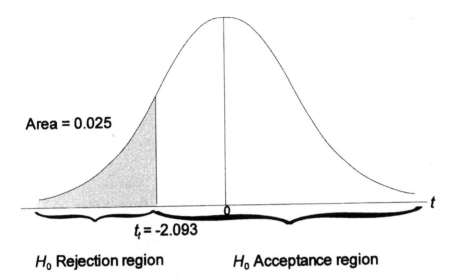

$$t_t = -2.093$$

H_0 Rejection region H_0 Acceptance region

FIGURE 13   Acceptance and rejection regions (Example 3, step 4).

XV. TEST FOR THE DIFFERENCES BETWEEN TWO MEANS (INDEPENDENT SAMPLES)

Example 4. Two antimicrobial products are compared for efficacy. The results are summarized:

Product 1	Product 2
$n_1 = 36$	$n_2 = 40$
$s_1 = 10.2$	$s_2 = 15.4$
$\bar{x}_1 = 86.3$	$\bar{x}_2 = 92.4$

Are the products' antimicrobial properties statistically different from one another?

Step 1.   State the hypotheses.
Because we are looking for a difference in the performance of products (either larger or smaller), the test hypothesis is $\mu_1 \neq \mu_2$, a two-tail test.

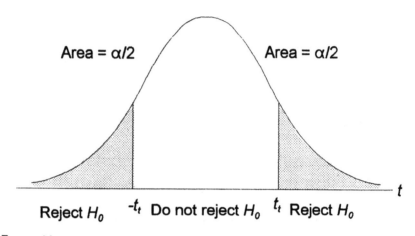

FIGURE 14   Acceptance and rejection regions (Example 4, step 4).

So:

$$H_0: \mu_1 = \mu_2 \quad \text{or} \quad \mu_1 - \mu_2 = 0$$

$$H_A: \mu_1 \neq \mu_2 \quad \text{or} \quad \mu_1 - \mu_2 \neq 0$$

Step 2. Set α and determine n. Because this problem has two samples, there are two *ns*: n_1 and n_2.

Thirty-six (36) zones were read for product 1 and forty (40) for product 2, so $n_1 = 36$ and $n_2 = 40$. Let us set $\alpha = 0.05$.

Step 3. Write out the test statistic.

$$t_c = \frac{\bar{x}_1 - \bar{x}_2}{\sqrt{S_1^2/n_1 + S_2^2/n_2}}$$

which is approximately distributed as Student's t for n_1+n_2 large.

Step 4. Formulate the decision rule. Find the tabled critical values for a two-sided t-test at level α with *df* degrees of freedom. Call these critical values $\pm t_t$ (Fig. 14). Note that, if the sample sizes are not equal, the smaller of the samples, minus 1, is used; in this case, $36 - 1 = 35$ df.

Decision rule: If t_c (t calculated) is greater than t_t or less than $-t_t$, reject H_0.

Step 5. Perform the calculations.

$$t_c = \frac{86.3 - 92.4}{\sqrt{(10.2)^2/36 + (15.4)^2/40}} = \frac{-6.1}{\sqrt{2.89 + 5.929}} = \frac{-6.1}{2.97} = -2.05$$

t_t with 35 df $= 2.030$

Step 6. Determine the conclusion.
Because $t_c < -t_t (-2.05 < -2.030)$, reject H_0 at $\alpha = 0.05$.

3

Exploratory Data Analysis

Once an experiment has been conducted, but before performing any statistical tests, it is a good idea to get a "feel" for the data collected. This can be effectively accomplished by using exploratory data analysis, or EDA. John W. Tukey, a famed statistician, at the level of R. A. Fisher, W. G. Cochran, W. S. Gossett (the "Student"), S. Siegel, and F. Mosteller, initially developed this concept. Tukey first presented this work in his book *Exploratory Data Analysis* [14] and later in *Data Analysis and Regression*, which was coauthored with Frederick Mosteller [15].

EDA is a straightforward, practical way of evaluating data without prior assumptions about the data. This allows the data themselves to help the researcher better understand them and, thereby, better select the appropriate parametric or nonparametric procedure to be used in the statistical analysis. Yet, EDA goes beyond this in that it helps the researcher to choose a specific statistical method to analyze the data and know why that specific statistical method has been chosen. This may seem like a small issue, but because there are often multiple ways to analyze data, to be able to analyze them optimally is important. Researchers need to ground the statistical method chosen based on the data's distribution. That is, one fits the statistical method to the data, not the data to the method.

EDA will enable one, through practice, to ascertain whether a data set derived from a small number of samples is distributed approximately normally. And it must be remembered that observations collected in applied research are rarely distributed in a perfectly symmetrical, bell-shaped, "normal" distribution. Data never fit a statistical distribution exactly. Instead, the data are usually "messy."

When a sample appears nonnormal, one can often transform, or reexpress,* the data to make them more normal. This procedure is an important aspect of EDA. For example, if a data set is skewed (piled up on one side of the curve with long tailing on the other side), a data reexpression can be performed to normalize the data. Or, if the sample is bimodal (has two peaks instead of one) EDA procedures can flag the researcher to investigate this problem further. Perhaps the data were unknowingly drawn from two populations, not one. For example, if blood pressure readings are taken from a sample of available people, one can often detect a bimodal distribution. This can be the result of selecting both males and females under the assumption that they are from a single population when they are really from two different populations, one for each sex.

In addition, many times a sample's outer edges, or "tails," extend beyond what is considered a normal distribution; i.e., there are enough data values beyond $\pm 3\sigma$ or $\pm 4\sigma$ to cast doubt on the presumption that the data are normal. They *straggle* more than they should according to statistical theory [14]. Yet, these straggler values—sometimes single, sometimes multiple—can reveal valuable hidden features contained in the data. For example, the antimicrobial efficacy ($\log_{10}$ microbial count) data in human trials of a preoperative skin prepping solution often have straggler values (also known as "outliers") that are either very large or very small, relative to the data's central tendency. Generally, upon investigation, this is not an anomaly related to the degerming characteristics of the antimicrobial solution but is a phenomenon both of bacterial populations normally residing on the skin surfaces and of skin sampling methods themselves. Even so, the normal distribution allows values beyond $\pm 3\sigma$ to be included in the population. In fact, 0.3% of values theoretically are beyond three standard deviations from the mean. So, by chance, one of these rare values may have been collected in the sample, even through 95% of the values are contained within $\pm 2\sigma$ of the mean. But these extreme values can also represent an error, such as a recording error or a calculation error in a specific dilution level, for example. EDA can be of immense help to a researcher in quickly identifying these extreme values. The researcher, then, must determine why these data were extreme. Did they occur by chance? Are they the result of some error? Or are they naturally occurring values that may provide unexpected insight into the problem being studied? This identification process is a challenge for the researcher.

Now, let us preview four general EDA operations useful for the researcher:

---

*I use the terms "transform" and "reexpress" as they apply to data interchangeably in this work.

1. *EDA data displays* provide a graphical depiction of the whole data set, thus enabling the researcher to visualize easily data clumping and data dispersion as well as the shape, "gappy-ness," tailing, and any extreme values. In short, they assist the researcher to understand quickly how the data are oriented to one another.

2. *EDA residual analyses* are important because they help the researcher see how well the data fit the model (i.e., how close the observed values are to the values predicted by the statistical model) in terms of the size and distribution of e_i. This information will be of concern to us, beginning in Chap. 4 and continuing through the remainder of the book.

$$e_i = x_i - \bar{x}$$

where e_i = random variation or statistical error
         x_i = actual value
         $\bar{x}$ = predicted value or mean

In the regression chapter, Chap. 11, we will estimate a regression function. If that function adequately portrays the actual collected data, the differences between each observed (collected) value and the predicted value will be minimal and random. When the predicted values do not portray the observed data adequately, a distinct, nonrandom data pattern is often observed in the residual values. The researcher can then reexpress the data and reevaluate the residual values for minimal spread and a random pattern.

3. *Data Reexpressions*, or transformations are a possible "fix" for data sets that are not approximately normal. For example, the data can often be reexpressed in another scale to make them normal.* Generally, such reexpressions are simple mathematical operations, such as the square root ($\sqrt{Y}$), the logarithmic value ($\log_{10} Y$ [base 10] or $\ln Y$ [natural]), or the reciprocal value ($1/Y$). The data transformation is usually performed, and the results, call them Y_i', are reevaluated, generally through another residual analysis. If the residual values ($Y_i' - \hat{Y}_i'$) are randomly distributed about zero, the process was adequate. If not, another reexpression iteration can be performed.

4. *Resistance*, or robustness, of a statistic can be checked using EDA to determine whether a single value, or a few extreme values, has had

---

*In general, reexpressions are first applied to the response, or dependent variable, y. If this is not satisfactory, the independent variable, x, can be transformed. Sometimes it is necessary to transform both x and y.

undue influence on the results of a statistical analysis. This is particularly useful for small sample sizes, where an extreme value can have much influence on the statistical parameters (e.g., $\bar{x}$ and s).

Finally, it is important to recognize that use of these four EDA tools together will maximize their efficiency. For example, in the situation where there are several extreme values (i.e., very different from the other data in the set), a data display, such as the stem-and-leaf display, will portray them quickly. A residual analysis will also portray this situation, not in terms of the actual numbers but in differences (e_i) between the observed and predicted values. And, if the data are skewed—piled to the left (smaller values) or piled to the right (larger values) with a long tail on the opposite end—reexpressing the data, in most cases, will be useful in making the data more normal in their distribution.

Finally, although EDA calculations are generally simple, in practice, they are tedious and time consuming to perform. The use of statistical software, particularly if large data sets are involved, is nearly mandatory. Fortunately, there are many software packages (e.g., SPSSX®, SAS®, MiniTab®) that contain many useful EDA application subroutines. By far the most user-friendly package is MiniTab, which we will use in tandem with the paper-and-pencil statistical analyses performed in this book. Let us now look at some individual EDA applications.

I. STEM-AND-LEAF DISPLAYS

As the applied researcher is aware, and as we have discussed, data sets (known as "batches" in EDA) come in variously shaped distributions. It is useful to know the shape of the data set(s) to ascertain that the data are normally distributed, etc., prior to conducting a parametric statistical test. A stem-and-leaf display is a data-ordering and presentation procedure that provides a convenient and direct way to become acquainted with the data. When a data set contains only a few values, a stem-and-leaf display is simple to construct with pencil and paper. Larger data sets are more conveniently displayed by using a computer.

The stem-and-leaf display was first presented by John Tukey [14] and is widely used throughout the statistical field. It is a type of frequency distribution that combines the leftmost digit(s) of each data value (stem) with the next digit to the right (leaf) simultaneously in an ordered manner. Individual data values are also easy to recover from the display* because, unlike the

---

*The recovered value may be only a two- or three-digit "approximation" to the original value if some digits on the right were truncated (see step 1 in the example that follows).

case of histograms, where data are grouped into categories and *only* the category frequencies are plotted, the numerical values do not disappear.

Specifically, the stem-and-leaf display enables a researcher to see:

1. How wide the data batch is (its range)
2. Where, within the data batch, the values are *concentrated* and where there are gaps, if any
3. Whether there are single or multiple modes (peaks)
4. How symmetrical or asymmetrical the data batch is
5. Whether any values are extreme, or stragglers, as Tukey described them

These important characteristics of the data usually go unnoticed and unchecked by those who merely gather data and "crank" them through a statistical analysis. But, by making EDA the first procedure in a statistical analysis (*after* the study has been designed and after the data have

TABLE 1 Thickness Levels of Biofilm Residue in μm

Run	Amount of residue left
1	4.305
2	7.210
3	5.161
4	8.204
5	8.191
6	6.502
7	6.307
8	5.211
9	11.701
10	9.801
11	8.213
12	2.051
13	10.133
14	4.221
15	4.305
16	5.261
17	4.305
18	7.159
19	6.793
20	5.201

been collected), the preceding five aspects can be examined and dealt with, if necessary.

A. Construction Procedure

Let us work an example to understand better how a stem-and-leaf display is constructed. Suppose a researcher has performed a series of measurements to determine the amount of biofilm residue left on a glass beaker's surface after a certain chemical cleaning treatment has been completed. Table 1 presents the collected data. Let us organize these data into a stem-and-leaf display.

Step 1. Choose the stems and leaves. The researcher has some flexibility here. For example, looking at the first value, 4.305, there are a number of ways to present it.

"Stem" leading component		"Leaf" trailing component
4		3
	or	
43		0
	or	
430		5

The number of digits assigned to the stem portion is arbitary. However, the leaf portion contains only one digit, and that is the digit immediately following the last stem digit. For example, if the number is 4.305 and the researcher decides to use a one-digit stem, that stem is 4, and its leaf is 3, and the "05" portion of 4.305 is truncated or dropped, giving

Stem	Leaf
4	3

Taking the data batch from Table 1 as an example, we will now construct the stem-and-leaf display, shown in Fig. 1. We will assign the stems the values to the left of the decimal point and will designate the *first* values to the right of the decimal point to be the leaves. (The other digits to the right of the decimal point are ignored.)

Step 2. The data are ordered in ascending order, and the stems are written in a column from smallest to largest to the left of the dividing line. The leaves are written to the right of the dividing line, beginning at the bottom and working up. Notice that we include all possible stem values even if no values occurred in the data for that stem. Where there are multiple identical values for the stem, the stem is not rewritten but, instead, an additional leaf value is shown. For example, if there are two values, 4.305 and 4.221, the stem for both is 4, the leaf for 4.305 is 3, and the leaf for 4.221 is 2. The display for these two values is 4|23. The leaf values are also written in ascending order. Same value leaves are similarly handled. For example, the three values 4.31, 4.31, and 4.30 would be displayed as 4|333. Clearly, every value in a data batch will have one leaf value.

By examining the MiniTab computer output in Fig. 2, one can see, as in the pencil-and-paper stem-and-leaf display in Fig. 1, that there is a data gap at stem "3." There are not enough data, however, to determine whether this gap is a significant feature of the data. Notice, also, that the MiniTab output provides a depth column. On both sides of the data set, the first value is termed "1," the second "2," and so forth. The median is found in the stem–leaf column and is the midvalue.

There is an interesting pattern at stem "8," subtly suggesting that the data are bimodal (two peaks). Again, there are not enough data to tell. So

Stem	Leaf
2	0
3	
4	2333
5	1222
6	357
7	12
8	122
9	8
10	1
11	7

FIGURE 1 Stem-and-leaf display.

Stem-and-Leaf Display $n = 20^*$

Leaf Unit = 0.10

Depth**	Stems	Leaves
1	2	0
1	3	
5	4	2333
9	5	1222
(3)	6	357
8	7	12
6	8	122
3	9	8
2	10	1
1	11	7

* n = sample size = 20
** this column, the depth column, is displayed by MiniTab®. It enables one to find the stem-leaf row where the median resides.

FIGURE 2   Stem-and-leaf display (MiniTab).

one is left with the question, "Is it possible that the mode at the stem 8 value is an anomaly, a random occurrence, or a distinct phenomenon unknown to the researcher?"

In performing research, one is often confronted with questions that cannot be answered directly. All one can do is be watchfully aware, looking for unusual features that might, for example, indicate that the data are not normal.

II. LETTER-VALUE DISPLAYS

Complementing the stem-and-leaf display is the letter-value display, which enables the researcher to examine data symmetry even more closely. The stem-and-leaf display provides useful, initial insight into data structure, but the letter-value display extends this view specifically for determining whether the data are skewed, focusing on the spread of the data between various points. The basic procedure is to divide a group of data in half at the median, then halve these two groups, halve the resulting groups, etc.

A. Construction Procedure

The first operation in constructing a letter-value display is to find the median of the ordered set of data.* The median (middle value) of a group of ordered data, with an odd sample size n, is the middle data value. A set of data in which n is an even number has a middle *pair* of numbers, and the average of these two values is the median.

Calculating the *depth* of the median is also important. Depth is *not* the median value; rather, it is the position of the median in the ordered data set.[†] The depth of the median is customarily written as $d(M)=(n+1)/2$, where M = median and n = sample size. When n is odd, $d(M)$ is a whole number; when n is an even number, the depth of the median is the average of two depth values. If $d(M)=8$, the median is the 8th ordered value in the data set. If $d(M)=10.5$, the median is the average of the 10th and 11th ordered values.

Note that the median divides a data batch in half whether n is odd or even. In computing a letter-value display, these two half batches are split in half again; the split points are called the *hinges*, denoted by the letter H. So, a data batch has one median, M, and two hinges, H, which divide the batch into, roughly, quarters.

In finding the depth of the hinges, we begin with the median's position, $d(M)$. The calculation is much like that for the depth of the median except that we drop any fractional value from $d(M)$ and add 1. Hence, the formula for the depth of the hinges is $d(H)=([d(M)]+1)/2$, where the square brackets around $d(M)$ mean "greatest integer portion of" and indicate that any fractional portion of $d(M)$ is truncated, or dropped.

Note that hinges are similar to quartiles[‡] in that both, along with the median (which is the second quartile), divide the data set into quarters. However, because of the difference in the way they are calculated, the hinges may be closer to the median than the first and third quartiles are.

The next step in letter-value display construction is to find the middle values for the outer data quarters. They are approximately an eighth of the way in from each end of the ordered data batch and are denoted E for eighth. The computational formula for computing the depth of eighths is $d(E)=([d(H)]+1)/2$, where the square brackets again remind us to drop the

---

*This method is the same as that discussed for stem-and-leaf plots, except that here we are working with the ordered raw data.

[†]Recall that depth can be measured either from below or from above.

[‡]The first or lower quartile can be calculated as the median of the observations below the location of the batch median, and the third or upper quartile is the median of the observations above the location of the batch median.

fractional portion (if there is one) of the depth of the hinge value and use only the greatest integer portion of $d(H)$.

The letter value in the tails beyond the eighths is used less often in pencil-and-paper procedures but is commonly computed in software programs. These D points lie midway between the E points and the ends of the data string.* Their depths are computed exactly as the depths of E and H were: $d(D)=([d(E)]+1)/2$.

An example using the data in Table 1 for constructing a letter-value display is provided in Table 2.

The depth of the median, $d(M)$, is first computed using the formula:

$$d(M) = \frac{n+1}{2} = \frac{20+1}{2} = 10.5$$

First, the data from Table 1 are ordered from smallest to largest, and then their depths are recorded. (Recall from the stem-and-leaf discussion that depths are counted "from below" for the smaller values and "from above" for the larger values, i.e., from the smallest value forward to the middle value in the data set and from the largest value backward to the middle value in the data set.)

Because the sample size n is even, we must add the two central data values (at depths of 10 and 11) from either end and divide by 2 to find the data value with the 10.5 depth position. The two values at depths 10 and 11, respectively, are 6.502 and 6.307 (counted from above) or 6.307 and 6.502 (counted from below); in either case, their average is $(6.502 + 6.307)/2 = 6.405$ (rounded), which is the median value of the data.

Now, let us find the depth of the hinges, $d(H)$.

$$d(H) = ([d(M)]+1)/2$$

$$= ([10.5]+1)/2^{\dagger}$$

So $\quad d(H) = (10+1)/2 = 5.5$

Again, the two values associated with depths 5 and 6 are averaged. Remember, there are two hinges, an upper hinge and a lower hinge, so we must

---

*The ends of the data string, the *extremes*, i.e., the minimum and maximum values, are said to have depth 1. Thus, each subsequent depth is halfway between the previous depth and 1, the depth of the extreme.

†Note that the fractional portion of $d(M)$ is truncated.

TABLE 2 Construction of a Letter-value Display

Depths of letter values for calculating display ($n=20$)	Depth	Data values			Letter value
	1	2.051			
$d(D) = (3 + 1)/2 = 2$	2	4.221	→	4.221	D
$d(E) = (5 + 1)/2 = 3$	3	4.305	→	4.305	E
	4	4.305			
	5	4.305			
$d(H) = (10 + 1)/2 = 5.5$	5.5		→	4.733	H
	6	5.161			
	7	5.201			
	8	5.211			
	9	5.261			
	10	6.307			
$d(M) = (20 + 1)/2 = 10.5$	10.5		→	6.405	M
	10	6.502			
	9	6.793			
	8	7.159			
	7	7.210			
	6	8.191			
$d(H) = (10 + 1)/2 = 5.5$	5.5		→	8.198	H
	5	8.204			
	4	8.213			
$d(E) = (5 + 1)/2 = 3$	3	9.801	→	9.801	E
$d(D) = (3 + 1)/2 = 2$	2	10.133	→	10.133	D
	1	11.701			

average the values with depths 5 and 6 from above and average the values with depths 5 and 6 from below:

$(8.204 + 8.191)/2 = 8.198,$ rounded = upper hinge value

$(5.161 + 4.305)/2 = 4.733$ = lower hinge value

With the hinge values found, now let us determine the depths of the eighths:

$$d(E) = ([d(H)] + 1)/2$$

$$= ([5.5] + 1)/2$$

$$= (5 + 1)/2 = 3$$

Because the depth of the eighths is a whole number, all we have to do is count three values from above for the upper eighth and three values from below for the lower eighth (Table 2).

9.801 is the upper eighth value.
4.305 is the lower eighth value.

Finally, let us determine the depth of the D value,

$$d(D) = ([d(E)] + 1)/2$$

$$= ([3] + 1)/2$$

$$= (3 + 1)/2 = 2$$

Because the depth of E is a whole number, we have to count only two values from above for the upper D value and two values from below for the lower D value.

10.133 is the upper D value.
4.221 is the lower D value.

The letter-value display data computed from Table 2 can now be put into the letter-value display format (Table 3). In producing this table, we need to compute the midsummaries (midhinge, mideighth, mid-D, and midextreme or midrange), by averaging the appropriate upper and lower values. The $H, E,$ and D spreads are merely the distance between the upper and lower letter values; the distance between the extremes is called the *range*.

It is far easier to let a computer's software compute and table letter-value displays once one knows and *senses* what is happening. Table 4 presents a MiniTab computer output of a letter-value display.

TABLE 3   Letter-value Display

Letter	Depth	Lower	Upper	Mid[a]	Spread[b]
M	10.5		6.405	6.405	
H	5.5	4.733	8.198	6.465	3.465
E	3.0	4.305	9.801	7.053	5.496
D	2.0	4.221	10.133	7.177	5.912
Extreme	1.0	2.051	11.701	6.876	9.650

[a]Mid is midpoint between the upper and lower values, (lower + upper)/2; for H, (4.733 + 8.198)/2 = 6.465.
[b]Spread is distance between upper and lower values (e.g., H spread = 8.198 − 4.733 = 3.465).

TABLE 4   MiniTab Letter-value Display

Letter	Depth	Lower	Upper	Mid	Spread
N	20				
M	10.5		6.405	6.405	
H	5.5	4.733	8.198	6.465	3.465
E	3	4.305	9.801	7.053	5.496
D	2	4.221	10.133	7.177	5.912
a	1	2.051	11.701	6.876	9.650

[a]The extreme values of the batch have no letter label; they are labeled with only their depth, 1.

Using the letter-value display, the symmetry or skewness of a sample data set can be determined by comparing the "mid" (midsummary) column values with one another, that is, comparing the median value with the mid-hinge, with the mideighth, with the mid-D, and with the midpoint of the two extreme values, the midrange.

If the data are symmetrical, the midsummary values will be close to the median value. If the midsummary values become progressively larger as we move from M to H to E to D to the extremes, the data are skewed to the right, or larger values. If the midsummary values become progressively smaller, the data are skewed to the left, or smaller values of the data batch.*

Looking at the midsummary values in Table 4, we see 6.405, 6.465, 7.053, 7.177, and 6.876. Because these values are increasing, up to 7.177, the data are apparently skewed to the right, but then this trend ceases at 7.177 and recedes to 6.876. The skewness of this sample set is not that significant, and anomalies are expected in small data sets such as this. Hence, a transformation of the data to make them more symmetrical would probably not be worthwhile. I would conclude that the data are approximately symmetrical. But, with an n of only 20, there are too few data points to be sure.

One can also learn about variability of the data batch from the "spread" column. The spread is simply the difference between the pair of upper and lower letter values, which typically increases from letter value to letter value as we move outward from the median. The last spread (depth 1) is the range of the entire data batch. The greater the spreads (range of data within each

---

*Skewed distributions are shown in Fig. 13. The easy way to remember which way the data are skewed is to think "skew, few." If the data right skew, there are only a few values on the right; i.e., there is a long right tail. If the data left skew, there are few values on the left, so there is a long left tail.

letter-value pair), the greater the variability of the data batch. Finding spread analyses truly useful will require hands-on practice.

When using the letter-value display, use the stem-and-leaf display with it to get a more comprehensive view. Notice that the data in the stem-and-leaf display (Figs. 1 and 2) are slightly skewed to the right because there are several large values but no small values (except 2.0) to "balance" the display of the data set. The data are "bunched up" at stems 4 and 5. There is no tail on the left because there is only one datum with a stem smaller than 4. The value 2.051 may represent something unique about the data batch. Why is the 2.051 value present? Without the 2.051 value, the data set would clearly be skewed to the right. The researcher will want to keep this in mind as the evaluation progresses. At present, this question cannot be answered.

It is in this "fuzzy" area that the researcher employing statistics has a far greater advantage in understanding what is occurring than does a mathematical statistician. The data represent phenomena in the researcher's expertise, not in that of the statistician!

If the researcher suspects that the smallest value (2.051) may be erroneous, she or he may decide to do statistical analyses with and without that data point. Or, at this point, it may be useful to transform or reexpress the data to normalize them. However, on a personal note, I would use a nonparametric method for data analysis, thereby sidestepping issues of skewness.

The letter-value display can be used to evaluate how close a particular symmetrical sample distribution is to the normal or Gaussian distribution.* The researcher compares the spreads in the letter-value display with the corresponding spreads for the standard normal distribution, which has a mean of zero and a standard deviation of 1. The H, E, and D spreads for the standard normal distributions are:

Letter value	$N(0,1)$ spread
H	1.349
E	2.301
D	3.068

If we assume that the data are approximately normal with mean μ and standard deviation σ, the data spread values divided by the $N(0, 1)$ spread values should provide estimates of σ.

---

*If the data were reexpressed to attain greater symmetry, the spreads of the reexpressed data would be used.

The formulae would be as follows:

$$S_H = (\text{data value of } H \text{ spread})/1.349$$

$$S_E = (\text{data value of } E \text{ spread})/2.301$$

$$S_D = (\text{data value of } D \text{ spread})/3.068$$

If the data resemble a normal distribution, all three of these quotients should be approximately equal (because they each estimate σ):

$$S_H \approx S_E \approx S_D$$

If the quotients grow—increase—as we move from H to E to D, the tails of the data are heavier than the tails of the normal curve.* If the quotients shrink, the tails of the data are lighter.

Let us perform these calculations on the data in Table 3:

$$S_H = 3.465/1.349 = 2.569$$

$$S_E = 5.496/2.301 = 2.389$$

$$S_D = 5.912/3.068 = 1.927$$

Because $S_H = 2.569$, $S_E = 2.389$, and $S_D = 1.927$ are not approximately equal, the data do not appear to be from a normal distribution. The S values shrink, so the tails are lighter (have less probability) than the tails of a normal distribution (Fig. 3). Personally, I would consider these data "normal enough" for most applications, particularly pilot studies. If I were concerned, I would merely increase the sample size, n, and check the new data for symmetry and normality.

If it is common practice in one's field to report data in the original scale, then a reexpression of the skewed data, particularly if skewness is not severe, will just confuse the situation. Perhaps one will apply a parametric method that relies on data normality but inform readers that the sample data are, in fact, skewed. Or, if the data are seriously skewed, the researcher will opt for a nonparametric method. Whatever the case, it is the researcher's conscious decision how best to deal with the data. This is far better than merely gathering data and mindlessly cranking them through a statistical analysis to report significance.

Statistics, to a large degree, are a form of communication and not an absolute decree. However, when a researcher chooses a statistic to support

---

*Heavier tails mean that there is more probability in the tails than the standard normal distribution. Figure 6 shows the t-distribution with 4 df and the standard normal distribution. All t-distributions have heavier tails than the standard normal distribution.

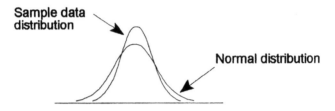

FIGURE 3   Sample data distribution vs. normal distribution.

a preconceived outcome, this action is not a legitimate use of statistics or the research process.

III. BOXPLOT

It is often helpful to have a clear, visual picture of where the middle of a sample batch of data lies and how spread out the data are, but without a lot of other detail. The middle point of a data batch is rarely problematic—unless the data distribution is multimodal—but the outermost data or tails can be. Hence, one is often more interested in the tail regions, particularly if extreme values, or outliers (also known as "strays"), are present.

Outliers are values so small or large—i.e., extreme—that they dramatically stand away from the rest of the data batch, sometimes many standard deviations away. Outliers can result from research peculiarities as well as from measuring errors, recording errors, procedural errors, and data entry errors. Having outlier values flagged visually is an advantage of the boxplot display. Once outliers have been identified, one can study them in greater detail and, if they are errors, correct them. Of course, not all outliers are errors. Outliers often reflect unusual or unexpected outcomes in a study and, at that, may be extremely valuable. Before performing actual statistical method calculations, the cause of an outlier should be investigated and identified as an error in recording, etc., or a unique phenomenon.

Sometimes one will be unable to identify the source of an outlier and may wish to remove it from a data set to enhance the power of a statistical test by reducing the data variability. In order to deal with such outliers with some type of legitimacy, the researcher needs a rule of thumb for when to leave the extreme values in a data batch or remove them as extraneous values. We can do this using EDA, without resorting to advanced statistical procedures. This is because boxplots utilize H (hinge) values, as calculated for the letter-value display, as a critical construction component.

A. Construction Procedure

Two calculations are made, for both the *upper* and *lower* portions of the box-plot display, called the inner and outer "fences." These fences define boundaries, and data outside the boundaries are labeled outliers. The computations are fairly straightforward.

Upper inner fence = upper hinge $+ (1.5 \times H$ spread)

Lower inner fence = lower hinge $- (1.5 \times H$ spread)

The outer fence also has upper and lower values.

Upper outer fence = upper hinge $+ (3 \times H$ spread)

Lower outer fence = lower hinge $- (3 \times H$ spread)

Data values beyond the inner fences are termed *outside* values and values beyond the outer fences are called *far outside* values. The data values that are not outside the inner fences, but are closest to them, are called *adjacent* values.

B. Boxplot Calculations

For the data in Table 1, displayed in stem-and-leaf form in Fig. 2 and summarized in the letter-value display (Table 3), we note that the hinge values are 4.733 and 8.198 with an H spread of 3.465. So the inner fence values are:

Lower inner fence = lower hinge $- (1.5 \times H$ spread)

$$= 4.733 - (1.5 \times 3.465)$$

$$= -0.465$$

Upper inner fence = upper hinge $+ (1.5 \times H$ spread)

$$= 8.198 + (1.5 \times 3.465)$$

$$= 13.395$$

The outer fence values are:

Lower outer fence = lower hinge $- (3 \times H$ spread)

$$= 4.733 - (3 \times 3.465)$$

$$= -5.662$$

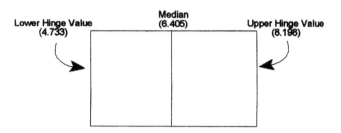

FIGURE 4   Preliminary sketch of skeletal boxplot showing only median and hinges.

$$\text{Upper outer fence} = \text{upper hinge} + (3 \times H \text{ spread})$$
$$= 8.198 + (3 \times 3.465)$$
$$= 18.593$$

The adjacent values are the most extreme data values that are within the inner fence values; in this example, they are 2.051 and 11.701.

An easy way to make a boxplot display by hand is to begin with a *skeletal boxplot*. A skeletal boxplot illustrates the "five-number summary;" i.e., it shows only the maximum and minimum data values (the extremes), the hinges,* and the median. It is constructed by drawing a box between the hinges (4.733 and 8.198) and depicting the median (6.405) as a solid line through the box (Fig. 4). To finish the skeletal boxplot, draw dashed lines from the hinges to the extremes (2.051 and 11.701). These dashed lines are called "whiskers" (Fig. 5). (Boxplots are also known as "box-and-whiskers" plots.)

A (modified) boxplot is similar to a skeletal boxplot except that we extend the dash marks (whiskers) out to the *adjacent values* (2.051 and 11.701), which are within the lower and upper inner fence values, −0.465 and 13.395, respectively. (In this example, the extremes are also the adjacent values.) The fences, by convention, are not marked.

Values outside the inner fence should be individually highlighted. Values lying outside the outer fence values should be very prominent. In this example, no values exceed the inner fences, so this step is not necessary. But suppose that two other values were present, say 14.0 and 20. (Ignore the fact that the median, hinges, etc. would all be changed by adding these two points

---

*Some texts use the first and third quartiles and the interquartile range instead of the hinges and the *H* spread. The slight difference, if any, between hinge and quartile values will not be distinguishable in a boxplot.

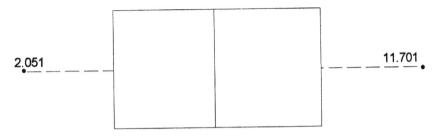

FIGURE 5 Skeletal boxplot with whiskers.

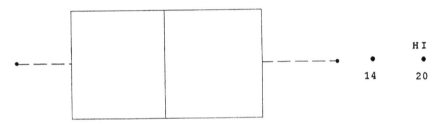

FIGURE 6 Boxplot with outliers.

to the data.) The value 14.0 is outside the upper inner fence (13.395) and 20 is outside the upper outer fence (18.593) (Fig. 6).*

It is far easier to generate a boxplot with a computer program. Software packages such as MiniTab and SAS have special commands for a boxplot display. Figure 7 provides a character-based boxplot generated from the data in Table 1 using a standard MiniTab routine.

Notice that the dotted whiskers extend to the adjacent values within the inner fence (2.051 and 11.701); "I" marks the hinge values (4.733 and 8.198). The median is denoted " +." No values exceed the inner fence or outer fence boundaries, so none are identified.

In addition, in initial data exploration, it is often useful to compare multiple groups tentatively. The boxplot offers the researcher a convenient way of doing so (Fig. 8).

But what does one compare? Our eyes tend to focus on the hinges as well as the whiskers, looking naturally at boxplots to categorize those that do and do not overlap. That procedure is useful, but a researcher usually

*The values outside the outer fences are often labeled "HI" or "LOW," depending upon their direction. The value 14 is "outside" and the value 20 is "far outside." Both are potential outliers and need to be investigated.

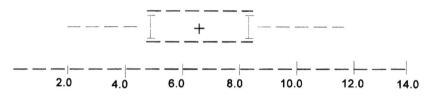

FIGURE 7   Boxplot.

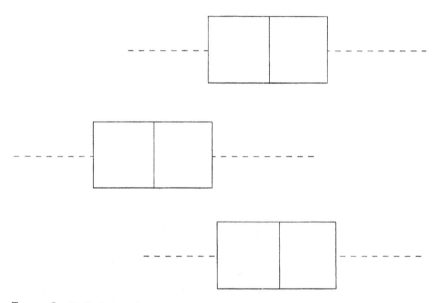

FIGURE 8   Multiple boxplots.

applies a little more formal method. McGill et al. [16] presented a useful way of performing multiple boxplot comparisons. The authors created special intervals around the medians in boxplots and then used the overlap or nonoverlap of these special intervals to develop a test of significance for the difference between the *two* populations whose samples are displayed in the boxplots. The end points of the intervals shown in the boxplot display are called notches.* These notches are usually located within the box itself, but

---

*Why these are called notches will not be apparent from the figures that follow. However, the illustrations in McGill et al. [16] show boxes with "dents" or "notches" (similar to what might be carved into the edge of a block of wood with a pocket knife). The resulting notched box resembles an hourglass, which, in our examples, would be lying on its side.

if the sample median is close to a hinge, a notch (interval end point) may be located outside the box along a whisker.

This, then, is the hypothesis test using notched boxplots. *Two samples* (batches or groups) whose notched intervals do *not* overlap indicate that the two populations (represented by these samples) are significantly different at, roughly, $\alpha = 0.05$. (Technically, this comes down to a test at, roughly, $\alpha = 0.05$ of H_0: population one's median = population two's median vs. H_A: population one's median $\neq$ population two's median, but, obviously, if the population medians are different, so are the populations.)

Notice that this is a comparison test of two populations. If notched boxplots are used to compare more than two groups, the researcher needs to understand that this already crude test will become even more crude. However, I find it very useful, particularly when grounded in one's field of expertise. This is also the purpose of EDA: to explore the data and get a feel for it, not to use what has been suggested by exploratory analysis to reach decisions regarding the research questions. The decision process comes much later, after a model for the data is selected, after the necessary model assumptions have been verified, after the method of analysis is selected, and after the analysis is done.

The notch calculation is:

$$\text{Median} \pm 1.58 \times (H \text{ spread})/\sqrt{n}$$

where 1.58 is the constant expressing, in part, the relationship between the H-spread and population standard deviation,* and $n =$ sample size. From the data in Table 3, the notches are:

$$\text{Lower notch} = 6.405 - 1.58(3.465/\sqrt{20})$$
$$= 6.405 - 1.224$$
$$= 5.181$$

---

*Technically, the notches on a notched boxplot should be used to compare only two boxes. For the researcher using the boxplot as a preliminary tool, this is a bit restrictive. But, as McGill et al. [16] presented it, a 95% confidence level is applied strictly to only two samples. With the formula: *notches = median* $\pm (1.58 \times$ *hinges-spread*$)/\sqrt{n}$, the factor, 1.58, combines the H spread and the population standard deviation, the variability of the same median, and the factor used in setting the confidence limits. It is well known that the H spread/1.349 provides a crude estimate of the standard deviation, σ, particularly for large samples, from a normal distribution. Similarly, in large samples, the variance of the population, σ^2, is $\pi/2$ times the variance of the samples, s^2. This tends to hold only for large sample sizes theoretically, but it has also been shown to be a surprisingly accurate measure of a wide variety of nonnormal distributions.

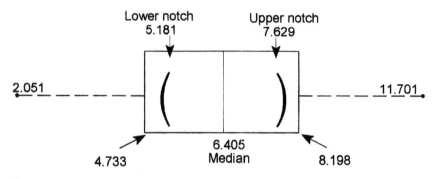

FIGURE 9   Boxplot with notches.

$$\text{Upper notch} = 6.405 + 1.58(3.465/\sqrt{20})$$

$$= 6.405 + 1.224$$

$$= 7.629$$

Figure 9 presents this boxplot with notches added. Figure 10 provides a MiniTab computer output of the notched boxplot.

Multiple boxplots, when notched and generated *on the same scale*, can be rapidly checked for evidence that the populations they represent are the same or are different (Fig. 11). Technically, only two groups should be compared. But when this is used as a preliminary screening method, comparisons beyond two may be surprisingly accurate.

From Fig. 11, one can see that the three boxplots vary a great deal in hinge locations, whiskers, and extreme or outlier values. Yet, a quick comparison can be made by just observing whether the notches overlap. The intervals of *A* and *C* overlap, so the populations from which they were drawn are not significantly different. Intervals in *A* and *B* do not overlap—their populations differ significantly in median values—and sample *C* overlaps both *A* and *B*. Although much more needs to be done in evaluating the data, one gets a relatively accurate indicator of where the population medians are relative

FIGURE 10   Boxplot with notches.

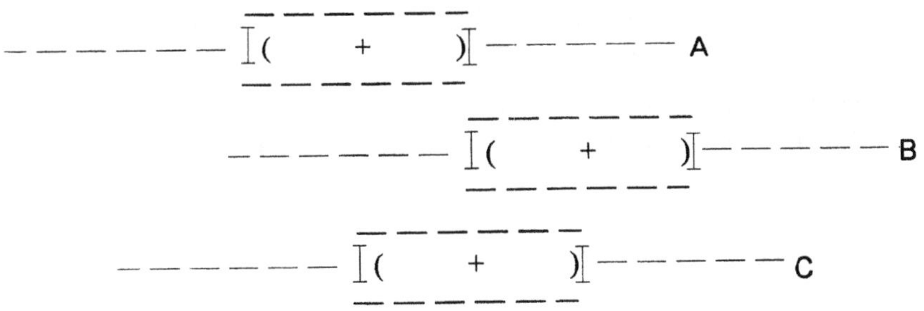

FIGURE 11   Multiple boxplots with notches.

to one another right at the beginning of the EDA process. The boxplot, then, provides the researcher information immediately about the data and the populations they represent.

IV. INTEGRATION

Now that we have discussed three major exploratory data analysis displays, it is important that they—all three of them—are employed in an integrated manner [17]. The stem-and-leaf and the letter-value displays, as well as the boxplot with notches, are reproduced in Fig. 12 to demonstrate one way of doing this.

By comparing the three EDA outputs simultaneously, one gets a very comprehensive perspective on the data set with just a few minutes of study. In the stem-and-leaf display, the data appear approximately normal, but there is a slight skewing of the data to the right (at H, E, and D) until one views the depth 1 values (letter-value display).

Here, the data really are not gappy enough to be a concern, nor do they appear to be multimodal (stem-and-leaf). Data are all clustered within the inner fences, and the median value is 6.405 (boxplot). There are no outliers (boxplot).

By just taking this brief time for examination, the researcher is more intimate with the data and better understands the data.

A. Nonnormally Distributed Data

There are many situations in which the shape of a data batch is clearly nonnormal. The researcher then has to make a decision:

1. Leave the data in the original form and, essentially, ignore the problem as related to parametric analysis;

2. Use a distribution-free method—a nonparametric method; or
3. Reexpress the data.

One may wonder why data that are nonnormally distributed would be left that way. Most often, this occurs because of *communication* and

Stem-and-leaf Display

1	2	0
1	3	
5	4	2333
9	5	1222
(3)	6	357
8	7	12
6	8	122
3	9	8
2	10	1
1	11	7

Letter-value Display

	DEPTH	LOWER	UPPER	MID	SPREAD
$n = 20$					
M	10.5	6.405		6.405	
H	5.5	4.733	8.198	6.465	3.465
E	3	4.305	9.801	7.053	5.496
D	2	4.221	10.133	7.177	5.912
	1	2.051	11.701	6.876	9.650

Boxplot

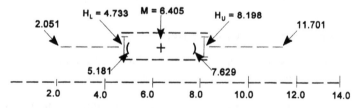

FIGURE 12   Stem-and-leaf, letter-value, and boxplot displays.

consistency. Researchers must communicate information, not only to fellow researchers but also to management, investors, regulatory agencies, and even politicians. Trying to describe the tensile strength of a new product in terms of a "reciprocal square root" transformation will probably result in frustration. A simplified portrayal of the data is needed.

In addition, if one is comparing the effectiveness of one treatment with that of another treatment where studies involving one of the treatments have been published in a technical journal, the researcher will often opt to perform not only the experiment but also the statistical data analysis in the same way as in the published study. This is so even if the conditions underlying the method of an analysis were not met and a different technique should have been used. The researcher may opt not to change methods so as not to "muddy the water."

Other times, a researcher will leave the data in nonnormal form and use a distribution-free, or nonparametric, method. But, in applied research, many studies are conducted on a very small scale, and the researcher wants to maximize power as well as more easily find potentially better products, processes, etc. In this case, data transformation is the best option. Parametric tests are more powerful than nonparametric tests, and transforming the data to achieve normality is better than ignoring the problem altogether.

B. Reexpressions of Data

Making nonnormal data normal by reexpression is fairly simple, particularly in skewed data conditions (Fig. 13). However, this is not the case for multimodal distributions (Fig. 14).

For example, a bimodal distribution is often encountered when data for males and females are mixed together. In situations like this, it is better to disentangle the subpopulations and treat them separately.

In performing reexpressions, in practice, it is more practical to use a statistical computer program because tedious calculations are often

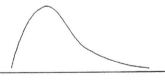

Skewed to the right   Skewed to the left

FIGURE 13   Skewed data.

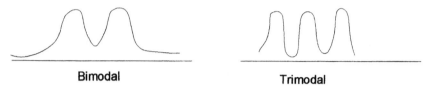

Bimodal

Trimodal

FIGURE 14   Multimodal distributions.

TABLE 5   Ladder of Powers

Use	Power	Reexpression	Expression name
For data skewed to the left	⋮	⋮	⋮
	3	x^3	Cubed
	2	x^2	Squared
Non-reexpressed data	1	x^1	Raw
For data skewed to the right	1/2	$\sqrt{x}$	Square root
	0^a	log x	Log transformation
	−1/2	$-1/\sqrt{x}$	Reciprocal root
	−1	$-1/x$	Reciprocal
	−2	$-1/x^2$	Reciprocal square
	−3	$-1/x^3$	Reciprocal cube
	⋮	⋮	⋮

[a]For all $a \neq 0, a = 1$, and there is no point in reexpressing each datum as 1. When we order the powers based on the strength of their effect, log falls in this relative position.

involved. Reexpressions are best handled methodically via a "scale of powers" (Table 5) [18].

Generally, one begins with the current data scale, called power 1, or power = 1.* If the data batch is skewed to the right (larger values), a power reexpression of less than 1 will pull out the left (smaller) values and push in the right (larger) values (Fig. 15). When a data batch is skewed to the left, the reexpression should be greater than the power of 1. This will push in the left (smaller) values and pull out the right (larger) values (Fig. 16). The farther one goes in either direction from $p = 1$, the more abruptly the data batch will be changed.

*$a^1 = a$ for all a.

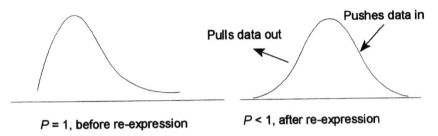

P = 1, before re-expression   P < 1, after re-expression

FIGURE 15   Reexpessing skewed-to-the-right sample data.

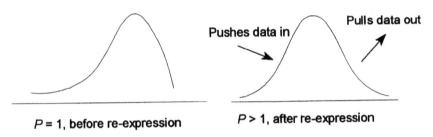

P = 1, before re-expression   P > 1, after re-expression

FIGURE 16   Reexpressing skewed-to-the-left sample data.

An effective way to find the best reexpression is to perform several re-expressions using various powers on the data and print out letter–value displays. [Recall that if the "mid" (midsummary) column values increase in size, the data are skewed to the right or larger end. If the mid column values become progressively smaller, the data are skewed to the left or smaller values. The mid column values should be about the same size or fluctuate randomly if the data are symmetrical.] The process is iterative, and whether one starts at a lower or greater power depends on the direction of skew (Table 5).

If one is working by hand, time can be saved by reexpressing only a portion of the data. The only values needing reexpression are the letter values. When the depth of a letter value involves $1/2$, the two values on which the letter value is based need reexpression. Once this is done, new mids and spreads can be calculated.

If positive and negative values are found in data batches, reexpression becomes more challenging. Because letter values are determined entirely by their depth in an ordered batch, if the order is disturbed, that reexpression cannot be used. So, if $a > b$ and both are positive, then $a^p > b^p$ for any positive power, p, and $-a^p > -b^p$ for any negative p.

TABLE 6   A Data Batch of $n = 30$ Observations

0.79	1.75	0.82	1.21	1.96	1.21
0.48	1.44	3.38	2.21	3.01	3.10
1.52	2.11	0.53	1.62	1.32	0.33
0.60	0.82	2.82	1.88	1.19	1.36
4.76	2.49	0.97	1.90	0.91	2.06

However, if either a or b or both are negative, power reexpressions will not preserve the order.*

Also, when the numbers in a data batch are not all positive (i.e., greater than zero), some reexpression operations will not be possible. For example, one cannot find $\sqrt{-2}$, and one cannot reexpress a zero with a $\log_{10}$ reexpression. Yet, one can add a constant to the value before transformation. For example, one could add $1/4$ or 0.25 to each value at the start.

$$x' = \log(x + 0.25), \text{ when } x = 0, \text{the log reexpression will be that}$$
of 0.25, a permissible operation.

Data that are all negative can be made positive by multiplying by -1 and then applying a reexpression to the resulting positive number.

Let us look at an example to see how reexpression works (Table 6). Figure 17 provides a stem-and-leaf display of Table 6.

Clearly, the data are skewed to the right (larger values). Looking at Fig. 18, a letter-value display, one can see the midsummary values increasing consistently, showing that the data are clearly skewed to the larger values.[†]

Because the data are skewed to the right, we look at Table 5 of power reexpressions and see that the power needed is less than 1. So $1/2$, 0, and $-1/2$ reexpressions are performed with the square root, $\log_{10}$, and reciprocal root, respectively. Table 7 provides the reexpressed values.

---

*Example: $a > b > 0$; rule: for $p > 0$, $a^p > b^p$.
Example: $9 > 4 > 0$. Let $p = 1/2 > 0$; then, $9^{1/2} > 4^{1/2}$ (i.e., $\sqrt{9} > \sqrt{4} = 3 > 2$). Or, let $p = 2 > 0$; then, $9^2 > 4^2 = 81 > 16$.
Example: $a > b > 0$; rule: for $p < 0$, $-a^p > -b^p$.
Example: $9 > 4 > 0$. Let $p = -1/2 < 0$, then $9^{-1/2} < 4^{-1/2} = 1/9^{1/2} < 1/4^{1/2} = 1/\sqrt{9} < 1/\sqrt{4} = 1/3 < 1/2$ but $-1/3 > -1/2$ (i.e., $-0.333 > -0.500$).
Recall that, if both numbers are negative, the one closer to zero is larger.
[†]The values that halve the tail areas outside a D are called C. The data values beyond C each constitute $1/32$ of the total number of values.

leaf unit = 0.10   n = 30

2	0	34
9	0	5678899
15	1	122334
15	1	567899
9	2	0124
5	2	8
4	3	013
1	3	
1	4	
1	4	7

FIGURE 17   Stem-and-leaf display of data.

	DEPTH	LOWER	UPPER	MID	SPREAD
n = 30					
M	15.5		1.48	1.48	
H	8.0	0.910	2.110	1.510	1.200
E	4.5	0.695	2.915	1.805	2.220
D	2.5	0.505	3.240	1.872	2.735
C	1.5	0.405	4.070	2.238	3.665
	1	0.330	4.760	2.545	4.430

FIGURE 18   Letter-value display.

Table 8 presents the reexpressed values in letter-value displays. The first reexpression, the square root, helped normalize the distribution as shown by a less pronounced incremental increase in the "mids."

The $\log_{10}$ transformation removed the skew to the larger values, overcorrecting the data to make them skewed to the smaller values. This can be seen in the mid values now incrementally decreasing.

The $-1/\sqrt{x}$ transformation overcorrected more than the $\log_{10}$ transformation.* The researcher may opt to pick the $\log_{10}$ reexpression or opt for

TABLE 7   Reexpressions of Raw Data

n	x	$\sqrt{x}$	$\log_{10}x$	$-1/\sqrt{x}$
1	0.79	0.88882	−0.102373	−1.12509
2	0.48	0.69282	−0.318759	−1.44338
3	1.52	1.23288	0.181844	−0.81111
4	0.60	0.77460	−0.221849	−1.29099
5	4.76	2.18174	0.677607	−0.45835
6	1.75	1.32288	0.243038	−0.75593
7	1.44	1.20000	0.158362	−0.83333
8	2.11	1.45258	0.324282	−0.68843
9	0.82	0.90554	−0.086186	−1.10432
10	2.49	1.57797	0.396199	−0.63372
11	0.82	0.90554	−0.086186	−1.10432
12	3.38	1.83848	0.528917	−0.54393
13	0.53	0.72801	−0.275724	−1.37361
14	2.82	1.67929	0.450249	−0.59549
15	0.97	0.98489	−0.013228	−1.01535
16	1.21	1.10000	0.082785	−0.90909
17	2.21	1.48661	0.344392	−0.67267
18	1.62	1.27279	0.209515	−0.78567
19	1.88	1.37113	0.274158	−0.72932
20	1.90	1.37840	0.278754	−0.72548
21	1.96	1.40000	0.292256	−0.71429
22	3.01	1.73494	0.478566	−0.57639
23	1.32	1.14891	0.120574	−0.87039
24	1.19	1.09087	0.075547	−0.91670
25	0.91	0.95394	−0.040959	−1.04828
26	1.21	1.10000	0.082785	−0.90909
27	3.10	1.76068	0.491362	−0.56796
28	0.33	0.57446	−0.481486	−1.74078
29	1.36	1.16619	0.133539	−0.85749
30	2.06	1.43527	0.313867	−0.69673

TABLE 8 Letter-value Displays

Letter	Depth	Lower	Upper	Mid	Spread
		$\sqrt{x}$			
$n = 30$					
M	15.5	1.216		1.216	
H	8.0	0.954	1.453	1.203	0.499
E	4.5	0.832	1.707	1.269	0.875
D	2.5	0.710	1.800	1.255	1.089
C	1.5	0.634	2.010	1.322	1.376
	1	0.574	2.182	1.378	1.607
		$\log_{10}x$			
$n = 30$					
M	15.5	0.170		0.170	
H	8.0	−0.041	0.324	0.142	0.365
E	4.5	−0.162	0.464	0.151	0.627
D	2.5	−0.297	0.510	0.106	0.807
C	1.5	−0.400	0.603	0.102	1.003
	1	−0.481	0.678	0.098	1.159
		$-1/\sqrt{x}$			
$n = 30$					
M	15.5	−0.822		−0.822	
H	8.0	−1.048	−0.688	−0.868	0.360
E	4.5	−1.208	−0.586	−0.897	0.622
D	2.5	−1.408	−0.556	−0.982	0.853
C	1.5	−1.592	−0.501	−1.047	1.091
	1	−1.741	−0.458	−1.100	1.282

a reexpression power between the square root $(1/2)$ and $\log(0)$, such as the $1/4$ power. But, given that the data batch has only $n = 30$ observations, such fine-tuning is usually not productive.

V. CONCLUSION

It is important to learn how to use EDA adequately and make it part of each analysis. By performing EDA at the outset, one can usually gain an understanding of the data that can be achieved in no other way.

---

*Recall that, when all the values are negative, the one closest to zero is the largest. Here, the midnumbers are *decreasing*.

4

Two-Sample Tests

I. BASIC EXPERIMENTAL PRINCIPLES

As discussed previously, three basic tools in the experimental design process are *replication, randomization*, and *blocking*. We will begin using them in this chapter and continue using them throughout the book. Recall that replication refers to repeating experimental runs in order to collect multiple measurements of the experimental phenomenon of interest. The replication process enables one to estimate the true mean value of a population with both greater precision and greater accuracy. It also allows estimation of the magnitude of experimental error. Randomization of experimental units and/or treatments is a precaution against bias. Each experimental unit, then, is equally likely to be assigned any one of several treatments. For example, virtually all statistical methods require that observations (or experimental errors) be independently distributed random variables, and randomization makes this assumption valid. Finally, blocking is a technique used to increase the precision of an experiment by controlling for an extraneous variable within a population sample. Blocks consist of sample items grouped to be more homogeneous with respect to that variable. For example, a simple block may combine microbial counts from the left and right sides of a test subject used in a preoperative skin preparation evaluation. This is because one would expect the population counts to be more similar in numbers on the left and right sides of an individual than counts among different individuals. The samples within a block undergo the experimental treatments with randomization occurring only within that block, and posttreatment results are compared with each other only within that block. In our simple example using two products, each would be assigned randomly to either the left or right side of the subject. This process reduces experimental error, making the statistical test more powerful—that is, more likely to reject a null hypothesis when it is false.

To use the statistical approach effectively in designing and analyzing an experiment, it is necessary to have a clear idea in advance of exactly what is to be studied, how it is to be represented by the data collected, and how those data are to be collected. The researcher should also have at least a general idea of how the data are to be analyzed. Let us expand this discussion [17].

1. *Recognition of and statement of the problem.* This may seem an obvious point, but in practice, it is often not simple to recognize what the problem is, how to measure it, and how to know what one thinks is measured actually is measured. Therefore, a clear statement of the problem, how to measure it, and how to validate the measurement of it is necessary before performing any experimentation.

2. *Choice of factors and levels.* The experimenter must explicitly identify and select the variables—independent and dependent—to be investigated in the experiment. The independent variables must be interval or ratio measures, and the dependent variable must be continuous (or approximately continuous data) in parametric statistics. The dependent variable(s) in nonparametric statistics may be nominal, ordinal or interval. One must also select the ranges over which the independent variables are to be varied. These levels may be chosen specifically or selected at random from the set of all possible factor levels (random effects model).

3. *Selection of a dependent variable.* In choosing a dependent or response variable, it is important that the response measured really provides the information that is wanted about the problem under study. This is a big challenge in many research situations.

4. *Choice of experimental design.* We will cover a number of experimental designs in this text. If a researcher takes the time to learn how to apply them, the selection of the appropriate design is rather straightforward. Initially, the experimenter will have to decide between parametric and nonparametric methods. In parametric statistics, when two sample groups with unknown population variances are compared, a Student's *t*-test is used. This test will be subdivided into the two independent samples and matched-pairs cases. For experiments comparing more than two samples, analysis of variance generally will be used. Blocking is analogous in these models to matched-pair Student's *t*-tests. When there is

trending involved over time, regression analysis will be used. And for nonparametric applications, analogs of the parametric methods will be used.

5. *Performing the experiment.* The experimenter must assure that randomization, blocking, and replication are carried out according to the experimental design's requirements, which are often quite specific. If these are not carried out appropriately, the entire statistical rationale undergirding the experiment is invalid.

6. *Data analysis.* In recent years, the computer has played an ever-increasing role in data analysis. There are currently a number of excellent statistical software packages available for statistical computing. We will employ MiniTab®. Graphical techniques, as we have seen in EDA, are particularly helpful in data analysis.

An important part of the data analysis process is *model adequacy checking* through the use of residual plotting, for example, to assure that the model accurately describes the data. In this book, we will learn to become intimate with the data so that we can better assess the statistical model's adequacy in describing the data. We will not merely plug values into a computer and crank out results.

7. *Conclusions and recommendations.* Once the data have been analyzed, the experimenter will use statistical inference to draw conclusions from the experiment's results. The conclusion may suggest that a further round of experiments be conducted because experimentation is often an iterative process, with an experiment answering some questions and simultaneously posing others. In presenting the results and conclusions, the experimenter should minimize unnecessary statistical terminology and jargon and, instead, present the information as simply as possible; the technical details can appear in an appendix in the final, written report. The use of graphical displays is a very effective way of presenting important experimental results to nonscientists.

II. TWO-SAMPLE COMPARISONS

There are two situations in which the researcher is interested in the differences between effects instead of the effects themselves: (1) the comparison of two independent groups (samples) and (2) the comparison of related or matched groups. Each of the two situations involves comparing two sets of sample data. One sample is generally designated the test group and the other, the control. The test group has undergone the treatment condition that is the main focus of interest. Its effect is judged relative to the response of the other group, the control group. The control group undergoes the standard treatment or no treatment at all. However, the two-sample comparison procedures can also be used to compare two new or separate treatments, products, or procedures or the differences in response when one group is measured two times, usually before and after a treatment process. The latter procedure is referred to as a pre-post measures design or a repeated-measures design.

Graphical representations of the experimental design are useful to clarify what the researcher is doing. For example, suppose a researcher has developed a new house paint that the researcher believes is superior to the standard paint, withstanding greater heat before peeling. Ten test paint panels and 10 control paint panels will be selected at random, placed in a 375°F oven for 48 hours, and then removed. The chipping pressure will then be measured for each panel.

A schematic depiction of this study is:

(R) A_1 O_1
(R) A_2 O_2

where (R) represents randomization, signifying that the panels were randomly selected, in this case, from the same population
(A_i) represents the independent variable, which in this case is the paint; $i = 1$, if test paint, or 2, if control paint (standard)
(O_i) represents the dependent variable (also known as the response variable), degree of paint peeling measurement at a specific pressure

Notice that this design does not identify a specific test to use—a two-sample t-test, a matched-pair t-test, or a nonparametric test, such as the Wilcoxon–Mann–Whitney test. The researcher can decide this beforehand, in such cases as a matched-pair test or, later, based on the EDA evaluation.

Suppose an immunologist wants to determine whether a curing process for a specific vaccine results in a longer shelf life for the vaccine than does the control (no process). The study schema is:

(R) A_1 O_1
(R) O_2

where (R) signifies that the bulk vaccine solution was randomly assigned to test and control groups
(A_1) represents the treatment (curing process) (note: only the treatment group undergoes the curing process)

(O_i) represents the observed variable (shelf life); $i=1$, if test group, or 2, if control group

This structure can also be used for pretest/posttest measurements on one sample:

Pretest		Posttest
O_1	A	O_2

where (O_i) represents the dependent variable; $i=1$, if pretest measurement, or 2, if posttest measurement

(A) represents the treatment (note: in this case, product was not randomly assigned, so an R is not present)

In this case, a measurement was performed prior to treatment. Once the pretreatment measurement occurred, the treatment was applied, and then the shelf life was remeasured.

This structure can be expanded to more complex studies. For example:

(R) A_1 O_1
(R) A_2 O_2
(R) O_3

or

(R) A_1 O_{11} O_{12} O_{13}
(R) O_{21} O_{22} O_{23}

or

(R) A_1 O_{11} O_{12} O_{13}
(R) A_2 O_{21} O_{22} O_{23}
(R) A_3 O_{31} O_{32} O_{33}
(R) O_{41} O_{42} O_{43}

III. TWO-SAMPLE TESTS

One of the most useful and powerful statistics in an applied researcher's toolbox is Student's two-sample t-test. As previously stated, there are two general types: (1) independent and (2) matched pair. We will now discuss the independent case, which is composed of two different tests. The first is used when the variances differ, and the second is used when the variances are assumed equal. In this book, we will focus on using the t-distribution instead of the Z-distribution. That is because it is more appropriate for small sample sizes than the Z table. And, as the sample sizes increase (≥ 120), the t- and Z-distributions are identical.

The linear statistical model for the two-sample t-test is:

$$x_{ij} = \mu + \beta_i + \varepsilon_{ij}, \qquad i = 1, 2, j = 1, 2, \ldots, n \qquad (1)$$

where x_{ij} = individual observations for each sample j for the ith treatment

μ = the combined average treatment effect of the sample treatments

β_i = effect due to treatment 1, if $i = 1$, or treatment 2, if $i = 2$

ε_{ij} = random or experimental error due to each treatment i at each sample j

A. Two-Sample t-Test, Independent Samples, Variances Not Equal ($\sigma_1^2 \neq \sigma_2^2$)

The two-sample t-test requires that both samples are randomly selected from normally distributed populations. Fortunately, the two-sample t-test is robust enough to tolerate considerable deviations from the normal distribution requirement, particularly if the sample sizes of the two samples, n_1 and n_2, are equal or nearly so. The greater the sample size differences between the two groups, the less efficient the two-sample t-test is. We will see this later in the chapter when we compute the sample sizes required to detect a specific significant difference, $\delta = |\mu_1 - \mu_2|$, in the population means. In addition, the two-sample t-test has been reported to be more robust in a two-tail application than in the upper or lower tail applications [19–21].

Note that the larger both the sample sizes n_1 and n_2 are, the more powerful the two-sample t-test is. Furthermore, if the underlying populations are found to be skewed and one does not want to utilize a scale transformation or a nonparametric statistic, it is reassuring to know that the two-tail t-test is not greatly affected by skewedness [19,22]. Even so, the experimenter must be wary of using a two-tail test on skewed data sets. This is particularly true, also, for small α values such as 0.05 or 0.01. The power* of the two-tail t-test is not seriously affected by skewed data but is affected in single-tail tests [19]. For small sample sizes, the actual power of the two-sample t-test has been

---

*Power is the ability of a statistic to reject correctly false null hypotheses.

shown to be somewhat less than the power computations suggest [19,23]. Finally, if the variances are unequal ($\sigma_1^2 \neq \sigma_2^2$), type I error will tend to be greater than the stated α level, but if the sample sizes are equal, the t-test is robust for moderate to large samples.

The two independent samples test assumes that the samples from one group are not related to those from the other group. Three test hypothesis conditions can be evaluated using the two-sample t-test in any of its three variations.

1. Upper tail

$H_0: \mu_1 \leq \mu_2$
$H_A: \mu_1 > \mu_2$
Reject H_0 if $t_c > t_{\text{tabled}}$ where
$t_c = t$-statistic calculated from the data
$t_{\text{tabled}} = t$-critical value (tabled)

2. Lower tail

$H_0: \mu_1 \geq \mu_2$
$H_A: \mu_1 < \mu_2$
Reject H_0 if $t_c < t_{\text{tabled}}$

3. Two-tail

$H_0: \mu_1 = \mu_2$
$H_A: \mu_1 \neq \mu_2$
Reject H_0 if $|t_c| \neq |t_{\text{tabled}}|$

Student's t-test statistic for two independent samples is:

$$t = \frac{\bar{X}_1 - \bar{X}_2}{\sqrt{(S_1^2/n_1) + (S_2^2/n_2)}} \qquad (2)$$

The term $\sqrt{(S_1^2/n_1)+(S_2^2/n_2)}$ provides an unbiased estimate of the combined variances, σ_{1+2}^2, where:

$$\bar{X}_1 = \text{sample mean for group 1} = \frac{\sum X_1}{n_1}$$

$$\bar{X}_2 = \text{sample mean for group 2} = \frac{\sum X_2}{n_2}$$

$$S_1^2 = \text{variance of sample one} = \frac{\sum (X_1 - \bar{X}_1)^{2*}}{n_1 - 1}$$

$$S_2^2 = \text{variance of sample two} = \frac{\sum (X_2 - \bar{X}_2)^2}{n_2 - 1}$$

The degrees of freedom = df = $n_1 + n_2 - 2$.

The two-sample t-test assumes that the samples were collected at random, that the data are normally distributed, but not that the variances are equal ($\sigma_1^2 \neq \sigma_2^2$).

Generally, it will not be necessary to utilize Student's t-test for independent samples and unequal variances, for most researchers assume variances are equal and pool them. This provides greater statistical power.

When the variances σ_1^2 and σ_2^2 are not assumed to be equivalent, a conundrum exists that statisticians call the Behrens–Fisher problem [24]. We have ignored the problem and merely used a procedure for evaluating two independent samples when variances are unequal. However, a number of statisticians would disagree and argue to use another procedure, Welch's approximate t-test [19].

The test statistic is the same as that presented in Eq. (2).

$$t_w = \frac{\bar{X}_1 - \bar{X}_2}{\sqrt{(S_1^2/n_1) + (S_2^2/n_2)}} \tag{2}$$

The computation of the degrees of freedom (df$'$), however, is not $n_1 + n_2 - 2$, but

$$df' = \frac{[(S_1^2/n_1) + (S_2^2/n_2)]^2}{(S_1/n_1)^2/(n_1 - 1) + (S_2/n_2)^2/(n_2 - 1)} \tag{3}$$

The degrees of freedom (df$'$) calculation usually does not result in an integer, so the fraction (decimal) portion of df is truncated. If $n_1 \neq n_2$ and the variance difference is great, t_w will provide a more powerful test than a standard two-sample t-test [Eq. (2)]. Also, Welch has suggested, to improve the test when $n_1 \neq n_2$, using $n_1 - 3$ and $n_2 - 3$ instead of $n_1 - 1$ and $n_2 - 1$ [Eq. (3)].

Some statisticians recommend actively comparing σ_1^2 and σ_2^2 for equivalence prior to conducting a t-test. However, because the two-sample pooled t-test is so robust and the variance (σ^2) comparison test performs

---

*When computing by hand, a simplified computational formula can be used:

$$s_i^2 = \left(\sum x_{ij}^2 - n\bar{X}^2 \right) / (n_i - 1)$$

poorly with nonnormal data, I do not recommend a test of the variance equivalence. Instead, I recommend the pooled two-sample t-test or, in cases of severe deviation from a normal distribution and/or severe nonequality of variances, a nonparametric test. The Wilcoxon–Mann–Whitney U-test is the one of choice and is discussed in Chap. 12.

B. Two-Sample Pooled t-Test, Independent Samples, Variances Equal $\sigma_1^2=\sigma_2^2$

When using a two-sample pooled t-test for independent samples, where we assume the variances are equal, the following formula is used:

$$t_c = \frac{\bar{X}_1 - \bar{X}_2}{S_{\bar{X}_1-\bar{X}_2}} \tag{4}$$

where $\bar{X}_1$ = sample mean for group 1
$\bar{X}_2$ = sample mean for group 2
$S_{\bar{X}_1-\bar{X}_2}$ = the pooled standard deviation = $\sqrt{\frac{S_p^2}{n_1} + \frac{S_p^2}{n_2}}$

where

$$S_p^2 = \frac{SS_1 + SS_2}{(n_1 - 1) + (n_2 - 1)}$$

or

$$S_p^2 = \frac{SS_1 + SS_2}{df_1 + df_2}$$

where

$$SS_i = \text{sum of squares} = \sum_{i=1}^{n}(x_i - \bar{x})^2$$

df_i = degrees of freedom = $n_i - 1$

Example 1:   A chemist wishes to test two chemical extraction methods for efficiency. Method 1 is a new method, and method 2 is the standard. Ten extraction runs with each of the two methods are conducted via random assignment. The researcher wants to know whether method 1 is "better" than method 2, that is, whether more ingredient volumes, in microliters, are extracted by method 1 than by method 2. The data for extractions using the two methods are presented in Table 1.

For computational ease, we will use the six-step procedure for all of our testing.

TABLE 1 Data for Chemical Extractions Using Two Methods

n	Method 1 = x_1	Method 2 = x_2
1	152	151
2	153	*[a]
3	149	156
4	162	155
5	165	157
6	168	161
7	157	158
8	178	168
9	161	149
10	186	174

[a]Sample 2 of method 2 was lost; its position is represented by an asterisk, not a 0.

Six-Step Procedure

Step 1. Formulate the test hypothesis, beginning with H_A.
Because we are determining whether method 1 is greater in extraction efficiency than method 2 (the standard), we will set this up as an upper tail test.

Let μ_1 = true extraction mean for method 1
μ_2 = true extraction mean for method 2 (the standard)
H_0: $\mu_1 \leq \mu_2$
H_A: $\mu_1 > \mu_2$

Step 2. Specify sample sizes n_1 and n_2 and the α-level for significance of difference.

$n_1 = 10$

$n_2 = 9$

Set $\alpha = 0.05$ (or any other α the researcher chooses).
Step 3. Select the test statistic. We assume here that the variances are equal.

$$t_c = \frac{\bar{X}_1 - \bar{X}_2}{S_{\bar{X}_1 - \bar{X}_2}}$$

Step 4. Specify the decision rule (Fig. 1).

t_{tabled} (Student's t table, Table B) $= t_t = t_{(\alpha, n_1 + n_2 - 2)} = t_{(0.05, 10 + 9 - 2)} = t_{(0.05, 17)} = 1.740$

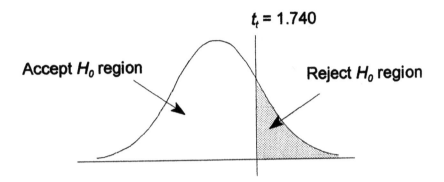

$t_t = 1.740$

Accept H_0 region

Reject H_0 region

FIGURE 1   Acceptance and rejection regions (Example 1, step 4).

Decision rule:

If $t_c > t_t$, reject H_0 at $\alpha = 0.05$, where $t_t = 1.740$.

Step 5.   Calculate test statistic:

$$t_c = \frac{\bar{X}_1 - \bar{X}_2}{S_{\bar{X}_1 - \bar{X}_2}}$$

$$\bar{X}_1 = \frac{152 + 153 + 149 + \cdots + 161 + 186}{10} = \frac{1631}{10} = 163.10$$

$$\bar{X}_2 = \frac{151 + 156 + 155 + \cdots + 149 + 174}{9} = 158.78$$

$$SS_1 = (152 - 163.10)^2 + (153 - 163.10)^2 + \cdots + (161 - 163.10)^2$$

$$+ (186 - 163.10)^2 = 1240.90$$

$$SS_2 = (151 - 158.78)^2 + (156 - 158.78)^2 + \cdots + (149 - 158.78)^2$$

$$+ (174 - 158.78)^2 = 503.56$$

$$S_p^2 = \frac{SS_1 + SS_2}{n_1 - 1 + n_2 - 1}$$

$$S_p^2 = \frac{1240.90 + 503.56}{9 + 8} = 102.62$$

$$S_{\bar{X}_1 - \bar{X}_2} = \sqrt{\frac{S_p^2}{n_1} + \frac{S_p^2}{n_2}} = \sqrt{\frac{102.62}{10} + \frac{102.62}{9}}$$

$$S_{\bar{X}_1 - \bar{X}_2} = 4.65$$

$$t_c = \frac{\bar{X}_1 - \bar{X}_2}{S_{\bar{X}_1 - \bar{X}_2}}$$

$$t_c = \frac{163.10 - 158.78}{4.65} = 0.93$$

Step 6. Because *t*-calculated is less than *t*-tabled (0.93 < 1.74), one cannot reject the H_0 hypothesis at $\alpha = 0.05$. The new method of extraction is not significantly better than the old method at $\alpha = 0.05$.

In addition, this *t*-test can be computed using a formula sometimes easier to perform by pencil-and-paper methods.

$$t_c = \frac{\bar{X}_1 - \bar{X}_2}{\sqrt{\frac{(n_1-1)S_1^2 + (n_2-1)S_2^2}{n_1 + n_2 - 2}}}$$

The pooled two-sample *t*-test can also be computed using a computer software package. When using a software package, it is important to check

TABLE 2   MiniTab Output of Data in Table 1

POOLED TWO-SAMPLE T FOR C1 VS C2

	N	MEAN	STDEV	SEMAN
c_1	10	163.1	11.7	3.7
c_2	9	158.78	7.93	2.6

95 PCT C1 FOR MU C1-MU C2:[a] (−5.5, 14.1)
TTEST MU C1 = MU C2 (VS NE): T = 0.93 P=0.37 DF=17
POOLED STEDEV = 10.1

where:
$c_1 = x_1$; $c_2 = x_2$
T = *t*-test calculated value
P = *p*-value
DF = $n_1 + n_2 - 2$

[a] $\mu_1 - \mu_2 = \bar{X}_1 \pm \bar{X}_2 \pm t_{\alpha/2} S_{x_1 - x_2}$.

the computer output and the hand calculation output to ensure that they are equivalent. The MiniTab® package uses the same formulae as were used to compute both the two-sample pooled t-test and the confidence interval around the difference between the two means. Let us apply MiniTab® to computation of the data presented in Table 1. Table 2 presents the output of the MiniTab® computation.

Notice in Table 2, the software version of the two-sample pooled t-test, that the software package computed the t-test as an $\bar{x}_1 - \bar{x}_2$ confidence interval, $-5.5 \le \mu \le 14.1$, which includes 0, so we know that the H_0 hypothesis cannot be rejected. Notice, too, that a p value is provided in the MiniTab® program. It means that, given that the H_0 hypothesis is correct, one can expect to observe a t-calculated (t_c) value at least as extreme as 0.93, 37% of the time. The probability of $t_c \ge 0.93 | H_0$ true $| = 0.37$. This is much greater than an $\alpha = 0.05$, so one is fairly certain that no difference exists between the populations.

C. Confidence Interval Method to Detect a Difference between Populations

The same conclusion could have been drawn by performing a 95% confidence interval procedure for $\mu_1 - \mu_2$. Technically, however, only a two-tail test can be computed in this way. The formula is:

$$\mu_1 - \mu_2 = \bar{X}_1 - \bar{X}_2 \pm t_{\alpha/2} S_{\bar{X}_1 - \bar{X}_2} \tag{5}$$

where $n_1 = 10, n_2 = 9$,

$$S_p^2 = \frac{SS_1 + SS_2}{(n_1 - 1) + (n_2 - 1)} = \frac{1240.90 + 503.56}{9 + 8} = 102.62, \text{ and}$$

$$S_{\bar{X}_1 - \bar{X}_2} = \sqrt{\frac{S_p^2}{n_1} + \frac{S_p^2}{n_2}} = \sqrt{\frac{102.62}{10} + \frac{102.62}{9}} = 4.65$$

For $t_{\alpha/2} = t_{0.025}$ at df $= n_1 + n_2 - 2 = 10 + 9 = 17$, Student's t table (Table B) shows $t_{0.025,17} = 2.11$. 95% CI$= \bar{X}_1 - \bar{X}_2 \pm t_{\alpha/2,df} S_{\bar{X}_1 - \bar{X}_2} = (163.10 - 158.78) \pm 2.11(4.65) = 4.32 \pm 9.81$. Therefore $-5.49 \le \mu_1 - \mu_2 \le 14.13$. Notice that, in the 95% interval range, zero is included. Whenever zero is included, the H_0 (null) hypothesis cannot be rejected at the $\alpha = 0.05$ level of significance.

Note: The same result can be achieved using a simplifying modification of Eq. (5).

$$\bar{X}_1 - \bar{X}_2 \pm t_{(\alpha/2, n_1 + n_2 - 2)} \sqrt{\frac{(n_1 - 1)S_1^2 + (n_2 - 1)S_2^2}{n_1 + n_2 - 2}}$$

IV. CONFIDENCE INTERVAL FOR EACH SAMPLE $\bar{X}$ GROUP

Recall that the computation for one population mean interval estimate is:

$$\bar{X} - t_{\alpha/2}\frac{S}{\sqrt{n}} \leq \mu \leq \bar{X} + t_{\alpha/2}\frac{S}{\sqrt{n}}, \qquad df = n - 1$$

In the two-sample situation, estimating a confidence interval on the two population means is similar. For situations where $\sigma_1^2 = \sigma_1^2$ (variances of population 1 and population 2 are the same), the confidence interval for either μ_1 or μ_2 is computed using the pooled variance, S_p^2, rather than either S_1^2 or S_2^2, as the best estimate of σ_{1+2}^2.

$$\bar{X}_i - t_{\alpha/2}\sqrt{\frac{S_p^2}{n_i}} \leq \mu_1 \leq \bar{X}_i + t_{\alpha/2}\sqrt{\frac{S_p^2}{n_i}} \approx \bar{X}_i \pm t_{\alpha/2}\sqrt{\frac{S_p^2}{n_i}}, \quad \text{where} \qquad (6)$$

$$S_p^2 = \frac{SS_1 + SS_2}{(n_1 - 1) + (n_2 - 1)}$$

with $n_1 + n_2 - 2$ degrees of freedom

From Example 1, let us compute a 95% confidence interval for the means in samples 1 and 2.

Sample 1 (x_1):

$$S_p^2 = \frac{1240.90 + 503.56}{9 + 8} = 102.62$$

for $\mu_1, \bar{X}_1 \pm t_{\alpha/2}\sqrt{S_p^2/n}$, where

Student's t tabled value (Table B) $=$

$$t_{\alpha/2, n_1 + n_2 - 2} = 2.11$$

$$= 163.10 \pm 2.11\sqrt{\frac{102.62}{10}}$$

$$= 163.10 \pm 2.11(3.20)$$

$$= 163.10 \pm 6.76$$

$$156.34 \leq \mu_1 \leq 169.86$$

Sample 2 (x_2):

$$\text{For } \mu_2, \quad 158.78 \pm 2.11\sqrt{\frac{102.62}{9}} = 158.78 \pm 6.76$$

$$152.02 \leq \mu_2 \leq 165.54$$

Notice that the confidence intervals for μ_1 and μ_2 overlap. This is to be expected because no difference exists between the sample group means.

The previous computation is very useful when the H_0 hypothesis is rejected. In cases such as this example, when the H_0 hypothesis was not rejected, an estimate of the common mean is often of more value. This is because where $\mu_1 = \mu_2$, the researcher is describing the same population. The best estimate of μ is a pooled estimate of the mean $\bar{X}_p$.

$$\bar{X}_p = \frac{n_1\bar{X}_1 + n_2\bar{X}_2}{n_1 + n_2} \tag{7}$$

$$= \frac{10(163.10) + 9(158.78)}{10 + 9} = \bar{X}_p = 161.05$$

So 161.05, the pooled estimate, is the best estimate of the common mean, μ.

The confidence interval for the common mean estimate when H_0 is not rejected is:

$$\bar{X}_p \pm t_{\alpha/2}\sqrt{\frac{S_p^2}{n_1 + n_2}} \tag{8}$$

$$161.05 \pm 2.11\sqrt{\frac{102.62}{10 + 9}}$$

$$161.05 \pm 2.11(2.32)$$

$$161.05 \pm 4.90$$

$$156.15 \leq \mu \leq 165.95$$

Hence, one may be 95% confident that the true mean of the population will be found in the preceding interval.

A. Sample Size Determination

Statistical estimation and hypothesis testing are designed primarily for protecting the researcher from making a type I (α) error but not from a type II (β) error [19,24]. The reason is that type I error is considered the more severe. Recall that type I error occurs when one rejects a true H_0 hypothesis—for example, stating that a new treatment process is better than the standard when really it is not. Conversely, type II error occurs when one accepts the H_0 hypothesis as true when it is actually false—that is, rejecting a new treatment process that really is more effective than the standard one.

For the applied researcher, a dynamic balance between α and β error prevention should be sought (25, 26, 27). This will enable one to maximize the likelihood of determining correctly whether or not some treatment process, for example, is or is not more effective. The ability of the statistic to do this is referred to as the *power* of the statistic.

There are several immediate things the investigator can do to increase statistical power. First, one can select the most efficient and powerful statistical model available. Second, one can increase the sample size, thereby enhancing the power of any statistic, reducing the probability of committing β error. One can also manipulate the α and β error levels. Recall that reducing the probability of making an α error (that is, decreasing the value of α) increases the probability of making a β error and vice versa. It is often helpful in a study having small sample sizes to increase the α value (e.g., from 0.05 to 0.10), thereby reducing the β error level. However, a larger study should be conducted subsequently to verify the conclusions made from a small pilot study.

Given this advice, it is important that one determine the sample sizes needed to ensure that, if a "significant difference" in sample group means exists, it will be picked up by the statistical model used. If not, one probably need not conduct the study, for it will not really contribute to the research effort.

A researcher must consider two other aspects in sample size determination: (1) the detection level between the two groups (i.e., the value $\delta = |\bar{X}_1 - \bar{X}_2|$) and (2) the variance ($S^2$) of the sample data. If an investigator requires very fine detection resolution to identify a small but real difference in sample means, a larger sample size, n, will be required than if the resolution of difference is larger. And, as well, the larger the variance (S^2) implicit in the sample data, the larger the number of samples one must collect within each set in order to demonstrate a significant difference between means that may exist.

The first issue (detection level) can often be addressed by requiring a specific preset numerical difference, δ, between the sample sets compared (i.e., $\delta = |\bar{X}_1 - \bar{X}_2|$). This simplifies a researcher's task considerably, particularly in the early stages of research, when one is screening for potential new and promising treatments, products, etc. Second, in controlled studies, a researcher usually has substantial knowledge about what the variance (S^2) of a particular kind of test data is. By refining techniques and, thereby, reducing common procedural error, the variance can often be further minimized and, to some degree, influenced and controlled.

By knowing these two parameters—the detection level and the sample variance—a researcher can easily determine the sample size required to detect a true difference between $\bar{X}_1$ and $\bar{X}_2$ *before* conducting a study. Let us begin our sample size determination by specifying the detection level required $|\mu_1 - \mu_2|$, remembering that the larger the sample sizes, the greater the ability to detect differences between sample means.

B. Sample Size and Power Computations for the Pooled Two-Sample *t*-Tests for Independent Means

Equation (9) can be used to estimate the sample size (estimated sample size $= n_e$) required, given specified confidence interval width, w, and variance, s^2.

$$n_e = \frac{2S_p^2 t_{\alpha/2,2(n-1)}^2}{(w/2)^2} \tag{9}$$

where:

$S_p^2 =$ the pooled variance $= \frac{SS_1 + SS_2}{n_1 - 1 + n_2 - 1}$

$t_{\alpha/2} =$ specific critical value from t table, with $n_1 + n_2 - 2$ [or $2(n-1)$ when $n_1 = n_2$] degrees of freedom, squared

$w =$ the data spread at the desired $1 - \alpha$ confidence level width

In order to determine the sample size, n, required, an iterative approach must be taken. The iterative process is quicker if the initial n "seed value" used to start the process is too high instead of too low, and it is always better, but not mandatory, that sample sizes be equal ($n_1 = n_2$). With each iteration, the estimate of n is successively improved.

Let us use the data in Example 1 to calculate the required sample size, n, for a 10-point spread in the confidence interval, so $w/2 = 5.0$. Recall $S_p^2 = 102.62$. Let us pick $n = 50$ to start the process, df $= 2(50-1) = 98$, and for $\alpha = 0.05$, $\alpha/2 = 0.05/2 = 0.025$, and $t_{0.25,98} = 1.984$. This is an iterative process, performed until the previous n_e calculated equals the present n_e. In case of a fraction, the n_e value is rounded up.

Step 1. Pick n (large). We will use 50, $t_{0.25,98} = 1.984$. Plug the required values into the n_e formula, and round up the answer to keep only the integer portion of n_e.

$$n_e = \frac{2(102.62)(1.984)^2}{(10/2)^2} = 32.32 \quad \text{(rounded up:} \quad 33)$$

Step 2. Next, use $n = 33$ as the entering value. The degrees of freedom equals $2(33-1) = 64$, $t_{0.25,64} = 1.998$

$$n_e = \frac{2(102.62)(1.998)^2}{(10/2)^2} = 32.77 \quad \text{(rounded up:} \quad 33)$$

Because this iteration reveals n_e to be 33, as did the first, we can stop here. In this case, only two iterations were required, and n_1 and n_2 will require at least 33 sample replicates each for a 95% confidence interval with a 10-unit spread, or ±5 units from the means at the 95% confidence level. Other examples may require more.

As previously stated, it is better to have the sample sizes equal, $n_1 = n_2$, but it is not a requirement. If one sample group must be constrained to a specific n, the other sample can be expanded to be able to differentiate them at a specific confidence interval width. The easiest way to do this is to let the known, fixed sample set equal n_1 and the unknown, adjustable one be n_2. We can determine n_2 by calculating

$$n_2 = \frac{nn_1}{2n_1 - n}$$

After calculating the appropriate n sample size from Eq. (9), use that value to represent n and solve for n_2. In addition, assume that n_1 can only be sample size $= 10$. Using Example 1 again, we determined the necessary sample size for $n = 33$.

$$n_2 = \frac{33(10)}{2(10) - 33} = -25.38$$

Notice $n_2 = -25.38$. If $(2n_1 - n) \leq 0$, then n_1 must be increased and/or α must be increased and/or the detection width increased so that n_2 is positive $(2n_1 > n)$.

We increased the sample size, n_1, in this example, but we could also increase $\alpha = 0.05$ to $\alpha = 0.10$ or 0.15 and increase the minimum detection width from 10 to 15 or 20 points to produce the same result without adding more replicates to n_1. However, we would lose statistical power.

n_1	$2n_1$	n	
2(10) =	20 <	33	too low sample size n_1
2(15) =	30 <	33	too low sample size n_1
2(16) =	32 <	33	too low sample size n_1
2(17) =	34 >	33	okay, the minimum number of replicates we can begin with is 17

$$n_2 = \frac{33(17)}{2(17) - 33} = 561$$

That number of n_2 samples is far too large. The researcher then decides to increase n_1 to 25.

$$n_2 = \frac{33(25)}{2(25) - 33} = 48.53 \text{ or } 49$$

This is far better.

So a sample size of $n_1 = 25$ will require a sample size $n_2 = 49$ in order to ensure that $|\mu_1 - \mu_2|$ is within a 10-point spread at a 95% confidence interval.

Notice that the statistical efficiency is eroded by uneven sample sizes. The researcher must keep this in mind, because many times in research, a control group sample size, n, is purposely set at a lower number. For example, if one is comparing a new drug with a control drug, 10 replicates may be collected with the test product and, to save time and money, 5 replicates are collected for the control product. This approach can greatly reduce the power of the statistical test, causing validity problems for the researcher.

C. Determining the Smallest Detectable Difference between Two Means

A common problem in conducting pilot studies based on small samples is a lack of statistical power that results, mainly, in committing type II error [19]. That is, it is difficult to detect a difference in the means, $\delta = |\bar{X}_1 - \bar{X}_2|$, when one really exists. This is also a problem in other practical applications, for example, when one uses small samples in quality control or assurance to verify that a process or product is not significantly different from a standard. In addition, problems may occur when a researcher tries to select the best one or two products of a group of products. Many times, testing of a group of products results in accepting a null hypothesis outcome (no difference) when one truly exists. Hence, it is important to know just what the statistical detection level is.

Let us review, for a moment, four factors that influence sample size requirements:

1. The detectable difference between population means ($\delta = |\mu_1 - \mu_2|$) is directly attributable to sample size. The smaller the difference between means, that is, the smaller the δ values, the larger the sample size must be to detect a difference. This detection limit value, δ, should be known by the researcher prior to conducting a test.
2. The sample variance, s^2, also directly influences the sample size required. The larger the sample variability or variance (s^2), the

larger the sample size needed to detect a specific δ level. And, generally speaking, for the two-sample t-test, the total variability of $\sigma_1^2 + \sigma_2^2$ estimated by S_1^2 and S_2^2 is less if the variances are equal $(S_1^2 = S_2^2)$ and can, therefore, be pooled (S_p^2).

3. The significance level set for type I (α) error also affects the sample size requirements. One can adjust the value of α downward from, say, 0.05 to 0.01, for greater insurance against type I (α) error, but in doing so, the probability of committing type II (β) error increases unless the sample size, n, is also increased.

4. The power of the statistical test, $1-\beta$ (its ability to detect a true difference in sample means when one exists), increases as the sample size increases. However, using a more powerful statistical test when possible—say a parametric instead of a nonparametric one—will generally increase the power without increasing the sample size.

D. δ Computation to Determine Detection Level between Two Samples

The formula to be used for determining the degree of detectable difference between sample sets of data is:

$$\delta \geq \sqrt{\frac{2S_p^2}{n}}(t_{\alpha/2,\,df} + t_{\beta,df}) \tag{10}$$

where δ = smallest difference that can be detected between the two sample means = $|\bar{x}_1 - \bar{x}_2|$.
$t_{\alpha/2}$ = standard significance level of α, either a two-tail test using $\alpha/2$ or a one-tail test using α
df = $n_1 + n_2 - 2$
t_β = significance level for β (type II) error
n = sample size
$S_p^2 = \frac{SS_1 + SS_2}{n_1 + n_2 - 2}$, df = $2(n - 1)^*$; $n = 33$, and $2(33-1) = 64$

Using the data in Example 1 again $\alpha = 0.05$, $\alpha/2 = 0.025$, $\beta = 0.10$ (that is, we have a $1 - \beta = 90\%$ probability of detecting true differences in sample means).

---

*Note: If $n_1 \neq n_2$, then df = $n_1 - 1 + n_2 - 1$.

Applying formula (10), the computation is carried out.

$$\delta \geq \sqrt{\frac{2(102.62)}{33}}(1.998 + 1.295) = 8.21 \quad \text{or rounded up, 9}$$

We note that, for a sample size of $33 = n_1 = n_2$, $\text{df} = 2(n - 1) = 64$, $S_p^2 = 102.62$, $\alpha/2 = 0.025$, and $\beta = 0.10$, the minimum detection level is 9 points, or $|x_1 - x_2| \geq 9$, if a significant difference is to be detected.

E. Power of the Pooled *t*-Test Prior to Conducting Experiment

When calculating the power of the statistical test, $(1 - \beta)$, prior to conducting the experiment, use Eq. (11). And it is usually wise to compute the power prior to conducting a study. Recall that the power of a test $(1 - \beta)$ is its ability not to make type II errors.

$$\phi = \sqrt{\frac{n\delta^2}{4S_p^2}} \tag{11}$$

where ϕ = critical value to find power $(1 - \beta)$ in Table A.4 (Power Tables). For *t*-tests, use Table A.4.1 where $v_1 = 1$.

n = sample size (see Note below)

δ = minimum detection level

$S_p^2 = \frac{SS_1 + SS_2}{n_1 - 1 + n_2 - 1}$ degrees of freedom for $\phi = n_1 + n_2 - 2$ or $2(n - 1)$, if $n_1 = n_2$

Note: When the sample sizes are unequal $(n_1 \neq n_2)$, use Eq. (12) (an unequal sample size correction factor) to calculate the n value.

$$n = \frac{2n_1 n_2}{n_1 + n_2} \tag{12}$$

Using the data from Example 1, let us assume $n_1 = n_2 = 10$ because that is our plan prior to conducting the test experiment. Because this is an estimate to be used before conducting the study, we can employ Eq. (11). Recall that we previously set $\delta = 10$ units and S_p^2 was 102.62. Therefore,

$$\phi = \sqrt{\frac{10(10)^2}{4(102.62)}} = 1.56$$

From Table A.4.1 (Power Tables) where $v_1 = 1$, and $v_2 = $ df $= n_1 + n_2 - 2 = 10 + 10 - 2 = 18$, use the α value 0.05 to determine the power of the test, $1 - \beta$. Find $\phi = 1.56$ on the power table for $\alpha = 0.05$, and ascend in a straight line to the corresponding value of v_2 (18). Then move all the way to the left most portion of the table to Read $1 - \alpha$ directly. The value 1.56 is too small to be found. This means that with a $\delta = 10$, $\alpha = 0.05$ and $S_p^2 = 102.62$ the power is very small. Let us adjust this using $\alpha = 0.01$. Here, we match $\phi = 1.56$ with the curved power line approximately $v_2 = 18$. Once this has been completed, again move to the left most portion of the table reading $1 - \beta$ directly. That value is about 0.58. So the power of the test is 0.58. The researcher will theoretically reject products that actually are effective, with 42% probability over the long run when $\alpha = 0.01$. Since this computation has been done prior to the experiment, the researcher can take action. Increase the sample size to reduce S_p^2 is the preferred way, and increase the value of δ, to reduce the detectable difference. Therefore, the β value corresponding to ϕ is 0.08. The power of the statistic is $1 - \beta = 1 - 0.08 \approx 0.92$.

V. POWER COMPUTATION AFTER THE EXPERIMENT HAS BEEN CONDUCTED

The power computations just presented must be computed prior to conducting an experiment. This is very important, for it is necessary to know the test's power so that the appropriate sample size is used. Yet, after the experiment has been run, it is also of value to determine or confirm what the power of the two-sample pooled t-test actually is, in terms of the probability of committing a type II error.

The power of the two-sample pooled t-test, computed after the experiment is run, can be estimated by:

$$\phi = \sqrt{\frac{nd^2 - 2S_p^2}{4S_p^2}} \tag{13}$$

where

$$S_p^2 = \frac{SS_1 + SS_2}{(n_1 - 1) + (n_2 - 1)}$$

$d = $ difference between sample means, or

$$\bar{X}_1 - \bar{X}_2$$

df $= n_1 + n_2 - 2$ where $\alpha = 0.01$ or $\alpha = 0.05$

$n = $ sample size when $n_1 = n_2$

If $n_1 \neq n_2$, then $n = (2n_1n_2)/(n_1 + n_2)$, the correction formula [Eq. (12)].

Using the data in Example 1, note that $n_1 \neq n_2$; one of our sample values was lost. Therefore, we will use the sample size correction factor [Eq. (12)].

$$n = \frac{2n_1n_2}{n_1 + n_2} = \frac{2(10)(9)}{10 + 9} = 9.47$$

Let $\alpha = 0.05$. The value of d computed is $163.10 - 158.78 = 4.32$, and $d^2 = 4.32^2 = 18.66$. This value will be too small to be useful for the same reason just discussed in IV. Suppose $d = 15$ and $d^2 = 225$.

$$S_p^2 = 102.62$$

$$\phi = \sqrt{\frac{9.47(225) - 2(102.62)}{4(102.62)}}$$

$$\phi = \sqrt{4.69} = 2.2$$

We again turn to the power tables, Table A.4.1 where $v_1 = 1$. Notice that α can be either 0.05 or 0.01 using these tables. The pooled sample degrees of freedom $(v_2) = n_1 + n_2 - 2$. Find the α graph to use, 0.05 or 0.01, and, at the bottom of the graph, find the value for ϕ. Again, trace that value straight up until it meets the line for degrees of freedom. Where they meet, draw a horizontal line to the vertical y axis of the table. This spot corresponds to $1 - \beta$, or the power of the statistic. We use $\alpha = 0.05$, so the left group of power curves is used. The computed value for ϕ at 0.05 is 2.2, corresponding to a df value of $n_1 + n_2 - 2 = 10 + 9 - 2 = 17$, which is v_2, for a power of ~ 0.58. This is not much power. The experimenter now runs a rather high risk of committing type II error.

In conclusion, it is important that the researcher acknowledges that sample sizes, confidence levels or widths, power, and detectable differences be viewed from a problematic perspective. As a researcher becomes more familiar and experienced with the methods and techniques used in the analysis, she or he will intuitively understand the significance of a particular parameter. Statistical computations are tools to assist a researcher, they do not determine what the research means, in and of themselves.

A. Differences between Variances

Later in this book, we will devote considerable time to learning to compare variances, σ^2, using several analysis of variance statistical methods, but for the time being, we will concentrate on two-sample pooled t-tests.

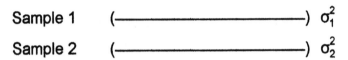

Sample 1   (————————————————) σ_1^2

Sample 2   (————————————————) σ_2^2

FIGURE 2   Equal variances of two populations.

Sample 1 (————————————————————————) σ_1^2

Sample 2   (—————) σ_2^2

FIGURE 3   Unequal variances.

When the variances are pooled in the two-sample pooled t-test, we assume variance equality ($\sigma_1^2 = \sigma_2^2$). We have noted earlier that comparing variances is not as powerful for revealing significant differences between populations as is a two-sample t-test. Yet, there are times in research when we really need to know whether the variability in one population is different from that of another. Take, for example, Fig. 2 and 3.

In Fig. 2, we have a graph of two variances of equal width. Figure 3, on the other hand, presents two samples with unequal variances (in width). A statistical power problem arises in situations where one variance is larger than the other. In a two-sample t-test, as long as σ_2^2 is located within the width of σ_1^2, the test would portray the samples as coming from the same population (Fig. 4).

Although it appears that samples 1 and 2 comes from the same population within the regions depicted in Fig. 4, intuitively, one can see a problem. The region of σ_1^2 is so large that one cannot readily see a difference in the two samples. One can see a biasing effect when $\sigma_1^2 \neq \sigma_2^2$ in that the relatively small variance, σ_2^2, will totally obscured by the larger one, σ_1^2, in analysis. In many cases, it would not be meaningful to compare the samples, particularly in situations with small sample sizes, because no meaningful difference could be detected. A better goal would be to equalize the variance, usually by increasing the sample sizes of both groups. The problem, however, will more than likely be a research issue, requiring a research solution, instead of a statistical one [19].

Sample 1 (————————————————————)σ_1^2

Sample 2 (————)↞(————)↞(————)σ_2^2

FIGURE 4   Positions of the samples relative to one another, in which they would be considered as coming from the same population.

Another option is to use an F-test to compare variances to ensure that they are equivalent, as required by the two-sample pooled t-test. There is heated debate as to the actual usefulness of this test, but we will consider it impartially.

The general approach to testing the variance in a two-sample t-test poses the hypothesis:

$$H_0: \sigma_1^2 = \sigma_2^2$$

$$H_A: \sigma_1^2 \neq \sigma_2^2$$

and the test is a variance ratio test: $S_i^2 / S_j^2 = F_c$.

The larger variance is placed in the numerator portion of the ratio because the F distribution is only an upper tail one.

$$F_c = \frac{S_2^2}{S_1^2}, \quad \text{given } S_2^2 > S_1^2$$

If $S_1^2 \approx S_2^2$, the quotient of the ratio will be near 1, where no difference is inferred.

Example 2: The data in Table 3 are microbial plate count values for *Escherichia coli* bacteria preserved either by freeze drying or by cryostorage.

TABLE 3   Microbial Plate Count Values

Group 1 freeze-dried	Group 2 −70°C
380	350
376	356
360	358
368	376
372	338
366	342
374	366
382	350
	344
	364
$\bar{x}_1 = 372.25$	$\bar{x}_2 = 354.40$
$n_1 = 8$	$n_2 = 10$
$df_1 = n_1 - 1 = 7$	$df_2 = n_2 - 1 = 9$
$S_1^2 = 54.214$	$S_2^2 = 142.044$
$F_c = 142.044/54.214 = 2.628$	

The experimenter wants to know whether the variances are significantly different.

$$H_0: \sigma_1^2 = \sigma_2^2, \ \alpha = 0.05$$

The F_{tabled} statistic has two values for the degrees of freedom, the one on the "top" for the numerator (v_1), the other to the left for the denominator (v_2), $F_{\alpha,v_1,v_2} = F_{\alpha,n_1-1;n_2-1}$.* Table A.3 contains the F distribution.

Using $\alpha = 0.05$, df for the numerator $v_1 = n_2 - 1 = 9$, and df for the denominator $v_2 = n_1 - 1 = 8 - 1 = 7$, we find the value, 3.68.

$$F_{0.05,9,7} = 3.68$$

Because F_c calculated (2.628) $< F_{\text{tabled}}$ (3.68), we cannot reject the H_0 hypothesis. That is, we cannot conclude that $\sigma_1^2 \neq \sigma_2^2$ at the $\alpha = 0.05$ level of significance.

A major problem with the variance test is that it is adversely affected by nonnormal populations, much more so than are two-sample t-tests.

VI. MATCHED-PAIR TWO-SAMPLE t-TEST

So far, the statistical methods we have discussed have been two independent-sample t-tests. We learned that it is better that they—the two sample sets—have the same variance so they can be pooled. This provides a more powerful test than when the variances cannot be pooled. Now we will discuss another variation of the two-sample t-test, the paired two-sample t-test. Pairing, a form of blocking, can be done when samples are related. In fact, the pair may be the same sample, as in a pre-post or before-and-after type of study design. The matched-pair t-test is statistically more powerful than both the pooled t-test and the nonpooled variance, independent-sample t-test. This is because the inherent variability between samples will be significantly reduced, a big advantage in that fewer replicates are needed to achieve comparable power [17,20,22].

Let us look at an example. Randomly selecting subjects from a population of patients to undergo either treatment A or treatment B is an example of an independent design approach. But, if each subject receives *both* treatments, a matched-pair design (that is, each subject is a block), the statistical analysis is more powerful than for the independent design. For example, in a preoperative skin preparation study design, if each study subject is a treatment *block* surgically prepped on one side of the abdomen near the umbilicus with product A and on the other side with product B, we have a case where we

---

*Note: The sample size of the larger S^2 value of the two is used as the n_1 value. So, if $n_2 = 10, v_1 = n_2 - 1 = 9$, if $n_1 = 8, v_2 = n_1 - 1 = 7$.

TABLE 4   Treatment of Randomly Selected Rats

1	2	3	4	5	6	7	8	9	10
A	A	A	B	A	A	A	B	A	A
B	B	B	A	B	B	B	A	B	B

can use the matched-pair two-sample t-test. This blocking technique is statistically a more powerful one than having x_1 number of patients treated with product A and x_2 number of patients with product B. In later chapters, blocking will continue to be very useful as we get into more complex designs.

Let us look at another example. If we select rats randomly from a colony of rats (different litters, age, facility, sex) and assign them treatment A or treatment B, we have an independent sampling design. If, on the other hand, we have a single litter of rats in the same pen, eating the same food, drinking the same water, and we wish to run an experiment to determine sexually determined responses, we could divide (block) the litter into males and females and derive meaningful data to which to apply the matched-pair, two-sample t-test.

If we had one metal strip, we could section it into 10 equal segments for 10 replicates, partition the 10 segments in half, and use treatment A on one half and treatment B on the other half of each of the 10 segments (Table 4). Or better yet, we could randomize each A or B placement by flipping a coin, where heads = treatment A in upper portion of the strip, and tails = treatment B in lower portion.

In the previous two-sample t-test section, we tested hypotheses of the two-tail test version in which two population means were either equal ($\mu_1 = \mu_2$) or not equal ($\mu_1 \neq \mu_2$). In the paired version of this test, we evaluate the difference ($\mu_1 - \mu_2 = \mu_d$). If $|\mu_d| > 0$, then we accept the alternative hypothesis ($\mu_1 \neq \mu_2$). If $\mu_d \approx 0$, we cannot reject the null hypothesis ($\mu_1 = \mu_2$).

The difference (d_i) between the ith paired treatments is calculated as:

$$d_i = x_{i_1} - x_{i_2}, \qquad i = 1, 2, \ldots, n$$

The average value difference is:

$$\mu_d = \frac{\sum(d_i)}{n} = \frac{\sum(x_{i_1} - x_{i_2})}{n}$$

Note, also, that we do not use the original measurements for the two samples in the paired t-test but instead use the difference for each sample.

The paired t-test is essentially a one-sample t-test. The paired t-test data are not under the same conditions of normality and equality as the variance found in the two-sample case; instead, the d_i values are assumed to be normally distributed. So, any exploratory data analyses are performed on the d_i values. We will discuss a nonparametric analog of the paired t-test in Chap. 12.

A. Setting up a Paired t-Test

Three test conditions are possible:

Two-tail:

H_0: $\mu_d = 0$

H_A: $\mu_d \neq 0$ Accept H_A if $|t_{\alpha/2}| > t_{\text{tabled}}$

Upper-tail:

H_0: $\mu_d \leq 0$

H_A: $\mu_d > 0$ Accept H_A if $|t_\alpha| > t_{\text{tabled}}$

Lower tail:

H_0: $\mu_d \geq 0$

H_A: $\mu_d < 0$ Accept H_A if $t_{-\alpha} < t_{\text{tabled}}$

The test statistic is:

$$t_c = \frac{\bar{d}}{S_d / \sqrt{n}}$$

where

$$\bar{d} = \frac{\sum d}{n}, \text{ and}$$

$$S_d = \left[\frac{\sum_{i=1}^{n}(d_i - \bar{d})^2}{n-1} \right]^{1/2^*} \quad \text{or } S_d = \left[\frac{\sum_{i=1}^{n} d_i^2 - \frac{1}{n}\left(\sum_{i=1}^{n} d_i\right)^2}{n-1} \right]^{1/2},$$

which is often easier to compute when using a hand calculator. If $|t_c| > t_{\text{tabled}}$, accept H_A.

---

*Note: $x^{1/2} = \sqrt{x}$.

TABLE 5 Blood-clotting Times for Mice, in Seconds

n	Females (x_1)	Males (x_2)	$d = x_1 - x_2$
1	44	46	−2
2	43	34	9
3	29	44	−15
4	34	37	−3
5	10	18	−8
6	47	22	25
7	42	42	0
8	17	33	−16
9	58	41	17
10	36	62	−26

Example 3: After an experimental clotting drug was administered to a genetically inbred colony of mice for 30 days, blood-clotting time was measured to determine whether there was a difference between clotting times for males and females. The researcher paired individuals of the two sexes on the basis of similar body weights. The data in Table 5 were collected for the clotting times in seconds.

Let us work this example using the six-step procedure:

Step 1. Formulate H_0 and H_A. We are interested in detecting a *difference* between clotting times of male and female mice. This is a two-tail test.

H_0: $\mu_1 = \mu_2$ μ_1 = female mice and H_A: $\mu_1 \neq \mu_2$ μ_2 = male mice

Step 2. Select α, and determine sample size. At this point we would calculate the sample size needed, power, and/or minimum detection limits, given that we knew or could accurately estimate S_d. We will not do this now, but the researcher in practice would.

$n_1 = n_2 = 10$ $\alpha = 0.01$ $df = n - 1 = 10 - 1 = 9$

Step 3. Select the test statistic. Because this is a paired *t*-test, the formula is:

$$t_c = \frac{\bar{d}}{S_d/\sqrt{n}} \tag{14}$$

Step 4. Present the decision rule (Fig. 5). $\alpha = 0.01/2 = 0.005$ and $n - 1 = df = 10 - 1 = 9$. $t_{t(0.005, 9)} = \pm 3.25$ because it is a two-tail test.

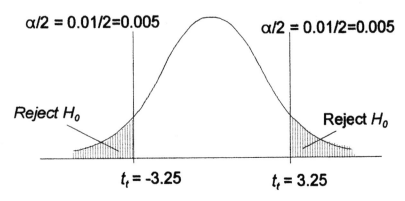

FIGURE 5   Decision rule.

Decision rule:
If t_c calculated is <-3.25 or >3.25, one must reject the H_0 hypothesis at $\alpha = 0.01$.

Step 5.   Compute the test statistic from the data in table 5.

$$\bar{d} = \frac{\sum d}{n} = \frac{-2 + 9 + \cdots + 17 - 26}{10} = -1.90$$

$$S_d = \left(\frac{\sum d^2 - (1/n)(\sum d)^2}{n-1} \right)^{1/2} \tag{15}$$

$$\sum d_i = -2 + 9 + \cdots + 17 + (-26) = -19$$

$$\sum d_i^2 = -2^2 + 9^2 + \cdots + 17^2 + (-26)^2 = 2229$$

$$S_d = \left(\frac{2229 - (1/10)(-19)^2}{10-1} \right)^{1/2} = 15.609$$

$$t_d = \frac{\bar{d}}{S_d/\sqrt{n}} = \frac{-1.9}{15.609/\sqrt{10}} = -0.385$$

Step 6.   Because $t_{calculated} = -0.385 > t_{tabled}(-3.25)$ and $t_{calculated} = -0.385 < t_{tabled}$ (3.25), the H_0 hypothesis cannot be rejected at $\alpha = 0.01$. No significant difference in blood-clotting times between males and females can be detected at the 0.01 level of significance.

Note that when using a paired *t*-test software model, MiniTab® in this case, the data utilized by the software are the difference between each matched pair, $x_1 - x_2 = d_j$ (Table 6).

TABLE 6   MiniTab Computer Input of d_i Values

Input									
−2	9	−15	−3	−8	25	0	−16	17	−26

TABLE 7   MiniTab Computer Output

	N	MEAN	STDEV	SE MEAN	T	P VALUE
Output						
MEAN	10	−1.9	15.609	4.936	−0.38	0.71

Table 7 provides the same results as the pencil-and-paper method used in Example 3. The *SE* in the output is the standard error of the mean $= S_{\bar{x}} = S_d/\sqrt{n} = 15.609/\sqrt{10} = 4.936$. The *P* value is the probability (71%) of observing a $t_{\text{calculated}}$ value $= 0.38$, or more extreme, given the H_0 hypothesis is true. This can be written as:

$$P(t) \geq 0.38 \text{ (given } H_0 \text{ is true)} = 0.71.$$

B. Confidence Interval for the Mean Differences: Paired *t*-Test

In the paired *t*-test example, because we work with *d* values, the confidence interval for the mean population difference, μ_d, is simply a confidence interval for the population of one mean, μ. Recall that the population μ is estimated from:

$$\mu = \bar{x} \pm t_{(\alpha/2, n-1)} S_{\bar{x}} \tag{16}$$

where $\mu =$ sample mean $\sum x_i/n$

$t =$ two-tail *t* value at $\alpha/2$, with $n-1$ degrees of freedom

$S_{\bar{x}} =$ standard error of the mean $s/\sqrt{n}$ or $\sqrt{s^2/n}$

The paired two-sample confidence interval is computed in much the same way, using the d_i values. The μ_d is estimated from:

$$\mu_d = \bar{d} \pm t_{(\alpha/2,n-1)} s_{\bar{d}} \tag{17}$$

where

$$\bar{d} = \frac{\sum d}{n}$$

t = two-tailed α level, $\alpha/2$, with $n - 1$ degrees of freedom

$$S_{\bar{d}} = \frac{S_d}{\sqrt{n}} \quad \text{or} \quad \sqrt{\frac{S_d^2}{n}}$$

For Example 3, the 95% confidence level for the mean difference is

$$\bar{d} \pm (t_{\alpha/2,n-1}) \frac{S_d}{\sqrt{n}} \tag{18}$$

where $t_{0.05/2=0.025,9 \text{ df}} = 2.262$ and $S = \frac{15.609}{\sqrt{10}} = 4.936$

$$-1.9 \pm 2.262(4.936)$$

$$-1.9 \pm 11.165$$

$$-13.065 \leq \mu_d \leq 9.265$$

The 95% confidence interval for the true difference, μ_d, is between -13.065 and 9.265. Note that, because 0 is included in the confidence interval, $-13.065 \leq \mu \leq 9.265$, one cannot reject the H_0 hypothesis at $\alpha = 0.05$.

C. Size Estimation of the Population Mean Contained in a Set Interval Using the Paired t-Test

For the paired t-test, the required sample size is computed as for a one-sample t-test with a predefined $\pm$ confidence interval width, d. The basic formula is:

$$n = \frac{S_d^2 t_{(\alpha/2,n-1)}^2}{d^2} \tag{19}$$

where

$$S_d^2 = \text{sample variance} = \frac{\sum(d - \bar{d})^2}{n - 1}$$

t = two-tail tabled value on Student's t-distribution for $\alpha/2$, $n - 1$ degrees of freedom

$d = 1/2$ the width of the confidence interval desired

The basic difficulty with Eq. (19) is that the degrees of freedom $(n - 1)$ depends upon a known n value, which, at this point, is unknown. However, as before, the solution can be determined by iteration. We "guesstimate" an initial n value, beginning with a larger sample size than we think is needed because using a larger n finds the appropriate value with fewer iterations than using a smaller n. As before, the reliability of the n value depends upon what the actual S_d^2 value is. As before, S_d^2 is improved—becomes smaller—with a larger sample size. And, as before, the calculated n value is rounded up to the next whole number, if a fraction is involved. Using the data from Table 4, the parameters are calculated in a three-step procedure following Eq. (19).

Step 1. Let's pick $n = 50$, so df $= 49$ with $\alpha = 0.05/2 = 0.025$, and $t(0.025, 49) = 2.021$. Let us set $2d = 10$ points, or $d = 5$.

$$n = \frac{S_d^2 t_{(\alpha/2, n-1)}}{d^2} = \frac{15.609^2 (2.021)^2}{5^2}$$

$n = 39.805$, or rounded up, 40

Step 2. The next interation will use $n = 40$, $n - 1 = 39$, $\alpha/2 = 0.05/2$, and $t(0.025, 39) = 2.042$.

$$n = \frac{15.609^2 (2.042)^2}{5^2} = 40.637, \text{ or rounded up, } 41$$

Step 3. Solve for $n = 41$, so $t_{(d/2; n-1)} = t_{(0.025, 40)} = 2.021$.

$$n = \frac{15.609^2 (2.021)^2}{5^2} = 39.806, \text{ or rounded up, } 40$$

Because the table degrees of freedom jump from 30 to 40, without including 31–39, the iterative power will continue to repeat from 40 to 41 and back to 40. When this pattern is seen, stop. The sample size required will be atleast 40 at $\alpha = 0.05$, with $S_d^2 = 15.609$, confidence interval width $= 10$.

D. Sample Size Determination of the Mean at Set a and β levels

The sample size needed for detecting the true mean with a probability of $1 - \alpha$, a specified β, and at a specified detection level, δ, is extremely useful. The detection level is very important at a specified pretest–posttest difference, $\mu_1 - \mu_2$. Equation (20) can be used for determining the sample size requirements.

$$n = \frac{S_d^2}{\delta^2}(t_{\alpha,n-1} + t_{\beta,n-1})^2 \tag{20}$$

Note that α can be a single or two-tail value.

$$S_d^2 = \text{sample variance} = \frac{\sum(d - \bar{d})^2}{n - 1}$$

t = two-tail or single-tail tabled value for α or β at

$\quad n - 1$ degrees of freedom

α = type I error significance level

β = type II error significance level

δ = specified detection level = $|\bar{x}_1 - \bar{x}_2|$.

The calculation is straightforward. Using the data from Table 5 and Eq. (20), the sample size is computed iteratively, again using an initial estimate higher than expected. Using a value higher than the actual number for the initial estimate finds the final n value more quickly than does a lower value.

$S_d = 15.609$

$\quad \alpha$, two-tail in this case for $\alpha = 0.05$, or $\alpha/2 = 0.025$

β = always a single tail, set at 0.10

δ = Let's set δ at a 10-point detection level for difference between males and females

Let us begin the iterative process with a large n, say $n = 50$.

Step 1. Let $n = 50$, so $n - 1 = 49$, the t_{tabled} value for $t_{\alpha/2,n-1} = t_{0.025,49} = 2.021$, the t_{tabled} value for $t_{\beta,n-1} = t_{0.10,49} = 1.296$. So

$n = \frac{15.609^2}{10^2}(2.021 + 1.296)^2 = 26.807$, or rounded up, 27

Step 2. Use the rounded up $n = 27$ to begin the next iteration. $n = 27, n - 1 = 26$, the t_{tabled} value for $t_{0.025,26} = 2.056$, the t_{tabled} value for $t_{\beta,n-1} = t_{0.10,26} = 1.315$

$n = \frac{15.609^2}{10^2}(2.056 + 1.315)^2 = 27.686$, or rounded up, 28

Step 3. Let $n = 28, n - 1 = 27$, so $t_{0.025,27} = 2.052$, and $t_{\beta,n-1} = t_{0.10,27} = 1.314$.

$$n = \frac{15.609^2}{10^2}(2.052 + 1.314)^2 = 27.604, \text{ or rounded up, } 28$$

Because iterations two and three are both 28 (when rounded up), we can stop computing. We need a minimum of 28 subjects for $\delta = 10$, $\alpha = 0.05$, $\beta = 0.10$, and $S_d = 15.609$. As before, we must depend upon S_d^2 being an accurate estimate of σ_d^2.

E. Minimum Detectable Differences

We can also compute the minimum detectable difference, δ_d, between x_1 and x_2 by rearranging terms in Eq. (20).

$$\delta_d = \sqrt{\frac{S_d^2}{n}}(t_{\alpha,n-1} + t_{\beta,n-1}) \tag{21}$$

As before, α can be a two-tail test $(\alpha/2)$ or a single-tail test (α). Using the information from the six-step procedure, as well as Eq. (21), the following δ_d is provided. No iteration is necessary, for we know what n is.

$$\delta_d = \sqrt{\frac{S_d^2}{n}}(t_{\alpha,n-1} + t_{\beta,n-1})$$

$$\delta_d = \sqrt{\frac{15.609^2}{28}}(2.052 + 1.314) = 9.929, \text{ or rounded up, } 10$$

Notice that δ was set at 10 in the previous calculation. That is, we can detect a minimum of 10 points between μ_1 and μ_2. To increase the detection level (reduce the difference) will require an increased sample size.

F. Power of the Paired t-Test

The probability of rejecting a false H_0 is the power of the test $(1-\beta =$ power). That can be determined by applying Eq. (22). Again, no iteration is necessary because we have solved for n previously. Note that the power of a test is greater for a one-tail than for a two-tail test.

$$t_{\beta,n-1} = \frac{\delta_d}{\sqrt{S_d^2/n}} - t_{\alpha,n-1} \tag{22}$$

Note that α can be a one-tail (α) or two-tail $(\alpha/2)$ test.

From the data used to generate the results of Eq. (22), the following derives.

$$t_{\beta,n-1} = \frac{10}{\sqrt{(15.609)^2/28}} - 2.052 = 1.338$$

Using Student's t table (Table B) with $n - 1$ df $= 27$, we see that $1.338 \approx 0.10$, that is, $\beta = 0.10$, and the power of the test $= 1 - \beta = 0.90$.

VII. FINAL COMMENTS

One challenge for researchers is to ensure that the statistics they use have been consciously chosen. If one had only to pick between a two-sample t-test for independent samples and a paired t-test for matched pairs, life would be easy. If the researcher, however, uses the stipulations we have already discussed in previous chapters as a fundamental guide, then she or he must think about the intended audience. If it is a statistically well-versed professional group, the appropriate design based on the conditions we have discussed can prevail. In my experience, this type of presentation is a rare event.

The researcher should also use practical, jargon-free communication to describe to investors, business management, and marketing personnel the statistical models used. This is often wise even when writing for many professional journals. Most of these groups have some knowledge of statistics, but often this begins and ends with the t-test. So, the majority of researchers' reports and discussions should maintain evaluations at the t-test level of complexity, particularly if the intent is to communicate rather than impress or, worse, confuse.

Many experiments will evaluate more than two sample sets. Technically, to do this, the t-test must be modified to account for multiple comparisons. In this case, the easiest way to do this is via confidence intervals.

Recall that the confidence interval for the population mean, μ, is:

$$\bar{X} \pm (t_{\alpha/2,n-1})\frac{s}{\sqrt{n}}$$

where $\bar{X} = \frac{\sum x}{n}$ or mean

$t =$ two-tail, tabled value for $\alpha/2, n - 1$ degrees of freedom

$s =$ standard deviation of sample set $\left(\frac{\sum(x-\bar{x})^2}{n-1}\right)^{1/2}$ or $\sqrt{\sum\frac{(x-\bar{x})^2}{n-1}}$

$n =$ sample size

However, the t-test is valid for only one two-sample comparison. Any more, and the true confidence level, $1 - \alpha$, is reduced by $(1 - \alpha)^k$, where k is the number of comparisons [20].

For example, at $\alpha = 0.05$, for one contrast, say, μ_1 vs. μ_2, the confidence level is

For one contrast: $(1 - 0.05)^1 = 0.950$

For two contrasts: $(1 - 0.05)^2 = 0.903$

For three contrasts: $(1 - 0.05)^3 = 0.857$

For four contrasts: $(1 - 0.05)^4 = 0.815$

For five contrasts: $(1 - 0.05)^5 = 0.774$

$\vdots$ $\vdots$

For k contrasts: $(1 - 0.05)^k$

There is an α' correction factor that should be used for multiple comparisons [20]:

$$\alpha' = 1 - (1 - \alpha)^k \tag{23}$$

where k = number of contrasts or comparisons
          α = standard set α
          α' = adjusted true significance level of all comparison tests used in the evaluation

Example 4: A researcher has six nutritional rations to evaluate for weight gain in broiler chickens after 8 weeks on the rations at full feeding. The six groups are designated A through F, with the final weights given, as in Table 8.

Note: Although technically, k contrasts are k contrasts and only k contrasts, I have repeatedly used k confidence intervals and compared all of them visually, which is more, technically, than one should do. I have not increased k to all possible combinations, for that provides a meaningless α. I have done this on a number of occasions without using the k correction factor, when it would merely serve to confuse the audience. The important point, however, is that this weakness should be presented to the audience.

TABLE 8   Example 4 Data

n	A	B	C	D	E	F
1	2.1	2.9	2.7	3.3	2.0	2.9
2	2.7	3.1	2.9	3.5	2.3	3.1
3	3.0	3.4	3.5	3.7	2.5	3.2
4	3.2	2.8	2.2	3.6	2.0	2.7
5	2.7	3.6	2.3	3.1	2.1	2.6
6	2.6	2.9	a	3.7	2.0	2.8
7	2.3	2.8	2.7	3.8	2.1	a
8	3.1	2.9	2.3	3.2	2.0	3.6
9	2.9	3.0	2.9	3.4	1.9	3.2
10	2.8	3.3	2.8	3.6	2.3	3.3
	$\bar{x}_A = 2.5$	$\bar{x}_B = 3.1$	$\bar{x}_C = 2.7$	$\bar{x}_D = 3.5$	$\bar{x}_E = 2.1$	$\bar{x}_F = 3.0$
	$S_A = 0.9$	$S_B = 0.3$	$S_C = 0.4$	$S_D = 0.2$	$S_E = 0.2$	$S_F = 0.3$
	$n_A = 10$	$n_B = 10$	$n_C = 9$	$n_D = 10$	$n_E = 10$	$n_F = 9$

[a] Missing value (chicken died).

In the current example, the procedure is as follows:

Step 1.   Because there are six groups (A through F), six confidence intervals are calculated at $\alpha/2 = 0.05/2, n - 1$ degrees of freedom. For groups A, B, D, and E: $\alpha = 0.05/2, n = 10, n - 1 = 9$, and $2.262 = t$. For groups C and F: $\alpha = 0.05/2, n = 9$, and $t_{0.025,8} = 2.306$.

$$\mu_A = 2.5 \pm 2.262 \ (0.9/\sqrt{10})$$
$$2.5 \pm 0.6$$
$$1.9 \le \mu_A \le 3.1$$

$$\mu_B = 3.1 \pm 2.262 \ (0.3/\sqrt{10})$$
$$3.1 \pm 0.2$$
$$2.9 \le \mu_B \le 3.3$$

$$\mu_C = 2.7 \pm 2.306 \ (0.4/\sqrt{9})$$
$$2.7 \pm 0.3$$
$$2.4 \le \mu_C \le 3.0$$

$$\mu_D = 3.5 \pm 2.262\ (0.2/\sqrt{10})$$
$$3.5 \pm 0.1$$
$$3.4 \le \mu_D \le 3.6$$
$$\mu_E = 2.1 \pm 2.262\ (0.2/\sqrt{10})$$
$$2.1 \pm 0.1$$
$$2.0 \le \mu_E \le 2.2$$
$$\mu_F = 3.0 \pm 2.306\ (0.3/\sqrt{9})$$
$$3.0 \pm 0.2$$
$$2.8 \le \mu_F \le 3.2$$

Step 2.   Plot the confidence intervals (Fig. 6). Notice that if the confidence interval boundaries do not overlap with those of another confidence interval, the groups will be considered different. Group D is the best of all for weight gain and is significantly different from all other groups. Clearly, all other groups (B, C, E, and F) are equivalent to A. Within that, group E is significantly different from and lower than groups B, C, and F.

Showing data in the form of Fig. 6 is often much better than trying to perform an ANOVA due to the complexity of explaining nonequivalent variances, etc. However, the 95% confidence level for this does not hold at 95%

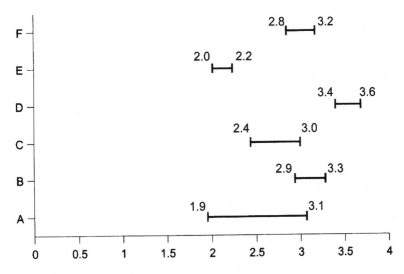

FIGURE 6   Plot of confidence intervals.

because of repealed contrasts. One must use the correction factor, $\alpha' = 1 - (1 - \alpha)^k$.

$$\alpha' = 1 - (1 - 0.05)^6 = 1 - 0.735 = 0.265$$

A value for α^* of 0.265 for all six confidence intervals is not particularly useful. If the researchers corrected for this by setting α at a very small number, e.g., 0.001, the effect would be to extend the confidence intervals out, making them wider. This has the effect of losing too much power, not being able to detect differences that may be there.

As stated, I have had very good practical luck with using multiple confidence intervals and not performing the α adjustments, particularly in small pilot comparisons. In addition, the researcher may want to protect against type I errors and be willing to have many type II errors to play it safe. I would not want to fly a plane with an α level of 0.05 for probability of failure. It should be more like $\alpha = 0.000001$. I would pay for replacing parts that are still good to achieve that safety edge.

Yet, in pilot studies, one often cannot justify using greater than an n of 5 due to budgets restraints. This puts tremendous pressure on the researcher to increase the power of the test. In certain cases, the researcher may use a paired t-test on data that are not really paired, to reduce the variance. The researcher, of course, is doing this for an intended reason (to increase the power) with too small a sample size. The researcher knows the statistical problems of this but can use wisdom gained from familiarity with the research field to help with the research conclusion. With that insight, this really is not naive use of the wrong model.

In many cases, I have been forced to use a small sample size to ensure that the test formulation is not different from the control. For example, many of our clients cannot justify the money required to detect the kind of discrete differences needed for assuring with high confidence that a difference truly does not exist between two formulations. For example, a client may change the color or fragrance of an antimicrobial product and want to validate that this action has caused no change in antimicrobial efficacy but wants to do this with five to eight replicates. Here again, I will do nearly anything to cut down on the variance in the actual testing and the statistic, including pairing. But this strategy is always explained in the statistical report, so the reader will understand the rationale.

Irrefutably, it is undesirable to use statistical inference to justify a bias. For example, if one wants to ensure that a fragrance change does not alter the product, and an n of 5 is used with a nonparametric statistic and an α of 0.01, the researcher has been not only negligent but also fraudulent. In such a case, it would be literally impossible to detect a difference if one is there, a β error by design. Unfortunately, statistical biasing such as this is all too prevalent.

The vast majority of statistics an applied research will encounter have now been discussed, and the researcher has the tools to peform most research comparisons. The rest of the book will essentially build on this knowledge.

5

Completely Randomized One-Factor Analysis of Variance

In the last chapter, I discussed Student's t-test and stated that I had favorable experiences using it for multiple sample comparisons. I also stated a problem with doing this. As the number of statistical comparisons increases, the $1 - \alpha$ level of significance decreases. For example, the 95% confidence level of the two-sample t-test drops to 85.7% (0.95^3) with three comparisons and 77.4% (0.95^5) with five comparisons. In Chap. 4 I provided a correction procedure to use to adjust α, when multiple t comparisons are to be performed, that will maintain the 95% confidence level when multiple comparisons are used. On the other hand, analysis of variance (ANOVA) models are designed specifically for multiple sample comparisons and should be employed, instead of multiple t-tests, unless there is a specific reason to use the t-test, such as presentation of the data to nonscientists.

I. ANALYSIS OF VARIANCE

The analysis of variance was first introduced by the British statistician Sir Ronald A. Fisher [25] (for whom the F-distribution is named). ANOVA methods are essentially a process for partitioning the total sum-of-squares variance into subcomponents that represent the treatment sum-of-squares variance and the random error sum-of-squares variance.

One-factor ANOVA designs appear in two forms—a completely randomized design and a randomized complete block design. These are analogous to the pooled two-sample t-test and the paired two-sample t-test, the difference being that instead of comparing means, we are comparing variances and usually more than two sample groups.

A. Completely Randomized Single-Factor Design

The order of each experimental test run is selected by a completely randomized selection process throughout the experiment, hence the name *completely randomized design*. The single factor means that only one parameter is of concern. For example, a researcher who is comparing the percentage of protein for weight gain in heavy-meat chickens may test five different levels of protein, say 10, 15, 20, 25, and 30%—all one factor. A factor is composed of treatments, so in this case there are five treatments of one factor, usually designated by A with a numerical subscript, 1 to k, indicating the number of treatments.

Within each treatment level are replicates that act in the same way as the replicates used in Student's t-test do: to increase accuracy and precision of the estimated parameters. As in the t-test, ANOVA replicates are also designated n.

The general linear model is:

$$y_{ij} = \mu + A_i + \epsilon_{ij} \qquad \begin{bmatrix} i = 1, 2, \ldots, k \text{ treatments} \\ j = 1, 2, \ldots, n \text{ replicates} \end{bmatrix} \qquad (1)$$

where

y_{ij} = the ith treatment and the jth replicate observation; the y_{ij} values are normally and independently distributed, having σ_ϵ^2 as the common error variance

μ = the common mean of all treatment samples

A_i = treatment effect for the ith treatment

ϵ_{ij} = random error = $y_{ij} - (\mu + A_i)$

There are five treatments [i.e., different levels of protein (the factor)]. The chickens in this experiment have been selected randomly from a group of 2000 chickens, age 1 week. Ten chickens will be assigned to each of the test ration groups and fed that ration for 8 continuous weeks. At the end of 8 weeks, the chickens will be weighed. Using a study design schema, the experiment is presented in Fig. 1.
where:

(R) represents that the chickens were randomly assigned to each of five groups. Each chicken was assigned only one treatment.

A_i is the independent variable: protein% of the feed.

O_i is the dependent variable: weight of the chickens after 8 weeks.

(R)	A_1	O_1
(R)	A_2	O_2
(R)	A_3	O_3
(R)	A_4	O_4
(R)	A_5	O_5

FIGURE 1   Experimental design schema.

B. Fixed-Effects and Random-Effects Models

In ANOVA designs, there are two basic types of models called fixed effects and random effects. Fixed-effects models are most commonly used by the applied researcher. For this model, the I_i values are set at specific, predetermined values. Figure 1 presents an example of a fixed-effects model because the researcher set the levels at 10, 15, 20, 25, and 30% protein. Hence, the scope of the researcher's conclusions will be limited to these levels: 10, 15, 20, 25, and 30% protein.

Suppose a researcher wants to compare five types of surgical scrub formulations for their antimicrobial efficacy. The researcher picks the top-selling products containing alcohol gel, parachlorometaxylenol (PCMX), triclosan, chlorhexidine gluconate (CHG), and iodine. This is a fixed-effects model comparing five products with one another. The researcher's conclusions are drawn not on the basis of all representative alcohol gel, PCMX, triclosan, CHG, and iodine products but only on those top sellers. To construct this as a random-effects model, the five product categories would entail random selection from all PCMX, CHG, triclosan, iodophor, and alcohol products available, instead of merely the top sellers. In a random-effects model, the I_is are randomly selected, not just assigned. We will discuss both models in this book, however, beginning with fixed-effects models.

C. Fixed-Effects Model (Model I)

In the fixed effects model, I_i represents the treatment effects (e.g., the chicken weights in the first example and the antimicrobial counts on the hands in the surgical scrub example). Note that the sum of treatment effects is 0.

$$\sum_{i=1}^{a} I_i = 0 \qquad (2)$$

Let us look at the construction of the chicken feed experiment, beginning with ANOVA configuration Table 1.

From ANOVA Table 1, we see that the sum of each treatment row equals $y_{1.}, y_{2.}, y_{3.}, \ldots y_5$, and the average of each total treatment row is $\bar{y}_{1.}, \bar{y}_{2.}, \ldots \bar{y}_{5.}$. The total of all treatments is $y..$, and the grand mean or mean of the treatment means is $y../N$ or $\bar{y}...$ So,

$$y_{i.} = \sum_{j=1}^{n} y_{ij} \quad \text{and} \quad \bar{y}_{i.} = \frac{y_{i.}}{n}, \quad \text{where } i = 1, 2, \ldots, a$$

$$y.. = \sum_{i=1}^{a} \sum_{j=1}^{n} y_{ij}$$

$\quad$ = the sum of each treatment set's replicate weight values

$\bar{y}.. =$ the grand treatment mean $= \dfrac{y..}{N}$

Note that N, the total sample size, is $(a \times n)$, or see Table 1, $5(10) = 50$.

In ANOVA problems, all hypothesis tests are two-tail tests that detect differences between any of the a treatments. The null hypothesis of a one-factor ANOVA is:

H_0: $\quad \mu_1 = \mu_2 \ldots \mu_a$. This means that the a treatment means are equivalent.

The alternative hypothesis is:

$\quad H_A$: $\mu_i \neq \mu_j$ for at least one pair. That is, at least one pair of treatment means differ.

TABLE 1 ANOVA Table

						Replicates							
		1	2	3	4	5	6	7	8	9	10	Total	Mean
Treatments	1 10%	y_{11}*	y_{12}	y_{13}	y_{14}	y_{15}	y_{16}	y_{17}	y_{18}	y_{19}	y_{110}	$y_{1.}$	$\bar{y}_{1.}$
	2 15%	y_{21}	y_{22}	y_{23}	y_{24}	y_{25}	y_{26}	y_{27}	y_2	y_{29}	y_{210}	$y_{2.}$	$\bar{y}_{2.}$
	3 20%	y_{31}	y_{32}	y_{33}	y_{34}	y_{35}	y_{36}	y_{37}	y_{38}	y_{39}	y_{310}	$y_{3.}$	$\bar{y}_{3.}$
	4 25%	y_{41}	y_{42}	y_{43}	y_{44}	y_{45}	y_{46}	y_{47}	y_{48}	y_{49}	y_{410}	$y_{4.}$	$\bar{y}_{4.}$
	5 30%	y_{51}	y_{52}	y_{53}	y_{54}	y_{55}	y_{56}	y_{57}	y_{58}	y_{59}	y_{510}	$y_{5.}$	$\bar{y}_{5.}$
												Total	$y..$	$\bar{y}..$

$a =$ number of treatments $= 5$
$n =$ number of replicates $= 10$
$N = a \times n = 50$
*Note: $y_{11} = y_{row, column}$; that is, $y_{11} =$ the value in row 1, column 1.

Note that, in the fixed-effects model, we speak of the means, μ_i, being equal in hypothesis-testing. In the random-effects model, we will compare equalities of variance, σ_i^2 in hypothesis-testing.

D. Decomposition of the Total Sum of Squares

There are two components that make up the total sum of squares in one-factor analysis of variance models. Recall that, in the last chapter, we defined the sum of squares as simply $\sum(x_i - \bar{x})^2$, the sum of the squared differences between the individual x_i values and the mean. The process is very similar in the ANOVA model.

$$SS_T = \text{sum of squares total} = \sum_{i=1}^{a} \sum_{j=1}^{n} (y_{ij} - \bar{y}..)^2$$

which is simply the summation of the squared differences between each y_{ij} value and the mean of the treatment means—the grand mean, $\bar{y}...$

The total variability, or total sum of squares (SS_T), can be decomposed into two components: the variability due to the treatments and the random variability, or error. This is written as:

$$SS_T = SS_{TREATMENT} + SS_{ERROR} \tag{3}$$

Mathematically, the decomposition is written

$$SS_T = \underbrace{\sum_{i=1}^{a} \sum_{j=1}^{n} (y_{ij} - \bar{y}..)^2}_{SS_{TOTAL}} = \underbrace{n \sum_{i=1}^{a} (\bar{y}_{i.} - \bar{y}..)^2}_{SS_{TREATMENT}} + \underbrace{\sum_{i=1}^{a} \sum_{j=1}^{n} (y_{ij} - \bar{y}_{i.})^2}_{SS_{ERROR}} \tag{4}$$

$SS_{TOTAL} = \sum_{i=1}^{a} \sum_{j=1}^{n} (y_{ij} - \bar{y}..)^2 = $ the sum of each individual y_{ij} minus the grand mean, the quantity squared

$SS_{TREATMENT} = n \sum (\bar{y}_{i.} - \bar{y}..)^2 = $ the sum of each treatment mean minus the grand mean, the quantity squared. Once that total has been computed, it is multiplied by n, the number of replicates.

$SS_{ERROR} = \sum_{i=1}^{a} \sum_{j=1}^{n} (y_{ij} - \bar{y}_{i.})^2 = $ the sum of each individual y_{ij} minus the specific treatment mean $\bar{y}_{i.}$, the quantity squared

The $SS_{TREATMENT}$ variable is a measure of variability *between* the a treatment groups. The SS_{ERROR} is a measure of variability *within* each treatment group.

Intuitively, if the H_0 hypothesis is correct, each $SS_{TREATMENT}$ and SS_{ERROR} component will provide a measure of "random" variability, or error, and they will, therefore, be equivalent when adjusted (divided) by their respective degrees of freedom.

$$\frac{SS_{TREATMENT}}{df} = \frac{SS_{ERROR}}{df}$$

or

$$\frac{SS_{TREATMENT}/df}{SS_{ERROR}/df} \approx 1$$

When $SS_{TREATMENT}$ is significant, it can be decomposed into a measure of both random error and the treatment effect, A. The SS_{ERROR} is composed only of error and cannot be further subdivided.

$$SS_{TREATMENT} = error + treatment\ effect\ A$$

$$SS_{ERROR} = error$$

Recall in Chap. 4 that the sum of square values was divided by the degrees of freedom; similarly:

SS_{TOTAL} has $N-1$ degrees of freedom
$SS_{TREATMENT}$ has $a-1$ degrees of freedom
SS_{ERROR} has $(N-a)$ degrees of freedom

Let us look at the error term more closely.

$$SS_E = \sum_{i=1}^{a} \sum_{j=1}^{n}(y_{ij} - \bar{y}_{i.})^2 = \sum_{i=1}^{a}\left[\sum_{v=1}^{n}(y_{ij} - \bar{y}_{i.})^2\right] \tag{5}$$

If the bracketed term is divided by $N-a$, it is of the form of sample variance described in Chap. 4, where $n-1$ is the denominator or degrees of freedom.

$$S_i^2 = \frac{\sum_{i=1}^{n}(y_{ij} - \bar{y}_{i.})^2}{n-1} \quad \text{where } i = 1, 2, \ldots, a \text{ and } j = 1, 2, \ldots, n. \tag{6}$$

In this ANOVA model, the a sample variances (number of treatments) are combined to give a single estimate of s^2, which has the form:

$$\frac{(n-1)S_i^2+(n-1)S_2^2+(n-1)S_3^2+\cdots+(n-1)S_a^2}{(n-1)+(n-1)+(n-1)+\cdots+(n-1)} = \frac{\sum_{i=1}^{a}\left[\sum_{j=1}^{n}(y_{ij}-\bar{y}_{i.})^2\right]}{\sum_{i=1}^{a}(n-1)} \tag{7}$$

$MS_{ERROR} = \frac{SS_E}{N-a} =$ the mean square error (MSE), the estimate of the common variance (σ^2) within each of the a treatments. It is the variability due to random error.

Also, if one computes the differences between the a treatment means and there is no treatment effect, the mean square treatment, $MS_{TREATMENT}$, is also an estimator of the common variance, MSE. The variability between those a means can be measured. The equation is:

$$MS_{TREATMENT} = \frac{n \sum_{i=1}^{a}(\bar{y}_{i.} - \bar{y}_{..})^2}{a-1} = \frac{SS_{TREATMENTS}}{a-1}$$

$$= \text{variability due to treatments}$$

When the treatment effect $= 0$, $MS_{TREATMENT} = MSE$.

When a significant treatment effect is noted, $MS_{TREATMENT} > MSE$, and when no significant treatment effect is noted, $MS_{TREATMENT} \approx MSE$. More formally, the expected values are:

$$E(MS_{TREATMENT}) = \underbrace{[\sigma^2]}_{\text{[Error term]}} + \underbrace{\frac{n \sum_{i=1}^{n} A_i^2}{a-1}}_{\text{[Treatment term]}} \qquad (8)$$

$$E(MS_{ERROR}) = \underbrace{\sigma^2}_{\text{[Error term]}} \qquad (9)$$

A most important aspect of the one-factor ANOVA is the complete randomization of the order of samples collected both within and between treatments. That is, each observation $(y_{11}, y_{12}, \ldots, y_{33})$ is as likely to be collected at this sample time as any of the other observations (Table 2). Let us take the example of a three-treatment, three-replicate model.

Using a random number generator, or nine pieces of paper, each representing one and only one y_{ij} sample randomly drawn from a box, suppose a researcher drew y_{22} for draw 1, y_{31} for draw 2, ... etc. (Table 3). The order of the runs in the experiment, then, is y_{21} first, y_{31} second, ... and y_{13} ninth. This ordering is important, for it defines why a completely randomized one-factor ANOVA is termed "completely randomized."

TABLE 2 Three-Treatment, Three-Replicate Model

| | Replicates | | |
Treatments	1	2	3
1	y_{11}	y_{12}	y_{13}
2	y_{21}	y_{22}	y_{23}
3	y_{31}	y_{32}	y_{33}

TABLE 3   Random Number Generator Results

Experimental Run Order	Observation
1	y_{22}
2	y_{31}
3	y_{12}
4	y_{32}
5	y_{11}
6	y_{23}
7	y_{33}
8	y_{21}
9	y_{13}

In performing a one-factor, completely randomized statistical design, an analysis of variance table must be constructed (Table 4).

Computing formulae for the sum of square are provided below:

$$SS_{TOTAL} = \sum_{i=1}^{a} \sum_{j=1}^{n} y_{ij}^2 - \frac{y_{..}^2}{N}$$

$$SS_{TREATMENTS} = \frac{1}{n} \sum_{i=1}^{a} y_{i.}^2 - \frac{y_{..}^2}{N},$$

SS_{ERROR} is determined by subtraction:

$$SS_{ERROR} = SS_{TOTAL} - SS_{TREATMENTS}$$

TABLE 4   ANOVA Table for One-Factor, Completely Randomized Design, Fixed Effects

Source of variation	Sum of squares	Degrees of freedom	Mean square	$F_{CALCULATED}$
Treatment effect (between treatments)	$SS_{TREATMENTS}$	$a-1$	$\frac{SS_{TREATMENT}}{a-1} = MS_{TREATMENT}$	$F_c = \frac{MS_{TREATMENT}}{MS_{ERROR}}$
Random error (within treatments)	SS_{ERROR}	$N-a$	$\frac{SS_{ERROR}}{N-a} = MS_{ERROR}$	
Total	SS_{TOTAL}	$N-1$		

In order to determine whether at least one of the treatment means differs significantly from any other treatment mean, we will compute the test or F_c ratio:

$$F_c = \frac{SS_{TREATMENT}/(a-1)}{SS_{ERROR}/(N-a)}$$

$$= \frac{MS_{TREATMENT}}{MS_{ERROR}} \text{ with } a-1; N-a \text{ degrees of freedom} \qquad (10)$$

So, if $F_C > F_{tabled, (\alpha, a-1; N-a)}$, reject the H_0 hypothesis $\qquad (11)$

Let us now, using the six-step procedure, put all of this together in an example.

Cell culture media are produced by four different manufacturers and used to grow fibroblast tumor cells. Now a researcher wants to determine whether they differ in supporting tissue culture growth quality, which is measured as nitrogen content. Five replicates are to be performed using each of the four different media source samples. The following results were collected in terms of protein nitrogen, a cell culture metabolic by-product. The runs of each observation were completely randomized (Table 5).

Step 1.   Formulate the hypothesis:
H_0: $\mu_1 = \mu_2 = \mu_3 = \mu_4$ (the suppliers provide equivalent media to support cell culture growth)
H_A: The μ_i value differs in at least one medium. (Notice that this is a two-tail test, as are all ANOVA problems.)

Step 2.   If one were performing a pivotal study, one would want to calculate the minimum sample size required in each treatment to detect a specific difference between means (microliters of nitrogen) at set, acceptable β and α error levels. Because this is but a small pilot study, this will not be done. We will set the sample size as $n = 5$ for each group and the significance level, $\alpha = 0.05$.

TABLE 5   Completely Randomized Observations of Four Different Media

	Replicates					Totals	Averages
Suppliers	1	2	3	4	5	y_i	$\bar{y}_i$
1	100	100	99	101	100	500	100.00
2	101	104	98	105	102	510	102.00
3	107	103	105	105	106	526	105.20
4	100	96	99	100	99	494	98.80
						$y.. = 2030$	$\bar{y}.. = 101.50$

Step 3. Choose the appropriate statistic. We will choose a one-factor, completely randomized design.

Step 4. Formulate the decision rule.

The degrees of freedom for the $F_{T(\alpha, a-1; N-a)}$ is $a - 1$ for treatment effect (numerator), $N - a$ for random error (denominator).

$n =$ sample size $= 5$

$N = a \times n = 4 \times 5 = 20$

$a - 1 = 4 - 1 = 3$

$N - a = 20 - 4 = 16$

In the F table (Table A.3) at $\alpha = 0.05$, find the numerator value of $a - 1 = 3$ and the denominator value of $N - a = 16$, and read their corresponding value, which is 3.24. So if F_c (calculated) is greater than 3.24 ($F_C > F_T$), reject the H_0 hypothesis at $\alpha = 0.05$; at least one of the supplier's formulas differs in cell culture growth abilities.

Step 5. Conduct the experiment. Then EDA is performed on the collected data to assure that one-factor ANOVA is appropriate. Basically, this is to assure the data are normally distributed and the error is random. We will discuss this in more detail at the end of the chapter. If the data are not, perhaps a nonparametric analysis, such as the Kruskal–Wallis, should be used. If the data are okay, the computations are performed.

$$SS_{TOTAL} = \sum_{i=1}^{4} \sum_{j=1}^{5} y_{ij}^2 - \frac{y_{..}^2}{N}$$

$$= 100^2 + 101^2 + 107^2 + \cdots + 102^2 + 106^2 + 99^2 - \frac{(2030)^2}{20}$$

$$= 206,214 - 206,045 = 169.00 \tag{12}$$

$$SS_{TREATMENT} = \left(\frac{1}{n} \sum_{i=1}^{4} y_{i.}^2\right) - \frac{y_{..}^2}{N}$$

$$= \frac{1}{5}(500^2 + 510^2 + 526^2 + 494^2) - \frac{(2030)^2}{20}$$

$$= 206,162.40 - 206,045 = 117.40 \tag{13}$$

SS_{ERROR} is determined by subtraction:

$$SS_{ERROR} = SS_{TOTAL} - SS_{TREATMENT}$$
$$= 169.00 - 117.40 = 51.60 \qquad (14)$$

$$\text{Mean square (treatment)} = \frac{SS_{TREATMENT}}{a-1} = \frac{117.40}{3} = 39.133$$

$$\text{Mean square (error)} = \frac{SS_{ERROR}}{N-a} = \frac{51.60}{16} = 3.225$$

$$F_{CALCULATED} = \frac{MS_{TREATMENT}}{MS_{ERROR}} = \frac{39.133}{3.225} = 12.134$$

Next, the appropriate values are placed in the ANOVA Table 6, using the format presented in Table 4.

Step 6. Because $F_{calculated}$ (12.134) > F_{tabled} (3.24), reject the H_0 hypothesis at $\alpha = 0.05$.

Performing the same computation via MiniTab software provides Table 7. In this MiniTab example, "FACTOR" represents treatments, the cell growth media, and P value = probability value, which is $P(F_C \geq 12.13\ H_0$ true) = 0. That is, the probability of computing an F_C value of 12.13 or larger, given that the null hypothesis is true, is about zero.

The one-factor ANOVA model is a robust statistic, reliable even when there is considerable heterogeneity of variances, as long as the sample sizes (n) of the individual treatments are equal or close to equal [9]. The assumption that the individual a_i sample sets come from normal populations with equivalent variances has been evaluated using, for example, Bartlett's test for homogeneity. However, that test has been argued to be inefficient in this capacity, as well as being adversely affected by nonnormal sample sets [19, 21, 26].

However, if the n_i are quite different in size, the probability of α (type I) error can differ significantly from the stated α level. If larger variances are associated with the larger sample sizes in each treatment group, the

TABLE 6   ANOVA of Table 5

Source of variation	Sum of squares	Degrees of freedom	Mean square	F calculated
Treatment effect	117.40	3	39.133	12.134
Random error effect	51.60	16	3.225	
Total	169.00	19		

TABLE 7   MiniTab Output

Analysis of variance

Source	DF	SS	MS	F	P
Factor	3	117.40	39.13	12.13	0.000
Error	16	51.60	3.23		
Total	19	169.00			

probability of α will be less than the stated α value, and if associated with smaller samples, the probability will be greater than the stated α. The validity of the ANOVA is affected only slightly by considerable deviations from normality as n increases.

E. The Unbalanced Design

When the sample sizes n are not equal, the design is said to be unbalanced. The one-factor, completely randomized design may still be used, but its calculation requires a slight modification.

The computations of SS_{TOTAL} and $SS_{TREATMENT}$ change.

$$SS_{TOTAL} = \sum_{i=1}^{a} \sum_{j=1}^{n_i} y_{ij}^2 - \frac{y_{..}^2}{N}$$

$$SS_{TREATMENT} = \sum_{i=1}^{a} \frac{y_{i.}^2}{n_i} - \frac{y_{..}^2}{N}$$

where $N = \sum_{i=1}^{a} n_i$

$$SS_{TOTAL} = SS_{TREATMENT} - SS_{ERROR}$$

Everything else is the same, degrees of freedom, ANOVA table, etc.

F. Parameter Estimation

Recall that for the one-factor, completely randomized design, the linear model was presented in Eq. (1)

$$y_{ij} = \mu + A_i + \epsilon_{ij}$$

where μ, the common population mean, is estimated by $\bar{y}_{..}$ *, and the treatment effect, A_i, by:

$$A_i = \bar{y}_{i.} - \bar{y}_{..} \quad \text{for treatments 1 through } a \tag{15}$$

---

*Technically, these are one set of an infinite number of solutions. Neither μ nor A_i are estimable by themselves (i.e., they must be combined—$\mu + A_i$).

A confidence interval for each of the ith treatment means ($\hat{\mu} = \mu + A_i$) can be determined by an equation similar to that which we used in the last chapter for determining the confidence interval for $\hat{\mu}$, which was $\bar{x} \pm t_{\alpha/2,df}, s\sqrt{n}$. For the ANOVA model, however, σ^2 is estimated by MSE, with the error being normally and independently distributed with a mean of μ and variance of σ^2/n. That is, the error terms of each $y_{i.}$ are NID $(\mu_i, \sigma^2/n)$.

The $100(1 - \alpha)$ confidence interval of the ith treatment group is computed as:

$$\hat{\mu}_i = \bar{y}_{i.} \pm t_{(\alpha/2,N-a)}\sqrt{\frac{\text{MSE}}{n}} \tag{16}$$

The $100(1 - \alpha)$ confidence interval for the difference between any two treatment means is $\mu_i - \mu_j$, or

$$\hat{\mu}_i - \hat{\mu}_j = \bar{y}_i - \bar{y}_j \pm t_{(\alpha/2,N-a)}\sqrt{\frac{2\text{MSE}}{n}} \tag{17}$$

Let us calculate Eqs. (16) and (17). Recall that

$$\begin{aligned}
&\bar{y}_{..} = 101.5 && \text{MSE} = 3.225 \\
&\bar{y}_{1.} = 100 && N - a = 20 - 4 = 16 \\
&\bar{y}_{2.} = 102 && \alpha = 0.05 \\
&\bar{y}_{3.} = 105.2 && t_{0.05/2,16} = 2.12 \\
&\bar{y}_{4.} = 98.80
\end{aligned} \tag{18}$$

$$\hat{\mu}_1 = \bar{y}_{1.} \pm 2.12\sqrt{\frac{3.225}{5}}$$

$$= 100 \pm 2.12\sqrt{\frac{3.225}{5}} = 100 \pm 1.703$$

$$= 98.297 \le \hat{\mu}_1 \le 101.703$$

$$\hat{\mu}_2 = \bar{y}_{2.} \pm 2.12\sqrt{\frac{3.225}{5}}$$

$$= 102 \pm 2.12\sqrt{\frac{3.225}{5}}$$

$$= 102 \pm 1.703$$

$$= 100.297 \le \hat{\mu}_2 \le 103.703$$

$$\hat{\mu}_3 = \bar{y}_{3.} \pm 2.12\sqrt{\frac{3.225}{5}}$$

$$= 105.2 \pm 2.12\sqrt{\frac{3.225}{5}}$$

$$= 105.2 \pm 1.703$$

$$= 103.497 \leq \hat{\mu}_3 \leq 106.903$$

$$\hat{\mu}_4 = \bar{y}_{4.} \pm 2.12\sqrt{\frac{3.225}{5}}$$

$$= 98.8 \pm 2.12\sqrt{\frac{3.225}{5}}$$

$$= 98.8 \pm 1.703$$

$$= 97.097 \leq \hat{\mu}_4 \leq 100.503$$

Let us now find the $100(1 - \alpha)$ confidence interval for the difference between $\hat{\mu}_3$ and $\hat{\mu}_4$, or $\hat{\mu}_3 - \hat{\mu}_4$.

$$\hat{\mu}_3 - \hat{\mu}_4 = \bar{y}_{3.} - \bar{y}_{4.} \pm t_{(\alpha/2, N-a)}\sqrt{\frac{2MSE}{n}} \tag{19}$$

$$= 105.2 - 98.8 \pm 2.12\sqrt{\frac{2(3.225)}{5}}$$

$$= 6.400 \pm 2.408 = 3.992 \leq \hat{\mu}_3 - \hat{\mu}_4 \leq 8.808$$

Note: Recall that, when means ($\hat{\mu}_i$) are subtracted, the standard deviations (σ_i^2) are summed.

So the 95% confidence interval for $\hat{\mu}_3 - \hat{\mu}_4$ is 3.992 to 8.808. Notice that, because 0 is not included in the 95% confidence interval, there is a significant difference between μ_3 and μ_4 at $\alpha = 0.05$.*

G. Computer Output

Using a software package (MiniTab in this case), the 95% confidence interval output of the four treatments is reproduced in Table 8.

Note that the 95% confidence intervals are determined as they were in Chap. 4, without pooling them. However, the pooled standard deviation,

---

*A $100(1 - \alpha)$ confidence interval can also be constructed for the individual treatments, A_i, using Eq. (15) ($T_i = \bar{y}_{i.} - \bar{y}_{..}$) and the variance estimation about the mean using the formula:
$A_i = \bar{y}_{i.} - \bar{y}_{..} \pm t_{(\alpha/2, N-a)}\sqrt{\frac{MSE}{n}}$

TABLE 8   95% Confidence Intervals for the Four Treatments

LEVEL	N	MEAN	STDEV	INDIVIDUAL 95 PCT CI'S FOR MEAN BASED ON POOLED STDEV
				--------+----------+----------+----------
c1	5	100.00	0.71	(-----*-----)
c2	5	102.00	2.74	(-----*-----)
c3	5	105.20	1.48	(-----*-----)
c4	5	98.80	1.64	(-----*-----)
				--------+----------+----------+----------
POOLED STDEV =		1.80		99.0 102.0 105.0

1.80, is $\sqrt{MSE}$. The confidence intervals for the entire ANOVA model, as performed for the data in Table 5, can be computed as $\hat{\mu}_1 \pm t_{(\alpha/2, N-a)} 1.80/\sqrt{n}$.

We have learned to obtain individual confidence levels for the $\hat{\mu}_i$, as well as the difference between $\hat{\mu}_i$ and $\hat{\mu}_j$. But the researcher runs into the same problem discussed in Chap. 4—when multiple contrasts are performed, the level of the actual α increases in size. So, to compare treatment means, once we have detected a significant F value, we must use a different approach, that of contrasts.*

H. Orthogonal Contrasts (Determined Prior to Experiment)

Orthogonal contrasts can be determined by the investigator if the specific contrasts—the treatment means to be compared—are selected *prior* to conducting the experiment and, therefore, before knowing its outcome. This requires some background of the data to be really useful.

In addition, only $a - 1$ contrasts can be performed. For example, using data from Table 5, suppose the researcher, before running the experiment, chose these $a - 1$ ($= 4 - 1 = 3$) contrasts:

$$\begin{array}{ll} C_i = \text{Contrast} & \text{Hypothesis} \\ C_1 = \bar{y}_{1.} - \bar{y}_{4.} = 0 & \mu_1 = \mu_4 \\ C_2 = \bar{y}_{2.} - \bar{y}_{3.} = 0 & \mu_2 = \mu_3 \\ C_3 = \bar{y}_{1.} - \bar{y}_{2.} - \bar{y}_{3.} + \bar{y}_{4.} = 0 & \mu_1 + \mu_4 = \mu_2 + \mu_3 \end{array} \quad (20)$$

In other words, the researcher has chosen to compare the mean of treatment 1 ($\bar{y}_{1.}$) with the mean of treatment ($\bar{y}_{4.}$) and the mean of treatment 2 ($\bar{y}_{2.}$) with the mean of treatment 3 ($\bar{y}_{3.}$), as well as both the means of treatments 1 and 4 ($\bar{y}_{1.}, \bar{y}_{4.}$) with both the means of treatments 2 and 3 ($\bar{y}_{2.}, \bar{y}_{3.}$).

---

*If a significant F value has not been computed, there is no need to perform contrasts because $\mu_1 = \mu_2 = \cdots \mu_a$. The compared sample means are all equal.

Orthogonal contrasts are independent contrasts in that one contrast is not affected by another. "Orthogonal" is an algebraic term; two straight lines are said to be orthogonal if they are perpendicular to one another. Lines that are perpendicular to one another have negative reciprocal slopes (Fig. 2). Recall that a slope is rise/run $= \Delta y / \Delta x = (y_2 - y_1)/(x_2 - x_1)$. If line a has a slope of $3/1$, then a line perpendicular to it, b, has a slope of $-1/(3/1)$, or $-1/3$.

Contrasts require a linear combination that will utilize coefficients, c_i, as well as the treatments means $\bar{y}_i$. When the sample sizes are equal, the contrasts are orthogonal if they equal zero. Each contrast has one degree of freedom. The sum of the contrasts is:

$$\sum_{i=1}^{a} c_i = 0 \tag{21}$$

The linear combination is of the form:

$$c_n = \sum_{i=1}^{a} c_i y_i. \tag{22}$$

where c_n cannot $> a - 1$. So, at most, there can be only three contrasts in our previous example because there were four treatments. There can be no more contrasts than the degrees of freedom $(a - 1)$ for the treatment term.

Let us return to our conjectural contrasts based on data from Table 5. We can perform $a - 1 = 4 - 1 = 3$ contrasts. The actual contrast calculations are performed on the y_i (the sum of the values in each treatment, *not* the $\bar{y}_i$ treatment mean (Table 9). Let us first construct a table of orthogonal coefficients (Table 10). Remember, this orthogonal contrast computation requires equal replicate sample sizes or that $n_1 = n_2 = \cdots n_a$.

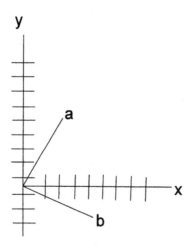

FIGURE 2   Perpendicular lines have negative reciprocal slopes.

TABLE 9   The Sum of the Values
in Each Treatment

$$C_1^* = Y_1 - Y_4$$
$$C_2 = Y_2 - Y_3$$
$$C_3 = Y_1 - Y_2 - Y_3 + y_4$$

*C_i=Contrast.

Step 1.   Make orthogonal coefficient table.

Recall that $y_1 = 500, y_2 = 510, y_3 = 526$, and $y_4 = 494$ (from Table 5).

Step 2.   Apply the equation $\sum_{i=1}^{a} c_i y_i$ to each contrast, based on Table 10:

$$c_1 = +1(500) + 0(510) + 0(526) - 1(494) = 6.00$$
$$c_2 = +0(500) + 1(510) - 1(526) + 0(494) = -16.00$$
$$c_3 = +1(500) - 1(510) - 1(526) + 1(494) = 42.00$$

Step 3.   The sum of squares, balanced design, for each contrast is calculated:

$$SS_c = \frac{\left(\sum_{i=1}^{a} c_i y_i\right)^2}{n \sum_{i=1}^{a} c_i^2} \tag{23}$$

$$SS_{c_1} = \frac{(6.00)^2}{5[1^2 + 0^2 + 0^2 + (-1)^2]} = \frac{36}{10} = 3.60$$

$$SS_{c_2} = \frac{(-16.00)^2}{5[0^2 + 1^2 + (-1)^2 + 0^2]} = \frac{256}{10} = 25.60$$

$$SS_{c_3} = \frac{(-42.00)^2}{5[1^2 + (-1)^2 + (-1)^2 + 1^2]} = \frac{1764}{20} = 88.20$$

Note that the sum of the three sum of squares contrasts (3.60 + 25.60 + 88.20) equals 117.40, which equals SS$_{TREATMENT}$. Each contrast has 1 degree

TABLE 10   Table of Orthogonal Coefficients

	y_1	y_2	y_3	y_4	$\sum_{i=1}^{a} c_i$
C_1^*	+1	0	0	-1	0
C_2	0	+1	-1	0	0
C_3	+1	-1	-1	+1	0

*C_i = Contrast

of freedom, and its mean square value is compared with (divided by) the mean square error term to generate F_C values in an expanded ANOVA table (Table 11).

Clearly, the researcher sees that at $\alpha = 0.05$, the treatment effects are different:

$\mu_1 = \mu_4$ The null hypothesis cannot be rejeted at $\alpha = 0.05$.

$\mu_2 \neq \mu_3$ The null hyposthesis is rejected at $\alpha = 0.05$.

$\mu_1 + \mu_4 \neq \mu_2 + \mu_3$ The null hypothesis is rejected at $\alpha = 0.05$

I. Unbalanced Designs

An unbalanced design is one that accommodates unequal sample sizes in the treatment groups. Orthogonal contrasts can still be made. Recall that Eq. (24) for the sum of squares for each balanced contrast was:

$$SS_c = \frac{\left(\sum_{i=1}^{a} c_i y_i.\right)^2}{n \sum_{i=1}^{a} c_i^2}$$

For the unbalanced design, everything is the same throughout, except that the equation is modified at the denominator.

Instead of $n \sum_{i=1}^{a} c_i^2$, the denominator becomes $\sum_{i=1}^{a} n_i c_i^2$. The entire equation is:

TABLE 11   ANOVA with Orthogonal Contrasts, Expansion of Table 5

Source of variance	Sum of squares	Degrees of freedom	Mean square	$F_{calculated}$	F_{tabled}[a]	Significant(S) or Not Significant (NS)
Treatment effect orthogonal contrasts	117.4	3	39.133	12.134	3.24	S
$C_1: \mu_1 = \mu_4$	3.60	1	3.60	1.116	3.24	NS
$C_2: \mu_2 = \mu_3$	25.60	1	25.60	7.938	3.24	S
$C_3: \mu_1 + \mu_4 = \mu_2 + \mu_3$	88.20	1	88.20	27.349	3.24	S
Random error	51.60	16	3.225			
Total	169.00	19				

[a] $F_{tabled} = F_{0.05, 3, 16} = 3.24$.

$$SS_c = \frac{\left(\sum_{i=1}^{a} c_i y_{i\cdot}\right)^2}{\sum_{i=1}^{a} n_i c_i^2} \tag{24}$$

which is merely an adjustment to correct for the unequal sizes of n_i. Note that

$$\sum_{i=1}^{a} n_i c_i^2 = n_1 c_1^2 + n_2 c_2^2 + \cdots + n_a c_a^2$$

II. POWER (ϕ) OF THE ONE-FACTOR ANALYSIS PRIOR TO CONDUCTING THE TEST

In Chap. 4, we learned how to compute the power for two-sample t-tests. Recall that the power of a statistic $(1 - \beta)$ is its ability to detect a true alternative hypothesis—that is, accept a true H_A hypothesis when it is true. The power of a one-factor, completely randomized ANOVA before the study is conducted the equation to employ is:

$$\phi_c = \sqrt{\frac{n \sum_{i=1}^{a} (\mu_i - \mu)^2}{a s^2}} \tag{25}$$

ϕ_c = Phi-calculated, used to find power in Table A.4.

where n = the replicate sample size

s^2 = the variance, estimated by MSE

a = the number of treatment groups to be tested

μ = the overall average population "common" value (estimated by $\bar{y}..$)

μ_i = the population average for each treatment group (estimated by $\bar{y}_{i\cdot}$)

Note that

$$\mu = \frac{\sum_{i=1}^{a} \mu_i}{a} = \frac{\sum_{i=1}^{a} \bar{y}_{i\cdot}}{a} = \bar{y}..$$

To find the tabled value of the power of the statistic, ϕ_T, go to Table A.4 (power tables) and find ϕ_c at $v_1 = a - 1$, $v_2 = a(n - 1)$, and α. This will make it possible to determine the power of the statistic $(1 - \beta)$ when conducted with a specific sample size n.

Let us calculate the power of the statistic for the data in Table 5.

a = number of group = 4
n = replicates per group = 5
s^2 = estimate of σ^2 = MSE = 3.225
$\alpha = 0.05$
v_1 = df = $a - 1 = 3$
v_2 = df = $a(n - 1) = 4(4) = 16$

$$\phi_C = \sqrt{\frac{n\sum_{i=1}^{a}(\mu_i - \mu)^2}{as^2}} = \sqrt{\frac{n\sum_{i=1}^{a}(\bar{y}_{i\cdot} - \bar{y}_{\cdot\cdot})^2}{a(MSE)}}$$

$$\mu = \bar{y}_{\cdot\cdot} = \frac{\sum_{i=1}^{a}\bar{y}_{i\cdot}}{n} = \frac{100 + 102 + 105.20 + 98.80}{4} = 101.50$$

$$\phi_C = \sqrt{\frac{5[(100-101.5)^2+(102-101.5)^2+(105.2-101.5)^2+(99.8-101.5)^2]}{4(3.225)}}$$

$$\phi_C = \sqrt{7.39} = 2.72$$

Notice that when $v_1 = 3$, $v_2 = 16$, $\alpha = 0.05$, and MSE = 3.225, $\phi_c = 2.72$ and 6 the tabled power value is (Table A.4.3), $1 - \beta$, is > 0.99, so clearly "an n of 5" with an anticipated ϕ_c of 2.72 is sufficient.

An alternative and very common way to determine power is to specify a desired detection level difference, δ. Unlike the previous equation, this equation gives the power of the statistic at a specific detection level.

$$\phi_C = \sqrt{\frac{n\delta^2}{2as^2}} \tag{26}$$

where δ = minimum detectable difference (i.e., the minimum difference between mesh values a researcher wants to be able to detect), say 5 nitrogen points

a = number of groups = 4
n = replicates = 5
s^2 = estimate of σ^2 = MSE = 3.225
$\alpha = 0.05$
v_1 = df = $a - 1 = 4 - 1 = 3$
v_2 = df = $a(n - 1) = 4(4) = 16$

Again, using the data from Table 5:

$$\phi_C = \sqrt{\frac{5(5^2)}{2(4)3.225}} = 2.201$$

From Table A.4.3, with $v_1 = 3$, $v_2 = 16$, $\alpha = 0.05$, and $\phi_C = 2.201$, we find the power value $(1 - \beta) \approx 0.93$, which is very good for β error detection.

Note that when a small detectable difference is desired, the power of the statistic generally drops, often dramatically. The power of the statistic, $1 - \beta$, is 0.93, which means there is a $1 - 0.93 = 0.07$, or 7% chance of committing a type II error (stating that a significant difference does not exist when one does) at a detectable difference of 5 points.

Note, however, that the previous two power estimates are, in practice, conducted before a test is conducted. Hence, one could not use a computed σ^2 value because it would be unknown. The value of σ^2, however, often can be estimated from previous experimental knowledge.

Once the experimental part of completely randomized ANOVA *has been conducted*, a different power calculation equation should be used. It is wise to determine the power of the statistic at this time, particularly if H_0 has not been rejected.

The formula for finding the power of the one-factor ANOVA is:

$$\phi_C = \sqrt{\frac{(a - 1)MS_{TREATMENT} - MS_{ERROR}}{a(MSE)}} \tag{27}$$

Using data from Table 5:

$a = 4$
$MS_{TREATMENT} = 39.133$
$MS_{ERROR} = 3.225$
$v_1 = a - 1 = 3$
$v_2 = a(n - 1) = 4(5 - 1) = 16$
$\alpha = 0.05$

$$\phi_C = \sqrt{\frac{3(39.113 - 3.225)}{4(3.225)}} = 2.889$$

From Table A.4.3, we see that, where $\alpha = 0.05$, $v_1 = 3$, $v_2 = 16$, and $\phi_C = 2.889$, the power, $(1 - \beta)$, is $\sim >0.99$, meaning there is less than 1 chance in 100 of committing a type II error.

A. Sample Size Requirement

Generally, a researcher determines the sample size required by setting the α and β levels and estimating σ^2. As with the two-sample t-tests, the sample size estimate is performed by iteration.

In sample size determination, the same formula used for the power of the statistical test "prior" to conducting it can be used [Eq. (26)]. Simply stated, one performs iterations until ϕ_c corresponds to the desired $1-\beta$ value.

Again using data from Table 5, let's assume we do not know how many replicates to use. Recall σ^2, or MSE $= 3.225$, which ordinarily would not be known, but we will use it anyway. Also, $v_1 = a - 1 = 3$, $\alpha = 0.05$, $\delta = $ minimum detectable difference between group means, which we will set at 3 points, and let us set $\beta = 0.20$.

Let us begin with a sample size of 3 ($n = 3$) as our initial estimate. Hence, the v_2 value is $a(n-1) = 4(3-1) = 8$.

$$\phi_C = \sqrt{\frac{n\delta^2}{2as^2}} = \sqrt{\frac{3(3)^2}{2(4)(3.225)}} = 1.023$$

Using Table D3, where $v_1 = 3$, $v_2 = 8$, $\alpha = 0.05$, we find that with an $\phi_c = 1.023$, Table D is in Appendix the power $(1 - \beta)$ is ≈ 0.27, which makes $\beta = 0.73$, which is too large. We need to find the sample size where the power of the test, $1 - \beta$, is close to 0.80.

Next, the researcher increases the estimate of n to, say, $n = 4$. The parameters remain the same, except that the v_2 changes. $v_2 = a(n-1) = 4(4-1) = 12$.

$$\phi_C = \sqrt{\frac{4(3)^2}{2(4)(3.225)}} = 1.181$$

Consult Table D3 with $v_1 = 3$, $v_2 = 12$, $\alpha = 0.05$ and a ϕ_c of 1.181. The power $1 - \beta = 0.35$ and $\beta = 0.65$, which is still too large.

For the next iteration, the researcher selects $n = 6$.
$v_1 = 3$, $v_2 = a(n-1) = 4(6-1) = 20$, $\alpha = 0.05$.

$$\phi_C = \sqrt{\frac{6(3)^2}{2(4)(3.225)}} = 1.447$$

The ϕ_C value corresponds to $(1 - \beta)$, at about 0.63, making $\beta \approx 0.37$, which is still too large. The researcher next sets $n = 10$ and recomputes. $v_1 = 3$, $v_2 = a(n-1) = 4(10-1) = 36$, $\alpha = 0.05$.

$$\phi_C = \sqrt{\frac{10(3)^2}{2(4)(3.225)}} = 1.868$$

which provides a power $(1 - \beta)$ of ≈ 0.87 or a β of ≈ 0.13, which is smaller than needed. The researcher next decreases n to 9.

$$v_1 = 3, \quad v_2 = 4(9 - 1) = 32, \quad \alpha = 0.05.$$

$$\phi_C = \sqrt{\frac{9(3)^2}{2(4)(3.225)}} = 1.772$$

which provides a power $(1 - \beta)$ of ≈ 0.80 and a β of ≈ 0.20, which is the level desired.

Notice that in this example, the detectable difference (δ) value of 3 drove the sample size way up. If the researcher thinks this is too many replicates, she or he can, of course, adjust it by increasing α, β, and/or δ.

B. Minimum Detectable Differences Between Treatment Means (δ)

As with the two-sample t-tests, the researcher can specify α, β, and n and estimate s^2. The minimum detectable difference can then be determined. The researcher needs to only find ϕ_T from Table A.4 and plug it into the equation:

$$\delta = \sqrt{\frac{2as^2\phi_T^2}{n}} \tag{28}$$

In this example, let us again use the data from Table 5. $s^2 = MSE = 3.225$, $n = 5$, and $a = 4$, so $v_1 = a - 1 = 3$, $v_2 = a(n - 1) = 4(5 - 1) = 16$, $\alpha = 0.05$. $\beta = 0.20$, and $1 - \beta = 0.80$.

From Table D3, we find $\phi_T = 1.81$, which corresponds to $1 - \beta$ of 0.80, so

$$\delta = \sqrt{\frac{2(4)3.225(1.81)^2}{5}} = 4.112$$

Hence, the detectable difference is about 4.112 points.

C. Power of One-Factor, Completely Randomized (Random Effects) ANOVA

The power $(1 - \beta)$ for the random-effects model (which will be discussed in greater detail later) can be determined from:

$$F_{(1-\beta,v_1,v_2)} = \frac{v_2 S^2(F_{\alpha,v_1,v_2})}{(v_2 - 2)MS_{\text{TREATMENT}}} \tag{29}$$

We use the data from Table 5, which is technically wrong, because they are fixed-effect data, but we will use them to demonstrate the procedure.

$$MS_{\text{TREATMENT}} = 39.113$$

$$s^2 = MSE = 3.225$$
$$v_1 = a - 1 = 4 - 1 = 3$$
$$v_2 = a(n-1) = 4(5-1) = 16$$
$$F_{\alpha = 0.05, \, 3, \, 16} = 3.24 \text{ (from } F \text{ distribution Table A.3)}$$
$$F_{(1-\beta,v_1,v_2)} = \frac{16(3.225)(3.24)}{(16-2)(39.113)} = 0.305$$

The value, 0.305, in this calculation, provides a probability value of the power $1 - \beta$.

D. Orthogonal Contrasts—Discussion

Orthogonal contrasts are extremely useful in applied research, particularly in that the power of the contrast is greater, at any given α level, than any of the contrasts that are determined after the experimental runs have been completed. Many researchers penalize themselves by relying on "canned" software programs to provide contrasts, which can often be too conservative for the researcher's requirements. That is, they generally require that treatment effect differences between the treatment means be relatively large in order to be detected. This can be very problematic for the researcher limited, all too often, to low sample sizes and with significant variability in the data. To help avoid this situation, the researcher must do everything possible to reduce variability within the treatment groups themselves, use orthogonal contrasts whenever possible, and increase the α level from, say, 0.05 to 0.10 for preliminary studies aimed at detecting differences between treatments.

Finally, even when beneficial, but to maintain consistency in reports, the researcher will want to consider not using orthogonal contrasts when attempting to replicate an experiment in which the original researcher used a different treatment comparison procedure, such as Scheffe's test or the LSD test. However, it may be beneficial to run orthogonal contrasts in this situation to contrast the results.

E. Bonferroni Multiple Comparison Procedure

This procedure, like orthogonal contrasts, is very useful not only in pairwise comparisons but also in more complex contrasts, as long as they are stipulated *prior to* conducting the study. The Bonferroni method is also beneficial in that it is not limited, like orthogonal contrasts, to $a - 1$ comparisons. The Bonferroni multiple contrast procedure also is applicable for unequal, as well as equal, sample sizes and can be used for single or multiple confidence estimation.

The Bonferroni procedure uses confidence intervals to evaluate significance. In pairwise comparisons where, say, y_i and y_j are compared, if the α level confidence interval of $y_i - y_j$ includes 0, there is no significant difference between the treatments.

The following is the general form of the Bonferroni method:

$$L \pm BS(L) \tag{30}$$

where $L =$ linear combination

$B = t(\alpha/2(g) : N - a) =$ modification of the t tabled procedure
$S(L) = \text{MSE} \sum_{i=1}^{a} c_i^2/n_i$, which is the variability of the linear combination and $\sum c_i = 0$
$g =$ number of linear combination contrasts made.*

Let us use the data from Table 5 to demonstrate the Bonferroni method. This time we will let $\alpha = 0.01$, which is the α level for all four linear combinations to be evaluated. Recall that MSE $= 3.225, N = 20, a = 4,$ and $n_1 = n_2 = n_3 = n_4 = 5.$

Let us call

$L_1 = \bar{y}_1 - \bar{y}_2$ (linear combination 1), which compares group 1 and group 2

$L_2 = \bar{y}_3$ (linear combination 2), which will provide a $1 - \alpha$ confidence interval for group 3

$L_3 = \frac{\bar{y}_1 + \bar{y}_2}{2} - \frac{(\bar{y}_3 + \bar{y}_4)}{2}$ (linear combination 3), which compares groups 1 and 2 with groups 3 and 4

$L_4 = \bar{y}_3 - \frac{\bar{y}_1 + \bar{y}_2 + \bar{y}_4}{3}$ (linear combination 4), which compares group 3 with the average of groups 1, 2, and 4

---

*With the Bonferroni method, the α is portioned among the (g) contrasts; i.e., each contrast has α/g confidence.

Let's begin with determining $B = t_{\alpha/2(g); N-a}$, where $g = 4$ and $\alpha = \alpha/2(4) = 0.01/8 = 0.001$.

$$B = t_{(0.001; 20-4)} = t_{(0.001, 16)} = 3.686, \text{from the student's t Table A.2}$$

$$L_1 = \bar{y}_1. - \bar{y}_4. \pm BS(L)$$

$$L_1 = 100 - 98.80 \pm 3.686\sqrt{3.225\left(\frac{1^2}{5} + \frac{1^2}{5}\right)} = 1.20 \pm 4.187$$

$$L_1 = -2.987 \leq \mu_1 - \mu_2 \leq 5.387$$

Because zero is included in the 99% confidence interval, $\mu_1 - \mu_2 = 0$, we cannot conclude that a difference between μ_1 and μ_2 exists at $\alpha = 0.01$. But note that this is a simultaneous 99% CI for all contrasts considered.

$$L_2 = \bar{y}_3. \pm BS(L)$$

$$L_2 = 105.20 \pm 3.686\sqrt{\frac{3.225}{5}} = 105.20 \pm 2.960$$

$$L_2 = 102.240 \leq \mu_3. \leq 108.160$$

Note that the L_2 is merely a 99% simultaneous confidence interval for the treatment mean $(\bar{y}_3)$.

Turning our attention to a more complex linear combination, let us solve L_3. The process looks intimidating, but with patience, it will become clear.

$$L_3 = \frac{\bar{y}_1. + \bar{y}_2.}{2} + \frac{(\bar{y}_3. + \bar{y}_4.)}{2} \pm BS(L)$$

$$= \frac{100 + 102}{2} - \frac{105.2 + 98.8}{2}$$

$$\pm 3.686\sqrt{3.225\left(\frac{\left(\frac{1}{2}\right)^2}{5} + \frac{\left(\frac{1}{2}\right)^2}{5} + \frac{\left(-\frac{1}{2}\right)^2}{5} + \frac{\left(-\frac{1}{2}\right)^2}{5}\right)}$$

$$L_3 = -1 \pm 3.686\sqrt{3.225(0.2000)}$$

$$L_3 = -3.960 \leq \mu_1 + \mu_2 - (\mu_3 + \mu_4) \leq 1.960$$

Hence, because the contrast interval L_3 includes 0, we cannot conclude that $\mu_1 + \mu_2 - (\mu_3 + \mu_4)$ are significantly different pairs at $\alpha = 0.01$ for the simultaneous contrasts.

New for contrast L_4

$$L_4 = \bar{y}_{3.} - \frac{(\bar{y}_{1.} + \bar{y}_{2.} + \bar{y}_{4.})}{3}$$

$$L_4 = 105.20 - \frac{(100 + 102 + 98.8)}{3}$$

$$\pm 3.686 \sqrt{3.225 \left(\frac{1^2}{5} + \frac{\left(\frac{-1}{3}\right)^2}{5} + \frac{\left(\frac{-1}{3}\right)^2}{5} + \frac{\left(\frac{-1}{3}\right)^2}{5} \right)}$$

$$L_4 = 1.515 \le \mu_3 - \frac{\mu_1 + \mu_2 + \mu_4}{3} \le 8.351$$

Because zero is not included in the L_4 combination, μ_3 is significantly different from $(\mu_1 + \mu_2 + \mu_4/3)$ at $\alpha = 0.01$ for the simultaneous contrasts.

F. Multiple Test Comparisons via Critical Values

Multiple two-tail test comparisons can be made on the basis of critical values. The two-tail hypotheses are of the form:

$H_0: L = 0$

$H_A: L \ne 0$

Use the Student's t-test calculated values compared with the Student's t-test tabled value.

$t_c = t$ - test computed $= L/S(L)$

where

$$S(L) = \sqrt{MSE \sum_{i=1}^{a} \frac{c_i^2}{n_i}}, \quad \text{as before}$$

$t_t = t$-test tabled value $= t_{(\alpha/2g; N-a)}$
$g = $ number of comparisons made

If $|t_c| > t_{t(\alpha/2g, N-a)}$, conclude $H_A: L \ne 0$.

Again using the data from Table 5 and $\alpha = 0.01$, we will perform the same linear contrasts (L) as just performed, except that we will not compute L_2 because L_2 was only one parameter providing a confidence interval. Hence, $g = 3$, $\alpha/2(g) = 0.01/2(3) = 0.002$, and t at $\alpha = 0.002$, 16 df ≈ 3.469.

$H_0: \mu_1 = \mu_2$

$H_A: \mu_1 \neq \mu_2$

$L_1 = \bar{y}_{1.} - \bar{y}_{4.} = 100 - 98.8 = 1.2$

$t_c = \dfrac{1.2}{\sqrt{3.225(\frac{12}{5} + \frac{12}{5})}}$

$t_c = 1.06$

Because $t_c(1.06) \not> t_t(3.469)$, we cannot conclude $\bar{y}_{1.} \neq \bar{y}_{2.}$ at $\alpha = 0.01$. Hence, the null hypothesis cannot be rejected.

$L_3 = \dfrac{\bar{y}_{1.} + \bar{y}_{2.}}{2} - \dfrac{(\bar{y}_{3.} + \bar{y}_{4.})}{2}$

$L_3 = \dfrac{100 + 102}{2} - \dfrac{105.2 + 98.8}{2} = -1.000$

$t_c = \dfrac{-1.000}{\sqrt{3.225\left((\frac{1}{2})^2/5 + (\frac{1}{2})^2/5 + (-\frac{1}{2})^2/5 + (-\frac{1}{2})^2/5\right)}}$

$t_c = -1.245$

Because $t_c(|-1.245|) \not> t_t(3.469)$, one cannot reject H_0 at $\alpha = 0.01$.

In linear contrast 4 (L_4), we have:

$H_0: \mu_3 = \dfrac{\mu_1 + \mu_2 + \mu_4}{3}$

$H_A : \mu_3 \neq \dfrac{\mu_1 + \mu_2 + \mu_4}{3}$

$L_4 = 105.2 - \dfrac{(100 + 102 + 98.8)}{3} = 4.933$

$L_4 = \dfrac{4.933}{\sqrt{3.225\left(\frac{1}{5} + (-\frac{1}{3})^2/5 + (-\frac{1}{3})^2/5 + (-\frac{1}{3})^2/5\right)}}$

$L_4 = \dfrac{4.933}{0.927} = 5.319 = t_c$

Because $t_c |5.321| > t_t(3.469)$, reject H_0 at $\alpha = 0.01$.

As stated, the Bonferroni method of multiple contrasts is very useful as long as the linear combinations one wants to calculate are determined *prior to* conducting the test. The Bonferroni contrasts are simultaneous for all contrasts considered (at the α level). Using more contrasts lowers the power. In practice, because the Bonferroni procedure tends to be less powerful (more conservative) in rejecting H_0 than the orthogonal contrasts we previously viewed, it is perhaps more attractive when there is an overriding desire to prevent type I error. This will increase type II error, however, which can be problematic, particularly in pilot studies. Generally, however, the Bonferroni comparison tends to be more powerful than the other contrasts that can be performed after the data from a study have been analyzed. Note, however, that if all possible contrasts are to be computed, the Tukey method (to be discussed) provides more power. And when the contrasts performed are close in number to a, or fewer, the Bonferroni method is more powerful than the Scheffe method (also to be discussed).

Some authors [26] suggest that one compute using all of the methods—the Bonferroni, the Scheffe, and the Tukey—and choose the one that appears most advantageous. This, in my opinion, often leads in practice to massaging the data, trying to support a preexisting experimental bias. There must be criteria stronger than a tight confidence interval for selecting one procedure over another.

G. Holm Simultaneous Test Procedure

The Holm test procedure is a modification of the Bonferroni test procedure and can improve the power of the family of tests [26]. It, too, is applicable when pairwise comparisons of means or linear combinations, or a combination of these, are used. And, as in the Bonferroni procedure, the linear contrasts, comparisons, or the mixture of these must be determined prior to conducting the study.

The Holm procedure can be applied to equal or unequal sample sizes. As in the Bonferroni procedure, the researcher will set g as the number of contrasts to perform. This procedure, like the Bonferroni procedure, will evaluate g contrasts using the hypothesis form.

H_0: $L = 0$

H_A: $L \neq 0$, where L is a linear combination

Hypothesis testing for each contrast (as it would be, also, for the Bonferroni method) is of the form $L_i / S(L_i)$. Each of the contrasts (t_c), following the Bonferroni procedure, is compared with the t tabled value with $N - a$ degrees of freedom to find the P value.

The Holm procedure, relying on P values, becomes tricky when the P value is very small and the t-calculated value large because then the t-tabled values are not exact. In addition, the P values are tested using the formula $\alpha/(g - k + 1)$ for contrasting the $k + 1$ smallest P values.

If the P value calculated is $< \alpha/(g - k + 1)$, reject H_0. If the P value calculated is $\geq \alpha/(g - k + 1)$, one cannot reject H_0. The Holm procedure computes the test procedures, obtaining a P value for each. It then modifies the level that the P value is compared with in order to increase the power of the statistical procedure. By this process, the Holm procedure may be able to detect significant differences in compared values that cannot be determined using the Bonferroni procedure without increasing the sample sizes [26]. This can be of real value to the researcher performing pilot studies or any other study where one desires to detect differences in contrasts with relatively small sample sizes.

This author has used this procedure and Dunnett's test (to be described later) for comparing a control product with $a - 1$ other products. The advantage of the Holm procedure over Dunnett's is increased statistical power [26]. The disadvantage of having to set up contrasts prior to conducting the study is not really applicable in control versus test contrasts. If the researcher wishes to compare the control with the $a - 1$ other test conditions, these are known prior to conducting the study. Where problems can arise is in trying to determine differences between test groups *prior* to conducting the study. One does not want to increase g frivolously because each contrast increases the value of α of the test procedure (e.g., 0.05 to 0.10). In small pilot studies, this can be a real problem.

One way in which I have countered the problem is to keep the test products or treatments no greater than three, plus a control. Often, I find that two test products with one control is even better.

A disadvantage, however, is that confidence intervals cannot be determined using this method. Some authorities recommend using the Bonferroni confidence interval procedure when using the Holm simultaneous test procedure [26]. However, this can result in a nonsignificant confidence interval for a contrast deemed significant by the Holms procedure. Each researcher must work within the constraints given to him or her.

The Holm procedure first requires that the researcher conduct a series of two-tail P-value tests, which are then ranked in ascending order (lowest P value = number one rank, second lowest = second rank, ... highest P value = highest rank value). The lowest P value (rank 1) is then compared with the value $\alpha/(g-1+1)$ (where g = number of comparisons) to determine whether to accept or reject H_0. As with the Bonferroni method, if the H_0 hypothesis is rejected for the rank 1 P value, the researcher moves to the next rank (rank 2), which is compared with the value $\alpha/(g - 2 + 1)$. If H_0 is accepted, the testing procedure is stopped. If not, the researcher moves to rank 3 and compares that rank with the value $\alpha/(g - 3 + 1)$ and so on. Remember that, once the H_0 hypothesis is accepted, no further comparisons are made because any subsequent ones will not reject H_0. Like the Bonferroni procedure, this procedure, taken as a whole family of contrasts, will be equivalent to α. Hence, the more tests performed, the more likely one is to commit a type II error. That is because the more tests that are conducted, the greater the difference must be to reject H_0.

Using the data from Table 5 and letting α again equal 0.05, let us construct contrasts using the Holm procedure.

$$L_1 = \bar{y}_{1.} - \bar{y}_{2.}$$

$$L_2 = \frac{(\bar{y}_{1.} + \bar{y}_{2.})}{2} + \frac{(\bar{y}_{3.} + \bar{y}_{4.})}{2}$$

$$L_3 = \bar{y}_{3.} - \frac{(\bar{y}_{1.} - \bar{y}_{2.} + \bar{y}_{4.})}{3}$$

where $\alpha = 0.05$, $\bar{y}_{1.} = 100$, $\bar{y}_{2.} = 102$, $\bar{y}_{3.} = 105.20$, and $\bar{y}_{4.} = 98.80$.

Let us compute the mean differences first:

$$L_1 = 100 - 102 = -2$$

$$L_2 = \frac{100 + 102}{2} - \frac{105.2 + 98.8}{2} = -1$$

$$L_3 = 105.2 - \frac{100 + 102 + 98.8}{3} = 4.933$$

Let us next compute the standard deviations of the contrasts, $S(L_i)$:

$$S(L_i) = \sqrt{\text{MSE} \sum \frac{c_i^2}{n_i}}$$

$$S(L_1) = \sqrt{3.225\left(\frac{1^2}{5} + \frac{-1^2}{5}\right)} = 1.136$$

$$S(L_2) = \sqrt{3.225\left(\frac{\left(\frac{1}{2}\right)^2}{5} + \frac{\left(\frac{1}{2}\right)^2}{5} + \frac{\left(-\frac{1}{2}\right)^2}{5} + \frac{\left(-\frac{1}{2}\right)^2}{5}\right)} = 0.803$$

$$S(L_3) = \sqrt{3.225\left(\frac{1^2}{5} + \frac{\left(-\frac{1}{3}\right)^2}{5} + \frac{\left(-\frac{1}{3}\right)^2}{5} + \frac{\left(-\frac{1}{3}\right)^2}{5}\right)} = 0.927$$

$$t_{c1} = L_1/S(L_1) = -2/1.136 = -1.761$$
$$t_{c2} = L_2/S(L_2) = -1/0.803 = -1.245$$
$$t_{c3} = L_3/S(L_3) = 4.933/0.927 = 5.321$$

TABLE 12 Holm Contrast Table

Contrast t_i	L_i	$S(L_i)$	t calc	P val	Rank	Rank order	P value in rank order (A)	$\alpha/g - k+1$[a] (B)	Conclusion
1	-2	1.136	-1.761	0.08	2	1	0.0002	0.017	Because $A < B$, accept H_A
2	-1	0.803	-1.245	0.24	3	2	0.08	0.025	Because $A > B$, accept H_0
3	4.933	0.927	5.321	0.0002	1	3	0.24		H_0 stop—no more can be significant

[a]Computation for $\alpha/g - k+1$, where g = number of linear contrasts = 3
$k = 1$ (test 1) and $\alpha/(g - 1+1) = 0.05/(3 - 1+1) = 0.05/3 = 0.017$
$k = 2$ (test 2) and $\alpha/(g - 2+1) = 0.05/(3 - 2+1) = 0.05/2 = 0.025$

The next step is to find the P value * on Student's t distribution (Table B) for each of the t_c values computed, with $N - a$ degrees of freedom. We must also multiply this value by 2 because the tabled value has been divided by 2 in the fraction $\alpha/2$.

This procedure is summarized in Table 12.

As can be seen, the only significant contrast was the third, $\bar{y}_3. - \dfrac{(\bar{y}_1. + \bar{y}_2. + \bar{y}_4.)}{3}$. The readers are urged to work some problems comparing the Bonferroni method with the Holm procedure to gain knowledge of their comparative effects and choose on their own which to use.

The Holm procedure can be extremely useful and is recommended for situations in which more than $a - 1$ contrasts are to be used. (25,27).

III. DISCUSSION CONCERNING BOTH GENERAL ORTHOGONAL CONTRASTS AND THE BONFERRONI AND HOLM PROCEDURES

When comparing no more than $a - 1$ groups, I prefer the general orthogonal contrasts. These are relatively easy-to-use procedures that logically portion the treatment sum of squares in a way that is easy for any audience to understand, with respect to an ANOVA table.

When one must compare more than $a - 1$ contrasts, I prefer the Bonferroni and Holm methods to any of the orthogonal contrasts. I generally prefer the Holm contrast procedure over the Bonferroni in that it is more powerful. However, I strongly urge the reader to choose wisely what contrasts will be computed, for the power of the statistic drops relative to the number of contrasts. This is particularly noticeable for studies with small sample sizes—many industrial experiments—where, ironically, the main goal is to detect significant differences between groups. One may also consider, in preliminary studies with low sample sizes, increasing α to 0.10. If one is performing small-scale studies, however, to identify a treatment (or treatments) that is highly significantly different (better) from the control, one should use an α of at least 0.05 and a posterior test such as those to be described, particularly Dunnett's, that contrasts test versus control.

---

*The P value is the probability of calculating a t_c value at least as large as the one calculated, given the H_0 hypothesis is true.

p value$_1$ (where $t_{c1} = -1.761$, df $= 16$) $\approx 0.04 \times 2 = 0.08$

P value$_2$ (where $t_{c2} = -1.245$, df $= 16$) $\approx 0.12 \times 2 = 0.24$

P value$_3$ (where $t_{c3} = 5.321$, df $= 16$) $\approx 0.0001 \times 2 = 0.0002$

IV. COMPARISONS MADE AFTER EXPERIMENTS ARE CONDUCTED

In practice, particularly if the experiment is covering new territory, a researcher will not know which contrasts to perform prior to conducting the study. Fortunately, a variety of methods can be used to compare and contrast the treatments after experimentation is completed. Those that we will discuss include:

> Scheffe's method
> Newman–Keuls test
> LSD (least significant difference) test
> Tukey's test
> Dunnett's comparisons
> Duncan's new multiple range test

A. Scheffe's Method

In many situations, the experimenter will not know which contrast comparisons should be made prior to conducting the experiment. This is usually the case in exploratory experimentation. Or the experimenter may be interested in more than $a - 1$ contrasts, which cannot be handled using orthogonal contrasts.

The Sheffe method can be used to test multiples of two groups such as $\mu_1 - \mu_2 \neq 0$ for H_A. Unfortunately, this type of comparison is less sensitive (less power) than the Newman–Keuls or the Tukey test. Often, the Scheffe test is apt to commit a type II error (stating that $\mu_1 - \mu_2 = 0$ when actually $\mu_1 - \mu_2 \neq 0$). Because of this, Scheffe's test is not generally recommended for multiple two-group testing. It is better applied in multiple comparisons comparing, say, $(\mu_1+\mu_2+\mu_3)/3 - \mu_4 = 0$ or $\mu_1+\mu_2 - \mu_3 - \mu_4 \neq 0$.

Both two-sample contrasts and multiple contrasts having greater than two samples will be demonstrated here.

The general hypothesis is:

H_0: $\mu_i - \mu_j = 0^*$

H_A: $\mu_i - \mu_j \neq 0$

Suppose k contrasts in the treatment means are to be conducted for a treatments.

---

*This hypothesis can also be written as:
H_0: $\mu_i = \mu_j$
H_A: $\mu_i \neq \mu_j$

$$T_c = \text{treatment contrasts}$$

$$T_c = C_1\mu_1 + C_2\mu_2 + C_3\mu_3 + \cdots C_a\mu_a \quad \text{and} \quad \mu = \mu_1, \mu_2, \ldots \mu_k$$

(31)

The actual contrasts will be made, however, substituting $\bar{y}_{i.}$ for μ_i. The standard error of the contrast is:

$$S_{c_i} = \sqrt{MSE \sum_{i=1}^{a} \left(\frac{c_i^2}{n_i}\right)}$$

(32)

where n_i = number of observations per ith treatment.

Each C value $(C = c_1\bar{y}_1 + c_2\bar{y}_2 + \cdots c_a\bar{y}_a)$ is to be compared to

$$S_\alpha = S_{c_i}\sqrt{(a-1)F_{\alpha,(a-1,N-a)}}$$

(33)

To test the contrast, T_c differs significantly from 0, we utilize C. If $|C| > S_\alpha$, the H_0 hypothesis is rejected.

Let us use the data from Table 5 to demonstrate how to set up contrasts. The procedure can be conveniently written in four steps.

Step 1. Set up all contrasts in null (H_0) hypothesis terms.
Step 2. Determine standard error for the contrasts (Sc_i).
Step 3. Determine the tabled S_α values.
Step 4. Make comparison table for $|C_i|$ vs. S_α.

Example 1: Suppose the researcher wants to conduct the following contrasts in H_0 terms; the null hypothesis would be:

$$Tc_1 = \mu_1 - \mu_2 = 0, \quad \text{or} \quad \mu_1 = \mu_2$$
$$Tc_2 = \mu_3 - \mu_4 = 0, \quad \text{or} \quad \mu_3 = \mu_4$$
$$Tc_3 = \mu_2 - \mu_3 = 0, \quad \text{or} \quad \mu_2 = \mu_3$$
$$Tc_4 = \mu_1 + \mu_2 - \mu_3 - \mu_4 = 0, \quad \text{or} \quad \mu_1 + \mu_2 = \mu_3 + \mu_4$$

Step 1. Contrast $1 = C_1 = \bar{y}_{1.} - \bar{y}_{2.}$
$C_1 = 100 - 102 = -2$
Contrast $2 = C_2 = \bar{y}_{3.} - \bar{y}_{4.}$
$C_2 = 105.20 - 98.80 = 6.40$
Contrast $3 = C_3 = \bar{y}_{2.} - \bar{y}_{3.}$
$C_3 = 102 - 105.20 = -3.2$
Contrast $4 = C_4 = \bar{y}_{1.} + \bar{y}_{2.} - \bar{y}_{3.} - \bar{y}_{4.}$
$C_4 = 100 + 102 - 105.20 - 98.80 = -2$

Step 2.   Determine standard error for the contrasts.

$$S_{c_i} = \sqrt{MSE \sum_{i=1}^{a} \left(\frac{c_i^2}{n_i}\right)}$$

$$S_{c_1} = \sqrt{3.225\left(\frac{1^2}{5} + \frac{1^2}{5}\right)}$$

$$S_{c_1} = 1.136$$

$$S_{c_2} = \sqrt{3.225\left(\frac{1^2}{5} + \frac{1^2}{5}\right)}$$

$$S_{c_2} = 1.136$$

$$S_{c_3} = \sqrt{3.225\left(\frac{1^2}{5} + \frac{1^2}{5}\right)}$$

$$S_{c_3} = 1.136$$

$$S_{c_4} = \sqrt{3.225\left(\frac{1^2}{5} + \frac{1^2}{5} + \frac{1^2}{5} + \frac{1^2}{5}\right)}$$

$$S_{c_4} = 1.606$$

Step 3.   Find the tabled S_α values in the F tables. From the F distribution table (Table A.3), with $\alpha = 0.05$, $a - 1 = 4 - 1 = 3$, and $N - a = 20 - 4 = 16$, $F_{(0.05, 3, 16)} = 3.24$.

$$S_{\alpha,i} = S_{c_i}\sqrt{(a-1)F_{\alpha,a-1;N-a}}$$

$$S_{(0.05,1)} = 1.136\sqrt{3(3.24)} = 3.542$$

$$S_{(0.05,2)} = 1.136\sqrt{3(3.24)} = 3.542$$

$$S_{(0.05,3)} = 1.136\sqrt{3(3.24)} = 3.542$$

$$S_{(0.05,4)} = 1.606\sqrt{3(3.24)} = 5.007$$

The $S_{\alpha i}$ values are compared with C_i values. If $|C_i| > S_{\alpha i}$, reject H_0, the null hypothesis at α.

Step 4.   Make comparison table (Table 13).

TABLE 13   **Comparison Table**

Comparison	C_i	$|C_i|$	$S_{\alpha, i}$	$|C_i| > S_{\alpha, i}$
$\bar{y}_{1.} - \bar{y}_{2.}$	-2	2	3.542	No, accept H_0
$\bar{y}_{3.} - \bar{y}_{4.}$	6.4	6.4	3.542	Yes, reject H_0
$\bar{y}_{2.} - \bar{y}_{3.}$	-3.2	3.2	3.542	No, accept H_0
$\bar{y}_{1.} + \bar{y}_{2.} - \bar{y}_{3.} - \bar{y}_{4.}$	-2	2	5.007	No, accept H_0

Using the Scheffe method, one can test all possible contrasts. This author's recommendation, however, is to use the Scheffe method when comparing more than two samples at a time. When only contrasting pairs of treatments, use the Newman–Keuls or the Tukey test. In this case, only $\bar{y}_1 + \bar{y}_2 - \bar{y}_3 - \bar{y}_4$ would qualify.

Confidence intervals can be computed, too, using the Scheffe procedure for two or more than two samples. For two-sample comparisons, the formula for a $100(1 - \alpha)$ confidence interval, where $\mu_{i.} - \mu_{j.} = \bar{y}_{i.} - \bar{y}_{j.}$, is:

$$\bar{y}_{i.} - \bar{y}_{j.} \pm S_\alpha(S_{c_i}) \tag{34}$$

where

$$S_{c_i} = \sqrt{MSE \sum_{i=1}^{a} \left(\frac{c_i^2}{n_i}\right)}$$

For more than two samples, the general formula for a $100(1 - \alpha)$ confidence interval is:

$$\sum c_i \bar{y}_{i.} \pm S_\alpha(S_{c_i}) \tag{35}$$

Let us look at 95% confidence intervals for contrasts, as follows, noting to the right of the "equal" signs how each of the contrasts also can be expressed in a "short-hand" notation.

contrast $1 = \mu_1 - \mu_3 = S_{c_{1-3}}$

contrast $2 = \mu_1 + \mu_2 - \mu_3 - \mu_4 = S_{c_{1+2-3-4}}$

contrast $3 = \mu_1 - \dfrac{\mu_2 + \mu_3 + \mu_4}{3} = S_{c_1 - \left(\frac{2+3+4}{3}\right)}$

Recall $S_\alpha = S_{c_i}\sqrt{(a-1)F_{\alpha,(a-1,N-a)}}$ for $\alpha = 0.05$, with degrees of freedom 3, 16.

Hence, $S_\alpha == S_{c_i}\sqrt{3F_{0.05,(3,16)}} = S_{c_i}\sqrt{3(3.24)} = 3.118$

Contrast confidence interval 1:

$$\bar{y}_{1.} - \bar{y}_{3.} \pm S_\alpha(S_{c_{1-3}}) = 100 - 105.20 \pm 3.118 S_{c_{1-3}}, \quad \text{and}$$

$$S_{c_{1-3}} = \sqrt{MSE \sum_{i=1}^{a} \left(\frac{c_i^2}{n_i}\right)} = \sqrt{3.225\left(\tfrac{1^2}{5} + \tfrac{1^2}{5}\right)} = 1.136$$

$-5.2 \pm 3.118(1.136)$
-5.2 ± 3.541
$-8.741 \le \mu_1 - \mu_3 \le -1.659$

Contrast confidence interval 2:

$$\bar{y}_{1.} + \bar{y}_{2.} - \bar{y}_{3.} - \bar{y}_{4.} \pm S_\alpha(S_{c_{1+2-3-4}}) = 100 + 102 - 98.8$$

and

$$S_{c_{1+2-3-4}} = \sqrt{3.225\left(\frac{1^2}{5} + \frac{1^2}{5} + \frac{-1^2}{5} + \frac{-1^2}{5}\right)} = 1.606$$

$$-2.00 \pm 3.118(1.606)$$
$$-2.00 \pm 5.008$$
$$-7.008 \le \mu_1 + \mu_2 - \mu_3 - \mu_4 \le 3.008$$

Contrast confidence interval 3:

$$\bar{y}_{1.} - \frac{\bar{y}_{2.} + \bar{y}_{3.} + \bar{y}_{4.}}{3} \pm S_\alpha S_{c_1 - \left(\frac{2+3+4}{3}\right)} = 100 - \frac{102 + 105.20 + 98.80}{3} \pm 3.118\left(S_{c-i\left(\frac{2+3+4}{3}\right)}\right),$$

and

$$S_{c_i} = \sqrt{3.225\left(\frac{1^2}{5} + \frac{\left(\frac{-1}{3}\right)^2}{5} + \frac{\left(\frac{-1}{3}\right)^2}{5} + \frac{\left(\frac{-1}{3}\right)^2}{5}\right)} = 0.927$$

$$= -2 \pm 3.118(0.927)$$
$$= -2 \pm 2.890$$
$$= -4.89 \le \mu_1 - \frac{\mu_2 + \mu_3 + \mu_4}{3} \le 0.890$$

B. Newman–Keuls Test

This test was originally devised by Newman in 1939 and later modified by Keuls in 1952. It has also been referred to as the Student–Newman–Keuls (SNK) test [2,27,28]. The Newman–Keuls is a powerful contrast test, tending to conclude significant differences more often than its sister, the Tukey test. However, it is more conservative for type I error than Duncan's contrast procedure [28]. A number of authors have criticized it and have recommended against it because of falsely declaring significant differences at a greater rate probability than α [3,19,21]. Hence, although it is powerful, for situations in which a type I error is to be avoided, it may be wise to substitute the Tukey test. The procedure for the Newman–Keuls test is as follows:

1. Order the a means in ascending order.
2. Refer to the ANOVA table (Table 6 in our example) and find degrees of freedom $(N-a)$ and value for MSE.
3. Compute *SE* (standard error) of each mean, where $SE = S_{\bar{y}_i} = \sqrt{MSE/n_i}$

Note: When the values of n_i are equal, *SE* will be the same for each n_i.

4. Go to the Studentized tables (Table A.12) for $\alpha = 0.01$, or 0.05, and using $(N-a)$ as error degrees of freedom, list the $a-1$ tabled ranges corresponding to $p = 2, 3, \ldots, a$. The table value is of the form qα(p,f)

5. Multiply these *ranges* by $SE = S_{\bar{y}_i}$ for the $a - 1$ values to obtain the Studentized range value (SRV).

6. Beginning with the largest mean value ($\bar{y}_i$) versus smallest, one compares with SRV at $p = a$; the largest versus the second smallest is then compared to $p = a - 1$, and so on. Once the largest value has been compared with $p = 3$, the process begins again. The second largest $\bar{y}_i$ is compared with the smallest SRV at $p = a - 1$, then the second smallest, and so forth until $p = 2$. The process is continued until the $a(a - 1)/2$ possible pairs have been compared. If the two means being compared are equal, no significant difference is determined.

Let us do this procedure using our own example data.

Step 1. Order the a test means in ascending order:

$$a = 4 = \begin{array}{cccc} 98.80 & 100 & 102 & 105.20 \\ \bar{y}_4 & \bar{y}_1 & \bar{y}_2 & \bar{y}_3 \end{array}$$

Step 2. Determine the degrees of freedom for the value of MSE.
MSE $= 3.225$, and degrees of freedom $= N - a = 20 - 4 = 16$

Step 3. Compute the standard error for each mean.

$$S_{\bar{y}_i} = \sqrt{\frac{3.225}{5}} = 0.803$$

Note: Because the n value is the same for each group $S_{\bar{y}_i}$ is the same, too.

Step 4. Using the Studentized range table (Table L) at $\alpha = 0.05$ and degrees of freedom $= N - a = 16$, (where "F" on the studentized range value equals n $-$ 2, or the degree of freedom), list the $a - 1$ tabled ranges corresponding to $p = 2, 3, 4$.

$$p = 2 \quad 3 \quad 4$$

Studentized range values (table A.12) $\quad = \quad 3.0 \quad 3.65 \quad 4.05$

Step 5. Multiply these ranges by $SE = S_{\bar{y}_i} = 0.803$

$$3(0.803) = 2.409 = SRV \quad \text{for } p = 2$$
$$3.65(0.803) = 2.931 = SRV \quad \text{for } p = 3$$
$$4.05(0.803) = 3.252 = SRV \quad \text{for } p = 4$$

Step 6. Beginning with the largest $\bar{y}_i$ versus the smallest $\bar{y}_i$, at $p = a$, then the largest to second smallest at $p = a - 1$, and so on, until $p = 2$ and the process begins with the second largest $\bar{y}_i$ until the $4(3)/2 = 6$ contrasts are compared.

Figure 3 presents the above results graphically in confidence interval (CI) style.

SR value	Conclude
$\bar{y}_{3.} - \bar{y}_{4.} = 105.2 - 98.80 = 6.400 > 3.252$	$\mu_3 > \mu_4$
$\bar{y}_{3.} - \bar{y}_{1.} = 105.2 - 100.0 = 5.200 > 2.931$	$\mu_3 > \mu_1$
$\bar{y}_{3.} - \bar{y}_{2.} = 105.2 - 102.0 = 3.200 > 2.409$	$\mu_3 > \mu_2$
$\bar{y}_{2.} - \bar{y}_{4.} = 102.0 - 98.80 = 3.200 > 2.931$	$\mu_2 > \mu_4$
$\bar{y}_{2.} - \bar{y}_{1.} = 102.0 - 100.0 = 2.000 < 2.409$	$\mu_2 = \mu_1$
$\bar{y}_{1.} - \bar{y}_{4.} = 100.0 - 98.80 = 1.200 < 2.409$	$\mu_1 = \mu_4$

So, at $\alpha = 0.05$:

μ_3 is significantly larger than the other three mean value, because the μ_3 CI does not overlap μ_1, μ_2 and μ_4.

μ_2 is larger than μ_4, is not different from μ_1, and is smaller than μ_3.

μ_1 is not significantly different from μ_2 or μ_4, but is smaller than μ_3.

The Newman–Keuls test is very useful for comparing all possible $a(a-1)/2$ contrast pair s. It is particularly useful in small pilot studies, where small sample sizes are the rule, to explore and screen multiple treatments. For example, in one situation, in the author's experience, it worked well in the process for selection of impregnated preoperative/precatheter insertion swabs tested on human subjects. The cost of the project was well over \$25,000 just for screening, with the goal of finding the "best" swab. "Best" was to be the swab that demonstrated the greatest reductions in skin microorganisms. If several were reasonably equivalent, the cheaper or cheapest would be selected. Only five subjects were used for each swab configuration, and the variability of the test was 0.99 $\log_{10}$ or nearly ± 1

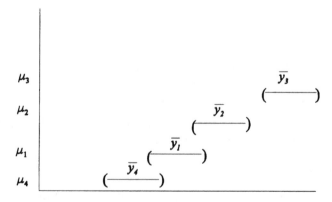

FIGURE 3   Contrast comparisons.

$\log_{10}$ of microorganisms. A rank-ordering (nonparametric) selection procedure was going to be used, but several of the decision makers were not versed in nonparametric analyses. Instead, ANOVA with the Newman–Keuls test was used, providing extremely useful information that was subsequently confirmed in a larger antimicrobial efficacy evaluation used in the drafting of a New Drug Application submitted to the Food and Drug Administration (FDA).

C. Least Significant Difference (LSD) Test

Another approach to comparing all pairs of means after the experiment has been conducted is the least significant difference, or LSD, test. The LSD test is a modification of the pooled two-sample t-test. Recall from Chap. 4 that the t statistic had the form

$$t_c = \frac{\bar{x}_1 - \bar{x}_2}{\sqrt{S_p^2(1/n_1 + 1/n_2)}}$$

The LSD comparison is similar in the denominator to the t statistic.

$$\sqrt{\text{MSE}\left(\frac{1}{n_1} + \frac{1}{n_2}\right)}, \quad \text{where MSE} = S^2 \tag{36}$$

The actual LSD comparison process is quite simple.

$$\text{If } |\bar{y}_{i.} - \bar{y}_{j.}| > \left(t_{(\alpha/2, N-a)}\sqrt{\text{MSE}\left(\frac{1}{n_i} + \frac{1}{n_j}\right)}\right) \tag{37}$$

the researcher can reject the H_0 hypothesis and conclude that the two group means compared are significantly different at the stated α level. The student's t table (table A.2) is used in this computation.

The LSD formula, when $n_i \neq n_j$, is

$$t_{(\alpha/2, N-a)}\sqrt{\text{MSE}\left(\frac{1}{n_i} + \frac{1}{n_j}\right)} \tag{38}$$

but, if the design is balanced, that is, $n_i = n_j$, Eq. (38) can be simplified to:

$$t_{(\alpha/2, N-a)}\sqrt{\frac{2\text{MSE}}{n}} \tag{39}$$

Because the example presented in Table 5 is a balanced design, we will use Eq. (39). The test statistic is

TABLE 14 LSD Procedure Contrasts

Contrasts	Significant if $\|\bar{y}_i - \bar{y}_j\| > LSD$	Significant = S Not significant = NS
$\|\bar{y}_{1.} - \bar{y}_{2.}\| = 100.0 - 102.0 =$	$2 < 2.408$	NS
$\|\bar{y}_{1.} - \bar{y}_{3.}\| = 100.0 - 105.2 =$	$5.2 > 2.408$	S
$\|\bar{y}_{1.} - \bar{y}_{4.}\| = 100.0 - 98.80 =$	$1.2 < 2.408$	NS
$\|\bar{y}_{2.} - \bar{y}_{3.}\| = 102.0 - 105.2 =$	$3.2 > 2.408$	S
$\|\bar{y}_{2.} - \bar{y}_{4.}\| = 102.0 - 98.80 =$	$3.2 > 2.408$	S
$\|\bar{y}_{3.} - \bar{y}_{4.}\| = 105.2 - 98.80 =$	$6.4 > 2.408$	S

$$|\bar{y}_{i.} - \bar{y}_{j.}| > t_{(\alpha/2, N-a)} \sqrt{\frac{2MSE}{n}}$$

where

$$LSD = t_{(\alpha/2, N-a)} \sqrt{\frac{2MSE}{n}} = t_{(\frac{0.05}{2}, 20-4)} \sqrt{\frac{2(3.225)}{5}} = 2.120(1.136) = 2.408$$

Continuing our work with data from Table 5, there are $a(4-1)/2 = 4(3)/2 = 6$ possible contrasts that can be made.

Table 14 presents these contrasts using the LSD procedure. Plotting these contrasts, provides a visual understanding of how they relate to one another (Fig. 4).

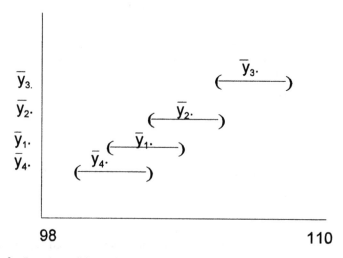

FIGURE 4 Rough confidence intervals, for the LSD procedure contrasts.

So $\bar{y}_3$ is greater than $\bar{y}_{2.}, \bar{y}_{1.}$ and $\bar{y}_{4.}$;
$\bar{y}_{2.}$ is less then $\bar{y}_{3.}$, equal to $\bar{y}_{1.}$, and greater than $\bar{y}_{4.}$;
$\bar{y}_{4.}$ is not less than $\bar{y}_{1.}$, but less than $\bar{y}_{2.}$ and $\bar{y}_3$.

The LSD method is a commonly used contrast offered on many computer software packages. It can also be easily computed using the pencil-and-paper procedure just shown. However, risk of type I (α) error can be pronounced using the LSD method, just as with the Newman–Keuls procedure. The LSD method is progressively more prone to α error as a becomes larger. One frustrating anomaly is that, when a is relatively large, with low sample sizes, n, and relatively high MSE, an F-test, as part of ANOVA, may be significant, but the LSD contrasts fail to detect any significant differences. This occurs because the LSD method compensates for all possible contrasts, not just one or two, which lowers the power. Hence, as a increases, the probability of concluding that no significant difference exists between $\bar{y}_{i.}$ and $\bar{y}_{j.}$ when, in actuality, it does, α error also increases. In practice, try to keep the comparisons to no more than three or, at the most, four.

D. Tukey's Test

The Tukey test, like the Newman–Keuls test, is based on a Studentized range statistic. The computation procedure is straightforward and useful for pairwise comparison of the means. Procedurally, as in the LSD method, where all $a(a-1)/2$ pairwise mean contrasts are made, the critical value, α is determined on the basis of all possible contrasts. As long as sample sizes are equal, the family confidence level is $100(1-\alpha)$ for all contrasts. When sample sizes are not equal, the significance level of the Tukey test is greater than $100(1-\alpha)$, or more conservative for making type I error [26]. This is very important, for the Tukey test is unsurpassed for studies where committing a type II error is not as critical as committing a type I error.

The procedure requires the use of a table of percentage points (q_α) of the Studentized range statistic to derive $q_{\alpha(p,f)}$ (Table A.12), where $p = a =$ number of sample groups, and $f = N - a$ (total number of observations less number of groups). This provides the critical acceptance value for all pairwise comparisons. Again, the Tukey test compares means $|\bar{y}_i - \bar{y}_j|$. If their absolute difference is greater than $T_c = q_{\alpha(p,f)} S_{\bar{y}_i}$, the hypothesis is rejected at α.

In the Tukey test, only one p value is used to determine q_α, not $a - 1$ value of p.

$$S_{\bar{y}_i} = \text{standard error of the mean} \sqrt{\frac{S^2}{n}} = \sqrt{\frac{\text{MSE}}{n}} \qquad (40)$$

Let us use the data from Table 5 and demonstrate the procedure.

$q_{\alpha(p,f)} = q0.05(a, N - a) = q_{0.05(4,16)} = 4.05$ from Table L.

Recall MSE $= 3.225$

$$S_{\bar{y}_i} = \sqrt{\frac{3.225}{5}} = 0.803 \qquad (41)$$

$T_c = 4.05(0.803) = 3.252$

Again, construct a contrast table of all $a(a-1)/n$ combinations (Table 15).

Notice from Table 15 and Fig. 5 that $\bar{y}_3.$ is not greater than $\bar{y}_2.$, but is greater than $\bar{y}_1.$ and $\bar{y}_4.$; $\bar{y}_2.$ is not less than $\bar{y}_3.$ not greater than $\bar{y}_1.$ or $\bar{y}_4.$; $\bar{y}_1.$ is equivalent to $\bar{y}_2.$ and $\bar{y}_4.$, but less than $\bar{y}_5.$; $\bar{y}_4.$ is equivalent to $\bar{y}_1.$ and $\bar{y}_2.$ but less than $\bar{y}_3.$

In many of the clinical trial studies I have performed, the use of Tukey contrasts has been extremely valuable when it is less desirable to commit a type I error than to commit a type II error. For example, in evaluating a series of surgical scrub formulations, the critical point of the research is to ensure that a significant difference—an indication of "better"—would mean that a product is *clearly* better, which the Tukey test ensures because of its conservative properties. I have also found it useful in research and development, particularly when, for example, a new formulation is compared with the standard formulation, and it is important that the new formulation be markedly better if one is going to replace the standard with a new one. But it is important to note that, if a product is worse than the standard, it will be more difficult to detect using the Tukey test, which could be problematic.

The Tukey procedure is prone to misuse. For example, at one firm for which I consulted, the Tukey contrast was used to ensure that batches of the manufactured drug did not go out of tolerance. As long as the Tukey test showed that the batch manufacturing process was not different at the

TABLE 15 Contrast Table

Mean difference	T_c	Significant $=$ S Not significant$=$NS[a]
$|\bar{y}_1. - \bar{y}_2.| = |100 - 102| =$	$2 < 3.252$	NS
$|\bar{y}_1. - \bar{y}_3.| = |100 - 105.2| =$	$5.2 > 3.252$	S
$|\bar{y}_1. - \bar{y}_4.| = |100 - 98.80| =$	$1.2 < 3.252$	NS
$|\bar{y}_2. - \bar{y}_3.| = |102 - 105.2| =$	$3.2 < 3.252$	NS
$|\bar{y}_2. - \bar{y}_4.| = |102 - 98.80| =$	$3.2 < 3.252$	NS
$|\bar{y}_3. - \bar{y}_4.| = |105.2 - 98.8| =$	$6.4 > 3.252$	S

[a]If $|\bar{y}_i - \bar{y}_j| > T_c$ test is significant at α, or if $|\bar{y}_i - \bar{y}_j| \leqslant T_c$ test is not significant at α.

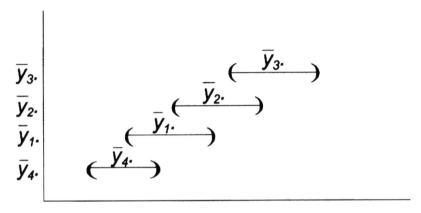

FIGURE 5   Tukey test (plotted roughly).

$\alpha = 0.05$ level of significance, the batch was considered in tolerance. This way of using the Tukey test was exceptionally liberal, for it is more difficult to detect true out of tolerances, and the analysts would be prone to say the process was in control when it really was not. It is also likely to be a poor test (i.e., lower power by design).

The Tukey test is a standard contrast option in many statistical software packages. Table 16 provides a MiniTab printout of the Tukey test. Notice that it is the same as the hand computation.

E. Dunnett's Comparison (Test Versus Control)

In many kinds of experimentation, an investigator is interested in testing a group of products compared with a control. Generally, the control is a "standard," such as the standard treatment, standard product, etc. Often the researcher is interested in developing a product better than the standard. For example, drug A may be a firm's major product in a specific category. Researchers work to create new drugs that perform better than drug A. In this developmental process, they compare new formulations with the standard (drug A). In order to replace drug A, a new drug must be significantly better.

In one prime example of this, the author's group worked on the development of a new generation of a triclosan–alcohol antimicrobial handwash formulation. The standard product was 62% ethanol without triclosan. Three new ethanol test product prototypes had been developed containing the antimicrobial agent, triclosan, at incremental levels. The goal was to find

TABLE 16 MiniTab Tukey Output (Provides the Same Information as the Hand Calculation)

Tukey's pairwise comparisons
Family error rate = 0.0500
Individual error rate = 0.0113
Critical value = 4.05

	Intervals for (column level mean) − (row level mean)		
	1	2	3
2	5.253[a]		
	1.253 NS		
3	− 8.453	− 6.453 NS	
	− 1.947 S	0.053	
	0.053		
4	− 2.053	− 0.053	3.147
	4.453 NS	6.453 NS	9.653 S

[a] $|\bar{y}_1 - \bar{y}_2|$ at a 95% confidence interval. If 0 is intersected, no significant difference is present (NS). If 0 is not intersected, the comparison is significant (S) at $\alpha = 0.05$.

a triclosan–alcohol product that had greater antimicrobial effectiveness than the alcohol alone. Employing Dunnett's test on this project proved highly useful.

The test procedure is straightforward. There are a treatments in the experiment, and the researcher will evaluate the $a - 1$ treatment groups, compared with the control group, using either a two-tail or a one-tail test. Dunnett's test utilizes Table M for two-tail and one-tail tests at both $\alpha = 0.05$ and 0.01.

The first step is to establish the value, $d_{\alpha(a-1, f)}$, where $a - 1$ is the number of treatments compared with control and $f = N - a =$ total number of observations minus number of treatments.

The formula for contrasts having the same sample sizes ($n_i = n_j$) is

$$S_{\bar{y}_i} = \sqrt{\frac{2MSE}{n}} \tag{42}$$

For pairs where $n_i \neq n_j$, the formula is

$$S_{\bar{y}_i} = \sqrt{MSE\left(\frac{1}{n_i} + \frac{1}{n_j}\right)} \tag{43}$$

Let us use "c" to denote the control group, and the $a - 1$ mean contrasts will have the form:

$$|\bar{y}_{i.} - \bar{y}_c|, \qquad i = 1, 2, \ldots, a - 1$$

The decision rule is that if

$$|\bar{y}_i - \bar{y}_c| > d_{\alpha(a-1,f)}\sqrt{\frac{2\text{MSE}}{n}} \tag{44}$$

reject H_0 at α, where:

$$f = N - a$$

Using the data in Table 5 again to demonstrate the procedure, MSE = 3.225, and $\bar{y}_1$ is the control = $\bar{y}_c$, let us calculate Dunnett's comparison.

Let us perform a two-tail test. Looking in Table M, $\alpha = 0.05/2, a - 1 = 3$, $f = 16$, $d_{\alpha(a-1,f)} = d_{(0.05/2)(3,16)} = 2.59$. Because the n_is are all equal,

$$S_{\bar{y}_i} = \sqrt{\frac{2\text{MSE}}{n}} = \sqrt{\frac{2(3.225)}{5}} = 1.136$$

Therefore, $d_{\alpha/2(a-1,f)}\sqrt{2\text{MSE}/n} = 2.59(1.136) = 2.942$. A table (Table 17) can then be constructed for Dunnett's comparison of the three treatment means ($\bar{y}_2, \bar{y}_3, \bar{y}_4$) with the control ($\bar{y}_1$). From these contrasts, we see that, at $\alpha = 0.05$, only $\bar{y}_3$ is significantly different from the control group $\bar{y}_1$.

Let us now do an example for a one-tail test. We will construct a one-way Dunnett comparison that uses, again, Table A.13 where $d_{\alpha(a-1,f)} = d_{0.05(3,16)} = 2.23$.

Computing using the same methods, we will discover, again, that the only significant contrast was $\mu_3 - \mu_1$, so $\mu_2 \leq \mu_1$, $\mu_3 > \mu_1$, and $\mu_4 \leq \mu_1$, at the 0.05 level of confidence.

Note: When comparing treatments with a control, the control group should preferably have a larger sample size, n, than the other $a - 1$ treatments.

The ratio of n_c to n_i should ideally be

$$\frac{n_c}{n_i} = \sqrt{a}, \quad \text{where } a = \text{number of groups tested} \tag{45}$$

TABLE 17   Dunnett's Table

Mean contrast	S = Significant NS = Not significant
$|\bar{y}_2 - \bar{y}_1| = |102 - 100| = 2 < 2.942$	NS
$|\bar{y}_3 - \bar{y}_1| = |105.2 - 100| = 5.2 > 2.942$	S
$|\bar{y}_4 - \bar{y}_1| = |98.8 - 100| = 1.2 < 2.942$	NS

TABLE 18   MiniTab Output

Dunnett's intervals for treatment mean minus control mean
Family error rate = 0.0500
Individual error rate = 0.0196
Critical value = 2.59
Control = level 1 of C1

	Level	Lower	Center	Upper	—+——+——+——
					+——
$\bar{y}_2$	2	−0.942	2.000	4.942	(——*——)
$\bar{y}_3$	3	2.258	5.200	8.142	(——*——)
$\bar{y}_4$	4	−4.142	−1.200	1.742	(——*——)

In our example, $\sqrt{4} = 2$, so $n_c/5 = 2$, and $n_c = 10$. Hence, 10 replicates should be run in the control group when 5 are run in the other $a - 1$ groups.

Confidence intervals can be constructed for the $a - 1$, $\bar{y}_i - \bar{y}_c$ groups.

$$\mu_i - \mu_c = \bar{y}_i - \bar{y}_c \pm d_{\alpha/2,(a-1,f)}\sqrt{\frac{2MSE}{n}} \quad \text{for groups where } n_i = n_j$$

or

$$\sqrt{MSE\left(\frac{1}{n_i} + \frac{1}{n_j}\right)} \quad \text{for groups where } n_i \neq n_j.$$

Using the MiniTab format, the confidence intervals appear as in Table 18. Note that the confidence interval on $\mu_3 - \mu_c$, the one significant contrast, does not include zero.

F. Duncan's New Multiple Range Test

This is a popular procedure for comparing all $a(a - 1)/2$ possible pairs of means. The test can be used for both equal and unequal sample sizes, and the procedure is quite straightforward.

The a mean values are first ordered in ascending order, and then the standard error of the mean is computed for each of the means. For groups where the sample sizes are equal, Eq. (46) is used.

$$S_{\bar{y}_i} = \sqrt{\frac{MSE}{n}} \tag{46}$$

If the sample sizes are not equal, n' must be computed, which is a (total number of treatments) divided by the sum of the reciprocals of the n_i values, and this replaces n in Eq. (46). The formula for computing the value of n' is:

$$n' = \frac{a}{\sum_{i=1}^{a}(1/n_i)} \qquad (47)$$

In addition, the researcher must obtain range values, $r_{\alpha(p,f)}$ for $p = 2$, $3, \ldots, a$, where $\alpha =$ significance level and $f =$ number of degrees of freedom, which is $N - a$. The range values must then be converted to a set of $a - 1$ least significant ranges for $p = 2, 3, 4, \ldots, a$. This is done by calculating:

$$R_p = (r_{\alpha(p,f)})S_{\bar{y}_i} \qquad (48)$$

for $p = 2, 3, \ldots, a$, where $r_{\alpha(p,f)}$ values are found in Table E for $\alpha = 0.05$ and 0.01. Then the observed differences between means are evaluated, beginning by comparing the largest with the smallest, which is then compared with the least significant range value, R_p.

The next step is to determine the difference between the largest and second smallest and compare it with the range R_{a-1}. The process is continued until the differences of all possible $a(a-1)/2$ pairs of means have been evaluated. If an observed difference is greater than the corresponding least significant range value, the researcher concludes that the mean pairs are different, that is, rejects H_0 at α.

To eliminate any decisional contradictions, no difference between a pair of means is considered significant if the two means involved lie between two other means that are not significantly different.

Let us compute Duncan's multiple range test using, again, the data from Table 5.

Step 1. The $\bar{y}_i$ values are arranged in ascending order.

Values of $\bar{y}_i$	Values of $\bar{y}_i$ in ascending Order	
$\bar{y}_1 = 100$	$\bar{y}_4 = 98.80$	MSE $= 3.225$, as before, and $n_1 = n_2 = n_3 = n_4 = n_5 = 5$ Let us set $\alpha = 0.05$.
$\bar{y}_2 = 102$	$\bar{y}_1 = 100$	
$\bar{y}_3 = 105.2$	$\bar{y}_2 = 102$	$S_{\bar{y}_i} = \sqrt{\frac{MSE}{n}} = \sqrt{\frac{3.225}{5}} = 0.803$
$\bar{y}_4 = 98.80$	$\bar{y}_3 = 105.2$	

Step 2. The $a - 1$, R_p values are computed beginning with R_2 and ending with R_a.

The computations of $R_p = r_{\alpha(p,f)} S_{\bar{y}_i}$, where $p = 2, 3, 4$ and $f = N - a = 20 - 4 = 16$ are

$R_2 = r_{0.05(2,16)} = 3.0$, and $3.0(0.803) = 2.409$
$R_3 = r_{0.05(3,16)} = 3.15$, and $3.15(0.803) = 2.530$
$R_4 = r_{0.05(4,16)} = 3.23$, and $3.23(0.803) = 2.594$

Step 3. The largest versus smallest means are compared with the largest R_p value. The largest and second smallest mean values are compared with the second largest R_p value. Finally, the largest versus the third smallest mean values are compared with the third largest R_p value. Then the process is repeated, using the second largest mean compared with the smallest mean.

$\bar{y}_{i.} - \bar{y}_{j.}$

3 vs. 4 $= 105.2 - 98.80 = 6.400 > 2.594\,(R_4)$; because $\bar{y}_3 - \bar{y}_4 > R_4$, reject H_0

3 vs. 1 $= 105.2 - 100 = 5.20 > 2.530\,(R_3)$;   because $\bar{y}_3 - \bar{y}_1 > R_3$, reject H_0

3 vs. 2 $= 105.2 - 102 = 3.20 > 2.409\,(R_2)$;   because $\bar{y}_{3.} - \bar{y}_{2.} > R_2$, reject H_0

2 vs. 4 $= 102 - 98.80 = 3.20 > 2.530\,(R_3)$;   because $\bar{y}_{2.} - \bar{y}_{4.} > R_3$, reject H_0

2 vs. 1 $= 102 - 100 = 2 < 2.409\,(R_2)$;   because $\bar{y}_{2.} - \bar{y}_{1.} < R_2$, cannot reject H_0

1 vs. 4 $= 100 - 98.80 = 1.2 < 2.409\,(R_2)$;   because $\bar{y}_{1.} - \bar{y}_{4.} < R_2$, cannot reject H_0

Notice that group 3 is significantly different from the other groups, and group 2 is different from group 4, but not group 1.

Please note that Duncan's multiple range test requires an increasingly greater difference between mean groups to detect differences as the number of treatment groups, a, increases. And, it should be noted that Duncan's multiple range test and the LSD test will provide identical results. The α set is the α level for all $a(a - 1)/2$ paired comparisons.

Duncan's multiple range procedure is quite powerful in that it detects differences that are different, given that the a value is not big. This condition needs to be known if a researcher is performing, say, a screening study where one must guard against type II error as well as type I error. In this case, only a few test treatments should be contrasted ($a \leq 4$).

In choosing any of these tests of contrast, it is important that one balance α (type I) and β (type II) error levels. One can do this by specifying the α level and computing the power $(1 - \beta)$ of the statistic used, based on the detectable difference requirements and the σ^2 estimate. With the two values α and β, one can perform some theoretical modeling to determine whether the α and β levels are acceptable. If one loosens α from, say, 0.05 to 0.10, the β level will tighten from, say, 0.25 to 0.20. This procedure can be very useful in designing adequate studies.

V. ADEQUACY OF THE ONE-FACTOR ANOVA

The one-factor, completely randomized ANOVA makes the assumption that the errors [the actual y_{ij} value minus the predicted $\bar{y}_{ij}$ $(e_{ij} = y_{ij} - \bar{y}_{ij})$] are independently and normally distributed with a mean of 0 and an unknown but constant variance, σ^2 [NID$(0,\sigma^2)$]. The data gathered are also expected to be normally distributed and randomly collected. In addition, as previously discussed, the model requires a completely randomized method of sampling all N samples.

However, in the field, the researcher will generally find the e_{ij}s not to be exactly [NID$(0,\sigma^2)$] but to be approximately so. The use of exploratory data analysis (EDA) will help the researcher determine whether to use the one-factor, completely randomized design. If the stem-and-leaf display, the letter-value display, and the boxplot display show the data to be skewed, nonlinear, etc., it may be wise to use a nonparametric statistic, such as the Kruskal–Wallis model, in place of the one-factor, completely randomized ANOVA. We will discuss nonparametric statistics in Chap. 12.

Yet, use of a nonparametric approach is not always a choice for the researcher. For example, if one needs more power than a nonparametric test provides, one is essentially forced to use an ANOVA model. Also, the ANOVA may be chosen because decision makers receiving the information may understand it better than a nonparametric statistic.

When one does choose to use the one-factor, completely randomized ANOVA, it is a good idea to check the model's adequacy. Adequacy includes normality, variance equivalence, and residual analysis for randomness and outliers.

VI. ASSESSING NORMALITY

Perhaps the easiest way to do this is use a stem-and-leaf display and letter-value display for each of the i treatment groups' data and their error terms— that is, the actual y_{ij} values, and the error value for each group, $y_{ij} - \bar{y}_i = e_{ij}$.

The most common problem in normality assumptions is a violation of normality due to extreme or "wild" values (outliers) relative to the main body of data. If the outlier value is not an actual reading but an error, it is better removed, given that it truly is a traceable error. If that cannot be determined, I find it useful to perform the analysis both with and without the outlier(s) in the data. This provides a dual but perhaps more correct world view—one that is more vague but real.

VII. ASSESSING VARIANCE EQUALITY

Variance equality is known as homoscedasticity, and nonequivalent variances are heteroscedastic. A number of tests are used to evaluate variance equality. One is to compare the variance and/or standard deviations of each of the a groups. The boxplot and the letter-value display are also applicable.

A. Bartlett's Test for Assessing Equality of Variances

One of the better and most popular tests is Bartlett's test for variance equality. It involves calculating a statistic that approximates a chi square (χ^2) distribution with $a - 1$ degrees of freedom. The hypothesis is:

H_0: $\sigma_1^2 = \sigma_2^2 = \cdots \sigma_a^2$

H_A: at least one of the variances is different from the others

The test statistic is:

$\chi_c^2 = 2.3026\, q/c$

where

$$q = (N - a)\log_{10} S_p^2 - \sum_{i=1}^{a}(n_i - 1)\log_{10} S_i^2 \tag{49}$$

$$c = 1 + \frac{1}{3(a - 1)}\left(\sum_{i=1}^{a}(n_i - 1)^{-1} - (N - a)^{-1}\right) \tag{50}$$

$$S_p^2 = \frac{\sum\limits_{i+1}^{a}(n_i - 1)S_i^2}{N - a}, \text{ and } S_i^2 = \text{sample variance for the } i\text{th group.}$$

$$\tag{51}$$

If the sample variances of the a treatments are significantly different from one another, the q value will become large, also making χ_c^2 large. H_0 is rejected when $\chi_c^2 > \chi_{\alpha(a-1)}^2$. The $\chi_{\alpha(a-1)}^2$ value is found in Table A.10.

It is important to recognize that Barlett's test is sensitive to nonnormal samples and should not be used if normality is doubtful. Hence, the researcher should perform EDA (stem-leaf and letter-value displays) to ensure that the data are approximately normal.

Using the data from Table 5, let us demonstrate the procedure.

Step 1. First, the sample variance for each data group is calculated.

$$S^2 = \frac{\sum_{i=1}^{a}(y - \bar{y})^2}{n-1}$$

and the variances for the four sets of data, S_1^2, S_2^2, S_3^2, and S_4^2 are 0.5,

7.5, 2.2, and 2.7, respectively, as calculated from $S_i = \frac{\sum_{i=1}^{n}(y_i - \bar{y})^2}{n-1}$

Step 2. Next, compute, S_p^2, q, and c:

$$S_p^2 = \frac{4(0.5) + 4(7.5) + 4(2.2) + 4(2.7)}{16} = 3.225$$

$$q = 16(\log_{10} 3.225) - [4\log_{10} 0.5 + 4\log_{10} 7.5$$
$$+ 4\log_{10} 2.2 + 4\log_{10} 2.7]$$

$$q = 2.745$$

$$c = 1 + \frac{1}{3(3)}[(4^{-1} - 16^{-1}) + (4^{-1} - 16^{-1}) + (4^{-1} - 16^{-1})]$$
$$+ (4^{-1} - 16^{-1})]$$

$$c = 1 + \frac{1}{9}[(0.25 - 0.063) + (0.25 - 0.063)$$
$$+ (0.25 - 0.063) + (0.25 - 0.063)]$$

$$c = 1.083$$

Step 3. Now calculate the Chi Square statistic and find $\chi^2_{T(\alpha, a-1)}$.

$$\chi_c^2 = 2.3026\left(\frac{2.745}{1.083}\right) = 5.836$$

$$\chi^2_{T(0.05,3)} = 9.49 \text{ from Table J, the Chi Square table}$$

Because $5.836 < 9.49$, one cannot reject H_0. It cannot be concluded that the variances are different at $\alpha = 0.05$.

B. Hartley Test For Assessing Equality of Variances

This method assumes that the values used in the study are independently distributed, of equal sample size, and that the error terms are random, or normally distributed [26]. The test is designed to detect the most extreme differences (largest vs. smallest variances), that is, if extremely large (significant) differences exist between the largest and the smallest group variances. Let us demonstrate the procedure using the data from Table 5. Let us set $\alpha = 0.05$, $a = 4$, and $n - 1 = 4$.

> *Step 1.* State the hypothesis.
> H_0: $\sigma_1^2 = \sigma_2^2 = \sigma_3^2 = \sigma_4^2$ (the variances are equal)
> H_A: the above is not true (at least one variance differs from the others)
> *Step 2.* Divide largest variance by smallest variance. Recall that the variances are $S_1^2 = 0.5$, $S_2^2 = 7.5$, $S_3^2 = 2.2$, and $S_4^2 = 2.7$.

$$H_c = \frac{\text{MAX } S_i^2}{\text{MIN } S_i^2} = \frac{7.5}{0.5} = 15.0$$

> *Step 3.* Decision rule:
> If $H_c \leq H_{1-\alpha(r, df)}$, accept H_0
> $H_c > H_{1-\alpha(r, df)}$, reject H_0

Using the Hartley method, we look at Table N. The table can be used for $\alpha = 0.05$ and 0.01, but in terms of $1 - \alpha$, $r = a$ and $df = n - 1$; so $H_{0.95(4, 4)} = 20.60$.

Because $H_C < H_T$, accept H_0; the four variances are equivalent at the $\alpha = 0.05$ level.

In practice, the Hartley test is exceptionally easy to compute and has served this researcher well as a decision-making tool, given that the sample sizes, n, are equal and normality can be assured. If normality is in question, the Hartley test becomes overly sensitive.

VIII. RESIDUAL ANALYSIS

In addition to checking normality and equality of variances, residual analysis should be conducted. In residual analysis, residuals are evaluated for trends, curvature, extreme points, lateral wedge shapes, or any other particular pattern.

A. Plot of Residuals in Time Sequence

It is important that residuals be plotted against the time order of data collection. This will be even more important in the two-factor ANOVA design.

However, suppose the researcher does not completely randomize the data collection (a requirement of the model) but instead collects the data in a pre-set way. This occurs all the time in practice. Suppose, for example, a researcher is evaluating the efficacy of protein sequencing at four separate temperatures: 60, 70, 80, and 90°C. More than likely, the researcher will collect the data at 60, then at 70, then at 80, and then at 90°C or, if not, in some ordered, temperature-related sequence. It is very doubtful that each sample will be selected in a completely randomized manner, going from 90°C to 60°C, etc. A time sequence plot is important because, for example, by the time the researcher evaluates the last sample group, the protein may have changed due to "fixing." This time-related problem must be detected to avoid

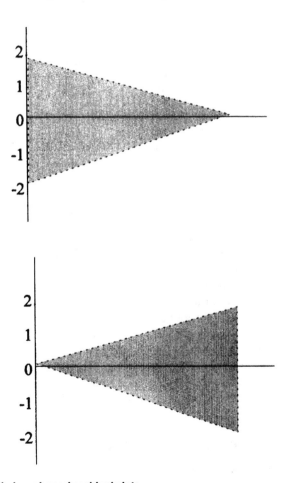

FIGURE 6   Wedge-shaped residual plots.

TABLE 19   Twenty Values from Table 5

n	Level	y_{ij}	$\bar{y}_i$	$e_{ij} = y_{ij} - \bar{y}_{i.}$
1	1	100	100.0	0.0
2	1	100	100.0	0.0
3	1	99	100.0	−1.0
4	1	101	100.0	1.0
5	1	100	100.0	0.0
6	2	101	102.0	−1.0
7	2	104	102.0	2.0
8	2	98	102.0	−4.0
9	2	105	102.0	3.0
10	2	102	102.0	0.0
11	3	107	105.2	1.8
12	3	103	105.2	−2.2
13	3	105	105.2	−0.2
14	3	105	105.2	−0.2
15	3	106	105.2	0.8
16	4	100	98.8	1.2
17	4	96	98.8	−2.8
18	4	99	98.8	0.2
19	4	100	98.8	1.2
20	4	99	98.8	0.2

concluding inadvertently that the fourth run group is different from the others because of the temperature when actually it was "aging." This cannot be evaluated directly because the temperature effect and the fixing effects are confounded—mixed up. In this case, the experiment (treatments) ideally should be run two different times, the second time in a reverse of the original. For example, if one randomly chose the run order, 80, 60, 90, and 70, it would be wise to run one half of the replicates in that order, then the remainder in run order 70, 90, 60, and 80, and compare the same temperature groups to one another to ensure no change.

Time series plots are very useful for detecting drift in the variance. The most common observation is that the residuals take on a wedge shape (Fig. 6).

The tests for equivalence of variance would more than likely pick this up, but one will not realize a drift condition unless the e_{ij} values are plotted against time.

B.   Plot of Residuals Versus Fitted Value

This is perhaps the most important residual graph. Given that the statistical model is correct and the assumptions are satisfied, the graph should be struc-

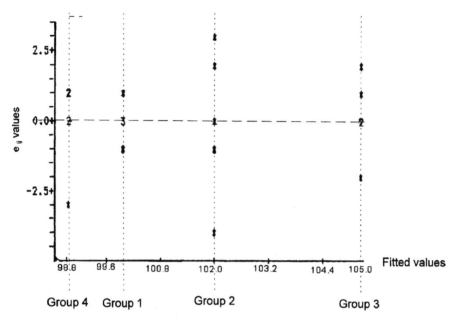

Note: a numeric value, rather than an asterisk, indicates the number of the values clustered at that point.

FIGURE 7 Residual versus fitted values.

tureless, with the central value located at 0. The graphic is constructed by plotting the error terms against the fitted values. Recall that error terms (e_{ij}) equal the actual minus the fitted values. The fitted value in each case is the sample group mean, $\bar{y}_i$. Therefore, $e_{ij} = y_{ij} - \bar{y}_i$. Table 19 displays the 20 values from Table 5.

Figure 7 provides a plot of the residuals versus the fitted values.

Notice that values for groups 1 and 2 are distributed much differently, which is to be expected for a small sample size such as $n = 5$. It is important that the researcher feel this variability intuitively as well as verify it visually. Because the variability may be of concern, a test is conducted to ensure equality of variance (Bartlett's or Hartley's, which we already did). It is clear, by this time, that much of the success in performing statistical analyses lies in the researcher's ability to deal with ambiguity—for in statistics, equivalence is always in terms of degrees, not absolute numbers.

Stem and Leaf Display

```
1    -4   0
1    -3
3    -2   81
5    -1   00
9    -0   1100
(5)   0   00118
6     1   0118
2     2   0
1     3   0
```

Letter Value Display

MTB > lval c3

	Depth	Lower	Upper	Mid	Spread
N=	20				
M	10.5	0.000		0.000	
H	5.5	-0.600	1.100	0.250	1.700
E	3.0	-2.200	1.800	-0.200	4.000
D	2.0	-2.800	2.000	-0.400	4.800
	1	-4.000	3.000	-0.500	7.000

Box Plot with Notches

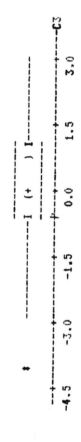

FIGURE 8   EDA of residual values (stem and leaf, letter value, and boxplot).

C. Exploratory Data Analysis (EDA)

The next step in residual analysis is to perform exploratory data analysis tests on the residuals, particularly the stem-and-leaf display and the letter-value display, although the boxplot with notches may also be useful. Figure 8 provides all three.

The stem-and-leaf display is approximately normal, with the − 4 value being slightly extreme. The letter-value display, at the midrange column, depicts the values trending to the lower end, meaning a slight skew to the left. Notice that the asterisk in the boxplot denotes an extreme value, which, again, is − 4, caused by 98, the eighth value in Table 18, which had a predicted value of 102. This value probably contributes more to the skewedness of the data than any other. It is an interesting value in that it is extreme by one whole number. Is this normal; can I determine its cause? It is something to be concerned about, a question the researcher must address, not so much from a statistical perspective but based on knowledge in one's specific field of research. If the data were more seriously nonnormal, the researcher could perform a variance stabilizing transformation, such as converting the values to ln or $\log_{10}$ scale, etc., processes discussed earlier in the EDA section (see Chap. 3).

D. Outliers

A common problem in data analysis is outlier values, which are very extreme values. They are so extreme that they just do not seem to fit the rest of the data set, particularly when evaluating residuals. We discussed this problem in Chap. 3. Once an outlier is discovered, the researcher must evaluate it closely. Is it a "typo," a measurement error, or a calculation error? Certainly, some are. But others cannot be determined one way or the other. In cases like this, it is often useful to perform the analysis with and without the outliers in the data sets. A very useful and easy computation toward this end is to standardize the residuals:

$$S_r = \frac{e_{ij}}{\sqrt{MSE}} \tag{52}$$

This can be accomplished for individual values with a pen and paper or for the entire data set using a computer. For example, for value 8 in Table 19, $e_{23} = -4$, and recalling MSE $= 3.225$ (Table 6).

$$S_r = \frac{-4}{\sqrt{3.225}} = -2.227$$

Recall that, in the normal distribution, 68% of the data fall within ±1 standard deviation, 95% within ±2 standard deviations, and 99% within

± 3 standard deviations. A deviation of greater than 3 and, certainly, any of 4 standard deviations should be considered a potential outlier. The value -2.227, as in this case, is extreme but is not really an outlier.

This author prefers to perform the outlier calculations with pen and paper. All too often, when the S_r values are a part of yet one more computer printout, it is just too easy to gloss over the data.

IX. RANDOM-EFFECTS (TYPE II) ANOVA

Up to this point, we have been discussing the fixed-effects ANOVA. Whether a model is fixed-effects or random-effects is determined when the treatment groups are selected. Recall that in our study at the beginning of this chapter, we selected four media suppliers. Had we selected the media suppliers at random, the model would have been a random-effects model.

It is important that the researcher clearly understand the difference between the fixed- and random-effects models. For the fixed-effects model, one can discuss the results of the experiment and its interpretation only in terms of and limited to the fixed treatment levels. For example, if I want to compare products based on five different antimicrobial compounds—chlorhexidine gluconate (CHG), povidone iodine (PVP), parachlorometaxylenol (PCMX), isopropyl alcohol (IPA), and triclosan—to determine which of the compounds is the best in terms of immediate kill, I must select each of the five representative compounds randomly from all available formulations within each compound group in order to apply a random-effects model. I can then state (generalize) how these compounds—not brands—compare with each other in terms of immediate antimicrobial properties. That is, I can infer general statements from specific evaluations.

The random-effects model is the same as the fixed-effects one, as a linear statistical model.

$$y_{ij} = \mu + A_i + \epsilon_{ij}, \quad \text{where } i = 1, 2, \ldots, n \tag{53}$$

However, the interpretation is different, for in the random-effects model, both A_i and ϵ_{ij} are random variables.

The variance component of each value, $V_{y_{ij}}$, consists of both the treatment variance portion, σ_A^2, and the error variance, σ^2, portion.

$$V_{y_{ij}} = \sigma_A^2 + \sigma^2$$

Both σ_A^2 and σ^2 are NID(0, σ^2). In addition, A_i and ϵ_{ij} are independent. The sum of squares, $SS_{TOTAL} = SS_{TREATMENT} + SS_{ERROR}$, continues to hold for the random-effects model. However, testing about the individual treatments is not useful. What is evaluated is that the treatment variances are equal. That is, the hypothesis-testing for random-effects models does not evaluate means but evaluates variances. If $\sigma_A^2 = 0$, all treatments are the same and have the same variance. Hence, H_0: $\sigma_A^2 = 0$, and H_A: $\sigma_A^2 \neq 0$ or $\sigma_A^2 > 0$.

The rest of the ANOVA evaluation for the completely randomized design is identical to that of the fixed-effects model. As before, when H_0 is true ($\sigma_A^2 = 0$), both MS_{ERROR} and $MS_{TREATMENTS}$ are unbiased estimators of σ^2 because the treatment effect variance is 0. That is, $E(MS_{TREATMENTS}) = \sigma^2$ and $E(MS_{ERROR}) = \sigma^2$. But when the H_A hypothesis is true, $E(MS_{TREATMENTS})$ is composed of both the treatment and error variance, $n\sigma_A^2 + \sigma^2$, and $E(MS_{ERROR}) = \sigma^2$.

The variance components, however, can be estimated as

$$\hat{\sigma}^2 = MSE \quad \text{and} \quad \hat{\sigma}_A^2 = \frac{MS_{TREATMENTS} - MS_{ERROR}}{n}$$

When the sample sizes are not equal, n is replaced by n^*, where

$$n^* = \frac{1}{a-1} \left[\sum_{i=1}^{a} n_i - \frac{\sum_{i=1}^{a} n_i^2}{\sum_{i=1}^{a} n_i} \right]$$

Using data from Table 6, where $n = 5$, MSE $= 3.225$, and $MS_{TREATMENT} = 39.133$,

$$\hat{\sigma}^2 = 3.225, \quad \text{and} \quad \hat{\sigma}_A^2 = \frac{39.133 - 3.225}{5} = 7.182$$

The treatment variance effect is 7.182, and the error variance effect is 3.225. Note that $E(MS_{TREATMENT}) = n\sigma_A^2 + \sigma^2 = 5 \times 7.182 + 3.225 = 39.135$.

The random-effects model does not have the requirement of normality because it yields estimates of $\sigma^2 + \sigma_A^2$, which provides the best minimum variance by means of an unbiased quadratic equation.

The error variance can be estimated by:

$$\frac{(N-a)MSE}{\chi_{\alpha/2,N-a}^2} \leq \sigma^2 \leq \frac{(N-a)MSE}{\chi_{(1-\alpha/2,N-a)}^2} \tag{54}$$

where χ^2 is the Chi-square value at $\alpha/2$ and $N-a$ degrees of freedom.

The variance confidence interval for the treatment variance is more difficult, well beyond the scope of this book.

6

One and Two Restrictions on Randomization

I. RANDOMIZED COMPLETE BLOCK DESIGN: ONE RESTRICTION ON RANDOMIZATION

A. Fixed-Effects Model

The randomized complete block design is different from a completely randomized design. Instead of randomly selecting each sample unit from all the N observations, randomization is conducted within the specific test group samples. This design is very useful when experimental units can be grouped meaningfully. Such a grouping is designated a *block*. The objective of blocking is to have the within-block units as uniform as possible. This is not a new concept, for we encountered it in pairing in Chap. 4 for the matched paired t-tests. Variability among the sample units in different blocks will be greater, on the average, than variability among the units in the same block. Ideally, the variability among experimental units is controlled so that the variation among blocks is maximized and the variability within minimized.

    The randomized complete block design is the ANOVA version of the paired two-sample t-test. For example, in skin sensitization studies, subjects may be recruited into a study in which 5 to 10 different products are applied on the same person. In this case, each person is a block, and each treatment product factor is a separate treatment group. Blocks can also be established in time and space. In a sequential study, measurements conducted on day one could be block 1, those on day two, block 2, and so on. In addition, if an experiment is on pieces of material, the pieces of material could be blocks.

The statistical model is:

$$y_{ij} = \mu + A_i + B_j + \epsilon_{ij} \tag{1}$$

where

μ = overall mean
i = treatments 1, 2, 3, ... a
j = blocks 1, 2, 3, ... b
A_i = the ith treatment effect
B_j = the jth block effect
ϵ_{ij} = the random error component, which is NID$(0, \sigma^2)$

Recall from Chap. 2 the discussion on randomization and blocking. Randomization of experimental units is conducted so that unknown and uncontrolled variability is not injected into the study in a *biasing* way, causing a researcher to think that a treatment effect is due to the treatment when really it is due to a bias in the study design.

Blocking is a technique used to control variability by creating individual blocks of data that are as homogeneous as possible. Examples of blocking include subjects (blocks) receiving multiple treatments that do not interact; an experiment using humans in blocks based on same weight class or liver function rates; blocks of animals based on same sex, weight, class, or litter; brands of cars (as blocks) when evaluating four different tire brands; a chemical reaction rate experiment involving four catalyst treatments using six different batches of chemical ingredients (blocks); or measuring the durability of six different paints (treatments) on each of five different wood coupons (blocks).

During the course of the experiment, all treatments or units in a block must be treated as uniformly as possible in all aspects other than the treatment. Any changes should be done throughout a complete block, not just to an individual component within a block. For example, if the y_{ij} values are known to be influenced by, say, the performance of a particular technician, the same technician should be used throughout the study, or at least for each block. Multiple technicians performing the same work should not be assigned a specific treatment in each block. Each technician should, instead, perform the experiment in each block or *randomly* assigned specific units within each block. In conclusion, what cannot be controlled should be randomized and what can be controlled should be blocked.

Note that Eq. (1) is additive; that is, if the first block effect increases the expected value by two units or points ($B_1 = 2$) and the treatment effect for the first treatment (A_1) is 4, this additive model assumes that the treatment effect is always 4 units and the block effect is always 2.

The schematic for the evaluation is similar to the completely randomized design, except that a parenthetical R, (R), is used to indicate that randomization was conducted only within each block. Suppose there are three treatments using four blocks. The schematic is (R) A_1O_1, (R) A_2O_2, and (R) A_3O_3, where

(R) designates randomization within each of the four blocks
A_i = treatment i of a (independent variable)
O_j = measured effect of treatment j (dependent variable)

Figure 1 provides a representation of the blocked study.
The treatment and block effects are defined as deviations from μ, so

$$\sum_{i=1}^{a} A_i = 0 \quad \text{and} \quad \sum_{j=1}^{b} B_j = 0 \tag{2}$$

As in the completely randomized design, the researcher is interested in testing the equality of the treatment means.

$H_0: \mu_1 = \mu_2 = \cdots \mu_n$
H_A: at least one mean is different from another

The design is computed in the same way whether the model is a fixed-effects (type I), random-effects (type II), or mixed (blocks random/fixed, treatments random/fixed) model. However, the notation is slightly expanded to account for another factor, blocks designated by b.

$y_{i.}$ = the total summation of all observations in the ith treatment
$y_{.j}$ = the total summation of all observations in the jth block
$N = ab$ = total number of observations

$$y_{i.} = \sum_{j=1}^{b} y_{ij} \quad \text{for } i = 1, 2, \ldots, a$$

and

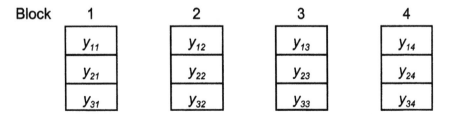

Block	1	2	3	4
	y_{11}	y_{12}	y_{13}	y_{14}
	y_{21}	y_{22}	y_{23}	y_{24}
	y_{31}	y_{32}	y_{33}	y_{34}

FIGURE 1 Blocked design.

$$y_j = \sum_{i=1}^{a} y_{ij} \quad \text{for } j = 1, 2, \ldots, b \tag{3}$$

Notice that $y.. = \sum_{i=1}^{a} \sum_{j=1}^{b} y_{ij} = \sum_{i=1}^{a} \bar{y}_{i.} = \sum_{j=1}^{b} y_j$, which is to be expected.

If one adds the treatment totals over the b blocks, or if one adds the block totals over the a treatments, the net result is $y..$.

In addition, $\bar{y}_{i.} = (y_{i.}/b), \bar{y}_j = (y_j/a)$ and $\bar{y}.. = (y../N)$, and the total sum of squares for the model $y_{ij} = \mu + A_i + B_j + \epsilon_{ij}$ is:

$$\underbrace{\sum_{i=1}^{a} \sum_{j=1}^{b}(y_{ij} - \bar{y}..)^2}_{\substack{\text{The difference of} \\ \text{each observation} \\ \text{from the grand} \\ \text{mean is composed} \\ \text{of}}} = \underbrace{b\sum_{i=1}^{a}(\bar{y}_i - \bar{y}..)^2}_{\substack{\text{the treatment} \\ \text{effect A}}} + \underbrace{a\sum_{j=1}^{b}(\bar{y}_{.j} - \bar{y}..)^2}_{\substack{\text{the block effect} \\ B}} + \underbrace{\sum_{i=1}^{a} \sum_{j=1}^{b}(y_{ij} - \bar{y}_{i.} - \bar{y}_j - \bar{y}..)^2}_{\text{the random error component}}$$

which can be expressed in sum-of-square terms as:

$$SS_{TOTAL} = SS_{TREATMENT} + SS_{BLOCK} + SS_{ERROR}$$

There are $N - 1$ degrees of freedom for SS_{TOTAL}, as before, and there are $a - 1$ degrees of freedom for $SS_{TREATMENT}$, $b - 1$ degrees of freedom for the SS_{BLOCK} component, and $(a - 1)(b - 1)$ degrees of freedom for the SS_{ERROR}.

In addition, the expected mean squares are as follows:

$$E(MS_{TREATMENT}) = \underbrace{\frac{\sigma^2}{}}_{\substack{\text{random} \\ \text{error}}} + \underbrace{\frac{b\sum_{i=1}^{a} A_{i.}^2}{a - 1}}_{\substack{\text{treatment} \\ \text{effect}}} \tag{4}$$

$$E(MS_{BLOCKS}) = \underbrace{\frac{\sigma^2}{}}_{\substack{\text{random} \\ \text{error}}} + \underbrace{\frac{a\sum_{j=1}^{b} B_j^2}{b - 1}}_{\substack{\text{block} \\ \text{effect}}} \tag{5}$$

$$E(MS_{ERROR}) = \sigma^2 \tag{6}$$

Hence, if the block effect is 0 and the treatment effect is 0, all three EMS values are estimated by σ^2.

The $F_{\text{calculated}}$ value for the treatment effect is:

$$F_c = \frac{\text{MS}_{\text{TREATMENT}}}{\text{MS}_{\text{ERROR}}} \tag{7}$$

The F_{tabled} value is: $F_{t(\alpha,a-1;(a-1)(b-1))}$.

If $F_c > F_t$, the H_0 hypothesis is rejected at the selected α value. The block effect is generally not tested. That is, $H_0\colon B_j = 0$ and $H_A\colon B_j \neq 0$. The block effect is assumed significant, or one would not undertake the blocking process.

Recall that the block effect limits randomization to being within each block, a restricted randomization. Box, Hunter, and Hunter [29] suggest that the block effect be evaluated as MS_B/MS_E, if the error terms are $\text{NID}(0,\sigma^2)$. Anderson and McClean [30], on the other hand, argue that the restricted randomization prevents the block effect test from being meaningful.

In practice, this author usually does not test the significance of the block effect but uses a suggestion of Montgomery [28] that, if the ratio MS_B/MS_E is significantly larger than 1, as anticipated, the block effect removes assignable error. However, if the ratio is near 1, the block effect is negligible. This should cause the experimenter to rethink the design, for if the block effect is near zero, one is wasting valuable degrees of freedom and reducing the detectability of the treatment effect. Perhaps the experimenter, in the next set of studies, would be well advised to randomize the order of observations completely and not block them. It is not wise to perform a completely randomized one-factor ANOVA on data collected with a restriction on the randomization, as in the randomized complete block design. Also, when the variability among experimental units within each block is large, a large MS_E term results. Hence, it is critical that the units within each block are uniform to provide the greatest power.

The ANOVA table for the randomized complete block design is presented in Table 1.

In practice, this ANOVA model computation is more easily performed using a software package, such as MiniTab, SAS, or SPSSX. However, we will perform it using pencil and paper. The computational formulae necessary are:

$$\text{SS}_{\text{TOTAL}} = \sum_{i=1}^{a}\sum_{j=1}^{b} y_{ij}^2 - \frac{y_{..}^2}{N} \tag{8}$$

$$\text{SS}_{\text{TREATMENTS}} = \frac{1}{b}\sum_{i=1}^{a} y_{i.}^2 - \frac{y_{..}^2}{N} \tag{9}$$

TABLE 1 Completely Randomized Block ANOVA

Source of variance	Sum of squares	Degrees of freedom	Mean square	F_C
Treatment	$SS_{TREATMENT}$	$a-1$	$\frac{SS_{TREATMENT}}{a-1}$	$\frac{MS_{TREATMENT}}{MS_{ERROR}}$
Blocks	SS_{BLOCK}	$b-1$	$\frac{SS_{BLOCK}}{b-1}$	
Error	SS_{ERROR}	$(a-1)(b-1)$	$\frac{SS_{ERROR}}{(a-1)(b-1)}$	
Total	SS_{TOTAL}	$N-1$		

$$SS_{BLOCKS} = \frac{1}{a}\sum_{j=1}^{b} y_{j}^2 - \frac{y_{..}^2}{N} \tag{10}$$

The error, as before, is found by subtraction.

$$SS_{TOTAL} - SS_{TREATMENT} - SS_{BLOCK} = SS_{ERROR}$$

Let us now work an example.

Example 1. A researcher studying nutritional formulations in mice blocked test animals per litter and evaluated three test formulations, *A*, *B*, and *C*. At the end of 3 months, after weaning, the mice were weighed. The researcher wants to know whether the formulations affected the mouse weights differently.

	Block				
Formulation	1	2	3	4	5
A	20	20	19	24	19
B	23	21	22	26	20
C	18	17	19	21	18

In practice, before any analysis is conducted, exploratory data analysis should be performed as described in Chap. 3.

First, let us observe the basic study design:

(R) A_1O_1
(R) A_2O_2
(R) A_3O_3

Notice that (R) means there is a restriction on randomization. In this case, randomization was performed only among the three treatments, per each of the five blocks. Treatment order within each block was randomized (Fig. 2).

The three mice within each litter were assigned randomly one of the three rations. The mice in each litter were tagged 1, 2, and 3.

Also notice that for each of the A_i treatments, there is one O_i weight measurement.

Let us now perform the problem computation using the six-step procedure:

Step 1. Formulate hypothesis:

H_0: $\mu_A = \mu_B = \mu_C$ There is no difference in weights in mice after 3 months of receiving the three different rations.

H_A: At least one of the rations produced a different weight gain than the others.

Step 2. The α level is set at 0.05, and the sample size is five per treatment.

Step 3. A randomized block design will be used in this evaluation.

Recall that in this blocking procedure we assume that it will make a difference, by reducing the degree of variability.

Step 4. Decision rule: If $F_c > F_{\text{tabled}}$, reject H_0, that the rations produced comparable weight gain. From Table A.3 (F-distribution), $F_T = F_{0.05,a-1;(a-1)(b-1)} = F_{(0.05,2,8)} = 4.46$

Step 5. Calculate the ANOVA parameters from ANOVA Table of Raw data (Table 2)

$$SS_{\text{TREATMENTS}} = \frac{1}{b}\sum_{i=1}^{3}y_{i.}^2 - \frac{y_{...}^2}{N} = \frac{1}{5}(102^2 + 112^2 + 93^2) - \frac{(307)^2}{15}$$

$$= \frac{1}{5}(31,597) - \frac{(307)^2}{15} = 6319.4 - 6283.267 = 36.133$$

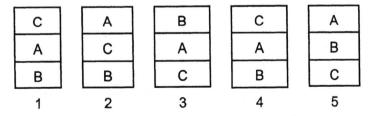

Block   1   2   3   4   5

FIGURE 2   Randomized treatment order within each block.

TABLE 2 ANOVA Table (Raw data)

Formulation	Litter 1	Litter 2	Litter 3	Litter 4	Litter 5	$y_{i.}$
			Block			
A	20	20	19	24	19	102
B	23	21	22	26	20	112
C	18	17	19	21	18	93
$y_{.j}$	61	58	60	71	57	$307 = y_{..}$
$a = 3$	$N = ab = 15$					
$b = 5$	$\alpha = 0.05$					

As the sum of square values are computed, they are arranged in an ANOVA Table for clarity (Table 3).

$$SS_{TOTAL} = \sum_{i=1}^{3}\sum_{j=1}^{5} y_{ij}^2 - \frac{y_{..}^2}{N} = (20^2 + 20^2 + 19^2 + \cdots + 21^2 + 18^2) - \frac{(307)^2}{15}$$

$$= 6,367 - \frac{(307)^2}{15} = 6,367 - 6,283.267 = 83.733$$

$$SS_{BLOCKS} = \frac{1}{a}\sum_{j=1}^{5} y_{j}^2 - \frac{y_{..}^2}{N} = \frac{1}{3}(61^2 + 58^2 + 60^2 + 71^2 + 57^2) - \frac{(307)^2}{15}$$

$$= \frac{1}{3}(18,975) - \frac{(307)^2}{15} = 6325 - 6283.267 = 41.733$$

$$SS_E = SS_{TOTAL} - SS_{TREATMENT} - SS_{BLOCK}$$

$$= 83.733 - 36.133 - 41.733 = 5.867$$

Step 6. Decision:

$$F_C = \frac{MS_{TREATMENT}}{MS_{ERROR}} = \frac{18.067}{0.733} = 24.648$$

Because $F_{calculated}(24.534) > F_{tabled}(4.46)$, reject H_0. At least one formulation differs from the other two at $\alpha = 0.05$.

Also, although the experimenter did not to test the block effect, she or he can intuitively see that the ratio, $10.433/0.736 = 14.175$, is considerably greater than 1. This points to the benefit of using a randomized block design in that the error term is reduced considerably by blocking.

TABLE 3 ANOVA Table

Source of variance	Sum of squares	Degrees of freedom	Mean square	F_C
Treatment	36.133	2	18.067	24.648
Blocks	41.733	4	10.433	
Error	5.867	8	0.733	
Total	83.733	14		

$SS_E = SS_{TOTAL} - SS_{TREATMENT} - SS_{BLOCKS};\ 83.733 - 36.133 - 41.733 = 5.867$

Let us now review a computer printout of this ANOVA, using MiniTab (Table 4). Note that the F_C value is not calculated and that the experimenter must do that. So, $18.067/0.733 = 24.648$ is the $F_{calculated}$ value.

MiniTab also provides an option for 95% confidence intervals on the μ_i treatment means, using the formula:

$$\bar{y}_{i.} \pm t_{\alpha/2;(a-1)(b-1)}\sqrt{\frac{MSE}{b}} \tag{11}$$

See Fig. 3.

B. Adequacy of Fixed-Effects Model

Exploratory data analysis (EDA) procedures should be conducted prior to performing the six-step ANOVA procedure. These include stem-and-leaf displays, letter-value displays, and boxplots to check for the normality of each sample $y_{i.}$ group, in terms of skewed data, multimodal data, and extreme values.

The assumption of equal variances between the test groups must be evaluated, as it was in Chap. 5. Following that, several residual plots are

TABLE 4 MiniTab ANOVA

Source	DF	SS	MS
Treatments	2	36.133	18.067
Blocks	4	41.733	10.433
Error	8	5.867	0.733
Total	14	83.733	

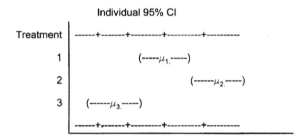

FIGURE 3   Confidence intervals.

useful. Table 5 provides a MiniTab computer printout of the actual data, the residuals, and predicted or fitted values.

     Figure 4 presents the residual data plotted against the three treatments. Nothing unusual is noted, and all the residual values appear to be distributed randomly about 0. In Fig. 5, plotting of the residuals against the blocks also shows the data to be centered randomly about 0. In Fig. 6, residuals plotted against the predicted (fitted) values also appear to be distributed randomly about 0. If interaction between the treatments and blocks was present, the residual versus fitted values would appear nonrandom.

TABLE 5   MiniTab Printout of Data

Row	y_{ij}	Treatment	Block	e_{ij}	$\hat{y}_{ij}$ = predicted value of y_{ij}
1	20	1	1	−0.266666	20.2667
2	20	1	2	0.733334	19.2667
3	19	1	3	−0.933332	19.9333
4	24	1	4	0.400000	23.6000
5	19	1	5	0.066668	18.9333
6	23	2	1	0.733334	22.2667
7	21	2	2	−0.266666	21.2667
8	22	2	3	0.066668	21.9333
9	26	2	4	0.400000	25.6000
10	20	2	5	−0.933332	20.9333
11	18	3	1	−0.466665	18.4667
12	17	3	2	−0.466667	17.4667
13	19	3	3	0.866667	18.1333
14	21	3	4	−0.799999	21.8000
15	18	3	5	0.866667	17.3333

y_{ij} = actual value and $\hat{y}_{ij}$ = predicted value.
$\hat{y}_{ij} = \bar{y}_{i.} + \bar{y}_{.j} - \bar{y}_{..}$, and $e_{ij} = y_{ij} - \hat{y}_{ij}$
Example for y_{11} : $\hat{y}_{11} = 20.333 + 20.400 - 20.467 = 20.266$ and $e_{11} = 20 - 20.266 = -0.266$.

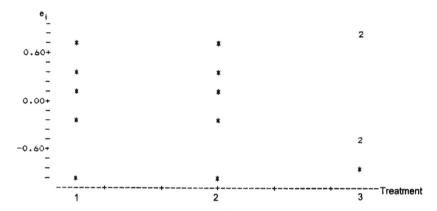

FIGURE 4   Residuals versus treatments.

That is, perhaps the negative residuals would occur with high or low $\hat{y}_{ij}$ values and the reverse with positive residual values. This has not occurred with these data.

It is also a good idea to run EDA tests (stem-and-leaf displays, letter-value displays, and boxplots) to get a different perspective on the residuals. Table 6 is a table of the data in stem-and-leaf format. Table 7 displays the residual values in letter-value format. Figure 7 provides the data in a boxplot format with notched display.

The data on the stem-and-leaf display (Table 6) portray a random/flat distribution with a slight, but not significant, piling of the data at the lower

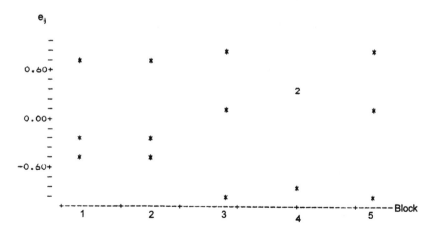

FIGURE 5   Residuals versus blocks.

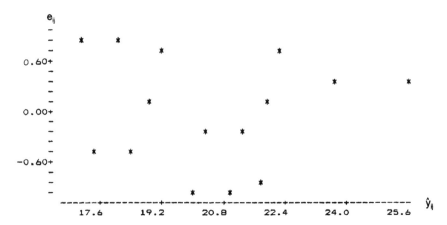

FIGURE 6   Residuals versus fitted.

value end. This is supported by the letter-value display, where a very slight skew to the lower portion of the data is noted. The boxplot provides a final view of the data, displaying nothing unusual. There is nothing to be concerned with about the data.

C.   Efficiency of the Randomized Block Design

Generally, the randomized block design is used in order to reduce the error term value by reducing inherent variability that cannot be traced to the treatment effect. The variability is the sum of random error and innate differences between the experimental units when no treatment is applied. This variability can often be reduced by blocking, but not always. And if blocking does not significantly reduce the error term's magnitude, it is

TABLE 6   Stem-and-Leaf Display (Leaf Unit = 0.10)

3	−0	998
3	−0	
5	−0	44
7	−0	22
7	−0	
(2)	0	00
6	0	
6	0	44
4	0	77
2	0	88

TABLE 7   Letter-Value Display

	Depth	Lower	Upper	Mid	Spread
N	15				
M	8.0		0.067		0.067
H	4.5	−0.467	0.567	0.050	1.033
E	2.5	−0.867	0.800	−0.033	1.667
D	1.5	−0.933	0.867	−0.033	1.800
	1	−0.933	0.867	−0.033	1.800

counterproductive because of a significant loss of degrees of freedom $[(a − 1)(b − 1)]$ as opposed to $N − a$. It is usually worthwhile to compute the relative efficiency of the randomized block design versus the completely randomized design. That relative efficiency equation is:

$$R = \frac{(df_{CB} + 1)(df_{CR} + 3)}{(df_{CB} + 3)(df_{CR} + 1)} \left(\frac{\sigma^2_{CR}}{\sigma^2_{CB}} \right) \tag{12}$$

where df_{CB} = degrees of freedom for the complete block design for MS_{ERROR}
df_{CR} = degrees of freedom for the randomized block design for MS_{ERROR}
σ^2_{CB} = MS_{ERROR} term for the complete block of design
σ^2_{CR} = MS_{ERROR} term for the completely randomized design

However, the computation for σ^2_{CR} was not done, for the model used was a complete block design. To compute the data via a completely randomized design, ignoring the block structure, will not work. Instead, it is better

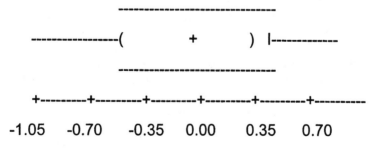

-1.05   -0.70   -0.35   0.00   0.35   0.70

FIGURE 7   Boxplot with notches.

to use an estimate of σ_{CR}^2, applying the Cochran–Cox method to calculate $\hat{\sigma}_{CR}^2$ [9,26].

$$\hat{\sigma}_{CR}^2 = \frac{(b-1)MS_{BLOCKS} + b(a-1)MS_{ERROR}}{ab-1} \tag{13}$$

Let us perform this comparison using the data in Example 1 (Table 2). Recall that $b = 5$, $a = 3$, MSE $= 0.733 = \sigma_{CB}^2$, and MS$_{BLOCKS}$ $= 10.433$. Therefore:

$$\hat{\sigma}_{CR}^2 = \frac{(5-1)10.433 + 5(3-1)0.733}{(15-1)} = 3.504$$

$$R = \frac{(df_{CB} + 1)(df_{CR} + 3)}{(df_{CB} + 3)(df_{CR} + 1)}\left(\frac{\hat{\sigma}_{CR}^2}{\sigma_{CB}^2}\right)$$

where:

$$df_{CB} = (a-1)(b-1) = (3-1)(5-1) = 8$$

$$df_{CR} = N - a = (a \cdot b) - a = (3 \cdot 5) - 3 = 12$$

$$\hat{\sigma}_{CR}^2 = 3.504$$

$$\sigma_{CB}^2 = 0.733$$

$$R = \frac{(8+1)(12+3)}{(8+3)(12+1)}\left(\frac{3.504}{0.733}\right) = 4.513$$

An R value of 4.513 means the complete block design was about 4.5 times more efficient than the completely randomized design would have been, which is very advantageous for the researcher.

In this researcher's experience, rarely does someone who works in the field block an experiment and find it inefficient compared with a completely randomized design. Therefore, whenever feasible, it is strongly recommended to block. The vast majority of studies are not funded sufficiently not to take advantage of the reduction in variability, which increases the power of the statistic, thereby allowing reduced sample size (blocks, in this case). In addition, the coefficient of determination, R^2, can be calculated to provide a direct estimate of the amount of variability in the data explained by both the treatment and block effects.

$$R^2 = \frac{SS_{TREATMENT} + SS_{BLOCK}}{SS_{TOTAL}} = \frac{36.133 + 41.733}{83.733} = 0.930$$

Thus, about 93% of the total variability in the data is explained by the treatment and block effects, indicating that the model provides a very good fit to the data.

D. Multiple Comparisons

As with the completely randomized design, to know that a difference exists in at least one group is not enough. The researcher needs to know which one or ones differ. With the fixed-effects model, the interest is in the treatment means, $\mu_{i.}$. As noted previously, the blocks are not evaluated.

The comparisons used in the completely randomized design (Chap. 5) can be used in evaluating the randomized complete block design, with several minor adjustments:

1. Substitute b (blocks) in place of n, as used in the completely randomized design.
2. The number of degrees of freedom for the error term is not as in the completely randomized design $N - a$ but is $(a - 1)(b - 1)$.

Also, note that the individual confidence intervals for each treatment mean can be calculated from:

$$\bar{y}_{i.} \pm t_{\alpha/2,(a-1)(b-1)} \sqrt{\frac{\text{MSE}}{b}} \tag{14}$$

and the difference between two means, similarly, can be calculated:

$$\bar{y}_{i.} - \bar{y}_{j.} \pm t_{\alpha/2,(a-1)(b-1)} \sqrt{\frac{2\text{MSE}}{b}} \tag{15}$$

Everything else is the same. It is important that the researcher return to Chap. 5 to review the multiple comparisons (a priori and a posteriori).

Let us perform the Tukey test on the data set in Example 1 (Table 2). Recall that

$T_\alpha = q_{\alpha(p,f)} S_{\bar{y}_{i.}}$.

$p = a = 3 =$ number of treatments.

$f = $ not $N - a$, as in the completely randomized design, but $(a - 1)(b - 1) = 8$.

$q = $ Studentized value in Table A.12. In using Table A.12, one can set α at 0.05 or 0.01 and find the corresponding p and f values to determine q.

$$S_{\bar{y}_{i.}} = \sqrt{\frac{\text{MSE}}{b}} = \sqrt{\frac{0.733}{5}} = 0.383$$

α: let's set it at 0.05.

Recall that:

$$\bar{y}_{1.} = 20.4, \quad \bar{y}_{2.} = 22.4, \quad \text{and} \quad \bar{y}_{3.} = 18.6, q_{0.05\,(3,8)} \text{ From table L} = 4.04$$

$$T_{0.05} = q_{0.05}(3,8)S_{\bar{y}_{i.}} = 4.04(0.383) = 1.547$$

Note: None of the $\bar{y}_{i.} - \bar{y}_{j.}$ is considered significant unless $|\bar{y}_{i.} - \bar{y}_{j.}| > 1.547$.

	S = Significant NS = Not significant
$\|\bar{y}_{1.} - \bar{y}_{2.}\| = \|20.40 - 22.40\| = 2.00 > 1.547$	S
$\|\bar{y}_{1.} - \bar{y}_{3.}\| = \|20.40 - 18.60\| = 1.80 > 1.547$	S
$\|\bar{y}_{2.} - \bar{y}_{3.}\| = \|22.40 - 18.60\| = 3.80 > 1.547$	S

Hence, using the Tukey test, the individual contrasts are significantly different from each other at the cumulative $\alpha = 0.05$ level of significance. A confidence interval placement of these data would appear as depicted in Fig. 8.

E. Random-Effects Model

The F-test procedure is the same for the random effects model if the treatments, or the blocks, or both treatments and blocks are random. However, the hypothesis for the random-effects model is concerned with the variance equivalence, not mean equivalence.

When the blocks are random (i.e., selected from the population of all blocks), it is expected that the comparisons among the treatments will be the same throughout the total population of blocks from which those used in the experiment were randomly selected. Given that the blocks are randomly selected from a population of all possible blocks, if the blocks then are independent variables, the treatment effect ($MS_{TREATMENT}$) is always free of block interaction. If there is obvious block–treatment interaction, the treatment tests are unaffected by the interaction, unlike the case of the fixed-effects model. The reason for this in the random-effects model is that both the MS_{ERROR} and $MS_{TREATMENT}$ terms contain the interaction effect, neutralizing it in the significance test [see Eqs. (16)]. When interaction is present in the random block effects model, the interaction is negated because:

$$MSE = \sigma^2 + AB$$

$$MS_{TREATMENT} = \sigma^2 + A + AB \tag{16}$$

where AB = interaction of treatments and blocks.

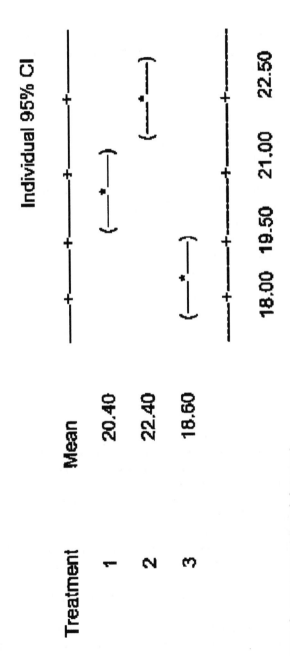

FIGURE 8   Confidence interval placement.

Careful thought by the researcher on preventing interaction between the blocks and treatment is probably the most effective way to prevent problems or, at least, to recognize potential impacts. Chapter 7 will discuss interaction in detail, for it is much more prevalent and troublesome in two-factor ANOVAs and beyond.

F. Sample Size Determination

As in the two-sample t-test and the completely randomized ANOVA design, it is important that the researcher realize the limits of his or her model's power, detection limits, and sample size requirements. In the randomized complete block design, the blocks are the same size. Hence, if one has a block size of 10, that is equivalent to an n of 10. This makes it particularly easy to use each of the methods for estimating sample size, power, and detection limits that were explained in Chap. 5 (completely randomized design) and also used in this section. However, as explained for multiple comparisons in this chapter, two adjustments are needed:

1. Substitute b (block) for any n used in the completely randomized design.
2. The number of degrees of freedom for the error term (denominator) is not $N - a$ but $(a - 1)(b - 1)$.

G. Missing Values

Many times in research, a sample observation is lost. A specimen is lost, a subject fails to report for a sample, or a test animal dies. As we saw in Chap. 5, a missing value in a completely randomized test presents no problem. However, when both blocks and treatments are evaluated, the design loses orthogonality because, for some blocks, the sum of the treatments, ΣA_i, no longer equals zero, and for some treatments, the sum of the blocks, ΣB_i, no longer equals zero. Therefore, the researcher must replace the one, or more, missing values with one(s) that minimizes SS_E.

Example 2: Let us look at one such approach. Using the data in Example 1, we generate the data for Example 2, where one of the litter 3 mice died, which we will label "X" (Table 8).

The first missing value replacement method the researcher can use is the derivative method: $d(\text{SSE})/dX$. In order to perform this, it is easier to code the data first by subtracting the average value (integer value, if the data are integers, or integers created by multiplying by factors of 10 to eliminate the decimal places) from all the observations, ignoring the

TABLE 8   Data for Example 2

Formulation	Litter				
	1	2	3	4	5
A	20	20	X^a	24	19
B	23	21	22	26	20
C	18	17	19	21	18

^{a}X = missing value.

missing value:

Step 1.

$$\frac{\sum y}{n} = \frac{20 + 20 + 24 + \cdots + 19 + 21 + 18}{14} = \frac{288}{14} = 20.571, \text{ or } 21$$

Step 2.   The second step is to subtract the average interval from the value and compute $y_{i.}$ and $y_{.j}$ values (Table 9). Recall that SS_E equals $SS_{ERROR} = SS_{TOTAL} - SS_{TREATMENT} - SS_{BLOCKS}$

So,

$$SS_E = \sum_{i=1}^{a}\sum_{j=1}^{b} y_{ij}^2 - \sum_{i=1}^{a}\frac{y_{i.}^2}{b} - \sum_{j=1}^{b}\frac{y_{.j}^2}{a} + \frac{y_{..}^2}{ab}$$

Let us now plug these values in and simplify algebraically

TABLE 9   Data in Example 2 with 21 Subtractions from Each Value

Formulation	Litter					$y_{i.}$
	1	2	3	4	5	
A	−1	−1	X^a	3	−2	x − 1
B	2	0	1	5	−1	7
C	−3	−4	−2	0	−3	−12
$y_{.j}$	−2	−5	x − 1	8	−6	$y_{..} = x − 6$

^{a}X = missing value.

$$= (-1)^2 + (-1)^2 + x^2 + 3^2 + (-2)^2 + 2^2 + 0^2 + 1^2 + 5^2 + (-1)^2$$

$$+ (-3)^2 + (-4)^2 + (-2)^2 + 0^2 + (-3)^2 - \frac{(x-1)^2 + 7^2 + (-12)^2}{5}$$

$$- \frac{(-2)^2 + (-5)^2 + (x-1)^2 + 8^2 + (-6)^2}{3} + \frac{(x-6)^2}{15}$$

$$= x^2 + 84 - \frac{(x+1^2) + 49 + 144}{5} - \frac{(x-1)^2 + 129}{3} + \frac{(x-6)^2}{15}$$

$$= x^2 + 84 - \frac{(x-1)^2 + 193}{5} - \frac{(x-1)^2 + 129}{3} + \frac{(x-6)^2}{15}$$

which is the simplified version of the preceding SS_E equation.

Now, let us take the first derivation of the SS_E equation.

$$\frac{d(SS_E)}{dx} = 2x - \frac{2(x+1)}{5} - \frac{2(x-1)}{3} + \frac{2(x-6)}{15} = 0$$

Next, using the lowest common denominator, we remove the fraction portion of the equation.

LCD is $15(2x) - 6(x+1) - 10(x-1) + 2(x-6) = 0$

$$30x - 6x - 6 - 10x + 10 + 2x - 12 = 0$$

$$16x = -8$$

$$x = \frac{-8}{16}$$

$$x = -0.5$$

Step 3. Convert -0.5 into full original value by adding 21: $21 + (-0.5) = 20.5$.

Step 4. Place 20.5 in the "X" position of the data table in Example 2 (Table 10).

Step 5. Perform the ANOVA losing 1 degree of freedom in the error term for the missing value. The error term for estimating the missing value is now $(a-1)(b-1) - 1$.

$$SS_{TOTAL} = \sum_{i=1}^{3} \sum_{j=1}^{5} y_{ij} - \frac{y^2_{..}}{N} = 20^2 + 20^2 + 20.5^2 + \cdots + 21^2 + 18^2$$

$$= 6426.25 - \frac{308.5^2}{15}$$

$$= 6426.25 - 6344.817 = 81.433$$

TABLE 10   Table with Missing Value Inserted into Litter 3, Treatment A

			Litter			
Formulation	1	2	3	4	5	$y_i.$
A	20	20	20.5	24	19	103.5
B	23	21	22	26	20	112
C	18	17	19	21	18	93
$y_j.$	61	58	61.5	71	57	$308.5 = y..$

$$SS_{\text{TREATMENT}} = \frac{1}{b}\sum_{i=1}^{3} y_i^2 - \frac{y^2..}{N} = \frac{1}{5}(103.5^2 + 112^2 + 93^2) - \frac{(308.5)^2}{15}$$

$$= 6381.05 - 6344.817 = 36.233$$

$$SS_{\text{BLOCKS}} = \frac{1}{a}\sum_{j=1}^{5} y_{ij}^2 - \frac{y^2..}{N} = \frac{1}{3}(61^2 + 58^2 + 61.5^2 + 71^2 + 57^2) - \frac{(308.5)^2}{15}$$

$$= 6385.750 - 6344.817 = 40.933$$

$$SS_E = SS_{\text{TOTAL}} - SS_{\text{TREATMENT}} - SS_{\text{BLOCKS}}$$

$$= 81.433 - 36.233 - 40.933 = 4.267 \quad (\text{Table 11})$$

$$F_T = F_{T\alpha[(a-1;(a-1)(b-1)-1)]}$$

$$F_T = F_{T0.05(2,7)} = 4.74$$

Because $F_C(29.7) > F_T(4.74)$, reject H_0 at $\alpha = 0.05$.

Note that the results are quite similar to those from the original problem. The SS_E was minimized, so it was less than that in the original problem, yet we lost a degree of freedom from the estimation of the missing value.

H. Approximate Method of Determining Missing Values

There is also an easier method based upon the differentiation of $d(SS_e)/dx$, where $x = (ay_{i.} + by_j' - y_..)/(a - 1)(b - 1)$, and

$y_{i.}'$ is the value of the treatment row, ignoring the missing value x.
$y_j'.$ is the value of the block column, ignoring the missing value.

TABLE 11 Revised ANOVA Table

Source of variance	Sum of squares	Degrees of freedom	Mean square	F_c
Treatment	36.233	2	18.117	29.700
Blocks	40.933	4	10.233	
Error	4.267	7[a]	0.610	
Total	81.433	13		

[a]$(a-1)(b-1) - 1 = (3-1)(5-1) - 1 = 7.$

$y'_{..}$ is the sum, $\sum y_{ij}$, ignoring the missing value.

Let us look at Example 2 and construct the tabled values, adding the rows and columns without the missing value (Table 12). Solving for x:

$$x = \frac{ay'_1 + by'_3 - y'_{..}}{(a-1)(b-1)}$$

$$= \frac{3(83) + 5(41) - 288}{(3-1)(5-1)}$$

$$= \frac{166}{8} = 20.75$$

The value 20.75 is plugged back into the original data set as in Table 10 and reworked. In addition, one degree of freedom is lost for each missing value in the SS_{ERROR} portion. Notice that the simplified approximation based upon the formula derived from dSS_ϵ/dx is nearly the same as for the actual differentiation, including the true value.

TABLE 12 Column and Row Totals Without the Missing Value X

Formulation	Litter					y_i
	1	2	3	4	5	
A	20	20	X	24	19	83
B	23	21	22	26	20	112
C	18	17	19	21	18	93
y_j	61	58	41	71	57	$288 = y'_{..}$

So, $y'_{.3} = 41, y'_{1.} = 83, y'_{..} = 288, a = 3,$ and $b = 5$

The differentiation methods can be used for more than one missing value. However, if that is the case, a computer-generated fit is the most practical. Most software packages have a general linear model (GLM) program that allows the calculation of the ANOVA model when one or more values are missing, making the model nonorthogonal.

An alternative that this researcher has found to be useful is to drop the entire block when one value is missing. Whereas some statisticians would argue that this is losing valuable data points, others would argue this is "dropping" data. The perspective of this author is that statistics are secondary to the experimenter's wisdom in his or her field. Statistical application should supplement his or her reason, not replace it. If it seems reasonable to drop an entire block, then do it. I find this is much better in practice than finding a theoretical value to plug into a series of values collected by research observation. The plugged-in value will minimize the contribution to error (SS_E), but it is not an actual observation. This is potentially a huge hole in applied research, particularly if the study is a small pilot study of, say, five blocks. One must ask whether they want to use actual data and lose a block (or more) or have a nice model that is more rooted in theory than in real observation.

I. GLM and Missing Values

The most practical way to perform the randomized complete block design with missing values is to use the GLM routine in a statistical software package such as SAS, SPSSX, or MiniTab. The GLM package will compute an ANOVA with missing values; however, they must be "full rank." That is, there must be enough values to estimate all the terms in the model. The software package will tell you whether there are data adequate for computing the model—you do not have to ascertain that.

When data are missing in a randomized complete block model, most commonly, the missing value is assigned an asterisk. The data for Example 2 are entered into the computer, one value for each treatment/block possibility. So, in the completely randomized ANOVA, the GLM model is:

$$Y = AB \tag{17}$$

where $A = 1$, if treatment A; $A = 2$, if treatment B; $A = 3$, if treatment C; $B = 1$, if block 1; $B = 2$, if block 2; $B = 3$, if block 3; $B = 4$, if block 4; $B = 5$, if block 5; and $Y = y_{ij}$.

Table 13 presents the $Y = AB$ computer input format. An asterisk is placed for the y_{ij} value of the first treatment (A) for the third block.

Table 14 provides the ANOVA using the GLM procedure with the missing value in treatment A, block 3. Notice that the ANOVA is essentially

TABLE 13   GLM Input for MiniTab

Y_{ij} C1	A = Treatment C2	B = Block C3
20	1	1
23	2	1
18	3	1
20	1	2
21	2	2
17	3	2
*[a]	1	3
22	2	3
19	3	3
24	1	4
26	2	4
21	3	4
19	1	5
20	2	5
18	3	5

[a]Missing value coded*.

TABLE 14   ANOVA Using the GLM Procedure with the Missing Value

MTB > GLM C1 = C2 C3
Analysis of variance for C1

Source	DF	SEQ SS[a]	ADJ SS	ADJ MS[b]	F	P
C2 (Treatments)	2	36.279	36.267	18.133	29.98	0.000
C3 (Blocks)	4	40.917	40.917	10.229	16.91[c]	0.001
Error	7	4.233	4.233	0.605		
Total	13	81.429				

[a]The sequential sum of squares value is computed by the software to minimize the SS_E term with the substituted value for the missing one. The sums of squares for the treatment, blocks, and total are essentially those appearing in Table 10, after the substitution of 20.5 was used for the missing value. The adjusted SS values are in the next column.

[b]The adjusted mean square values are merely the adjusted SS values divided by the degrees of freedom (a-1) for treatments and (b-1) for blocks. The error term degrees of freedom is based on $(a - 1)(b - 1)$ minus one degree of freedom for the missing value. Hence, the degrees of freedom for SS_E is $(a - 1)(b - 1) - 1$, or 7, as computed for Table 10.

[c]Notice that the block effect significance level was computed, which, as we learned in the beginning of this chapter, is not customarily done. It is done on the GLM routine, for this routine is based on a two-factor ANOVA. We merely ignore the second factor B and evaluate it as previously discussed in this chapter.

equivalent to the pencil-and-paper method using the actual derivative procedure or the formula based on the derivative procedure.

II. COMPUTATION OF INDIVIDUAL CONFIDENCE INTERVALS

Individual confidence intervals can be computed for the individual treatments using the denominator term $(a - 1)(b - 1) - k$, where k is the number of missing values. In practice, if k is greater than 1, the confidence levels become *too* hypothetical for practical use. In addition, the loss of one extra degree of freedom will inflate the confidence interval, particularly if the block number is small, say 5 to 10, as generally encountered in small studies. Again, in this author's opinion, it is more useful to ground confidence intervals in the data, not theory, so it is recommended that the entire block be dropped.

For determining the power of the test after the data have been collected, my recommendation is the same. The entire block for any treatment missing should be dropped. This is more conservative in preventing a type I error.

There are cases, however, where one is trying to determine whether a specific treatment has an advantage, and it is not a pivotal study. In those cases, the block may be saved by adding the derived missing value, then, perhaps, not removing the degree of freedom associated with estimating the missing value, as a hint toward the treatment's possible benefit. However, no claims should be made about the treatment's effect, for it is only one's gut feeling and must be checked out further.

By the way, any time one manipulates the data (e.g., estimating a missing value, $\hat{\sigma}^2$, or setting α or β at various levels, or removing or including extreme values), that process and its rationale must be annotated and thoroughly described in the background data report.

III. BALANCED INCOMPLETE BLOCK DESIGN

There are times when all the treatments cannot be replicated in each block. This author does not favor this type of experimentation, but it is necessary in some cases. In practice, an incomplete or unfilled block should not be sanctioned for a pivotal, determining study. In pilot or preliminary studies, this situation, however, is more acceptable. We will discuss the situation of a "balanced" design where each of the treatments is considered as important as another. In a balanced design that is incomplete, the expected data "gaps" are distributed evenly through the blocks such that all treatments have equivalent data loss.

For example, a block might be the abdomen region near the umbilicus used for preoperative skin-prepping evaluations. Anatomical space allows four samples, and that is it. Suppose a researcher wants to compare the antimicrobial effects of five products. The researcher could use a separate individual for each product, but that would be too expensive, and it would lose the blocking effect (same individual subject) of keeping the variability of the error term down. So, instead, she or he will use five products and five blocks (subjects) to keep it symmetrical.

The design could look like Table 15.

As in the case of the complete block design, there are a treatments and b blocks, each block contains k treatments, and each treatment is replicated r times in the design. There are N, or $a \times r$, or $b \times k$, total observations.

The statistical model has the same form as for the complete block design.

$$y_{ij} = \mu + A_i + B_j + \epsilon_{ij}$$

where

$\mu =$ common mean
$A_i =$ treatment effect for the ith treatment
$B_j =$ block effect for the jth block
$\epsilon =$ error term, which is NID(0, σ^2), as before

The sum of squares for the full effect is:

$$SS_{TOTAL} = \sum_{i=1}^{a} \sum_{j=1}^{b} y_{ij}^2 - \frac{y_{..}^2}{N}$$

We use the data from Table 15 and the six-step procedure:

Step 1.   Formulate the hypothesis:
H_0: $\mu_1 = \mu_2 = \mu_3 = \mu_4 = \mu_5$
H_A: One of the means differs from at least one other

TABLE 15   Symmetrical Block Design

Product (treatment)	Blocks (subjects)					$y_{i.}$
	1	2	3	4	5	
1	1.863	2.169	—	2.051	2.003	8.086
2	—	2.175	1.426	2.057	1.975	7.633
3	1.863	2.181	1.433	—	1.975	7.452
4	1.875	—	1.457	2.075	1.992	7.399
5	1.891	2.473	1.433	2.063	—	7.860
$y_{.j}$	7.492	8.998	5.749	8.246	7.945	38.430 = $y_{..}$

Step 2. The α level is set at 0.05, k = number of treatments in each block = 4, r = number of times each treatment is replicated = 4, a = number of treatments = 5, b = number of blocks = 5.

Step 3. A balanced, incomplete randomized block design will be used:

$$y_{ij} = \mu + A_i + B_j + \epsilon_{ij}$$

Step 4. Decision rule:

If $F_{calculated} > F_{tabled}$, reject H_0; the products are not equivalent at the $\alpha = 0.05$ level of significance.

Step 5. Perform calculations. SS_{TOTAL} is composed of $SS_{TREATMENT_{(Adj)}} + SS_{BLOCK} + SS_{ERROR}$ (Table 16). $SS_{TREATMENT}$ is adjusted because each treatment is represented in a different set of r blocks. The differences between unadjusted treatment totals, $y_{i.}, y_{2.}, \ldots y_{a.}$ are influenced by the differences between blocks.

The sum-of-squares treatment-adjusted calculation is:

$$SS_{TREATMENT_{(Adj)}} = \frac{k \sum_{i=1}^{a} Q_i^2}{\lambda a}$$

where k = number of treatments in each block
r = number of times each treatment is replicated
$\lambda = r(k-1)/(a-1)$ = number of times each pair of treatments in same block
Q = adjustment factor
Let us first compute the Q_i values.

$$Q_i = y_{i.} - \frac{1}{k} \sum_{j=1}^{b} n_{ij} y_{.j}, \qquad i = 1, 2, \ldots a$$

$$j = 1, 2, \ldots b$$
$$n_{ij} = 1, \text{ if treatment i appears in } jth$$
$$\text{block, and 0, if not}$$

TABLE 16 ANOVA Table

Source of variance	Sum of squares	Degrees of freedom	Mean square	F_C
Treatment (Adj)	$\frac{k \sum_{i=1}^{a} Q_i^2}{\lambda a}$	$a-1$	$\frac{SS_{TREATMENT(Adj)}}{a-1}$	$\frac{MS_{TREATMENT(Adj)}}{MS_{ERROR}}$
Blocks	$\frac{1}{k}\sum_{j=1}^{b} y_{.j}^2 - \frac{y_{..}^2}{N}$	$b-1$	$\frac{SS_{BLOCKS}}{b-1}$	
Error	By subtraction	$N-a-b+1$	$\frac{SS_E}{N-a-b+1}$	
Total	$\sum_{i=1}^{a}\sum_{j=1}^{b} y_{ij}^2 - \frac{y_{..}^2}{N}$	$N-1$		

$$Q_1 = y_1. - \frac{1}{4} \sum_{j=1}^{4} n_{11} y_{.1}$$

$$Q_1 = 8.086 - \frac{1}{4}[1(7.492) + 1(8.998) + 0(5.749) + 1(8.246) + 1(7.945)]$$

$$Q_1 = 8.086 - 8.170 = -0.084$$

$$Q_2 = y_2. - \frac{1}{4} \sum_{j=1}^{4} n_{22} y_{.2}$$

$$Q_2 = 7.633 - \frac{1}{4}[0(7.492) + 1(8.998) + 1(5.749) + 1(8.246) + 1(7.945)]$$

$$Q_2 = -0.102$$

$$Q_3 = y_3. - \frac{1}{4} \sum_{j=1}^{4} n_{33} y_{.3}$$

$$Q_3 = 7.452 - \frac{1}{4}[1(7.492) + 1(8.998) + 1(5.749) + 0(8.246) + 1(7.945)]$$

$$Q_3 = -0.094$$

$$Q_4 = y_4. - \frac{1}{4} \sum_{j=1}^{4} n_{44} y_{.4}$$

$$Q_4 = 7.399 - \frac{1}{4}[1(7.492) + 0(8.998) + 1(5.749) + 1(8.246) + 1(7.945)]$$

$$Q_4 = 0.041$$

$$Q_5 = y_5. - \frac{1}{4} \sum_{j=1}^{4} n_{55} y_{.5}$$

$$Q_5 = 7.860 - \frac{1}{4}[1(7.492) + 1(8.998) + 1(5.749) + 1(8.246) + 0(7.945)]$$

$$Q_5 = 0.239$$

Next compute λ

$$\lambda = \frac{r(k-1)}{a-1} = \frac{4(4-1)}{5-1} = 3$$

Finally we can compute $SS_{TREATMENT_{(Adj)}} = \dfrac{k \sum\limits_{j=1}^{a} Q_i^2}{\lambda a}$

$$= \frac{4([-0.084]^2 + [-0.102]^2 + [-0.094]^2 + [0.041]^2 + [0.239]^2)}{(3)(5)}$$

$$= 0.023$$

Next compute $SS_{BLOCKS} = \frac{1}{k} \sum\limits_{j=1}^{b} y_j^2 - \frac{y^2}{N}$

$$= \frac{1}{4}(7.492^2 + 8.9982^2 + 5.749^2 + 8.246^2 + 7.945^2) - \frac{(38.43)^2}{20}$$

$$= 1.473$$

Compute $SS_{TOTAL} = \sum\limits_{i=1}^{a} \sum\limits_{j=1}^{b} y_{ij} - \frac{y_{..}^2}{N}$

$$= 1.863^2 + 1.863^2 + 1.875^2 + \cdots + 1.975^2 + 1.992^2 - \frac{38.43^2}{20}$$

$$= 75.385 - 73.843$$

$$= 1.542$$

$$SS_{ERROR} = SS_{TOTAL} - SS_{TREATMENT_{(Adj)}} - SS_{BLOCKS}$$

$$SS_{ERROR} = 1.542 - 0.023 - 1.473 = 0.046$$

Table 17 provides the actual ANOVA table.
Step 6. Decision:

$$F_{T(\alpha, a-1; N-a-b+1)}$$

$$F_{T(0.05, 5-1; 20-5-5+1)}$$

$$F_{T(0.05, 4, 11)} = 3.36 \text{ (Table A.3, F distribution)} \quad \text{and} \quad F_C = 1.50$$

Because $F_C < F_T$, one cannot reject H_0 at the $\alpha = 0.05$ level of significance.

Note that, although the treatments were not significantly different statistically from one another, the blocking did reduce a significant amount of error. Without blocking, total error would have been $0.368 + 0.004 = 0.37$, and F_C would have been $0.004/0.37 = 0.01$, a much

TABLE 17 ANOVA Table

Source of variance	Sum of squares	Degrees of freedom	Mean square	F_C
Treatments(Adj.)	0.023	4	0.008	1.50
Blocks	1.473	4	0.368	
Error	0.046	11	0.004	
Total	1.542			

smaller value (and further removed from the possibility of showing any significant difference between treatments, had it existed) than the $F_C = 1.5$ that blocking provided. Based upon this ratio, it is safe for the investigator to assume the blocking effect was very significant in reducing the SS_E value. This can be evaluated further rather easily in the case of a type I fixed-effects model. Sometimes the researcher may want to determine the block effect. To do this, we must perform an alternative adjustment to the blocks because the design is not orthogonal. Hence, the sum of squares total is portioned as followed:

$$SS_{TOTAL} = SS_{TREATMENT} + SS_{BLOCK(Adj)} + SS_{ERROR}$$

Note that, in this case, $SS_{TREATMENTS}$ is unadjusted. If the design is symmetrical, $a = b$, a simple procedure will provide the $SS_{BLOCKS(Adjusted)}$ value.

In the case of symmetry,

$$Q'_j = y_j - \frac{1}{r} \sum_{i=1}^{a} n_{ij} y_{i.}, \qquad j = 1, 2, \ldots, b$$

and correspondingly,

$$SS_{BLOCKS(Adjusted)} = \frac{r \sum_{j=1}^{b} (Q'_j)^2}{\lambda b}$$

In addition, because $SS_{TREATMENT}$ is no longer adjusted, its formula is:

$$\frac{1}{k} \sum_{i=1}^{a} y_{i.}^2 - \frac{y_{...}^2}{N}$$

Using data from Table 15 and $a = b = 5$, $\lambda = 3$, and $r = 4$:

$$Q'_j = y_{j} - \frac{1}{r} \sum_{i=1}^{a} n_{ij} y_{i.}$$

$$Q'_1 = 7.492 - \frac{1}{4}(1[8.086] + 0[7.633] + 1[7.452] + 1[7.399] + 1[7.860])$$

$$Q'_1 = -0.207$$

$$Q'_2 = 8.998 - \frac{1}{4}(1[8.086] + 1[7.633] + 1[7.452] + 0[7.399] + 1[7.860])$$

$$Q'_2 = 1.240$$

$$Q'_3 = 5.749 - \frac{1}{4}(0[8.086] + 1[7.633] + 1[7.452] + 1[7.399] + 1[7.860])$$

$$Q'_3 = -1.837$$

$$Q'_4 = 8.246 - \frac{1}{4}(1[8.086] + 1[7.633] + 0[7.452] + 1[7.399] + 1[7.860])$$

$$Q'_4 = 0.502$$

$$Q'_5 = 7.945 - \frac{1}{4}(1[8.086] + 1[7.633] + 1[7.452] + 1[7.399] + 0[7.860])$$

$$Q'_5 = 0.303$$

$$SS_{TREATMENT} = \frac{1}{k} \sum_{i=1}^{a} y_{i.}^2 - \frac{y_{..}^2}{N}$$

$$= \frac{1}{4}(8.086^2 + 7.633^2 + 7.452^2 + 7.399^2 + 7.860^2)$$

$$- \frac{38.430^2}{20}$$

$$= 0.083$$

$$SS_{\text{BLOCKS(Adjusted)}} = \frac{r \sum_{j=1}^{b} (Q'_j)^2}{\lambda b}$$

$$= \frac{4([-0.207]^2 + [1.240]^2 + [-1.837]^2 + [0.502]^2)}{3 \times 5} + \frac{[0.303]^2)}{3 \times 5}$$

$$= 1.413$$

Table 18 presents the analysis.

Because F_C (88.25) $> F_T$ (3.36), reject H_0 at $\alpha = 0.05$. The blocks had a very significant reduction in assignable error. It should also be noted that $SS_{\text{TOTAL}} \neq SS_{\text{TREATEMENT(Adjusted)}} + SS_{\text{BLOCKS(Adjusted)}} + SS_{\text{ERROR}}$ due to the model lacking orthogonality.

A. Orthogonal Contrasts

Let us set up several contrasts. Recall that the five means are $\mu_1, \mu_2, \mu_3, \mu_4$, and μ_5. Each contrast carries one degree of freedom. So, $a - 1$ degrees of freedom are available to the researcher. Because $a = 5$, four contrasts are available.

1. Hypothesis

$H_0: \mu_1 = \mu_4$
$H_0: \mu_2 + \mu_4 = \mu_1 + \mu_3$
$H_0: 4\mu_3 = \mu_1 + \mu_2 + \mu_4 + \mu_5$
$H_0: \mu_3 = \mu_4$

TABLE 18   Analysis

Source of variance	Sum of squares	Degrees of freedom	Mean square	F_C
Treatments (adjusted)	0.023	4	0.006	1.50
Treatments (nonadjusted)	0.083	4		
Blocks (adjusted)	1.413	4	0.353	88.25[a]
Blocks (nonadjusted)	1.473	4		
Error	0.046	11	0.006	

[a]H_0: The block means are equal.
H_A: The block means differ.
$F_{T\ \text{BLOCKS (Adjusted)}\ (d;\ b-1,N-a-b+1)} = 88.25$ and $F_{T(\text{BLOCKS (Adjusted)})} = 3.36$.

2. Contrasts

The corresponding statistical contrasts to the hypotheses are:

$C_1 = y_1 - y_4.$

$C_2 = y_2. + y_4. - y_1. - y_3.$ or $-y_1. + y_2. - y_3. + y_4.$

$C_3 = 4y_3. - y_1. - y_2. - y_4. - y_5.$ or $-y_1. - y_2. + 4y_3. - y_4. - y_5.$

$C_4 = y_3. - y_4.$

Note: $\bar{y}_{i.}$ are not used in the contrasts, Q_i are.

$Q_1 = -0.084$ $Q_4 = 0.041$ $\lambda = 3$

$Q_2 = -0.102$ $Q_5 = 0.239$ $k = 4$

$Q_3 = -0.094$ $a = 5$

SS$_{\text{CONTRAST}}$

$$SS_{C_i} = \frac{k\left(\sum_{i=1}^{a} c_i Q_j\right)^2}{\lambda \sum_{i=1}^{a} c_i^2}$$

$$SS_{C_1} = \frac{4[1(-0.084)+0(-0.102)+0(-0.094)+(-1(0.041))+0(0.239)]^2}{3(5)[(1^2+(-1)^2]}$$

$SS_{C_1} = 0.0021$

$$SS_{C_2} = \frac{4[-1(-0.084) + 1(-0.102) + (-1(-0.094)) + 1(0.041)}{3(5)[(-1)^2 + 1^2 + (-1)^2 + 1^2]}$$
$$+ \frac{0(0.239)]^2}{3(5)[(-1)^2 + 1^2 + (-1)^2 + 1^2]}$$

$SS_{C_2} = 0.0009$

$$SS_{C_3} = \frac{4[-1(-0.084) + (-1(-0.102)) + 4(-0.094)] + [-1(0.041)]}{3(5)[(-1)^2 + (-1)^2 + 4^2 + (-1)^2 + (-1)^2]}$$
$$+ \frac{[-1(0.239)]^2}{3(5)[(-1)^2 + (-1)^2 + 4^2 + (-1)^2 + (-1)^2]}$$

$SS_{C_3} = 0.00295$

$$SS_{C_4} = \frac{4[0(-0.084)+0(-0.102)+1(-0.094)+(-1(0.041))+0(0.0239)]^2}{3(5)(1^2+(-1)^2)}$$

$$SS_{C_4} = 0.0024$$

Table 19 presents an ANOVA table with the four contrasts.

3. Contrasts

If the model is a random-effects model in the treatment, individual contrasts are irrelevant. Generally, however, both blocks and treatments are fixed and, occasionally, the blocks are random and the treatments fixed.

The methods from Chap. 5 can be used in this balanced, incomplete block design as well. If orthogonal contrasts are used, the treatment totals must be the adjusted ones (Q_i), not the total values ($y_{i.}$). The contrast sum of squares is:

$$SS_{CONTRAST} = \frac{k\left(\sum_{i=1}^{a} c_i Q_i\right)^2}{\lambda a \sum_{i=1}^{a} c_i^2} *$$

TABLE 19 ANOVA Table with Four Contrasts

Source of variance	Sum of squares	Degrees of freedom	MS	F_C
Treatments	0.023	4	0.006	1.00[a]
C_1	0.0021[a]	1	0.0021	
C_2	0.0009	1	0.0009	
C_3	0.00295	1	0.00295	
C_4	0.0024	1	0.0024	
Blocks	1.455	4	0.364	
Error	0.064	11	0.006	
Total	1.542			

[a]The $F_{calculated}$ values of the individual contrasts have not been computed. None are significant, because the treatment effect is not significant. Contrasts are never performed unless the treatment effects are significant. This contrast series was computed for demonstration purposes only. The degrees of freedom for each contrast are 1, and each is compared with the MSE term. For example, contrast 1 would have an F_C of $0.0021/0.006 = 0.35$. F_{tabled} would be $F_{(\alpha,1, N-a-b-1)}$ or for $\alpha = 0.05$, $F_{(0.05,1,11)} = 4.84$. Essentially, all other orthogonal contrasts can be constructed in the same way, using the Q_i (adjusted treatment values) in place of the $y_{i.}$ treatment total values.

Other contrast methods using all pairs of adjusted treatment effects are estimated from:

$$\hat{A}_i = \frac{kQ_i}{\lambda a}$$

The standard error of the adjusted treatment effect is:

$$S = \sqrt{\frac{k(\text{MSE})}{\lambda a}}$$

B. Nonorthogonal Contrasts

The researcher can also employ nonorthogonal contrasts—compare all pairs of adjusted means. Instead of utilizing a Q_i value, the researcher will instead use $\hat{A}_{i\prime} = kQ_i/\lambda a$ with the standard error $S = \sqrt{k(\text{MSE})/\lambda a}$ for balanced designs. Everything else is computed essentially the same way, as provided in Chap. 5.

Let us, however, for demonstration purposes, set up the computation of the least significant difference (LSD). Again, please note that the researcher would not determine individual pair contrasts unless there was a significant adjusted treatment effect (H_0 rejected). In addition, the determination of the appropriate contrast to use has been thoroughly described in Chap. 5. That rationale continues to hold.

1. Least Significant Difference (LSD) Contrast Method

Step 1. Compute the five adjusted treatment averages and S, using the MSE value from Table 18.

$$\hat{A}_1 = \frac{4(-0.084)}{3(5)} = -0.02240$$

$$\hat{A}_2 = \frac{4(-0.102)}{3(5)} = -0.02720$$

$$\hat{A}_3 = \frac{4(-0.094)}{3(5)} = -0.02507$$

$$\hat{A}_4 = \frac{4(0.041)}{3(5)} = 0.01093$$

$$\hat{A}_5 = \frac{4(0.239)}{3(5)} = 0.00648$$

$$S = \sqrt{\frac{k(\text{MSE})}{\lambda a}} = \sqrt{\frac{4(0.004)}{3(5)}} = 0.0327$$

$$LSD = t_{\alpha/2,(N-a-b+1)}\sqrt{\frac{k(\text{MSE})}{\lambda a}}^{*}$$

$$t_{(0.05/2,11)} = 2.201$$

$$LSD = 2.201(0.0327) = 0.07197$$

The $a(a-1)/2 = 5(4)/2 = 10$ contrasts are then carried out as previously explained in Chap. 5.

$\hat{A}_1 - \hat{A}_2 = -0.02240 - (-0.02720) = 0.0048 < 0.07197$

$^{\dagger}NSD$(not significantly different)

$\hat{A}_1 - \hat{A}_3 = -0.02240 - (-0.02507) = 0.00267 < 0.07197$

$^{\dagger}NSD$

$\hat{A}_1 - \hat{A}_4$ The remainder of the contrasts are performed
                        in the same manner

$\hat{A}_1 - \hat{A}_5$

$\hat{A}_2 - \hat{A}_3$

$\hat{A}_2 - \hat{A}_4$

$\hat{A}_2 - \hat{A}_5$

$\hat{A}_3 - \hat{A}_4$

$\hat{A}_3 - \hat{A}_5$

$\hat{A}_4 - \hat{A}_5$

IV. TWO RESTRICTIONS ON RANDOMIZATION

A. Latin Square Design

There are times when a researcher will want to restrict randomization beyond one block. For example, suppose a researcher is interested in evaluating the antimicrobial effectiveness of an antibacterial skin cleanser. Generally, the forearms can be used for this evaluation, two test sites per forearm

---

*The degrees of freedom $= N - a - b + 1$, which is the degrees of freedom of error term (MSE).
†Recall that if the absolute value of $|\hat{A}_i - \hat{A}_j| > LSD$, the contrast is significant at α, in this case, 0.05.

can be used (dorsal and anterior), and each test subject has two forearms. So a total of four product formulations can be evaluated.

A Latin square design procedure for this would be to restrict randomization within each person. That is, each of the four products would be evaluated on each person. However, experience shows that microbial populations vary between the dorsal and anterior aspects of the forearm, so a biasing effect is inherent in this design. A Latin square design restricts randomization in the subject site selection as well. Hence, each treatment will be assigned each site and each subject one time. That is, if subjects are rows and anatomical sites are columns, each product will be assigned each subject (row) and each site (column) one time.

The Latin square design is useful only in cases where the number of rows and columns equals the number of treatments (four subjects, four anatomical sites, and four products). Sometimes this is a problem, but a surprising number of times it is not. This author finds Latin square designs extremely useful for small pilot research and development studies. For larger, more pivotal experimental studies, it is less useful, as are all the more esoteric designs, for the simple problem of communication. If a researcher limits him or herself to the academic setting of basic research, it is not a problem. But research in industry is very different in that those funding the studies must be able to understand them. Most individuals in business, finance, management, quality assurance, regulatory agencies, and marketing and end users understand a t-test and, with some prompting, usually accept a one-factor ANOVA—completely random or random block design. But for more complicated studies—Latin squares, factorial experiments such as one-half fraction of the 2^k design, the general 2^{k-p} fractional factorial design, three factorial design, nested designs, split-plot designs, and response surface methods—this is not the case.

In this author's opinion, it is a waste of time to assign highly complex studies and expect many need-to-know individuals to understand them. It is important, then, to keep evaluations to the level of t-tests if at all possible, using multiple t-test correction factors as previously discussed.

In addition, the more complexity an experiment has, the more chance there is that the critical assumptions and model requirements will be violated.

Finally, when in doubt, it is not recommended that one turn a decision over to a statistical hypothesis. Instead, one needs to rely on innate wisdom in one's field of expertise. Who—as a researcher—has not worked with a statistician to design a very complex model that is seriously flawed because the researcher does not understand the statistics and the statistician does not understand the mechanisms involved in the research?

B. Latin Square Model

The basic Latin square model is:

$$y_{ijk} = \mu + y_i + y_j + y_k + \epsilon_{ijk} \tag{18}$$

where y_i = Row Effects $i = 1, 2, \ldots, p$
   y_j = Treatment Effects $j = 1, 2, \ldots, p$
   y_k = Column Effects $k = 1, 2, \ldots, p$
   y_{ijk} = the observation in the ith row, the kth column, in the jth treatment

Latin squares are row–column equal. Note that there is one and only one treatment j for each column k and each row i.

2 × 2	3 × 3	4 × 4
AB	ABC	ABCD
BA	BCA	BCDA
	CAB	CDAB
		DABC

A Latin square design, then, contains p rows, p columns, and p treatments. The number of observations in each $p \times p$ square is p^2. For example, a 3×3 square has $3^2 = 9$ observations. Rows and columns are generally numbered $1, 2, \ldots, p$. The treatments are labeled $A, B, \ldots, p$.
   The full Latin square analysis of variance model is:

$$SS_{TOTAL} = SS_{ROWS} + SS_{COLUMNS} + SS_{TREATMENTS} + SS_{ERROR}$$

$$\tag{19}$$

The degrees of freedom for the Latin square model are $p^2 - 1$. The usual assumption of the errors (ϵ_{ijk}) is that they are NID(0, σ^2) normal and independently distributed with a mean of 0 and a variance of σ^2.
   The model components are calculated by ANOVA procedures:

$$SS_{TREATMENTS} = \frac{1}{p} \sum_{j=1}^{p} y_{.j.}^2 - \frac{y_{...}^2}{N}$$

with $p - 1$ degrees of freedom where:

p = number of treatments
$y_{.j.}$ = jth treatment effect
$N = p^2$
$y_{...}^2$ = total j effect = total column and total row

$$SS_{\text{ROW EFFECT}} = \frac{1}{p} \sum_{i=1}^{p} y_{i..}^2 - \frac{y_{...}^2}{N}$$

where $y_{i..}^2$ = sum of squares of row effects, degrees of freedom = $p - 1$.

$$SS_{\text{COLUMN EFFECT}} = \frac{1}{p} \sum_{k=1}^{p} y_{..k}^2 - \frac{y_{...}^2}{N}$$

where $y_{..k}^2$ = sum of squares of column totals, degrees of freedom = $p - 1$.

$$SS_{\text{TOTAL}} = \sum_{i=1}^{p} \sum_{j=1}^{p} \sum_{k=1}^{p} y_{ijk}^2 - \frac{y_{...}^2}{N}$$

where y_{ijk}^2 = the sum of the squares of each of the p^2 values, degrees of freedom = $p - 1$.

$$SS_{\text{ERROR}} = SS_{\text{TOTAL}} - SS_{\text{TREATMENT}} - SS_{\text{ROW}} - SS_{\text{COLUMN}}$$

degrees of freedom $(p - 2)(p - 1)$

An ANOVA table constructed for the Latin square design is provided in Table 20.

To compute F_C, the mean square treatment effect is divided by the mean square error term. That is:

$$F_C = \frac{MS_{\text{TREATMENT}}}{MS_{\text{ERROR}}} \tag{20}$$

$F_{\text{tabled}}(F_T)$ is an F distribution with $(p - 1)$ degrees of freedom in the numerator and $(p - 2)(p - 1)$ degrees of freedom in the denominator (Tables A.3, A.6 distribution).

TABLE 20 ANOVA for the Latin Square Design

Source of variance	Sum of squares	Degrees of freedom	Mean square	F_C
Treatments	$\frac{1}{p}\sum_{j=1}^{p} y_{.j.}^2 - \frac{y_{...}^2}{N}$	$p - 1$	$\frac{SS_{\text{TREATMENT}}}{p-1}$	$\frac{MS_{\text{TREATMENT}}}{MS_{\text{ERROR}}}$
Row effect	$\frac{1}{p}\sum_{i=1}^{p} y_{i..}^2 - \frac{y_{...}^2}{N}$	$p - 1$	$\frac{SS_{\text{ROW}}}{p-1}$	
Column effect	$\frac{1}{p}\sum_{k=1}^{p} y_{..k}^2 - \frac{y_{...}^2}{N}$	$p - 1$	$\frac{SS_{\text{COLUMN}}}{p-1}$	
Error	$SS_{\text{TOTAL}} - SS_{\text{TREATMENT}}$ $SS_{\text{ROWS}} - SS_{\text{COLUMNS}}$	$(p - 2)(p - 1)$	$\frac{SS_{\text{ERROR}}}{(p-2)(p-1)}$	
SS_{TOTAL}	$\sum_{i=1}^{p} \sum_{j=1}^{p} \sum_{k=1}^{p} y_{ijk}^2 - \frac{y_{...}^2}{N}$	$p^2 - 1$		

$$F_{T(\alpha, p-1; (p-2)(p-1))} \tag{21}$$

The rows (MS_{ROWS}) and columns ($MS_{COLUMNS}$) can also be evaluated by dividing them by mean square error (MS_{ERROR}).

$$\frac{MS_{ROWS}}{MS_{ERROR}} \quad \text{and} \quad \frac{MS_{COLUMNS}}{MS_{ERROR}} \tag{22}$$

If the ratio is large, the blocking is effective. If not (the ratio is around 1), the blocking was not useful. In these cases, the ineffective block or row effect can be pooled with the error sum of squares to gain more degrees of freedom. But there is a danger because it means stating that there is no significant row or column effect, which was the reason for using a Latin square design that blocks in two directions.

Also, if a block or row effect is pooled with the error term, the researcher confounds random error with assignable error, which may or may not be problematic. This type of situation, however, is common in applied research. This author's suggestion is keep decision making grounded in the data and in the research field.

C. Randomization

Often, I am told that there is no need for randomization in a Latin square design. That is simply untrue. Randomization is important, and the following procedure ensures randomization:

Step 1. Randomly assign one blocking factor to rows, the other to columns.

Step 2. Then randomly assign levels of the row and then levels of the column.

Step 3. Then randomly assign products to the treatments.

Let us work an example.

Example 3: A researcher wants to conduct a pilot study to evaluate four new strengths of an antimicrobial skin cream lotion. The researcher will restrict randomization between subjects because each test subject will receive all four of the test products. Because there is a probable difference in microorganism baseline counts at each site, a second restriction on randomization will be enforced. That is, each anatomical site will be used by every product one time.

This will be a 4×4 Latin square design, where subjects will be the row effect, anatomical sites the column effect, and A, B, C, and D the treatment effect.

The basic design is presented in Table 21.

Let us use the six-step procedure as before.

TABLE 21   4 × 4 Latin Square Design

	1	2	3	4
1	A	B	C	D
2	B	C	D	A
3	C	D	A	B
4	D	A	B	C

Step 1.   Formulate the statistical hypothesis:

H_0: $\mu_A = \mu_B = \mu_C = \mu_D$

H_A: At least one of the treatments differs from the others.

Step 2.   Select the sample size appropriate for the Latin square design and α level. There are four products, which requires four anatomical sites and four subjects.

$$P = 4, \qquad p^2 = 16$$

Therefore, 16 subjects will be used in this design, and $\alpha = 0.05$.

Step 3.   The test statistic to be used is an ANOVA using the Latin square design.

$$y_{ijk} = \mu + y_i + y_j + y_k + \epsilon_{ijk}$$

where μ = common mean
y_i = ith row effect
y_j = treatment effect
y_k = column effect
y_{ijk} = individual observation
ϵ_{ijk} = random error—NID$(0, \sigma^2)$

Step 4.   Decision rule:
If $F_{calculated} > F_{tabled}$, reject H_0 at $\alpha = 0.05$.

Step 5.   Collect data and perform statistical evaluation.
Randomly assign row factor and column factor.
Randomly assign levels of the row and then column.
Randomly assign products to treatments.

Row factor randomly assigned anatomical site and column factor randomly assigned subjects. (Assigned by flip of coin for rows: tails = anatomical site, heads = subject.)
Randomly assign row level, then column level.

Row level: The four anatomical sites are then randomly assigned, each to one and only one row, by drawing labeled paper pieces from a box. The outcome is:

$$i = \begin{cases} 1, \text{ if lower right arm} \\ 2, \text{ if upper left arm} \\ 3, \text{ if lower left arm} \\ 4, \text{ if upper right arm} \end{cases}$$

Column effect: Next, the four subjects are randomly assigned to the row—each to one.

$$k = \begin{cases} 1, \text{ for subject JH} \\ 2 \text{ for subject RJ} \\ 3 \text{ for subject DP} \\ 4 \text{ for subject MJ} \end{cases}$$

Next, the four antimicrobial products (0.5, 1.0, 1.5, 2.0% PCMX) are randomly assigned one of the letter values. That is, the letters A–D are placed in one box, the levels 0.5, 1.0, 1.5, and 2.0% in another. The researcher draws one paper slip A–D and another 0.5–2.0%. The outcomes are matched and presented below.

$$j = \begin{cases} \text{A, if } 1.5\% \\ \text{B, if } 2.0\% \\ \text{C, if } 1.0\% \\ \text{D, if } 0.5\% \end{cases}$$

Next, the researcher conducts the study, using four products, four anatomical test sites, and four subjects. Baseline samples are taken, post-treatment samples are collected after 10 minutes of exposure, and these are plated on tryptic soy agar. Twenty-four hours later, the plates are counted; the $\log_{10}$ reduction values are presented in Table 22.

Treatment effect: Sum of squares treatment:

$$= \frac{1}{p} \sum_{j=1}^{p} y_{.j.}^2 - \frac{y_{...}^2}{N}$$

$$= \frac{1}{4}(10.375^2 + 9.600^2 + 10.000^2 + 11.825^2) - \frac{41.800^2}{16}$$

$$= \frac{1}{4}(439.631) - (109.203)$$

$$= 0.705$$

TABLE 22 Log₁₀ Values

	1	2	3	4	$y_{i..}$	Treatment totals $(y_{.j.})$
1	$A = 2.625$	$B = 1.925$	$C = 3.000$	$D = 3.300$	10.850	$A = y_{.1.} = 10.375$
2	$B = 2.775$	$C = 3.000$	$D = 2.575$	$A = 1.875$	10.225	$B = y_{.2.} = 9.600$
3	$C = 1.450$	$D = 3.050$	$A = 2.800$	$B = 3.425$	10.725	$C = y_{.3.} = 10.000$
4	$D = 2.900$	$A = 3.075$	$B = 1.475$	$C = 2.550$	10.000	$D = y_{.4.} = 11.825$
$y_{..k}$	9.750	11.050	9.850	11.150	41.800	$y_{...} = 41.800$

Row effect: Sum of squares rows:

$$= \frac{1}{p} \sum_{i=1}^{p} y_{i..}^2 - \frac{y_{...}^2}{N}$$

$$= \frac{1}{4}(10.850^2 + 10.225^2 + 10.725^2 + 10.000^2) - \frac{41.800^2}{16}$$

$$= \frac{1}{4}(437.299) - (109.203)$$

$$= 0.122$$

Column effect: Sum of squares columns:

$$= \frac{1}{p} \sum_{k=1}^{p} y_{..k}^2 - \frac{y_{...}^2}{N}$$

$$= \frac{1}{4}(9.750^2 + 11.050^2 + 9.850^2 + 11.150^2) - \frac{41.800^2}{16}$$

$$= \frac{1}{4}(438.510) - (109.203)$$

$$= 0.425$$

Error effect: Sum of squares error:

$$SS_{ERROR} = SS_{TOTAL} - SS_{COLUMN} - SS_{ROW} - SS_{TREATMENT}$$

$$SS_{ERROR} = 5.650 - 0.425 - 0.122 - 0.705 = 4.398$$

Total sum of squares:

$$= \sum_{i=1}^{p}\sum_{j=1}^{p}\sum_{k=1}^{p} y_{ijk}^2 - \frac{y_{...}^2}{N}$$

$$= (2.625^2 + 2.775^2 + \cdots + 3.425^2 + 2.550^2) - \frac{41.800^2}{16}$$

$$= (114.853) - (109.203)$$

$$= 5.650$$

The results are presented in Table 23.

Step 6. Apply decision rule: Because $F_C(0.321) < F_{T,0.05,3,6}$ (4.76), one cannot reject the H_0 hypothesis at $\alpha = 0.05$.

Clearly, the treatments are not significantly different as depicted by this Latin square design. However, from the researcher's background, she or he knows very clearly that four subjects are not enough to detect a significant difference, given that one exists. This type of reasoning is extremely important in the applied research situation—that is, drawing upon one's field experience instead of turning the decision-making process over to a statistical model, which is a model, not an extension of reality.

In addition, the row-to-error ratio $(0.041/0.733 = 0.056)$ is not intuitively significant, nor is the column-to-error ratio $(0.142/0.733 = 0.194)$. Recall that it needs to be much larger than 1, more on the side of about 5 in this case, to be significant.

D. Contrasts

As before, when significant differences exist between treatment groups, the investigator will want to determine which treatments or pairs of treatments differ. (The example following would not ordinarily be done and is for demonstration purposes only.)

TABLE 23 Results

Source of variance	Sum of squares	Degrees of freedom	Mean square	F_C
Treatment	0.705	3	0.235	0.321
Rows	0.122	3	0.041	
Columns	0.425	3	0.142	
Error	4.398	6	0.733	
Total	5.65			

V. ORTHOGONAL TREATMENT CONTRASTS

The orthogonal contrasts discussed in Chap. 5 still basically hold for Latin square design ANOVAs. Recall that for every contrast, one loses one degree of freedom. There are $p - 1$ degrees of freedom available. For Example 3, Table 22, there are $4 - 1 = 3$ possible contrasts.

Suppose the researcher determines that the treatment effects are significant and wants to know:

Hypothesis	Contrasts
$H_0: \mu_1 = \mu_4$	$C_1 = y_{.1.} - y_{.4.}$
$H_0: \mu_2 = \mu_3$	$C_2 = y_{.2.} - y_{.3.}$
$H_0: \mu_1 + \mu_4 = \mu_2 + \mu_3$	$C_3 = y_{.1.} - y_{.2.} - y_{.3.} + y_{.4.}$

From Table 22:

$$y_{.1.} = 10.375$$
$$y_{.2.} = 9.600$$
$$y_{.3.} = 10.000$$
$$y_{.4.} = 11.825$$

Because the Latin square is a balanced design, the sum of square contrasts is:

$$SS_{c_i} = \frac{\left(\sum_{j=1}^{p} c_j y_{.j.}\right)^2}{p \sum_{j=1}^{a} c_i^2}$$

$$SS_{c1} = \frac{[1(10.375) + 0(9.600) + 0(10.000) + (-1)(11.825)]^2}{4(1^2 + (-1^2))}$$

$$SS_{c1} = 0.26281$$

$$SS_{c2} = \frac{[0(10.375) + 1(9.600) + (-1)(10.000) + 0(11.825)]^2}{4(1^2 + (-1^2))}$$

$$SS_{c2} = 0.0200$$

$$SS_{c3} = \frac{[1(10.375) + (-1)(9.600) + (-1)(10.000) + 1(11.825)]^2}{4(1^2 + (-1^2))}$$

$$SS_{c3} = 0.42250$$

Table 24 presents an ANOVA table adjusted for contrasts, based on Table 23.

TABLE 24 Adjusted for Contrasts ANOVA Table Based on Table 23

Source of variance	Sum of squares	Degrees of freedom	Mean square	F_C
Treatment	0.705	3	0.235	0.321
C1	0.2628	1	0.2628[a]	
C2	0.0200	1	0.0200	
C3	0.4225	1	0.4225	
Rows	0.122	3	0.041	
Columns	0.425	3	0.142	
Error	4.398	6	0.733	
Total				

[a]Note that each of the $p - 1$ contrasts is compared with the error term. For example, to determine $F_{C(C1)} = 0.2628/0.733 = 0.3585$, and $F_{tabled} = F_{\alpha, 1, ((p-2)(p-1))}$ or $F_{\alpha(1,6)}$.

VI. NONORTHOGONAL CONTRASTS

For these contrasts determined after the experiment, nonorthogonal contrasts are used instead of orthogonal ones. Those described in Chap. 5 can be used for Latin square designs. For demonstration purposes, the least significant difference (LSD) will be used.

First, the mean treatment values are computed as in Chap. 5.

$$\bar{y}_{.1.} = \frac{10.375}{4} = 2.594$$

$$\bar{y}_{.2.} = \frac{9.600}{4} = 2.400$$

$$\bar{y}_{.3.} = \frac{10.000}{4} = 2.500$$

$$\bar{y}_{.4.} = \frac{11.825}{4} = 2.956$$

$$LSD = t_{\alpha/2,(p-2)(p-1)}\sqrt{\frac{2MSE}{p}}$$

Letting $\alpha = 0.05$, $t_{(0.025,6)} = 2.447$ (from table A.2)

$$LSD = 2.447\sqrt{\frac{2(0.733)}{4}} = 0.605$$

$$LSD = 2.447(0.605)$$

$$= 1.480$$

TABLE 25   MiniTab 4 × 4 Latin Square Design

Source	DF	Seq SS	Adj SS	Adj MS	F	P
C2 Row	3	0.1222	0.1222	0.0407	0.06[a]	0.981
C3 Column	3	0.4250	0.4250	0.1417	0.19	0.897
C4 Treatment	3	0.7053	0.7053	0.2351	0.32	0.811
Error	6	4.3975	4.3975	0.7329		
Total	15	5.6500				

[a]The F_C and p values for row and column are ignored.

So any pair $(|\bar{y}_{.i.} - \bar{y}_{j.}|)$ of means differing more than 1.480 are significantly different from each other at $\alpha = 0.05$. There will be $p(p-1)/2$ contrasts $= 4(3)/2 = 6$.

$$\bar{y}_{.1.} - \bar{y}_{.2.} = -|2.594 - 2.400| = 0.194 < 1.480\,\text{NSD}^*$$
$$\bar{y}_{.1.} - \bar{y}_{.3.} = -|2.594 - 2.500| = 0.094 < 1.480\,\text{NSD}$$
$$\bar{y}_{.1.} - \bar{y}_{.4.} = -|2.594 - 2.956| = 0.362 < 1.480\,\text{NSD}$$
$\bar{y}_{.2.} - \bar{y}_{.3.}$ The rest of the contrasts are performed in the same way.
$\bar{y}_{.2.} - \bar{y}_{.3.}$
$\bar{y}_{.2.} - \bar{y}_{.4.}$
$\bar{y}_{.3.} - \bar{y}_{.4.}$

Table 25 is a 4 × 4 Latin square design in MiniTab. Table 26 provides the complete data, which were input (columns C1 through C4), the predicted $\hat{y}$ values (C5), and the residual values (C6). MiniTab can also be used to compute the means and standard deviations of the treatment data (see Table 27). Note: The confidence interval computations for the $\bar{y}_{j.}$ are:

$$\bar{y}_{j.} \pm t_{\alpha/2,(p-2)(p-1)}\sqrt{\frac{MSE}{p}}$$

$$\bar{y}_{j.} \pm t_{0.025,6}\sqrt{\frac{0.7329}{4}}$$

(23)

It is always useful to perform a model adequacy check (Fig. 9)

Notice that the residual versus predicted values are not patterned. Figure 10 presents the residual versus the subject (column) plot, which is not extreme. Figure 11 provides the treatment versus residual plot, which

---

*NSD=not significantly different.

TABLE 26   Complete Data Minitab Display

Row	C1 y_{ijk}	C2 I	C3 j	C4 k	C5 $\hat{y}_{ijk}$	C6 $y - \hat{y} = e$
1	2.625	1	1	1	2.51875	0.106250
2	2.775	2	1	2	2.16875	0.606250
3	1.450	3	1	3	2.39375	−0.943750
4	2.900	4	1	4	2.66875	0.231250
5	1.925	1	2	2	2.65000	−0.725000
6	3.000	2	2	3	2.59375	0.406250
7	3.050	3	2	4	3.17500	−0.125000
8	3.075	4	2	1	2.63125	0.443750
9	3.000	1	3	3	2.45000	0.550000
10	2.575	2	3	4	2.75000	−0.175000
11	2.800	3	3	1	2.51250	0.287500
12	1.475	4	3	2	2.13750	−0.662500
13	3.300	1	4	4	3.23125	0.068750
14	1.875	2	4	1	2.71250	−0.837500
15	3.425	3	4	2	2.64375	0.781250
16	2.550	4	4	3	2.56250	−0.012500

again is not abnormal. Figure 12 presents the anatomical sites versus the residual. Figure 13 and Table 28 present the stem-and-leaf display and the letter-value display of the residuals. There is a gap in the data and a slight skew to the upper tail but not an excessive one.

VII. REPLICATION IN LATIN SQUARE DESIGNS

As useful as the Latin square design can be, its major flaw is the small sample size it uses. In the previous example, there were four products and four

TABLE 27   Mean Printout Chart

Treatment	Mean	Stdev
1	2.594	0.4281
2	2.400	0.4281
3	2.500	0.4281
4	2.956	0.4281

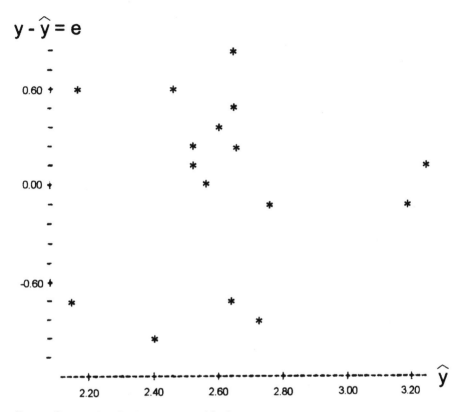

$y - \widehat{y} = e$

FIGURE 9   Predicted value versus residual.

anatomical sites, but the testing on only four subjects is not useful because there are no replicates. Hence, in cases in which different column effects (subjects) are used to increase the sample size but the same anatomical sites (row) and treatments are used, the ANOVA procedure needs to be modified. The modified ANOVA procedure is provided in Table 29, and Table 30 shows the basic format for data computation.

The model is:

$$y_{ijkl} = \mu + y_i + y_j + y_k + R_l + \epsilon_{ijkl}$$

where i = row factor, 1, 2, 3, 4 (Anatomical sites)

j = treatment 1, 2, 3, 4   1 = A, 2 = B, 3 = C, 4 = D

k = subject block 1, 2, 3, 4

l = replicate within subject block 1, 2, 3 (Each subject block contains n = 3 replicate subjects).

R = replicates

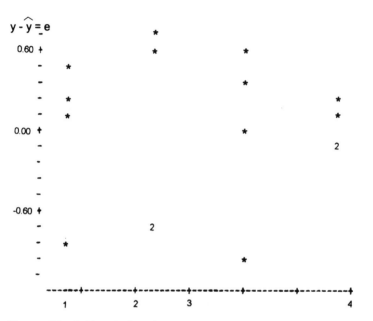

FIGURE 10   Subject (column) versus residual plot.

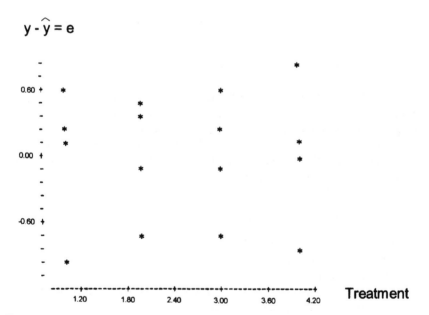

FIGURE 11   Treatment versus residual plot.

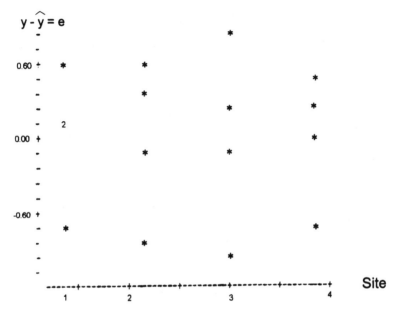

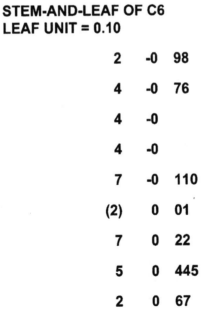

FIGURE 12   Anatomical sites versus residual plot.

STEM-AND-LEAF OF C6
LEAF UNIT = 0.10

2	-0	98
4	-0	76
4	-0	
4	-0	
7	-0	110
(2)	0	01
7	0	22
5	0	445
2	0	67

FIGURE 13   Stem-and-leaf display residual values.

TABLE 28 Letter-Value Display of Residual Value $Y - \hat{Y} = e$

	Depth	Lower	Upper	Mid	Spread
N	16				
M	8.5		0.087		0.087
H	4.5	−0.419	0.425	0.003	0.844
E	2.5	−0.781	0.578	−0.102	1.359
D	1.5	−0.891	0.694	−0.098	1.584
	1	−0.944	0.781	−0.081	1.725

Using the data in Table 30, let us compute the treatment value.
Treatments (j):

$$
\begin{aligned}
y_{.1..} \quad A &= 9.4 + 10.4 + 9.4 + 10 = 39.2 \\
y_{.2..} \quad B &= 11.2 + 11.6 + 10.9 + 11.2 = 44.9 \\
y_{.3..} \quad C &= 8.7 + 8.7 + 9.0 + 9.5 = 35.9 \\
y_{.4..} \quad D &= 6.5 + 7.7 + 7.9 + 7.9 = 30.0
\end{aligned}
$$

Replicates (l):

$$
y_{...1} = \text{rep1} = 3.3 + 3.5 + 2.9 + 1.8 + 4.0 + 3.0 + 2.8 + 3.5 + 2.9
$$

$$
+ 2.4 + 3.3 + 3.5 + 2.6 + 3.5 + 3.7 + 3.2 = 49.9
$$

TABLE 29 Modified ANOVA Table

Source of variance	Sum of squares	Degrees of freedom	Mean square	F_C
Treatments	$\frac{1}{np}\sum_{j=1}^{p} y_{.j..}^2 - \frac{y_{....}^2}{N}$	$p-1$	$\frac{SS_{TREATMENT}}{p-1}$	$\frac{MS_{TREATMENT}}{MS_{ERROR}}$
Rows	$\frac{1}{np}\sum_{i=1}^{p} y_{i...}^2 - \frac{y_{....}^2}{N}$	$p-1$	$\frac{SS_{ROWS}}{p-1}$	
Columns	$\frac{1}{p}\sum_{l=1}^{n}\sum_{k=1}^{p} y_{..kl}^2 - \sum_{l=1}^{n}\frac{y_{...l}^2}{p^2}$	$n(p-1)$	$\frac{SS_{COLUMNS}}{n(p-1)}$	
Replicates	$\frac{1}{p^2}\sum_{l=1}^{n} y_{...l}^2 - \frac{y_{....}^2}{N}$	$(n-1)$	$\frac{SS_{REPLICATES}}{n-1}$	
Error	$SS_{TOTAL} - SS_{TREATMENT}$ $- SS_{ROW} - SS_{COLUMN}$ $- SS_{REPLICATES}$	$(p-1)(np-1)$	$\frac{SS_{ERROR}}{(p-1)(np-1)}$	
Total	$\sum_{i=1}^{p}\sum_{j=1}^{p}\sum_{k=1}^{p}\sum_{l=1}^{n} y_{ijkl}^2 - \frac{y_{....}^2}{N}$	$np^2 - 1$		

TABLE 30 ANOVA Data

Anatomical sample site	Subject Block(k)																$y_{i...}$
	1				2				3				4				
	Rep$=l=$	1	2	3	Rep$=l=$	1	2	3	Rep$=l=$	1	2	3	Rep$=l=$	1	2	3	
1	B	3.3	3.0	3.1	C	4.0	3.7	3.9	D	2.9	3.0	3.1	D	2.6	2.8	2.5	37.9
2	C	3.5	3.9	3.8	D	3.0	2.8	2.9	A	2.4	2.8	2.7	A	3.5	3.4	3.1	37.8
3	D	2.9	3.0	2.8	A	2.8	2.5	2.4	B	3.3	3.2	2.9	B	3.7	3.9	3.6	37.0
4	A	1.8	2.0	2.7	B	3.5	3.4	3.5	C	3.5	3.6	3.8	C	3.2	3.3	3.0	37.3
$y_{..kl}$		11.5	11.9	12.4		13.3	12.4	12.7		12.1	12.6	12.5		13.0	13.4	12.2	$150 = y_{....}$
		$y_{..11}$	$y_{..12}$	$y_{..13}$		$y_{..21}$	$y_{..22}$	$y_{..23}$		$y_{..31}$	$y_{..32}$	$y_{..33}$		$y_{..41}$	$y_{..42}$	$y_{..43}$	

$y_{..2} = \text{rep2} = 3.0 + 3.9 + 3.0 + 2.0 + 3.7 + 2.8 + 2.5 + 3.4 + 3.0 + 2.8 + 3.2 +$
$3.6 + 2.8 + 3.4 + 3.9 + 3.3 = 50.3$

$y_{..3} = \text{rep3} = 3.1 + 3.8 + 2.8 + 2.7 + 3.9 + 2.9 + 2.4 + 3.5 + 3.1 + 2.7 + 2.9 +$
$3.8 + 2.5 + 3.1 + 3.6 + 3.0 = 49.8$

$$SS_{ROW} = \frac{1}{np} \sum_{i=1}^{p} y_{i..}^2 - \frac{y_{....}^2}{N}$$

$$= \frac{1}{3(4)} (37.9^2 + 37.8^2 + 37.0^2 + 37.3^2) - \frac{150^2}{48}$$

$$= 468.795 - 468.750 = 0.045$$

$$SS_{TREATMENT} = \frac{1}{np} \sum_{j=1}^{p} y_{.j.}^2 - \frac{y_{....}^2}{N}$$

$$= \frac{1}{3(4)} (39.2^2 + 44.9^2 + 35.9^2 + 30.0^2) - \frac{150^2}{48}$$

$$= 478.455 - 468.750 = 9.705$$

$$SS_{REPLICATES} = \frac{1}{p^2} \sum_{i=1}^{n} y_{...l}^2 - \frac{y_{....}^2}{N}$$

$$= \frac{1}{4^2} (49.9^2 + 50.3^2 + 49.8^2) - 468.750$$

$$= 468.759 - 468.750$$

$$= 0.009$$

$$SS_{COLUMN} = \frac{1}{p} \sum_{l=1}^{n} \sum_{k=1}^{p} y_{..kl}^2 - \sum_{l=1}^{n} \frac{y_{...l}^2}{p^2}$$

$$= \frac{1}{4} (11.5^2 + 11.9^2 + 12.4^2 + 13.3^2 +$$

$$12.4^2 + 12.7^2 + 12.1^2 + 12.6^2 + 12.5^2 +$$

$$13.0^2 + 13.4^2 + 12.2^2) - \left(\frac{49.9^2}{4^2} + \frac{50.3^2}{4^2} + \frac{49.8^2}{4^2} \right)$$

$$= 469.595 - 468.759$$

$$= 0.836$$

$$SS_{TOTAL} = \sum_{i=1}^{p}\sum_{j=1}^{p}\sum_{k=1}^{p}\sum_{l=1}^{n} y_{ijkl}^2 - \frac{y_{....}^2}{N}$$

$$= (3.3^2 + 3.0^2 + 3.1^2 + 3.1^2 + 3.1^2 + \cdots + 3.2^2$$

$$+ 3.3^2 + 3.0^2) - \frac{150^2}{48}$$

$$= 480.600 - 468.750 = 11.850$$

$$SS_{ERROR} = SS_{TOTAL} - SS_{TREATMENT} - SS_{ROW} - SS_{COLUMN}$$

$$- SS_{REPLICATES}$$

$$= 11.850 - 9.705 - 0.045 - 0.836 - 0.009$$

$$= 1.255$$

Next we construct an ANOVA table (Table 31).
$F_{tabled} = F_{(\alpha(p-1;(p-1)(np-1))} = F_{(0.05,3,33)} = 2.92$
Because $F_c(85.13) > F_T (2.92)$, reject H_0, $\alpha = 0.05$.

Clearly, employing $n = 3$ replicates in this Latin square design was use-ful. None of the ratios, SS_{ROW}/SS_{ϵ}, $SS_{COLUMN}/SS_{\epsilon}$, $SS_{REPLICATES}/SS_{\epsilon}$, were large. In fact, none were greater than 1. In the next experiment of this type, the researcher can ignore anatomical site-to-site differences. They were not significantly different. The researcher can also ignore the subject-to-subject differences. This might be a little tricky because there are extreme subject-to-subject differences in weight, sex, health, and age. But in this study, it was not significant. The replication effect was minimal in that we probably could have detected a difference with these data using four subjects, but this also has the disadvantage of having too few degrees of freedom to detect differ-ences using only four individuals as we saw in the last situation.

TABLE 31   ANOVA

Source of variation	Sum of squares	Degrees of freedom	Mean square	F_C
$SS_{TREATMENT}$	9.705	3	3.235	$\frac{3.235}{0.038} = 85.13$
SS_{ROW}	0.045	3	0.015	
SS_{COLUMN}	0.836	9	0.093	
$SS_{REPLICATES}$	0.009	2	0.005	
SS_{ERROR}	1.255	33	0.038	
SS_{TOTAL}	11.850			

In future studies, if the researcher ignored the anatomical differences, it would be easier to conduct this study using a random block design, subjects being the blocks and products being the treatments. Latin square values need to be collected in random order, so that order needs to be randomly determined.

Concerning missing values, it is a difficult topic. Because there are so few degrees of freedom in a standard Latin square design and the design is more useful for pilot studies, I recommend collecting the data for the squares prior to stopping the test. If the value for the square is flawed, it can be rerandomized, with the remaining needed square observations to complete the study.

If the study, however, has been completed before a missing value can be rerun, it must be a judgment call in the experiment to collect a new value or estimate the missing value. I have had far better luck collecting a new value, even though that value may be unconsciously biased. I strongly prefer collecting data—even when a possible bias is involved—instead of computing a theoretical value. For the rerun biased data, a researcher can use field and research experience to help determine its reasonableness. That cannot be done with a theoretical data point.

However, if the researcher would like to compute a theoretical data value, the procedure is nearly identical to the randomized block design. For a $p \times p$ standard Latin square the y_{ijk} value is estimated:

$$y_{ijk} = \frac{p(y'_{i..} + y'_{.j.} + y'_{..k}) - 2y'_{...}}{(p-2)(p-1)}$$

where p = number of squares
   $y'_{i..}$ = row total containing the missing value
   $y'_{.j.}$ = treatment group j total with missing value
   $y'_{..k}$ = column total with missing value

Example 4:   Drawing on Table 15, a standard 4×4 Latin square is given in Table 32.

The value in row 2 ($y_{2..}$), column 3 ($y_{.3}$), and treatment D ($y_{.4.}$) is missing. To estimate that missing value:

$$p = 4$$

$$y'_{i..} = 7.650$$

$$y'_{..k} = 7.275$$

$$y'_{.4.} = D = 2.900 + 3.050 + 3.300 = 9.25$$

$$y'_{...} = 39.225$$

TABLE 32   **Standard 4 × 4 Latin Square Design**

	1	2	3	4	
1	$A=2.625$	$B=1.925$	$C=3.000$	$D=3.300$	10.850
2	$B=2.775$	$C=3.000$	$D=X^a$	$A=1.875$	$7.650=y'_{2..}$
3	$C=1.450$	$D=3.050$	$A=2.800$	$B=3.425$	10.725
4	$D=2.900$	$A=3.075$	$B=1.475$	$C=2.550$	10.000
		$y_{..k}=7.275$			$39.225=y'_{...}$

$^a X =$ missing value.

Let us now predict the missing value:

$$\hat{y}_{243} = \frac{4(7.650 + 9.25 + 7.275) - 2(39.225)}{(4-2)(4-1)} = \frac{18.25}{6}$$

$$= 3.042$$

The value estimated to put into the Latin square for value $y_{243} = 3.042$. Recall that for this estimate, one degree of freedom for the error term is lost. The degrees of freedom for SS_{ERROR} are then $(p-2)(p-1)-1$, or $(4-2)(4-1)-1=5$, which is not many degrees of freedom to work with.

TABLE 33   **Row and Column Formulas**

Source		Sum of squares	Degrees of freedom
Rows not replicated		$\frac{1}{np}\sum_{i=1}^{p} y_{i...}^2 - \frac{y_{....}^2}{N}$	$p-1$
Rows replicated		$\frac{1}{p}\sum_{i=1}^{p}\sum_{i=1}^{p} y_{i...l}^2 - \sum_{i=1}^{n}\frac{y_{....l}^2}{p^2}$	$n(p-1)$
Columns not replicated		$\frac{1}{np}\sum_{k=1}^{p} y_{..k.}^2 - \frac{y_{....}^2}{N}$	$p-1$
Columns replicated		$\frac{1}{p}\sum_{i=1}^{n}\sum_{k=1}^{p} y_{...kl}^2 - \sum_{i=1}^{n}\frac{y_{....l}^2}{p^2}$	$n(p-1)$
SS_{ERROR}	By subtraction as before	When column or row replicated	$(p-1)(np-1)$
		When both column and rows replicated	$(p-1)[n(p-1)-1]$

The repeated replicate Latin square design can be adapted quickly for cases where the rows and/or columns are the replicated values. In that case, the row and column formulas are presented in Table 33.

The same calculation as for Table 23 is used for the treatments, replicates, total sum of squares, degrees of freedom, and mean square error.

In cases where data are missing, I have had better performance with collecting new data points. In fact, it is a good idea to be prepared to address any missing data points as they become known throughout the course of the study. If the value is lost when remaining square values need to be collected, that value's run time should be randomized and the remaining observations collected. Again, the emphasis is on collecting data grounded in one's field, not on theoretically constructed values unless there are no other choices.

Finally, whatever course the researcher took, that information needs to be provided to the readers so that they can make their own determination concerning the data, their presentation, and their interpretation.

VIII. INDIVIDUAL TESTS

After the ANOVA analysis and a significant treatment effect are noted, the researcher will want to determine which treatment groups differ from one another.

The methods from Chap. 5 for a completely randomized design can be used for the Latin square ANOVA evaluation with a few adjustments.

1. Substitute p in place of n in the completely randomized design in Latin squares.
2. The number of degrees of freedom for the error term will be used for the degrees of freedom in finding confidence intervals, etc.
3. Individual confidence interval values will use p in place of n for nonreplicated Latin squares and pn for replicated ones.[*]

We have now discussed and applied some pretty advanced statistical procedures. In the next chapter we will expand our ANOVA to include two factors.

---

[*]The individual confidence intervals for each mean can be calculated from:

$\bar{y}_{j.} \pm t_{\alpha/2,(p-2)(p-1)}\sqrt{\frac{MSE}{p}}$ for nonreplicated Latin squares

$\bar{y}_{j.} \pm t_{\alpha/2,(p-1)(np-1)}\sqrt{\frac{MSE}{pn}}$ for one block / row replicated

$\bar{y}_{j.} \pm t_{\alpha/2,(p-1)[(np-1)-1]}\sqrt{\frac{MSE}{pn}}$ for both block/row replicated

7

Completely Randomized Two-Factor Factorial Designs

For the investigator, factorial designs provide a greater dimension to statistical analysis than has previously been discussed. In factorial designs, at least two variable factors are evaluated. Recall that, in Chap. 6, the discussion focused on one experimental factor, one experimental factor with blocking in one direction (complete block design), and one experimental factor with blocking in two directions (Latin square design).

The researcher may ask, why not just compare one factor at a time? For example, if one wanted to compare (1) an antimicrobial product's efficacy relative to the concentration of the antimicrobial in several formulas as well as (2) the length of handwashing time, one could evaluate the concentration effects in one ANOVA and then evaluate the length of handwashing time in another ANOVA. However, any interaction affecting the product's efficacy related to both concentration and application time will probably not be discovered. This can present a major problem. Hence, the main advantage of a two-factor design over separate one-factor designs is detection of such interactions, when present.

In a two-factor design, the two factors are termed *main effects*. If one has factors A and B (application time $= A$ and antimicrobial concentration $= B$), these are the main effects. The selection of which effect is A or B is arbitrary and makes no difference. In general, the concept of comparison is quite simple. Suppose we have two factors, A and B, both having two levels, high and low. Figure 1 presents a display of this.

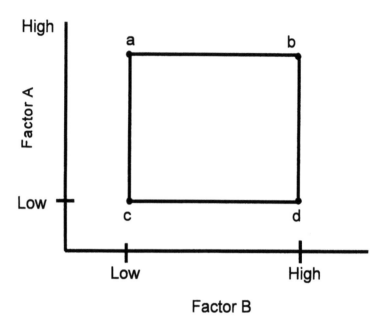

FIGURE 1   Display of high and low levels for factors A and B.

The high level for factor B is the average of $(b + d)/2$.
The low level average of factor B is $(a + c)/2$.
The average main effect of factor B is $\bar{B} = (b + d)/2 - (a + c)/2$.
The high-level average of factor A is $(a + b)/2$.
The low-level average of factor A is $(c + d)/2$.
The average main effect of factor A is $\bar{A} = (a + b)/2 - (c + d)/2$.

Let us now refine our view of a two-factor factorial. Suppose factor A is the length of application, 60 seconds and 30 seconds, and factor B is the antimicrobial concentration levels, high (20%) and low (5%).

Both factors A and B—the main effects—are independent variables. That is, factor A by itself does not influence factor B. But often, when products are applied in tandem, they have additive effects on the response variable (dependent variable), the microbial population (on $\log_{10}$ scale). Figure 2 portrays this.

As can be seen from Fig. 2, the antimicrobial properties and application times both determine the microbial populations that remain after treatment. The higher the concentration of the antimicrobial compound and the longer the application, the lower the microbial counts. When both the high concentration of antimicrobial compound and the longer time of application

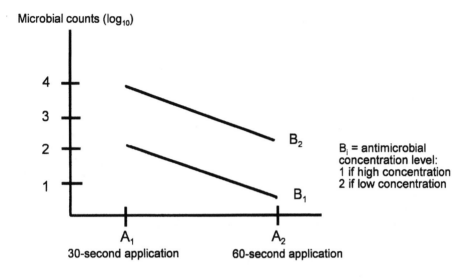

FIGURE 2   Independent variables' effects on response variable.

are used, the lowest microbial counts result. Clearly B_1 is more effective than B_2.

Notice that the shapes of B_1 and B_2 are parallel, or additive. That is, the change in efficacy from B_2 to B_1 is by a constant amount.

However, suppose that after using the products, the data in Fig. 2 were not observed, but instead the data in Fig. 3 were observed. Now we cannot discuss both main effects as one factor being better than another. Now we have *interaction* of the main effects. That is, we must take into consideration both main effects relative to each other. For example, B_2 is more effective than B_1 when applied for 30 seconds but less effective when applied for 60 seconds. Efficacy depends upon which time of application is used at what antimicrobial concentration. When interaction of main effects is present, main effects cannot be evaluated by themselves. They must be evaluated with respect to the other main effect.

The subject of interaction is a key advantage in using factorial designs. The interaction is often missed when an experimenter compares main effects one at a time—for example, using a one-factor ANOVA model for antimicrobial concentration and another for product application. In addition, significant interaction often masks the main effects. For example, consider the case in Fig. 4. Here we see that at factor A_1, B_1 is less effective than B_2. However, at

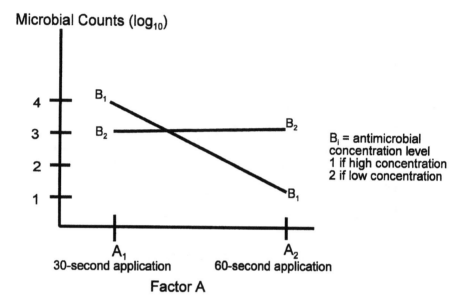

FIGURE 3   Interaction of main effects.

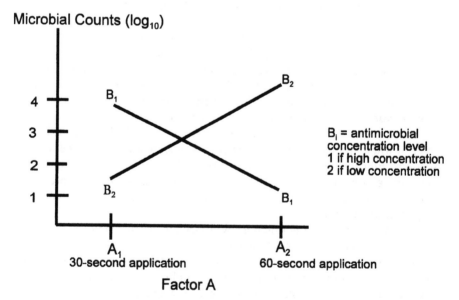

FIGURE 4   Factors *A* and *B* cancel each other out.

factor A_2, B_2 is less effective—by approximately the same amount B_1 was at factor A_1. The effects are clearly significant, but as main effects, factor A and factor B cancel each other out. Again, this interaction component can be discovered in factorial designs but will be missed in "one factor at a time" designs.

Other advantages of factorial designs include the following:

1. They are more experimental-unit efficient than one factor at a time.
2. They utilize the data more effectively than one-factor-at-a-time procedures.
3. As the factors increase beyond two, the points in one and two are more pronounced.

The use of factorial experimental designs is extremely important to the applied researcher. In pilot or small-scale studies where multiple independent values are used, an understanding of the principle is critically important. Probably the most versatile is the two-factor factorial model with various levels within each factor. Also, the concept of replication of each treatment at each level is very important.

A three-factor factorial design is also useful at times, but it is complex and more difficult to understand, not from a computation perspective but from one of data relevance and application. Any design beyond a three-factor factorial has little value in applied research conditions.

A linear regression model can be used to compute all factorial designs using dummy variables. However, this book uses an analysis of variance perspective, and the results are the same. Factorial or analysis of variance designs have qualitative independent variables. Regression generally has quantitative values for the independent variables but, with the adoption of dummy variables, can be designed to utilize qualitative variables.

I. TWO-FACTOR ANALYSIS OF VARIANCE (ALSO KNOWN AS A TWO-WAY ANALYSIS OF VARIANCE)

A. Fixed Effects

In the two-factor ANOVA model, there are two main effect variables, A and B, the interaction of the main effects, $A+B$, and the random error ε, all of which are measured.

The model is written as:

$$y_{ijk} = \mu + A_i + B_j + (AB)_{ij} + \epsilon_{ijk}$$

where y_{ijk} = the value of the ith A factor, the jth B factor, the ijth interaction factor, and the kth replicate within the treatments A and B

μ = the common mean

$A_i =$ the ith treatment in factor A

$B_j =$ the jth level in factor B

$(AB)_{ij} =$ the interaction between factors A and B

$\epsilon_{ijk} =$ the random error

B. Randomization

The randomization scheme of this model is important and is a completely randomized design. Suppose one is designing a study with two factors, A and B, factor A at three levels and factor B at two levels with two replicates per level (Table 1).

There are $a \times b \times n$ or $3 \times 2 \times 2 = 12$ observations. This design is also referred to as a 3×2 factorial design having three rows and two columns. The sampling order, as just stated, is completely random. That is, each y_{ijk} is as likely to be collected at any particular time as any other y_{ijk}. This is an extremely important restriction of this two-factor ANOVA design.

Let us now compare the one-factor completely randomized ANOVA, the complete block one-factor ANOVA, and the two-factor ANOVA, based upon the sum-of-squares computation.

Notice in Fig. 5A that the total sum of squares can be partitioned into the sum of squares treatment ($SS_{TREATMENT}$) and sum of squares error (SS_{ERROR}). Hence the model is additive. That is,

$$SS_{TOTAL} = SS_{TREATMENT} + SS_{ERROR}$$

Notice in Fig. 5B that the randomized block design is similar to the completely randomized design except that the error sum of squares (SS_E) is

TABLE 1   Two Factors at Three Levels with Two Replicates

		Factor B	
		1	2
Factor A	1	y_{111}	y_{121}
		y_{112}	y_{122}
	2	y_{211}	y_{221}
		y_{212}	y_{222}
	3	y_{311}	y_{321}
		y_{312}	y_{322}

Number of levels of $A = a = 3$.

Number of levels of $B = b = 2$.

Number of replicates per level $= n = 2$.

$y_{ijk} =$ the individual measurement observation, where $i =$ factor A (row effect), $j =$ factor B (column effect), $k =$ replicates 1, 2, and on to "n" (i.e., $k = 1, 2, \ldots, n$).

Completely Randomized One-Factor ANOVA

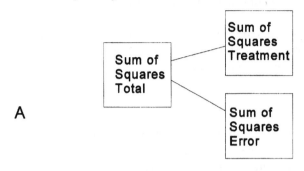

A

Complete Block Design

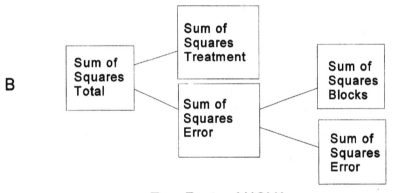

B

Two-Factor ANOVA

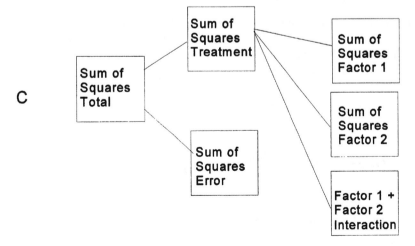

C

FIGURE 5   ANOVA designs.

further partitioned into SS$_{BLOCKS}$ and SS$_{ERROR}$. This makes the complete block design more efficient statistically (i.e., more powerful), for the random error is minimized.

Figure 5C portrays the two-factor ANOVA design. Notice that the treatment sum of squares is partitioned into both factors A and B and interaction between the factor components.

C. Hypotheses

There are three testable hypotheses in the two-factor factorial design. The first two ask whether there is a treatment effect. If yes, the treatment effect is not equal to zero. If no, the treatment effect is equal to zero. The third hypothesis asks whether there is an interaction between factors A and B. If not, the interaction effect is equal to zero.

1. Factor A $H_0: A_1 = A_2 = \cdots = A_a = 0$
             H_A: At least one $A_i \neq 0$
2. Factor B $H_0: B_1 = B_2 = \cdots = B_b = 0$
             H_A: At least one $B_j \neq 0$
3. Factor $A+B$ $H_0: (AB)_{ij} = 0$
     Interaction $H_A: (AB)_{ij} \neq 0$

Note: The hypothesis statement can just as easily be written as previously shown (i.e., factor A, H_0: $\mu_1 = \mu_2 = \cdots = \mu_a$ and factor B, $\mu_1 = \mu_2 = \cdots = \mu_b$).

D. Notation and Formula

Treatment A consists of the $y_{i..}$ values, $i = 1, 2, \ldots a$. Treatment B consists of the $y_{.j.}$ values, $j = 1, 2, \ldots b$. The interaction of treatments is $A + B = y_{ij.}$. The total value for the sum of the y_{ijk}s is designated $y_{....}$

The total model is written:

$$\text{Treatment } A: y_{i..} = \sum_{j=1}^{b} \sum_{k=1}^{n} y_{ijk}, \qquad \bar{y}_{i..} = \frac{y_{i..}}{bn}$$

$$\text{Treatment } B: y_{.j.} = \sum_{i=1}^{a} \sum_{k=1}^{n} y_{ijk}, \qquad \bar{y}_{.j.} = \frac{y_{.j.}}{an}$$

$$AB \text{ interaction}: y_{ij.} = \sum_{k=1}^{n} y_{ijk}, \qquad \bar{y}_{ij.} = \frac{y_{ij.}}{n}$$

$$\text{Total: } y\ldots = \sum_{i=1}^{a}\sum_{j=1}^{b}\sum_{k=1}^{n} y_{ijk}, \qquad \bar{y}\ldots = \frac{y\ldots}{abn}$$

$$SS_{TOTAL} = SS_{FACTOR\ A} + SS_{FACTOR\ B} + SS_{AB} + SS_{ERROR}$$

E. Degrees of Freedom

The degrees of freedom components for this model are presented in Table 2. The expected mean squares are:

$$E(MS_A)=E\left(\tfrac{SS_A}{a-1}\right)= \underbrace{\sigma^2}_{\substack{\text{Random} \\ \text{error} \\ \text{component}}} + \underbrace{\frac{bn\sum_{i=1}^{a} A_i^2}{a-1}}_{\substack{\text{Treatment } A \\ \text{effect}}} \tag{1}$$

$$E(MS_B)=E\left(\tfrac{SS_B}{b-1}\right)= \underbrace{\sigma^2}_{\substack{\text{Random} \\ \text{error} \\ \text{component}}} + \underbrace{\frac{an\sum_{j=1}^{b} B_j^2}{b-1}}_{\substack{\text{Treatment } B \\ \text{effect}}} \tag{2}$$

$$E(MS_{AB})=E\left(\frac{SS_{AB}}{(a-1)(b-1)}\right)= \underbrace{\sigma^2}_{\substack{\text{Random} \\ \text{error} \\ \text{component}}} + \underbrace{\frac{n\sum_{i=1}^{a}\sum_{j=1}^{b}(AB)_{ij}^2}{(a-1)(b-1)}}_{\substack{AB \text{ interaction} \\ \text{effect}}} \tag{3}$$

$$E(MS_E) = E\left(\frac{SS_E}{ab(n-1)}\right) = \underbrace{\sigma^2}_{\substack{\text{Random error} \\ \text{component}}} \tag{4}$$

TABLE 2. Degrees of Freedom

Effect	Degrees of freedom
Treatment A	$a-1$
Treatment B	$b-1$
$A \times B$ interaction	$(a-1)(b-1)$
Error	$ab(n-1)$
Total	$abn-1$

Notice that when the treatment or interaction effect is zero, the expected mean square is merely the random error (σ^2) component. The F_C tests for each main effect and the interaction are presented in Table 3.

F. Two-Factor ANOVA Analysis Strategy

For the researcher, the two-factor experimental design offers an advantage of detecting interaction between the two main effect factors, A and B. From a research perspective, interaction means that one cannot state unequivocally that one treatment is different from another. They differ in specific amounts but relative to the specific levels measured in each factor. Let me give you an example.

Say the researcher wants to compare two wash times (factor A), 1 minute and 2 minutes (Fig. 6). The researcher also wants to compare a handwash with bare hands only (no sponge brush) and with the use of a sponge brush. By plotting factor B in terms of $\log_{10}$ microbial counts remaining on the hands following the wash procedure versus wash times (factor A), the researcher can see graphically that interaction is present (nonparallel line). But so what?

The researcher now knows that factor A cannot be discussed with factor B without discussing the individual levels within each factor. She or he cannot say the use of a sponge brush in washing is more effective in reducing the microbial populations residing on the hands than is the nonsponge wash. Because interaction is present, statements must be conditional. The sponge and wash are equivalent at a 1-minute wash, but the sponge is better at 2 minutes than a barehand wash procedure in reducing microbial populations on the hands.

TABLE 3.   ANOVA Table for Two-Factor, ANOVA Fixed Model

Source of variance	Sum of squares	Degrees of freedom	Mean square	F_c	F_{tabled}
Treatment A	SS_A	$a-1$	$\frac{SS_A}{a-1} = MS_A$	$\frac{MS_A}{MS_E}$	$F_{\alpha[(a-1),ab(n-1)]}$
Treatment B	SS_B	$b-1$	$\frac{SS_B}{b-1} = MS_B$	$\frac{MS_B}{MS_E}$	$F_{\alpha[(b-1),ab(n-1)]}$
$A \times B$ interaction	SS_{AB}	$(a-1)(b-1)$	$\frac{SS_{AB}}{(a-1)(b-1)} = MS_{AB}$	$\frac{MS_{AB}}{MS_E}$	$F_{\alpha[(a-1)(b-1),ab(n-1)]}$
Error	SS_E	$ab(n-1)$	$\frac{SS_E}{ab(n-1)} = MS_E$		
Total	SS_T	$abn-1$			

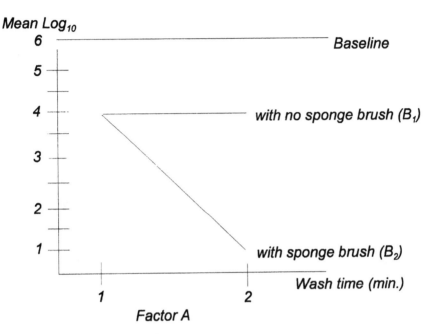

FIGURE 6   Treatment interaction.

Because of this situation, it makes no sense to perform a hypothesis test of the main effects when interaction is present. Hence, from a practical standpoint, when performing the hypothesis test, perform the interaction test first. If it is significant, there is no need to perform the main effects tests. However, it is important that one create a graphic display, such as Fig. 6, to see the interaction clearly.

Let us look at a similar model when no interaction is present (Fig. 7).

Notice, as depicted by parallel factor B lines on the two A time points, that the interaction is not significant. Here, the main effects are significant as blanket statements. One can state that factor B_1 (the use of the bristle brush) is more effective in reducing the microorganisms residing on the hands than a sponge brush wash (factor B_2) at both levels of factor A.

In summary, perform the interaction test first.

$H_0: (AB)_{ij} = 0$

$H_A: (AB)_{ij} \neq 0$

If the null hypothesis is rejected, one cannot, without restriction, test the two main effects, factors A and B. It is this researcher's practice not even

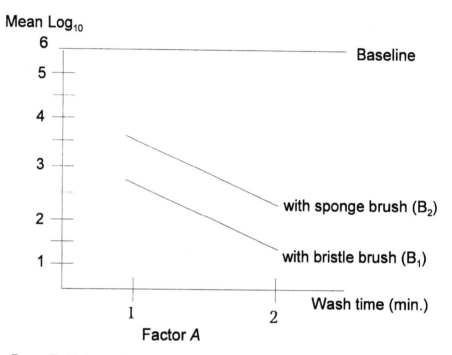

FIGURE 7   No interaction between treatments.

to test the main effects hypotheses because they are meaningless as independent tests. Instead, interpret what the data present by graphing the interaction, not just stating that the interaction hypothesis is significant at α.

G. Manual Computing Formulas

$$SS_{TOTAL} = \sum_{i=1}^{a}\sum_{j=1}^{b}\sum_{k=1}^{n} y_{ijk}^2 - \frac{y_{...}^2}{abn} \tag{5}$$

$$SS_A = \frac{1}{bn}\sum_{i=1}^{a} y_{i..}^2 - \frac{y_{...}^2}{abn} \tag{6}$$

$$SS_B = \frac{1}{an}\sum_{j=1}^{b} y_{.j.}^2 - \frac{y_{...}^2}{abn} \tag{7}$$

$$SS_{AB'} = \frac{1}{n}\sum_{i=1}^{a}\sum_{j=1}^{b}y_{ij.}^2 - \frac{y_{...}^2}{abn} \qquad \text{Step 1}$$

(8)

$$SS_{AB} = SS_{AB'} - SS_A - SS_B \qquad \text{Step 2}$$

$$SS_{ERROR} = SS_{TOTAL} - SS_{AB} - SS_A - SS_B \qquad (9)$$

Let us look at an example.

Example 1: Suppose a researcher has developed three different moisturizing lotion prototypes and wishes to evaluate how effective they are in maintaining skin moisture. The better the skin holds the moisture, the more intact the skin is. The total moisture content of the skin is measured in terms of electrical resistance in this design. The more resistance (the larger the number), the greater the amount of moisture held by the skin and the greater degree of moisturization. The researcher will use 48 human subjects in this study. There will be three different treatments comprising the moisture factor and two categories for the sex-of-subject factor. This design, then, has $3 \times 2 = 6$ categories, each replicated with eight subjects. The treatment assignments of 48 subjects are completely randomized, but the sex categories of male and female are predetermined. In actuality, males and females are not randomly assigned a sex category. They are, however, completely randomized in the run order of the study (Table 4).

Let us use the six-step procedure to test this example.

Step 1. Formulate the hypothesis.
$$y_{ijk} = \mu + A_i + B_j + (AB)_{ij} + \epsilon_{ijk}$$

Let rows be factor A, or sex; let columns be factor B, or moisturizing product.

Factor A: H_0: $\mu_{1.} = \mu_{2.}$ (females $=$ males in moisturization levels after treatment)

H_A: $\mu_{1.} \neq \mu_{2.}$ (females $\neq$ males in moisturization levels after treatment)

Factor B: H_0: $\mu_{1.} = \mu_{2.} = \mu_{3.}$ (moisturizer 1 $=$ moisturizer 2 $=$ moisturizer 3 in ability to moisturize the skin)

H_A: At least one of the moisturizers is different from the other two

Interaction: H_0: There is no significant interaction between factors A and B; $(AB)_{ij} = 0$

H_A: The above is not true; $(AB)_{ij} \neq 0$.

TABLE 4. Example 1 Data

		Moisturizers		
		1	2	3
Sex	Male	8 subjects	8 subjects	8 subjects
	Female	8 subjects	8 subjects	8 subjects

Step 2. In this case, the researcher assigned $\alpha = 0.05$ for each hypothesis

n = number of replicates = 8
a = number of categories of factor A = 2
b = number of categories of factor B = 3

Step 3. Identify the hypothesis test formula. There are three:

Treatment A: $\frac{MS_A}{MS_E} = F_C$. If $F_C > F_{tabled}$, reject H_0.

Treatment B: $\frac{MS_B}{MS_E} = F_C$. If $F_C > F_{tabled}$, reject H_0.

Interaction: $\frac{MS_{AB}}{MS_E} = F_C$. If $F_C > F_{tabled}$, reject H_0.

In this evaluation, the first F_C value calculated will be the interaction. If it is significant, the main effects need not be evaluated.

Step 4. Identify the tabled critical values at $\alpha = 0.05$.

Treatment A: $F_{T,\alpha,(a-1),ab(n-1)} = F_{T,0.05,(1,42)=4.08}$. If $F_C > 4.08$, reject H_0 at $\alpha = 0.05$.

Treatment B: $F_{T,\alpha,(b-1),ab(n-1)} = F_{T,0.05,(2,42)=3.23}$. If $F_C > 3.23$, reject H_0 at $\alpha = 0.05$.

Interaction: $F_{T,\alpha,(a-1)(b-1),ab(n-1)} = F_{T,0.05,(2,42)=3.23}$. If $F_C > 3.23$, reject H_0 at $\alpha = 0.05$.

Step 5. The next step is to conduct the study. In this study, skin moisturization measurements are conducted one individual at a time, using a completely randomized order. This has been conducted, and Table 5 presents the resultant data.

Once the data have been collected, the researcher should perform an EDA to become intimate with the data. Given that the researcher finds the data to be normal, etc., the actual ANOVA computation can be made (Table 6).

$$SS_A = \frac{1}{bn} \sum_{i=1}^{a} y_{i..}^2 - \frac{y_{...}^2}{abn}$$

$$= \frac{1}{3 \cdot 8}(744^2 + 618^2) - \frac{1362^2}{2 \cdot 3 \times 8} = 330.75$$

$$SS_B = \frac{1}{an} \sum_{j=1}^{b} y_{.j.}^2 - \frac{y_{...}^2}{abn}$$

$$= \frac{1}{2 \cdot 8}(372^2 + 436^2 + 554^2) - \frac{1362^2}{48} = 1065.50$$

$$SS_{AB'} = \frac{1}{n} \sum_{i=1}^{a} \sum_{j=1}^{b} y_{ij.}^2 - \frac{y_{...}^2}{abn}$$

$$= \frac{1}{8}(197^2 + 219^2 + 328^2 + 175^2 + 217^2 + 226^2) - \frac{1362^2}{48}$$

$$= 1746.25$$

$$SS_{AB} = SS_{AB'} - SS_A - SS_B$$

$$= 1746.25 - 330.75 - 1065.50 = 350.00$$

$$SS_{TOTAL} = \sum_{i=1}^{a} \sum_{j=1}^{b} \sum_{k=1}^{n} y_{ijk}^2 - \frac{y_{...}^2}{abn}$$

$$= (32^2 + 27^2 + 22^2 + 19^2 + 28^2 + 23^2 + 25^2 + 21^2 + \cdots$$

$$+ 26^2 + 30^2 + 32^2 + 29^2) - \frac{1362^2}{48}$$

$$= 41,014.00 - \frac{1362^2}{48}$$

$$SS_{TOTAL} = 2367.25$$

$$SS_{ERROR} = SS_{TOTAL} - SS_{AB} - SS_A - SS_B$$

$$= 2367.25 - 350.00 - 1065.50 - 330.75$$

$$SS_{ERROR} = 621.00$$

TABLE 5 Resultant Data of Example 1

y_{ij}, where $j = 1$ if group 1, 2 if group 2, 3 if group 3

Factor A — Sex $y_{i..}$	Factor B moisturizers 1		Factor B moisturizers 2		Factor B moisturizers 3		Total
1 if female	32	28	26	28	36	46	
	27	23	33	31	47	39	
	22	25	27	24	42	43	
	19	21	25	25	35	40	
	$y_{11.} = 197$		$y_{12.} = 219$		$y_{13.} = 328$		$y_{1..} = 744$
2 if male	18	16	25	27	24	26	
	22	19	32	31	27	30	
	20	24	26	27	33	32	
	25	31	24	25	25	29	
	$y_{21.} = 175$		$y_{22.} = 217$		$y_{23.} = 226$		$y_{2..} = 618$
$y_{.j.}$	372		436		554		1362
							$y_{...}$

TABLE 6.   ANOVA Table for Example 1

Source	Sum of squares	Degrees of freedom	Mean square	F_c	S = Significant NS = not significant
Factor A (sex)	330.75	1	330.75	22.369	S
Factor B (moisturization)	1065.50	2	532.75	36.021	S
Interaction A × B	350.00	2	175.00	11.832	S
Error	621.00	42	14.79		
Total	2367.25	48			

Interaction:
   H_0: Interaction between the main effects $= 0$; $(AB)_{ij} = 0$
   H_A: The above is not true; $(AB)_{ij} \neq 0$
   Because $F_C(11.832) > F_T(3.23)$, reject H_0.
Interaction between the main effects is significant. The next step is to
   graph the interaction effect, which appears in Fig. 8.
$\bar{y}_{ij.}$ = individual cell means of electrical resistance graphed in Fig. 8
$\bar{y}_{11.} = 197/8 = 24.63$
$\bar{y}_{12.} = 219/8 = 27.38$
$\bar{y}_{13.} = 328/8 = 41.00$
$\bar{y}_{21.} = 175/8 = 21.88$
$\bar{y}_{22.} = 217/8 = 27.13$
$\bar{y}_{23.} = 226/8 = 28.25$
Step 6.   Once we see that interaction between the main effects is present, we need to be careful in making blanket statements concerning
   the main effects.

The interaction is between sex and product 3. That is, product 3 is a
much better moisturizer (higher skin resistance means greater moisture-
holding ability) than products 1 or 2 when used with female subjects. Product
3, when used by males, is less dramatically effective than when used by
females. Products 1 and 2, on the other hand, appear to have no interaction
between them, providing roughly the same results (electrical resistance
readings) when used by males or females. In practice, one can still make
sense of the other two products, 1 and 2, relative to the sex factor from the
main effects tests.

   Let us evaluate the main factor effects, even though we know, from the
interaction, that blanket statements concerning the main effects (factors A
and B) for product 3 and sex cannot be made.

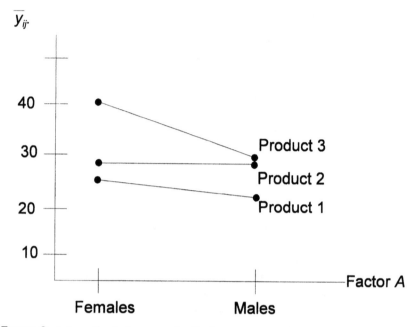

FIGURE 8   Interaction between main effects.

Factor A: H_0: Moisturization for females = moisturization for males
$\quad\quad\quad H_A$: The above is not true.
Clearly $F_C(22.369) > F_T(4.08)$, so the gender effect is significant at the $\alpha = 0.05$ level, but conditional.
Factor B: H_0: Product 1 = product 2 = product 3
$\quad\quad\quad H_A$: At least one product is different.
Clearly $F_C(36.021) > F_T(3.23)$, so the product effect is significant at $\alpha = 0.05$, but conditional.
I find that computing the main factor effects after interaction effects can be useful in explaining an experiment to nonstatisticians, given that the interaction is also discussed. But I find it even more useful to provide an explanation for the occurrence of the interaction component and then to follow up with certain treatment level comparisons, not all, to uncover differences between treatment levels, aside from the interaction.

H.   Multiple Comparisons

When the ANOVA model detects a difference between levels of main effect A and/or within levels of main effect B, comparisons can be made in a number of ways to determine which treatment within the main effects differs. The methods introduced in Chap. 5 and expanded in Chap. 6 can also be used for two-factor designs.

I. Orthogonal Testing

As discussed previously, a major benefit of the two-factor design is the ability to identify *interaction*. If interaction is detected, comparing levels within a main effect is useful but must be considered in light of the interaction. It is valuable to compute certain factor level differences to identify treatment level differences that are not interaction effects but valuable to the interpretation of data. We will compute all for demonstration purposes.

   Factor A. Looking at Example 1, where $a = 2$, we see that $a-1 = 2-1$ provides one degree of freedom for factor A and, therefore, only one contrast. But it is unnecessary to do that contrast because there were only two levels in factor A: male and female. They were significantly different.

   Factor B. There are two degrees of freedom for factor B $(b-1)$, so two orthogonal contrasts can be made.

   Factor B level totals are (from Table 5):

   Moisturizer $1 = y_{.1.} = 372$
   Moisturizer $2 = y_{.2.} = 436$
   Moisturizer $3 = y_{.3.} = 554$

   Let us make the following hypotheses and contrasts:

Hypothesis	Contrasts
$H_{01}: 2\mu_1 = \mu_2 + \mu_3$	$C_1 = 2y_{.1.} - y_{.2.} - y_{.3.}$
$H_{02}: \mu_2 = \mu_3$	$C_2 = -y_{.2.} + y_{.3.}$

So:

$$C_1 = 2(372) - (436) - (554) = -246$$
$$C_2 = -(436) + (554) = 118$$

The sum of squares contrast formula we have used before:

$$SS_C = \frac{\left(\sum_{j=1}^{b} c_j y_{.j.}\right)^2}{n \sum_{j=1}^{b} c_j^2}$$

Note that, because the sex factor is ignored, 8 males plus 8 females gives $n = 16$.

$$SS_{C_1} = \frac{(-246)^2}{16(2^2 + (-1)^2 + (-1)^2)} = 630.375$$

$$SS_{C_2} = \frac{118^2}{16(-1^2 + 1^2)} = 435.125$$

Rearranging the ANOVA table (Table 6), for factor B only, we construct Table 7.

Note that in Table 7, the orthogonal contrasts for factor B could have been different from those chosen, but only two can be computed because only two degrees of freedom are available ($b - 1 = 3 - 1 = 2$). These two were significant; that is, the H_0 hypothesis would be rejected at $\alpha = 0.05$.

J. Interaction

In cases such as this, where the interaction term is significant, the experimenter can set one of the factors, say factor B (moisturizer), to one of its levels and compare that level with the levels of factor A. For example, one could set factor B at product 2 and compare it for females and males. Currently, we will ignore this option as a viable orthogonal contrast procedure, for the chance of ever knowing what level of one main effect to set for comparisons of the levels of other main effects, a priori (prior to conducting the experiment), is essentially zero. But we will come back to this option later.

TABLE 7. ANOVA Table for Factor B Only

Source	Sum of squares	Degrees of freedom	Mean square	F_c	F_T[a]	S = significant NS = not significant[b]
Factor A (sex)	—	—	—	—	—	—
Factor B (moisturization)	1065.50	2	532.750	36.031	—	—
$C_1(2\mu_1 = \mu_2 + \mu_3)$	630.375	1	630.375	42.633[c]	4.08	S
$C_2(\mu_2 = \mu_3)$	435.125	1	435.125	29.428	4.08	S
Error	621	42	14.786			
Total	2752.0	46				

[a]F_T for the two contrasts is found in Table C, the F distribution table.
[b]The test statistic for these two contrasts is $F_{T(\alpha,1;ab(n-1))} = F_{T,(0.05,1;42)} = 4.08$. If $F_c > F_T$, reject H_0 at $\alpha = 0.05$.
[c]$42.633 = 630.375/14.786$.

When interaction is discovered, it is usually after the experiment has been conducted, so orthogonal contrasts are not applicable.

K. Bonferroni Procedure

The Bonferroni procedure can be used for pairwise comparisons if the comparisons desired are selected a priori [26]. The procedure is more effective (i.e., has greater statistical power) when only a few pairwise contrasts are made. It is important, however, to ensure that interaction between the main effects is not significant before one compares levels within main effects A and B, as we discussed previously.

Let us perform the Bonferroni procedure.

Factor A: Again, it is usually not useful to evaluate main effects when interaction is significant. Because there are only two levels of factor A, it is not necessary to compare them. Because the factor A effect was significant, the two levels within factor A are significantly different at the specified α level. If factor A was not significant, according to the F-test, the two levels would not be different from each other at the specified α level, so no contrasts would be necessary.

Factor B: In comparing levels of factor B, let us suppose the researcher wants to make three comparisons chosen *prior* to conducting the study. They are:

1. $H_0: \mu_1 = \mu_2$ or $\bar{y}_{.1.} - \bar{y}_{.2.}$
2. $H_0: \mu_1 = \mu_3$ or $\bar{y}_{.1.} - \bar{y}_{.3.}$
3. $H_0: \mu_2 = \mu_3$ or $\bar{y}_{.2.} - \bar{y}_{.3.}$

The test statistic to use in this procedure is precisely the one we used in both Chaps. 5 and 6.

$$t' = \frac{D}{S_D}, \quad \text{where } D = \left| \bar{y}_{.i.} - \bar{y}_{.j.} \right|$$

$$S_D = \sqrt{\frac{2\text{MSE}}{an}}$$

Decision rule: If $t' > t_{(\alpha/2g; ab(n-1))}$ (where g = number of contrasts), a significant difference exists between the pairs at α. Hence,

$$S_D = \sqrt{\frac{2\text{MSE}}{an}} = \sqrt{\frac{2(14.786)}{16}} = 1.36$$

$$t_1 = |\bar{y}_{.1.} - \bar{y}_{.2.}| = 23.250 - 27.250 = |-4| = 4$$

$$t_2 = |\bar{y}_{.1.} - \bar{y}_{.3.}| = 23.250 - 34.625 = |-11.375| = 11.375$$

$$t_3 = |\bar{y}_{.2.} - \bar{y}_{.3.}| = 27.250 - 34.625 = |-7.375| = 7.375$$

$t_{\alpha/2g;ab(n-1)}$ and $\alpha = 0.05, g = 3$, and $ab(n-1) = 42; t_{0.008(42)} = 2.80$

$$t_1 = \frac{D_1}{S_D} = \frac{4}{1.360} = 2.941 > 2.80 \quad \therefore \text{significant difference exists}$$

between $y_{.1.}$ and $y_{.2.}$ at $\alpha = 0.05$

$$t_2 = \frac{D_2}{S_D} = \frac{11.375}{1.360} = 8.364 > 2.80 \quad \therefore \text{significant difference exists}$$

between $y_{.1.}$ and $y_{.3.}$ at $\alpha = 0.05$

$$t_3 = \frac{D_3}{S_D} = \frac{7.375}{1.360} = 5.423 > 2.80 \quad \therefore \text{significant difference exists}$$

between $y_{.2.}$ and $y_{.3.}$ at $\alpha = 0.05$

L. Multiple Contrasts to Use After the Experiment Has been Run

In two-factor experiments, a posteriori contrasts are much more common than a priori ones because of the complication of the design.

M. Main Effects

If interaction is not significant and if the main effects are the relative variations within main effects, factors A and B can be compared. The procedures are identical to those used in Chaps. 5 and 6.

N. Interaction of the Main Effects

If significant interaction is present, the researcher can set a fixed level of a main effect and compare all or some of the other levels with each other. For example, one can set one level of A and compare all or some of the levels of B with each other. Or, one can compare the cell totals $(y_{ij.})$ that make up both main effects, A and B. As an example, using data from Table 5, this procedure will be demonstrated. Within each of the six cells are the eight replicated sums for both factors A and B. What is required, then, is to determine the sum value of each of the $y_{ij.}$ cells (Table 8).

TABLE 8. Sum Values Table

| Factor A (sex) | Factor B (moisturizer) | | | $y_{i..}$ |
	1 = Product 1	2 = Product 2	3 = Product 3	
1 = female	$y_{11.} = 197$	$y_{12.} = 219$	$y_{13.} = 328$	744
2 = male	$y_{21.} = 175$	$y_{22.} = 217$	$y_{23.} = 226$	618
$y_{.j.}$	372	436	554	$y_{...} = 1362$

Here the various $y_{ij.}$ totals can be compared with one another for differences between them. This procedure can be very useful to the experimenter, even when significant interaction is present.

Let us, however, begin with the main effect factor B to demonstrate how the computations are done. As before, there must be more than two levels of factor A or B for this to be useful. The researcher would then, as in Chaps. 5 and 6, perform the contrast procedure on both factors A and B, using two separate models, one for the row totals (factor A) and the other for column totals (factor B).

In our example, only factor B had greater than two levels, so only it will be compared. For factor A, we know already that the two levels, males and females, were significantly different at $\alpha = 0.05$.

Let us begin analysis of factor B using the Scheffe method, which is suitable for level comparisons a posteriori (after the experiment has been conducted).

O. Scheffe's Method

Recall that the Scheffe method can be used for comparing a number of different level contrasts but should not be used when comparing all the levels of a main effect with one another. Type I (α) error will be, at most, α for all of the level comparisons done. Most commonly, the mean levels of specific groups are compared from both main effects A and B.

The standard error of the contrast for factors A and B has the form:

$$S_C = \sqrt{MS_E \sum (c^2/n)} \tag{10}$$

where c is the number of hypothesized contrasts. The specific form for factor A is:

$$S_C = \sqrt{MS_E \sum_{i=1}^{a} \left(\frac{c_i^2}{n_i} \right)}$$

The specific form for factor B is:

$$S_C = \sqrt{MS_E \sum_{j=1}^{b} \left(\frac{c_j^2}{n_j}\right)}$$

For both factors A and B, the contrast has the form:

$$M = C_1\mu_1 + C_2\mu_2 + \cdots + C_m\mu_m$$

where M is the total number of contrasts. In practice, the $C_j = C_1\bar{y}_{.1.} + C_2\bar{y}_{.2.} + \cdots + C_b\bar{y}_{.b.}$ sample means ($\bar{y}$) are used in place of the population means (μ). The critical value to which C_j is evaluated in factor B is:

$$S_{\alpha_j} = S_{C_j}\sqrt{(b-1)F_{\alpha(b-1);(ab(n-1))}} \qquad (11)$$

The F value is found in Table A.3.

   Decision rule:
   If $|C_j| > S_{\alpha_j}$, reject H_0 hypothesis.
   Recall that

$$y_{.1.} = 372, \qquad \bar{y}_{.1.} = \frac{372}{16} = 23.250$$

$$y_{.2.} = 436, \qquad \bar{y}_{.2.} = \frac{436}{16} = 27.250$$

$$y_{.3.} = 554, \qquad \bar{y}_{.3.} = \frac{554}{16} = 34.625$$

Suppose the researcher wants to evaluate the following contrasts:

$$H_0: \mu_{.i.} = \mu_{.j.}$$

$$H_A: \mu_{.i.} \neq \mu_{.j.}$$

Three contrasts are possible:

1. $H_0: \bar{y}_{.1.} = \bar{y}_{.2.}; C_1 = \bar{y}_{.1.} - \bar{y}_{.2.} = 23.250 - 27.25.0 = -4.000$
2. $H_0: \bar{y}_{.2.} = \bar{y}_{.3.}; C_2 = \bar{y}_{.2.} - \bar{y}_{.3.} = 27.250 - 34.625 = -7.375$
3. $H_0: \bar{y}_{.1.} = \bar{y}_{.3.}; C_3 = \bar{y}_{.1.} - \bar{y}_{.3.} = 23.250 - 34.625 = -11.375$

$$S_{C_1} = \sqrt{14.786(1^2 + (-1)^2/16)} = 1.360$$

$$S_{C_2} = \sqrt{14.786(1^2 + (-1)^2/16)} = 1.360$$

$$S_{C_3} = \sqrt{14.786(1^2 + (-1)^2/16)} = 1.360$$

---

*To compare $\bar{y}_{i..}$ or the A treatment group, the S_α formula is $S_{\alpha_i} = S_{C_i}\sqrt{(a-1)F_{\alpha(a-1);(ab(n-1))}}$.

Let us set $\alpha = 0.05$:

$$S_{0.05,1} = S_{C_1}\sqrt{(b-1)F_{0.05,(b-1),ab(n-1)}}$$

$$F_{0.05,2,42} = 3.23 \quad \text{(from Table A.3)}$$

Therefore:

$$S_{0.05,1} = 1.360\sqrt{2(3.23)} = 3.457$$

$$S_{0.05,2} = 1.360\sqrt{2(3.23)} = 3.457$$

$$S_{0.05,3} = 1.360\sqrt{2(3.23)} = 3.457$$

If $|C_i| > S_{\alpha,i}$, the H_0 hypothesis is rejected at $\alpha = 0.05$.

$|C_1| = 4.00 > 3.457$; Reject H_0: $\mu_{.1} = \mu_{.2}$ at $\alpha = 0.05$
$|C_3| = 11.375 > 3.457$; Reject H_0: $\mu_{.1} = \mu_{.3}$ at $\alpha = 0.05$
$|C_2| = 7.375 > 3.457$; Reject H_0: $\mu_{.2} = \mu_{.3}$ at $\alpha = 0.05$

Note: In practice, comparing all possible pairs of means can be done with the Scheffe method, but this is generally not the most statistically efficient approach. It is more useful in these cases to use the least significant difference (LSD), Duncan's multiple range test, the Newman–Keuls test, or Tukey's test. However, Scheffe's test provides the researcher with more power and flexibility in comparing complex contrasts such as H_0: $\mu_1 + \mu_2 = \mu_3 + \mu_4$ or H_0: $3\mu_1 = \mu_2 + \mu_3 + \mu_4$.

P. Least Significant Difference (LSD)

Let us now look at a procedure designed to compare all possible combinations of means—the LSD procedure. Many statisticians recommend not using the LSD contrast method when the number of contrasts exceeds three because it can let type I error be much larger than the stated α level [21,23,24]. Nevertheless, it remains a commonly used test.

The LSD procedure is another contrast method to be used *after* the study has been conducted. Again, in contrasting row or column means (i.e., factor levels A or B) when interaction is present, the experimenter must be very careful. In all honesty, it would be better to compare the $\bar{y}_{ij}$ values, a combination of both A and B treatments, which is a procedure I shall discuss shortly. But for demonstration purposes, we shall continue contrasting levels within each of the main effect factors.

As before, the methods demonstrated in Chap. 5 hold for the two-factor factorial design. The computation of the LSD method is the same for the levels within the main effects except that one substitutes B for A and A for B. Because there are only two treatment levels in factor A, we already know from the ANOVA (Table 6) that the two levels within factor A (males and females) are significantly different.

The LSD method is used to compare each possible combination of mean pairs, μ_i and μ_j.

For unbalanced designs, $n_i \neq n_j$, the test is simply:

Factor A $\quad$ $\text{LSD} = t_{\alpha/2, ab(n-1)} \sqrt{MS_E \left(\dfrac{1}{an_i} + \dfrac{1}{an_i} \right)}$ $\qquad$ (12)

Factor B $\quad$ $\text{LSD} = t_{\alpha/2, ab(n-1)} \sqrt{MS_E \left(\dfrac{1}{bn_j} + \dfrac{1}{bn_j} \right)}$ $\qquad$ (13)

For balanced designs, $n_i = n_j$:

Factor A $\quad$ $\text{LSD} = t_{\alpha/2, ab(n-1)} \sqrt{\dfrac{2MS_E}{an}}$ $\qquad$ (14)

Factor B $\quad$ $\text{LSD} = t_{\alpha/2, ab(n-1)} \sqrt{\dfrac{2MS_E}{bn}}$ $\qquad$ (15)

The test contrast statistic is, if $|\bar{y}_i - \bar{y}_j| > \text{LSD}$, reject H_0 at α.

Let us work Example 1 for factor B:

$\bar{y}_{j.} = \bar{y}_{.1.} = 23.25$ $\qquad$ $\text{LSD} = t_{(0.05/2, 42)} \sqrt{\dfrac{2(14.786)}{16}}$

$\bar{y}_{.2.} = 27.50$ $\qquad$ and

$\qquad\qquad\qquad\qquad$ $\text{LSD} = (2.021) \sqrt{\dfrac{2(14.786)}{16}}$

$\bar{y}_{.3.} = 34.63$

$\qquad\qquad\qquad\qquad$ $\text{LSD} = 2.75$

The $b(b-1)/2 = 3 \times 2/2 = 3$ combinations possible are:

$$\text{LSD}$$

$\bar{y}_{.1.} - \bar{y}_{.2.} = |23.25 - 27.25| = 4.00 > 2.75$, significant

$\bar{y}_{.1.} - \bar{y}_{.3.} = |23.25 - 34.63| = 11.38 > 2.75$, significant

$\bar{y}_{.2.} - \bar{y}_{.3.} = |27.25 - 34.63| = 7.38 > 2.75$, significant

Hence, μ_1, μ_2, and μ_3 are significantly different from each other at $\alpha = 0.05$.

As one can see, the LSD method for the completely randomized two-factor factorial design is essentially the same as for the one-factor ANOVA except that there are two main effect factors, A and B, with which to contend.

If main effect A was more than two levels, the contrast analysis would be the same except that row means, instead of column means, would be used and a would be substituted for b.

Q. Duncan's Multiple Range Test

Duncan's multiple range test is also very useful in evaluating two-factor factorial designs. Contrasts can be performed on factor A's treatment level averages and factor B's treatment level averages. However, before doing this, the researcher will want to be assured that no significant two-way interaction is present.

In this example, because main effect A consisted of only two levels, the ANOVA table already determined that they were significantly different from one another. Hence, we will turn immediately to main effect B.

One first arranges the b treatment values in ascending order. In addition, the standard error of each factor is computed. When the sample sizes are equal, the formula is:

$$S_{\bar{y}_{j.}} = \sqrt{\frac{MS_E}{an}} \quad \text{(balanced)} \tag{16}$$

and when the sample sizes are not equal (unbalanced), one uses Eq. (16), replacing n with n', where:

$$n' = \frac{a}{\sum\limits_{i=1}^{a} (1/n_i)} \quad \text{(unbalanced correction factor)}$$

Note: For main effect A, the same basic formulas apply:

$$S_{\bar{y}_{i..}} = \sqrt{\frac{MS_E}{bn}} \quad \text{(balanced)}$$

and

$$n' = \frac{b}{\sum\limits_{j=1}^{b} (1/n_j)} \quad \text{(unbalanced correction factor)}$$

Recall that, for the $\bar{y}_{j.}$ value of factor B, we saw $\bar{y}_{.1.} = 23.250, \bar{y}_{.2.} = 27.250,$ and $\bar{y}_{.3.} = 34.625$, and these are already in ascending order.

For all three treatments: $S_{\bar{y}_{j.}} = \sqrt{\frac{MS_E}{16}} = \sqrt{\frac{14.786}{16}} = 0.961$

From Duncan's multiple range Table (Table A.5), one obtains the values of $r_\alpha(p, f)$ for $p = 2, 3, \ldots, b$. The α is 0.05, and $f =$ degrees of freedom for error term $ab(n - 1) = 42$.

This is followed by converting the ranges in a set of $b - 1$ ($a - 1$ if main effect A) least significant ranges for $p = 1, 2, \ldots, b$. The least significant range calculation is:

$$R_P = r_{\alpha(p,f)} S_{\bar{y}_{j.}} \quad \text{for } p = 2, 3, \ldots, b^*$$

The observed differences between the means are then tested, beginning with comparing the largest and the smallest, versus R_b (or R_a). Next, the largest is compared with the second smallest versus the $R_{(b-1)}$ (or $R_{(a-1)}$) value. The process is then continued until the differences of all possible $b(b - 1)/2$ pairs [or $a(a - 1)/2$] have been evaluated. If the observed pair difference is greater than the R_b (or R_a) value, the pair is significantly different at α.

No difference between a pair of means is considered significant if the values of two means involved lie between the values of a pair of means that are not significantly different.

For $R_2, r_{0.05(2,42)} = 2.86$ For $R_3 = r_{0.05(3,42)} = 3.01$

$R_2 = 2.86(0.961) = 2.748$ $R_3 = 3.01(0.961) = 2.893$

$$\text{Number of contrasts} = \frac{b(b - 1)}{2} = \frac{3(2)}{2} = 3 \text{ contrasts}$$

3 vs. $1 = 34.625 - 23.250 = 11.375 > 2.893 \, (R_3), \quad \text{significant}$

3 vs. $2 = 34.625 - 27.250 = 7.375 > 2.748 \, (R_2), \quad \text{significant}$

2 vs. $1 = 27.250 - 23.250 = 4.000 > 2.748 \, (R_2), \quad \text{significant}$

Hence, from Duncan's multiple range test, the researcher concludes that the three means are significantly different from one another at $\alpha = 0.05$.

Duncan's multiple range test requires greater differences between means to be significant as the number of contrasts increases. It is a relatively sensitive test, however, when only a few contrasts are calculated, as in this case.

R. Newman–Keuls Test

The application of this test is straightforward. Again, if the interaction is not significant, the test can be used for both factor levels A and B directly, but when significant interaction is present, the researcher should be very careful in interpreting significant results.

As before (Chaps. 5 and 6), the researcher calculates a set of specific critical values.

---

*For treatment A, the R_p value is computed as:
$R_P = r_{\alpha;(p,f)} S_{\bar{y}_{i.}} \quad \text{for } p = 2, 3, \ldots, a$

$$K_P = q_{\alpha(p,f)}S_{\bar{y}} \tag{17}$$

For factor A, the formula is:

$$K_P = q_{\alpha(p,f)}S_{\bar{y}_{i..}} \qquad p = 2, 3, \ldots, a, \ f = \text{df error term (MS}_E)$$

For factor B, the formula is:

$$K_P = q_{\alpha(p,f)}S_{\bar{y}_{.j.}} \qquad p = 2, 3, \ldots, b, \ f = \text{df error term (MS}_E)$$

Recall that factor A has only two values and, because a significant difference has already been demonstrated at $\alpha = 0.05$, there is no need to retest.

For factor B, the actual comparison is done in a way similar to the Duncan multiple range test.

The researcher's first computes:

$$K_P = q_{\alpha(p,f)}S_{\bar{y}_{.j.}}$$

where

$S_{\bar{y}_{.j.}} = \sqrt{\dfrac{\text{MS}_E}{an}}$ for, balanced designs

Note: For factor A, in balanced designs, use $S_{\bar{y}_{i..}} = \sqrt{\text{MS}_E/bn}$.

In cases where n values are different (unbalanced designs), substitute n' for n, where $n' = a/\sum_{i=1}^{a}(1/n_i)$.

Note: For factor A, in unbalanced designs, use $n' = b/\sum_{j=1}^{b}(1/n_j)$.

In our example for factor B: $S_{\bar{y}_{.j.}} = \sqrt{14.786/16} = 0.961$.

Next, arrange the $\bar{y}_{.j.}$ values (for a, the $\bar{y}_{i..}$) in ascending order:

$\bar{y}_{.1.} = 23.250$

$\bar{y}_{.2.} = 27.250$

$\bar{y}_{.3.} = 34.625$

For this example, $p = 2$ and 3, so $q_{\alpha(p,f)} = q_{(0.05)(2,42)} = 2.86$ and $q_{\alpha(p,f)} = q_{(0.05)(3,42)} = 3.44$.

Hence, where $K_p = q_{\alpha(p,f)}S_{\bar{y}_{.j.}}$, $K_2 = 2.86(0.961) = 2.748$, and $K_3 = 3.44(0.961) = 3.306$. The three possible treatment contrasts are:

3 vs. 1 $= 34.625 - 23.250 = 11.375 > 3.306$, ($K_p$), significant

3 vs. 2 $= 34.625 - 27.250 = 7.375 > 2.748$, ($K_p$), significant

2 vs. 1 $= 27.250 - 23.250 = 4.000 > 2.748$, ($K_p$), significant

Again, we see that each mean, $\bar{y}_{j.}$, is significantly different from every other mean at $\alpha = 0.05$.

S. Tukey Test

The Tukey contrast procedure for contrasting all mean level pairs for a two-factor factorial design, again, is straightforward. The requirement for main effect interaction (factors A and B) to be not significant remains important. When interaction is significant, as before, one cannot describe factor A and factor B effects independently.

As in Chaps. 5 and 6, the Tukey test considers any mean level pair difference (absolute) greater than T_α significant at α.

Recall:

$$T_\alpha = q_{\alpha(a,f)}S_{\bar{y}_{i.}} \qquad \text{for treatment } A \tag{18}$$

and

$$T_\alpha = q_{\alpha(b,f)}S_{\bar{y}_{j.}} \qquad \text{for treatment } B \tag{19}$$

All $a(a-1)/2$ or $b(b-1)/2$ mean level pairs are compared.

Again, for factor A, where $a = 2$, the two mean levels possible to compare were already determined significantly different at α via the main effect F-test, so no additional testing is necessary.

For factor B, $T_\alpha = q_{\alpha(b,f)}S_{\bar{y}_{j.}}$, where $b =$ number of levels of Factor B ($B = 3$), and $f =$ degrees of freedom for error term $= ab(n-1)$, the denominator for the Studentized range statistic table (Table L).

$$q_{\alpha(b,f)} = q_{0.05(3,42)} = 3.44$$

$$S_{\bar{y}_{j.}} = \sqrt{\frac{MS_E}{an}} = \sqrt{\frac{14.786}{16}} = 0.961$$

$$S_{\bar{y}_{j.}} = 0.961$$

$$T_\alpha = 3.44(0.961) = 3.306$$

Note: For factor A, the computation of $S_{\bar{y}_{i.}}$ is:

$$\sqrt{\frac{MS_E}{bn}}$$

Decision rule: If $\left| \bar{y}_{i.} - \bar{y}_{j.} \right| > T_\alpha$ reject H_0, that the mean pairs are equivalent at α.

For factor B, there are $b(b-1)/2 = 3(2)/2 = 3$ pairwise contrasts. They are:

3 vs. 1 $= |34.625 - 23.250| = 11.375 > 3.306$, significant

3 vs. 2 $= |34.625 - 27.250| = 7.375 > 3.306$, significant

2 vs. 1 $= |27.250 - 23.250| = 4.000 > 3.306$, significant

Hence, the three contrasts are significantly different at $\alpha = 0.05$.

T. Dunnett's Method (Test Versus Control Comparisons)

Recall from Chaps. 5 and 6 that Dunnett's contrast method is useful when one compares several treatment levels with one control. As before, it can be used effectively for both factors A and B, given that there is no significant interaction between the main effects. Otherwise, it should not be used or used only with extreme caution. We will perform the computation only for demonstration purposes because we did not designate a control prior to testing. And, as before, we will ignore factor A, for there are only two levels.

For factor B, let $\bar{y}_{.1.}$ = the control product. Then the researcher can test $b - 1$ contrasts ($a - 1$ for treatment A, given $a > 2$). The contrasts for our example involve $b - 1 = 3 - 1 = 2$ contrasts. They are:

$\bar{y}_{.2.} - \bar{y}_{.1.}$

$\bar{y}_{.3.} - \bar{y}_{.1.}$

The test contrast hypothesis is:

$H_0 : \mu_{.j.} = \mu_c$, where μ_c = mean for control level group estimated by $\bar{y}_{.1.}$

$H_A : \mu_{.j.} \neq \mu_c$

The Dunnett test, as in Chaps. 5 and 6, is straightforward:

$$\left| \bar{y}_{.i.} - \bar{y}_{.j.} \right| > d_{\alpha(b-1,f)}\sqrt{\frac{2MS_E}{an}} \quad \text{if balanced design } (n_i = n_j) \qquad (20)$$

$$\left| \bar{y}_{.i.} - \bar{y}_{.j.} \right| > d_{\alpha(b-1,f)}\sqrt{MS_E\left(\frac{1}{an_i} + \frac{1}{an_j}\right)} \quad \text{if unbalanced design } (n_i \neq n_j)$$

$$(21)$$

Note: In comparing factor A, the formulas are identical except that b is used instead of a in the denominator.

Using Example 1, again for factor B:

$\bar{y}_{.c.} = \bar{y}_{.1.} = 23.250$ is the control product

$\bar{y}_{.2.} = 27.250$

$\bar{y}_{.3.} = 34.625$

$MS_E = 14.786$

$n_1 = n_2 = n_3$,   so this experiment is balanced

$\left| \bar{y}_{.2.} - \bar{y}_{.1.} \right| = 27.250 - 23.250 = 4.000$

$\left| \bar{y}_{.3.} - \bar{y}_{.1.} \right| = 34.625 - 23.250 = 11.375$

$\sqrt{\dfrac{2MS_E}{an}} = \sqrt{\dfrac{2(14.786)}{16}} = 1.360$

$d_{\alpha(b-1,f)} = d_{(0.05)(2,42)} = 2.29$, from Dunnett's Table (Table A.13).

So,

$d_{\alpha(b-1,f)} \sqrt{\dfrac{2MS_E}{an}} = 2.29(1.360) = 3.114$

The contrast H_A decisions are:

If $\left| \bar{y}_{.j.} - \bar{y}_c \right| > 3.114$, reject H_0 at $\alpha = 0.05$, where $\bar{y}_{.j.} = \bar{y}_{.2.},\ \bar{y}_{.3.}$, and $\bar{y}_{.c.} = \bar{y}_{.1.}$
Because $\left| \bar{y}_{.2.} - \bar{y}_{.1.} \right| = 4.000 > 3.114$, reject H_0 at $\alpha = 0.05$
Because $\left| \bar{y}_{.3.} - \bar{y}_{.1.} \right| = 11.374 > 3.114$, reject H_0 at $\alpha = 0.05$

Both test group levels are significantly different from the control at $\alpha = 0.05$.

U. Comparing Factor A and B Combined Levels

Given that interaction is significant, it is often useful to compare factor $A \times B$ combination levels. Using Example 1, those combinations are as displayed in Table 9. From Table 5, we previously computed the factor $A \times B$ cell totals in Table 10.

The main difference between comparing the main effects $A \times B$ combination levels, as opposed to factor A or B levels, is that cell values are $y_{ij.}$, not $y_{i..}$ or $y_{.j.}$. The factor $A \times B$ comparisons of cell means can be very useful when interaction is present.

TABLE 9. Factor $A \times B$ Combinations

		Factor B—product formulations		
		1	2	3
Factor A	1 = female	A_1B_1 or C_{11}	A_1B_2 or C_{12}	A_1B_3 or C_{13}
	2 = male	A_2B_1 or C_{21}	A_2B_2 or C_{22}	A_2B_3 or C_{23}

For cell$_{ij}$, where i = row and j = column, cell$_{11}$ is the row 1, column 1 combination value, for example.

V. Orthogonal Contrasts (A Priori Selection of Contrasts)

From an applied perspective, the probability of knowing in advance which factor $A \times B$ combination levels to compare is very low, so we will not spend time computing these. However, both orthogonal linear combinations and the Bonferroni procedure can be used.

The main aspects are that:

The degrees of freedom for each contrast are 1, as described in earlier chapters.

The degrees of freedom for the error term are, as before, $ab(n-1)$.

The possible $A \times B$ combination levels to evaluate can become large very quickly because they are based on two effects, not just one, using the formula $(ab(ab-1)/2)$. In the present example (Example 1), this would be

$$\left(\frac{2 \times 3(2 \times 3 - 1)}{2} = 15 \right)$$

TABLE 10. Factor $A \times B$ Level Combinations

		Factor B — Product Formulations			
		1	2	3	$y_{i..}$
Factor A	1 = Female	$y_{11.} = 197$ $n = 8$	$y_{12.} = 219$ $n = 8$	$y_{13.} = 328$ $n = 8$	744
	2 = Male	$y_{21.} = 175$ $n = 8$	$y_{22.} = 217$ $n = 8$	$y_{23.} = 226$ $n = 8$	618
	$y_{.j.}$	372	436	554	$1362 = y$

The total degrees available for contrasts using the interaction degrees of freedom $= (a - 1)(b - 1) = (2 - 1)(3 - 1) = 2$. The Bonferroni procedure is useful only if the number of contrasts, g, is kept low because it balloons the interval width as the number of contrasts increases, making the test essentially useless.

In my opinion, it is really not useful, then, to compare factor $A \times B$ combination levels using the a priori orthogonal procedure.

W. A × B Contrasts Determined A Posteriori

Let us work through the interaction contrasts that can be used effectively by the researcher after the experiment has been conducted and interaction between the main effects factors A and B has been discovered.

1. Scheffe's Method

The Scheffe method can be used for $A \times B$ comparisons of means, but comparing all possible pairs of $A \times B$ means is not that statistically efficient with this method. Other "pairwise" tests should be used instead, such as the Newman–Keuls procedure.

We have already discussed the Scheffe method for contrasting levels within factor A or B. However, when $A \times B$ interaction is significant, the researcher will want to compare $A \times B$ means with one another. Looking at the C_{ij} mean values from Table 10, we have the following:

$$\frac{C_{ij}^*}{n} = \frac{A_1 B_1}{n} = \bar{y}_{11} = \frac{197}{8} = 24.625$$

$$\frac{A_1 B_2}{n} = \bar{y}_{12} = \frac{219}{8} = 27.375$$

$$\frac{A_1 B_3}{n} = \bar{y}_{13} = \frac{328}{8} = 41.000$$

$$\frac{A_2 B_1}{n} = \bar{y}_{21} = \frac{175}{8} = 21.875$$

$$\frac{A_2 B_2}{n} = \bar{y}_{22} = \frac{217}{8} = 27.125$$

$$\frac{A_2 B_3}{n} = \bar{y}_{23} = \frac{226}{8} = 28.250$$

---

*C_{ij} = Contrast pairs where $i = A$ and $j = B$.

The Scheffe procedure is best used for few, but more complicated contrasts. Suppose the researcher wants to perform two contrasts, C_1 and C_2.

Contrast 1: $H_0: \mu_{11.} - \mu_{12.} = 0$

$$H_A: \mu_{11.} - \mu_{12.} \neq 0$$

and a more complex contrast:
Contrast 2: Does $\mu_{11.} + \mu_{12.} + \mu_{13.} = \mu_{21.} + \mu_{22.} + \mu_{23.}$?
Or written as a test hypothesis,

$$H_0: \mu_{11.} + \mu_{12.} + \mu_{13.} - \mu_{21.} - \mu_{22.} - \mu_{23.} = 0$$

$$H_A: \mu_{11.} + \mu_{12.} + \mu_{13.} - \mu_{21.} - \mu_{22.} - \mu_{23.} \neq 0$$

Recall the critical value with which C_{ij} is compared:

$$S_{\alpha_i} = S_{c_i}\sqrt{(a-1)(b-1)F_{\alpha,(a-1)(b-1);ab(n-1)}}$$

where $S_{c_i} = \sqrt{MS_E\left(\sum c_{ij}^2/n\right)}$. The decision rule is:

If $|C_i| > S_{\alpha_i}$, reject H_0
So,

$$C_1 = |24.625 - 27.375| = |-2.750| = 2.750$$
$$C_2 = |24.625 + 27.375 + 41.000 - 21.875 - 27.125 - 28.250|$$
$$= 15.75$$

$$S_{c_1} = \sqrt{14.786\left(\frac{1^2 + (-1)^2}{8}\right)} = 1.923$$

$$S_{c_2} = \sqrt{14.786\left(\frac{1^2 + 1^2 + 1^2 + (-1)^2 + (-1)^2 + (-1)^2}{8}\right)} = 3.330$$

$C_1: H_0: \mu_{11.} - \mu_{12.} = 0$

$\qquad H_A: \mu_{11.} - \mu_{12.} \neq 0 \qquad \alpha = 0.05$

$$S_{\alpha_1} = S_{c_1}\sqrt{(a-1)(b-1), F_{0.05,(a-1)(b-1);ab(n-1))}}$$

$$= F_{(0.05,12;42)}. \text{ From Table A.3, } F = 3.23$$

$$S_{\alpha_1} = 1.923\sqrt{2(3.23)} = 4.888$$

Because $|C_1| = 2.750| < 4.888$, one cannot reject the H_0 hypothesis at $\alpha = 0.05$.

C_2: H_0: $\mu_{11.} + \mu_{12.} + \mu_{13.} - \mu_{21.} - \mu_{22.} - \mu_{23.} = 0$

H_A: $\mu_{11.} + \mu_{12.} + \mu_{13.} - \mu_{21.} - \mu_{22.} - \mu_{23.} \neq 0$ $\alpha = 0.05$

$S_{\alpha_2} = S_{c_1}\sqrt{(a-1)(b-1)}, F_{(0.05,(a-1)(b-1);ab(n-1))}$

$F_{(0.05,2;42)} = 3.23$

$S_{\alpha_2} = 3.330\sqrt{2(3.23)} = 8.464$

Because $|C_2 = (15.702)| > 8.464$, reject the H_0 hypothesis at $\alpha = 0.05$.

2. Least Significant Differencoe (LSD)

The least significant difference procedure is a most useful test when $A \times B$ interaction is significant and all possible pairwise comparisons of $\bar{y}_{ij.}$ means are desired. The total number of $A \times B$ $\bar{y}_{ij.}$ contrasts is:

$$\frac{ab(ab-1)}{2} \quad \text{or} \quad \frac{3 \times 2(3 \times 2 - 1)}{2} = 15$$

Recall that the LSD value is:

$$\text{LSD} = t_{(\alpha/2),ab(n-1)}\sqrt{\text{MS}_E\left(\frac{1}{n_{lk.}} + \frac{1}{n_{kl.}}\right)} \quad \text{for an unbalanced design, and}$$

(22)

$$\text{LSD} = t_{(\alpha/2),ab(n-1)}\sqrt{\frac{2\text{MS}_E}{n}} \quad \text{for a balanced design} \quad (23)$$

The test hypothesis is:

H_0: $\bar{y}_{lk.} - \bar{y}_{kl.} = 0$

H_A: $\bar{y}_{lk.} - \bar{y}_{kl.} \neq 0$

The decision rule is:
If

$$\left|\bar{y}_{lk.} - \bar{y}_{kl.}\right| > t_{(\alpha/2),ab(n-1)}\sqrt{\text{MS}_E\left(\frac{1}{n_{lk.}} + \frac{1}{n_{kl.}}\right)} \quad (24a)$$

for an unbalanced design

$$\left|\bar{y}_{lk.} - \bar{y}_{kl.}\right| > t_{(\alpha/2),ab(n-1)}\sqrt{\frac{2\text{MS}_E}{n}} \quad (24b)$$

for a balanced design, the H_0 hypothesis is rejected at α.

For our example, $\alpha = 0.05$. The design is balanced so:

$$\sqrt{\frac{2MS_E}{n}} = \sqrt{\frac{2(14.786)}{8}} = 1.923 \quad \text{and} \quad t_{(\alpha/2,ab(n-1))} = t_{(0.025,42)} = 2.021$$

$$LSD = t_{(\alpha/2,42)}\sqrt{\frac{2MS_E}{n}} = (2.021)(1.923) = 3.886$$

So, if $|\bar{y}_{lk.} - \bar{y}_{kl.}| > 3.886$, reject H_0 at $\alpha = 0.05$.

The 15 test combinations are as follows:

	S = significant NS = not significant
$\|\bar{y}_{11.} - \bar{y}_{12.}\| = 24.63 - 27.38 = 2.750 < 3.886$	NS
$\|\bar{y}_{11.} - \bar{y}_{13.}\| = 24.63 - 41.00 = 16.370 > 3.886$	S
$\|\bar{y}_{11.} - \bar{y}_{21.}\| = 24.63 - 21.88 = 2.750 < 3.886$	NS
$\|\bar{y}_{11.} - \bar{y}_{22.}\| = 24.63 - 27.13 = 2.500 < 3.886$	NS
$\|\bar{y}_{11.} - \bar{y}_{23.}\| = 24.63 - 28.25 = 3.620 < 3.886$	NS
$\|\bar{y}_{12.} - \bar{y}_{13.}\| = 27.38 - 41.00 = 13.620 > 3.886$	S
$\|\bar{y}_{12.} - \bar{y}_{21.}\| = 27.38 - 21.88 = 5.500 > 3.886$	S
$\|\bar{y}_{12.} - \bar{y}_{22.}\| = 27.38 - 27.13 = 0.250 < 3.886$	NS
$\|\bar{y}_{12.} - \bar{y}_{23.}\| = 27.38 - 28.25 = 0.875 < 3.886$	NS
$\|\bar{y}_{13.} - \bar{y}_{21.}\| = 41.00 - 21.88 = 19.120 > 3.886$	S
$\|\bar{y}_{13.} - \bar{y}_{22.}\| = 41.00 - 27.13 = 13.870 > 3.886$	S
$\|\bar{y}_{13.} - \bar{y}_{23.}\| = 41.00 - 28.25 = 12.750 > 3.886$	S
$\|\bar{y}_{21.} - \bar{y}_{22.}\| = 21.88 - 27.13 = 5.250 > 3.886$	S
$\|\bar{y}_{21.} - \bar{y}_{23.}\| = 21.88 - 28.25 = 6.370 > 3.886$	S
$\|\bar{y}_{22.} - \bar{y}_{23.}\| = 27.13 - 28.25 = 1.120 < 3.886$	NS

X. Using Approximate Confidence Intervals for the $\bar{y}_{ij.}$ Values

The value $\bar{y}_{13.}$ is different from all others, being the largest value; $\bar{y}_{23.}$ and $\bar{y}_{12.}$ are equivalent because their values overlap, based on all possible contrasts performed. Also, $\bar{y}_{12.}$ and $\bar{y}_{11.}$ are equivalent. Finally, $\bar{y}_{11.}$ and $\bar{y}_{21.}$ are equivalent.

Recall that as the number of contrasts increases, so doest type I error (rejecting a true H_0 hypothesis). So it is critical that the experimenter use his or her field knowledge to help determine the reliability of the pair-wise tests.

$y_{13.}$	(41)				
$y_{23.}$		(28.25)			
$y_{12.}$			(27.38)		
$y_{22.}$			(27.13)		
$y_{11.}$			(24.63)		
$y_{21.}$				(21.88)	

FIGURE 9A   Approximate confidence intervals: LSD test.

1. Duncan's Multiple Range Test for Interaction

As encountered previously, Duncan's multiple range test is useful for comparing all pairs of $\bar{y}_{ij.}$ means, whether the design is balanced or not. The procedure is like those we have done previously.

First, the $\bar{y}_{ij.}$ means are ranked in ascending order and the standard error of the mean is computed as:

$$S_{\bar{y}_{ij.}} = \sqrt{\frac{MS_E}{n}} \quad \text{for a balanced design} \tag{25a}$$

For an unbalanced design, the sample cell size, n, is replaced with

$$n' = \frac{(a-1)(b-1)}{\sum\limits_{j=1}^{b}\sum\limits_{i=1}^{a}(1/n_{ij})} \tag{25b}$$

The hypothesis used for each pairwise contrast is:

$$H_0: \mu_{lk.} - \mu_{kl.} = 0$$
$$H_A: \mu_{lk.} - \mu_{kl.} \neq 0$$

Decision rule:

If $(\bar{y}_{lk.} - \bar{y}_{kl.}) > r_{\alpha(p,f)}S_{\bar{y}_{lk.}}$, reject H_0 at α.

The computational procedure is very similar to that of the previous example when we were dealing with the main effects factors A and B, but now we compare combinations of $A \times B$ means, $\bar{y}_{lk.}$.

The means are first arranged in ascending order. Because this is a balanced design, the standard error of the mean is computed using Eq. (25a).

Combination		$A \times B$ mean		Value
A_2B_2	=	$\bar{y}_{21\cdot}$	=	**21.875**
A_1B_1	=	$\bar{y}_{11\cdot}$	=	**24.625**
A_2B_2	=	$\bar{y}_{22\cdot}$	=	**27.125**
A_1B_2	=	$\bar{y}_{12\cdot}$	=	**27.375**
A_2B_3	=	$\bar{y}_{23\cdot}$	=	**28.250**
A_1B_3	=	$\bar{y}_{13\cdot}$	=	**41.000**

$$S_{\bar{y}_{ij\cdot}} = \sqrt{\frac{14.786}{8}} = 1.360 \qquad (25a)$$

Let us set $\alpha = 0.01$. As before:

$$R_P = r_{\alpha(p,f)} S^*_{\bar{y}_{ij\cdot}}$$
$$p = 2, 3 \ldots, (a \cdot b) \text{ or } 2 \cdot 3 = 6, \text{ or } p = 2, 3, 4, 5, 6$$
$$f = ab(n-1) = 2 \cdot 3 \cdot 7 = 42$$
$$R_2 = r_{0.01(2,42)} 1.360 = 3.82(1.360) = 5.195$$
$$R_3 = r_{0.01(3,42)} 1.360 = 3.99(1.360) = 5.426$$
$$R_4 = r_{0.01(4,42)} 1.360 = 4.10(1.360) = 5.576$$
$$R_5 = r_{0.01(5,42)} 1.360 = 4.17(1.360) = 5.671$$
$$R_6 = r_{0.01(6,42)} 1.360 = 4.24(1.360) = 5.776$$

All possible contrasts $= \frac{ab\,(ab-1)}{2} = \frac{2 \cdot 3(2 \cdot 3 - 1)}{2} = 15$ total contrasts

Contrasts	S = significant NS = not significant
$\bar{y}_{13\cdot}$ vs. $\bar{y}_{21\cdot} = 41.000 - 21.875 = 19.125 > 5.766\ (R_6)$	S
$\bar{y}_{13\cdot}$ vs. $\bar{y}_{11\cdot} = 41.000 - 24.625 = 16.375 > 5.671\ (R_5)$	S
$\bar{y}_{13\cdot}$ vs. $\bar{y}_{22\cdot} = 41.000 - 27.125 = 13.875 > 5.576\ (R_4)$	S
$\bar{y}_{13\cdot}$ vs. $\bar{y}_{12\cdot} = 41.000 - 27.375 = 13.625 > 5.426\ (R_3)$	S
$\bar{y}_{13\cdot}$ vs. $\bar{y}_{23\cdot} = 41.000 - 28.250 = 12.750 > 5.195\ (R_2)$	S
$\bar{y}_{23\cdot}$ vs. $\bar{y}_{21\cdot} = 28.250 - 21.875 = 6.375 > 5.671\ (R_5)$	S
$\bar{y}_{23\cdot}$ vs. $\bar{y}_{11\cdot} = 28.250 - 24.625 = 3.625 < 5.576\ (R_4)$	NS
$\bar{y}_{23\cdot}$ vs. $\bar{y}_{22\cdot} = 28.250 - 27.125 = 1.125 < 5.426\ (R_3)$	NS
$\bar{y}_{23\cdot}$ vs. $\bar{y}_{12\cdot} = 28.250 - 27.375 = 0.875 < 5.195\ (R_2)$	NS
$\bar{y}_{12\cdot}$ vs. $\bar{y}_{21\cdot} = 27.375 - 21.875 = 5.500 < 5.576\ (R_4)$	NS
$\bar{y}_{12\cdot}$ vs. $\bar{y}_{11\cdot} = 27.375 - 24.625 = 2.750 < 5.426\ (R_3)$	NS
$\bar{y}_{12\cdot}$ vs. $\bar{y}_{22\cdot} = 27.375 - 27.125 = 0.250 < 5.195\ (R_2)$	NS
$\bar{y}_{22\cdot}$ vs. $\bar{y}_{21\cdot} = 27.125 - 21.875 = 5.250 < 5.426\ (R_3)$	NS
$\bar{y}_{22\cdot}$ vs. $\bar{y}_{11\cdot} = 27.125 - 24.625 = 2.500 < 5.195\ (R_2)$	NS
$\bar{y}_{11\cdot}$ vs. $\bar{y}_{21\cdot} = 24.625 - 21.875 = 2.750 < 5.195\ (R_2)$	NS

* Table A.5 is used for Duncan's multiple range test.›

$\bar{y}_{13.}$	(	41	)				
$\bar{y}_{23.}$			(	28.25	)		
$\bar{y}_{12.}$				(	27.375	)	
$\bar{y}_{22.}$				(	27.13	)	
$\bar{y}_{11.}$					(	24.635	)
$\bar{y}_{21.}$						(	21.88	)

FIGURE 10   Approximate confidence intervals: Duncan Multiple Range test.

In this case, $\bar{y}_{13.}$ is significantly greater than the other cell mean values; $\bar{y}_{23.}$ is equal to $\bar{y}_{12.}$, $\bar{y}_{22.}$, and $\bar{y}_{11.}$ but greater than $\bar{y}_{21.}$, and $\bar{y}_{12.}$, $\bar{y}_{22.}$, $\bar{y}_{11.}$, and $\bar{y}_{21.}$ are equivalent at $\alpha = 0.01$. Rough confidence intervals are provided in Fig. 10.

This test proved to be slightly less sensitive than the LSD test, but the Duncan multiple range test is quite powerful and is very efficient in detecting differences when they actually exist.

2.   Newman–Keuls Test Interaction

As we have seen in earlier chapters, this test is similar to the Duncan multiple range test. Recall that a set of critical values is computed using the formula:

$$K_p = q_{\alpha(p,f)} S_{\bar{y}_{ij.}} \qquad p = 2, 3, \ldots ab$$

For this example, $ab = 2 \times 3 = 6$; hence, $p = 1, 2, 3, 4, 5, 6$. $\alpha = 0.01$ (using 0.01 again) and the Studentized range table (Table A.12) is used to determine $q_{\alpha(p,f)}$.

$$S_{\bar{y}_{ij.}} = \sqrt{\frac{MS_E}{n}} = \sqrt{\frac{14.786}{8}} = 1.360 \tag{26}$$

Hypothesis testing: The hypothesis form for each pair of cell means tested is:

$$H_0: \mu_{ij.} - \mu_{ji.} = 0$$

$$H_A: \mu_{ij.} - \mu_{ji.} \neq 0$$

Decision rule: Reject H_0 if $\bar{y}_{ij.} - \bar{y}_{ji.} > K_p$.

The next step is to compute the K_p values:

$$K_P = q_{\alpha(p,f)}S_{\bar{y}_{ij}}.$$
$$K_2 = q_{(0.01)(2,42)}(1.360) = 3.82(1.360) = 5.195$$
$$K_3 = q_{(0.01)(3,42)}(1.360) = 4.37(1.360) = 5.943$$
$$K_4 = q_{(0.01)(4,42)}(1.360) = 4.70(1.360) = 6.392$$
$$K_5 = q_{(0.01)(5,42)}(1.360) = 4.93(1.360) = 6.705$$
$$K_6 = q_{(0.01)(6,42)}(1.360) = 5.11(1.360) = 6.950$$

The $A \times B$ cell treatment means $\bar{y}_{ij}.$ are listed in ascending order.

$$\bar{y}_{21.} = 21.875$$
$$\bar{y}_{11.} = 24.625$$
$$\bar{y}_{22.} = 27.125$$
$$\bar{y}_{12.} = 27.375$$
$$\bar{y}_{23.} = 28.250$$
$$\bar{y}_{13.} = 41.000$$

The largest value is compared with the smallest, the next with the smallest, and so on, up to the value ranked just above the largest value. The process is repeated with the second to the largest value, etc.

$$\frac{ab(ab-1)}{2} = \frac{2 \times 3(2 \times 3 - 1)}{2} = \frac{6 \times 5}{2} = 15 \text{ (number of possible contrasts)}$$

Using the same comparative strategy as with the Duncan multiple range test:

Contrasts	S = significant NS = not significant
$\bar{y}_{13.}$ vs. $\bar{y}_{21.} = 41.000 - 21.875 = 19.125 > 6.950$ (K_6)	S
$\bar{y}_{13.}$ vs. $\bar{y}_{11.} = 41.000 - 24.625 = 16.375 > 6.705$ (K_5)	S
$\bar{y}_{13.}$ vs. $\bar{y}_{22.} = 41.000 - 27.125 = 13.875 > 6.392$ (K_4)	S
$\bar{y}_{13.}$ vs. $\bar{y}_{12.} = 41.000 - 27.375 = 13.625 > 5.943$ (K_3)	S
$\bar{y}_{13.}$ vs. $\bar{y}_{23.} = 41.000 - 28.250 = 12.750 > 5.195$ (K_2)	S
$\bar{y}_{23.}$ vs. $\bar{y}_{21.} = 28.250 - 21.875 = 6.375 < 6.705$ (K_5)	NS
$\bar{y}_{23.}$ vs. $\bar{y}_{11.} = 28.250 - 24.625 = 3.625 < 6.392$ (K_4)	NS
$\bar{y}_{23.}$ vs. $\bar{y}_{22.} = 28.250 - 27.125 = 1.125 < 5.943$ (K_3)	NS
$\bar{y}_{23.}$ vs. $\bar{y}_{12.} = 28.250 - 27.375 = 0.875 < 5.195$ (K_2)	NS
$\bar{y}_{12.}$ vs. $\bar{y}_{21.} = 27.375 - 21.875 = 5.500 < 6.392$ (K_4)	NS
$\bar{y}_{12.}$ vs. $\bar{y}_{11.} = 27.375 - 24.625 = 2.750 < 5.943$ (K_3)	NS
$\bar{y}_{12.}$ vs. $\bar{y}_{22.} = 27.375 - 27.125 = 0.250 < 5.195$ (K_2)	NS
$\bar{y}_{22.}$ vs. $\bar{y}_{21.} = 27.125 - 21.875 = 5.250 < 5.943$ (K_3)	NS
$\bar{y}_{22.}$ vs. $\bar{y}_{11.} = 27.125 - 24.625 = 2.500 < 5.195$ (K_2)	NS
$\bar{y}_{11.}$ vs. $\bar{y}_{21.} = 24.625 - 21.875 = 2.750 < 5.195$ (K_2)	NS

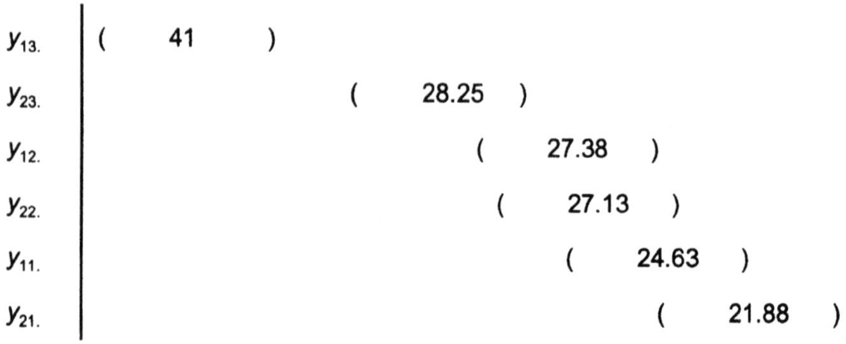

$y_{13.}$	(41)		
$y_{23.}$	(28.25)		
$y_{12.}$	(27.38)		
$y_{22.}$	(27.13)		
$y_{11.}$	(24.63)		
$y_{21.}$	(21.88)		

FIGURE 11   Approximate confidence intervals: Newman-Keuls test.

The conclusions reached are that $\bar{y}_{13.}$ is significantly larger than the other cell means and $\bar{y}_{11.}$, $\bar{y}_{12.}$, $\bar{y}_{21.}$, $\bar{y}_{22.}$, and $\bar{y}_{23.}$, are equivalent at $\alpha = 0.01$. Rough confidence intervals are provided in Fig. 11.

Notice that the Newman–Keuls test provides essentially the same information as the Duncan multiple range test, except that the former indicated no significant difference between $\bar{y}_{23.}$ and $\bar{y}_{21.}$, whereas the latter did. In general, the Newman–Keuls test is a little more conservative, meaning less powerful.

3. Tukey Test

This procedure was discussed earlier for main effects comparison. For AB cell mean comparisons, the procedure is similar.

The hypothesis for the Tukey test is:
$$H_0 : \mu_{ij.} - \mu_{ji.} = 0$$
$$H_A : \mu_{ij.} - \mu_{ji.} \neq 0$$

Reject H_0 if $|\bar{y}_{ij.} - \bar{y}_{ji.}| > T_\alpha$, where:

$$T_\alpha = q_{\alpha(p,f)} S_{\bar{y}_{ij.}} \quad \text{where } p = ab \text{ and } f = ab(n-1)$$

$$T_\alpha = q_{\alpha(ab;ab(n-1))} S_{\bar{y}_{ij.}}$$

The Studentized range table (Table L) is used for this.

The Tukey, being an all possible pairwise test, consists of $ab(ab-1)/2 = 15$ contrasts.

$$S_{\bar{y}_{ij.}} = \sqrt{\frac{MS_E}{n}} = \sqrt{\frac{14.786}{8}} = 1.360 \tag{27}$$

Using $\alpha = 0.05$

$$q_{\alpha(p,f)} = q_{\alpha(ab;ab(n-1))} = q_{0.05(6,42)} = 4.23, \quad \text{and}$$

$$T_\alpha = 4.23(1.360) = 5.753$$

Contrasts	S=significant NS=not significant
$\bar{y}_{13\cdot}$ vs. $\bar{y}_{21\cdot} = 41.000 - 21.875 = 19.125 > 5.753$	S
$\bar{y}_{13\cdot}$ vs. $\bar{y}_{11\cdot} = 41.000 - 24.625 = 16.375 > 5.753$	S
$\bar{y}_{13\cdot}$ vs. $\bar{y}_{22\cdot} = 41.000 - 27.125 = 13.875 > 5.753$	S
$\bar{y}_{13\cdot}$ vs. $\bar{y}_{12\cdot} = 41.000 - 27.375 = 13.625 > 5.753$	S
$\bar{y}_{13\cdot}$ vs. $\bar{y}_{23\cdot} = 41.000 - 28.250 = 12.750 > 5.753$	S
$\bar{y}_{23\cdot}$ vs. $\bar{y}_{21\cdot} = 28.250 - 21.875 = 6.375 > 5.753$	S
$\bar{y}_{23\cdot}$ vs. $\bar{y}_{11\cdot} = 28.250 - 24.625 = 3.625 < 5.753$	NS
$\bar{y}_{23\cdot}$ vs. $\bar{y}_{22\cdot} = 28.250 - 27.125 = 1.125 < 5.753$	NS
$\bar{y}_{23\cdot}$ vs. $\bar{y}_{12\cdot} = 28.250 - 27.375 = 0.875 < 5.753$	NS
$\bar{y}_{12\cdot}$ vs. $\bar{y}_{21\cdot} = 27.375 - 21.875 = 5.500 < 5.753$	NS
$\bar{y}_{12\cdot}$ vs. $\bar{y}_{11\cdot} = 27.375 - 24.625 = 2.750 < 5.753$	NS
$\bar{y}_{12\cdot}$ vs. $\bar{y}_{22\cdot} = 27.375 - 27.125 = 0.250 < 5.753$	NS
$\bar{y}_{22\cdot}$ vs. $\bar{y}_{21\cdot} = 27.125 - 21.875 = 5.250 < 5.753$	NS
$\bar{y}_{22\cdot}$ vs. $\bar{y}_{11\cdot} = 27.125 - 24.625 = 2.500 < 5.753$	NS
$\bar{y}_{11\cdot}$ vs. $\bar{y}_{21\cdot} = 24.625 - 21.875 = 2.750 < 5.753$	NS

In this case, $\bar{y}_{13\cdot}$ is significantly larger than the other cell means; $\bar{y}_{23\cdot}$ is equal to $\bar{y}_{11\cdot}$, $\bar{y}_{12\cdot}$, and $\bar{y}_{22\cdot}$ but greater than $\bar{y}_{21\cdot}$. Finally, $\bar{y}_{11\cdot}, \bar{y}_{12\cdot}, \bar{y}_{21\cdot}$, and $\bar{y}_{22\cdot}$, are equal at $\alpha = 0.05$. Note that these are the same results as derived from the Duncan multiple range test using $\alpha = 0.01$ (Fig. 12).

$y_{13\cdot}$	(41.00)
$y_{23\cdot}$	(28.25)
$y_{12\cdot}$	(27.38)
$y_{22\cdot}$	(27.13)
$y_{11\cdot}$	(24.63)
$y_{21\cdot}$	(21.88)

FIGURE 12 Approximate confidence intervals: Tukey test.

TABLE 11   Data in MiniTab format

n	Factor A	Factor B	y_{ijk}	$\bar{y}_{ij.}$	ϵ_{ijk}
1	1	1	32	24.625	7.375[a]
2	1	1	27	24.625	2.375
3	1	1	22	24.625	−2.625
4	1	1	19	24.625	−5.625
5	1	1	28	24.625	3.375
6	1	1	23	24.625	−1.625
7	1	1	25	24.625	0.375
8	1	1	21	24.625	−3.625
9	2	1	18	21.875	−3.875
10	2	1	22	21.875	0.125
11	2	1	20	21.875	−1.875
12	2	1	25	21.875	3.125
13	2	1	16	21.875	−5.875
14	2	1	19	21.875	−2.875
15	2	1	24	21.875	2.125
16	2	1	31	21.875	9.125
17	1	2	28	27.375	0.625
18	1	2	31	27.375	3.625
19	1	2	24	27.375	−3.375
20	1	2	25	27.375	−2.375
21	1	2	26	27.375	−1.375
22	1	2	33	27.375	5.625
23	1	2	27	27.375	−0.375
24	1	2	25	27.375	−2.375
25	2	2	27	27.125	−0.125
26	2	2	31	27.125	3.875
27	2	2	27	27.125	−0.125
28	2	2	25	27.125	−2.125
29	2	2	25	27.125	−2.125
30	2	2	32	27.125	4.875
31	2	2	26	27.125	−1.125
32	2	2	24	27.125	−3.125
33	1	3	36	41.000	−5.000
34	1	3	47	41.000	6.000
35	1	3	42	41.000	1.000
36	1	3	35	41.000	−6.000
37	1	3	46	41.000	5.000
38	1	3	39	41.000	−2.000
39	1	3	43	41.000	2.000
40	1	3	40	41.000	−1.000

(Continued)

TABLE 11   (Continued.)

41	2	3	24	28.250	−4.250
42	2	3	27	28.250	−1.250
43	2	3	33	28.250	4.750
44	2	3	25	28.250	−3.250
45	2	3	26	28.250	−2.250
46	2	3	30	28.250	1.750
47	2	3	32	28.250	3.750
48	2	3	29	28.250	0.750

$^a \epsilon_{ijk} = y_{ijk} - \bar{y}_{ij.}; 32.000 - (24.625) = 7.375.$

Y. Computer Printout

Before continuing, let us review a series of computer printouts of this two-factor factorial, completely randomized design. The computer output is a standard generalized linear model (GLM) routine, specifically as applied by the MiniTab software, which is extremely user-friendly.

In this model, C_1 (column 1) represents treatment factor A (sex) and C_2 represents treatment factor B (product). Also, C_3 represents the actual measured (dependent) variable y_{ijk}, C_4 is the specific $A \times B$ cell means, and C_5 is the residual difference between C_3 and C_4. Table 11 provides these data in MiniTab format.

Table 12 provides a printout of the two-factor factorial experiment, which is the same as depicted in Table 6, of the hand-computed example. The table is straightforward to read.

Table 13 provides the means $A(C_1)$ for the ith level of treatment A, the jth level of treatment $B(C_2)$, and the ith, jth level of Treatments A and $B(C_1 + C_2)$.

TABLE 12   Two-Factor Factorial Experiment Printout

Analysis of variance for C_3 Source	DF	Seq SS	Adj SS	Adj MS	F	P
C_1 (factor A)	1	330.75	330.75	330.75	22.37	0.000
C_2 (factor B)	2	1065.50	1065.50	532.75	36.03	0.000
$C_1 * C_2$ (Factor A $\times$ B)	2	350.00	350.00	175.00	11.84	0.000
Error	42	621.00	621.00	14.79		
Total	47	2367.25				

TABLE 13   Means for Treatment Levels

		Means for Factors C_i	
Factor A	$C_1 = A$		**Mean**
	1		31.00
	2		25.75
Factor B	$C_2 = B$		
	1		23.25
	2		27.25
	3		34.63
Factors $A \times B$	$C_1 * C_2 = A \times B$		
	1	1	25.63
	1	2	27.38
	1	3	41.00
	2	1	21.87
	2	2	27.13
	2	3	28.25

II. THE MODEL AND ITS ASSESSMENT

Before the researcher can make assumptions about the two-factor factorial model, it is important that its adequacy be evaluated. Recall that the linear statistical model is:

$$y_{ijk} = \mu + A_i + B_j + (AB)_{ij} + \epsilon_{k(ij)} \tag{28}$$

TABLE 14   Stem-and-Leaf Format

1	-6	0
4	-5	860
5	-4	2
10	-3	86321
18	-2	86332110
24	-1	863210
24	-0	311
21	0	1367
17	1	07
15	2	013
12	3	13678
7	4	78
5	5	06
3	6	0
2	7	3
1	8	
1	9	1

TABLE 15 Letter-Value Format

	Depth	Lower	Upper	Mid	Spread
N	48.0				
M	24.5		-0.687	-0.687	
H	12.5	-2.500	2.750	0.125	5.250
E	6.5	-3.750	4.813	0.531	8.563
D	3.5	-5.312	5.812	0.250	11.125
C	2.0	-5.875	7.375	0.750	13.250
	1.0	-6.000	9.125	1.563	15.125

where the $\epsilon_{k(ij)}$ values are normally and independently distributed with a μ of zero and a variance of σ_ϵ^2 [i.e., $NID(0, \sigma^2)$]. Also, $\epsilon_{ijk} = y_{ijk} - \bar{y}_{ij.}$ (the error term equals the actual value minus the predicted value).

As before, the researcher will first want to perform exploratory data analysis (EDA) on the ϵ_{ijk} residuals to get a sense of their distribution, which should be patternless. The stem–leaf display, letter-value display, and box-plot display are valuable here.

A. Stem–Leaf

Table 14 provides a display of the residuals in stem–leaf formats. The data do not appear to have any patterns.

B. Letter-Value Displays

The letter-value display (Table 15) of the residual data indicates that the data are skewed to the upper value or the right side of the bell curve. This can be seen by noticing that the "Mid" column is increasing after "D." This is not a serious problem but one of which the researcher will want to be aware.

C. Boxplot

The boxplot with notches is provided in Table 16. The data again appear to be spread out more toward the upper values (the right), but it is not a serious skew.

TABLE 16 Boxplot Format

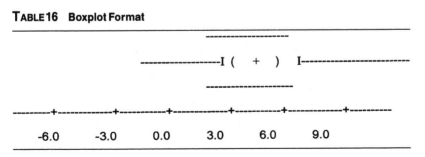

To get a better sense of the data, it is also useful to plot the residuals against the main treatment factors, A and B, as well as against the predicted values ($\bar{y}_{ij}$). Figure 13 provides a plot of main effects for factor A (where $1 =$ females and $2 =$ males) against the residual values. The residuals seem to be reasonably centered about 0.

Figure 14 presents a graph of the residuals compared with factor B, or the three levels of products.

The residuals for product 1 are spread out further than those for the other two, and those for product 3 are spread more than those for product 2. Yet, these disparities are not enough of a concern to perform a transformation of the dependent variable or to use a nonparametric statistic.

Figure 15 presents a plot of the residuals against the $\bar{y}_{ij}$ (estimated y values) or the $A_i \times B_j$ cell means. Again, the residuals do not appear to be seriously nonnormally distributed about zero.

Note: Because $\bar{y}_{22}$ (27.125) and $\bar{y}_{12}$ (27.375) are so close in value proximity, their ϵ_{ijk} values are superimposed.

D. Model Parameter Estimation

For the linear model:

$$y_{ijk} = \mu + A_i + B_j + (AB)_{ij} + \epsilon_{ijk} \tag{29}$$

the following estimations are useful:

$$\hat{\mu} = \bar{y}_{...} \tag{30}$$

$$\hat{A}_i = \bar{y}_{i..} - \bar{y}_{...}, \qquad i = 1, 2, \ldots, a \tag{31}$$

$$\hat{B}_j = \bar{y}_{.j.} - \bar{y}_{...}, \qquad j = 1, 2, \ldots, b \tag{32}$$

$$\left(\widehat{AB}\right)_{ij} = \bar{y}_{ij.} - \bar{y}_{i..} - \bar{y}_{.j.} + \bar{y}_{..}, \qquad i = 1, 2, \ldots, a, \text{ and } j = 1, 2, \ldots, b \tag{33}$$

E. Pooling the Interaction Term with the Error Term

Once the analysis of residuals has been completed and the researcher is comfortable with meeting the normality assumptions, etc., there is another decision to make. If the interaction of the two main effects, A and B, is not significant, some statisticians suggest that the interaction sum of squares and the error sum of squares be pooled.

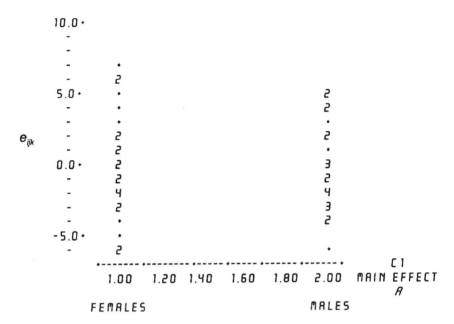

FIGURE 13 Residuals versus main effect A (sex).

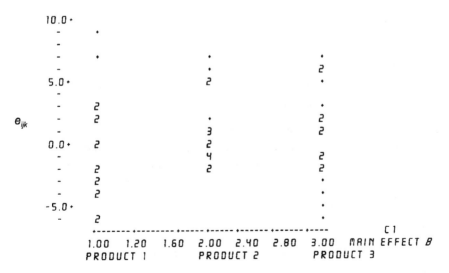

FIGURE 14 Residuals versus main effect B (product).

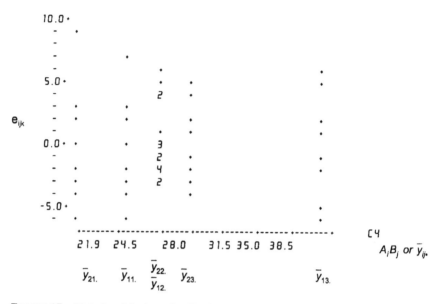

FIGURE 15   Plot of residuals and cell values.

Recall that the original linear model for the two-factor design is:

$$y_{ijk} = \mu + A_i + B_j + (AB)_{ij} + \epsilon_{ijk} \qquad (34)$$

If the interaction is not significant, the interaction essentially drops out, so the model becomes:

$$y_{ijk} = \mu + A_i + B_j + \epsilon_{ijk} \qquad (35)$$

In cases like this, the researcher does not have to recalculate the model in its entirety. Instead, the new $SS_{E_{(new)}}$ term is:

$$SS_{E_{(new)}} = SS_{AB} + SS_E \qquad (36)$$

That is, the sums of squares are merely added to each other (pooled).

The only other change is in the degrees of freedom. The degrees of freedom for $SS_{AB} = (a-1)(b-1)$ and the degrees of freedom for $SS_E = ab(n-1)$. These are simply added to one another:

$$df_{(new)} = df_{AB} + df_E$$

or

$$df_{(new)} = (a-1)(b-1) + ab(n-1) = nab - a - b + 1 \qquad (37)$$

Everything else is the same.

The pooling affects both the power of the statistical tests for main effects factors A and B and the level of significance.

Some statisticians recommend that pooling not be done, even if the interaction is not significant, unless:

1. Degrees of freedom value for the error term is small (i.e., 5 or less).
2. The test statistic ratio, MS_{AB}/MS_E, is very small (i.e., less than 2 at $\alpha = 0.05$).

These rules have the effect of limiting pooling to cases in which degrees of freedom being small for MS_E will be increased and ensures that pooling occur only in cases where interaction has a high probability of not being present at all.

However, it is critical that the researcher, at no time, use a smorgasbord of techniques to justify a preconceived bias. That is, a researcher must not simply compute a variety of statistical tests until some desired outcome is derived.

The fitted values for this model are:

$$\hat{y}_{ijk} = \bar{y}_{i..} + \bar{y}_{.j.} - \bar{y}_{...}$$

$$\hat{\mu} = \bar{y}_{...}$$

$$A_i = \bar{y}_{i..} - \bar{y}_{...} \qquad i = 1, 2, \ldots, a$$

$$B_j = \bar{y}_{.j.} - \bar{y}_{...} \qquad j = 1, 2, \ldots, b$$

F. Two-Factor ANOVA, One Observation per Cell

In practice, sometimes, the researcher can make only one measurement per cell because of the expense of the study or some other factor. In these cases, where no cell replication is done, $k = 1$ (as does n) and the linear model is:

$$y_{ij} = \mu + A_i + B_j + (AB)_{ij} + \epsilon_{ij} \qquad \begin{aligned} i &= 1, 2, \ldots, a \\ j &= 1, 2, \ldots, b \end{aligned} \qquad (38)$$

Notice that with only one observation within each cell, the error term (ϵ_{ij}) and the interaction term $(AB)_{ij}$ are confounded, or "mixed together." There is no way to retrieve the interaction term in this model. So, prior to using only one observation per cell, the investigator should be familiar with the system being studied to assure that no significant interaction between factors will occur. When that cannot be assured, it is critical that the experimenter take more than one observation per cell.

The analysis of variance for a two-factor completely randomized design, $n = 1$ is straightforward (Table 17).

TABLE 17 The Analysis of Variance for a Two-Factor Design with No Replication

Source of variance	Sum of squares	Degrees of freedom	Mean square	F_c	F_{tabled}
Treatment A	$\sum_{i=1}^{a} \frac{y_{i.}^2}{b} - \frac{y_{..}^2}{ab}$	$a-1$	$\frac{SS_A}{a-1} = MS_A$	$\frac{MS_A}{MS_E}$	$F_{\alpha[a-1;(a-1)(b-1)]}$
Treatment B	$\sum_{j=1}^{b} \frac{y_{.j}^2}{a} - \frac{y_{..}^2}{ab}$	$b-1$	$\frac{SS_B}{b-1} = MS_B$	$\frac{MS_B}{MS_E}$	$F_{\alpha[b-1;(a-1)(b-1)]}$
Error	Subtraction	$(a-1)(b-1)$	$\frac{SS_E}{(a-1)(b-1)} = MS_E$	MS_E	
Total	$\sum_{i=1}^{a}\sum_{j=1}^{b} y_{ij}^2 - \frac{y_{..}^2}{ab}$	$ab-1$			

Tukey has presented a test to help determine whether interaction actually is present when $n = 1$ [15,29].

$$SS_I = \frac{\left[\sum_{i=1}^{a}\sum_{j=1}^{b} y_{ij} y_{i.} y_{.j} - y_{..} \left(SS_A + SS_B + y_{..}^2/ab\right)\right]^2}{(ab)(SS_A)(SS_B)} \tag{39}$$

where y_{ij} = individual cell value
   $y_{i.}$ = ith row total (factor A)
   $y_{.j}$ = jth column total (factor B)
   $y_{..}$ = row or column totals

The test hypothesis is:

   $H_0 : AB = 0$ (interaction not significant at α)

   $H_A: AB \neq 0$

$$F_C = \frac{SS_I}{SS_E^*/[(a-1)(b-1)-1]}$$

$$SS_E^* = SS_E - SS_I$$

Decision rule:
   Reject H_0 if $F_c > F_{\alpha[1;(a-1)(b-1)-1]}$
   It is extremely dangerous for the researcher to rely on this interaction test if the researcher does not have solid field knowledge of the data, especially that no interaction is present. It is often not wise to omit one of the biggest advantages of a two-factor factorial model over a one-factor-at-a-

time analysis—nteraction—but that is what happens where there is only one observation per cell.

G. Power of the Test (Fixed Effects)

1. Power Calculated A Priori

The power of the test—two-factor factorial—is straightforward and is computed as previously described in Chaps. 5 and 6. We will perform it again for demonstration.

Factors A and B (main effects) are computed separately.

$$\phi = \sqrt{\frac{n' \sum_{m=1}^{k'}(\mu_m - \mu)^2}{k's^2}} \tag{40}$$

where $k' = a$ or b, depending upon the factor with which one is working
$n' = bn$, if factor A, or an, if factor B
$s^2 = MS_E$
$\mu = \frac{\sum_{m=1}^{k'}\mu_m}{k'}$ = grand population mean

Note: Assume that these example calculations were computed prior to running the F-tests for the two-factor factorial ANOVA.

2. Factor A

For this test, the researcher uses Table A.4, the power table. The necessary parameters to determine the power are:

$k' = a = 2$

$n' = bn = 3 \times 8 = 24$

$v_1 = k' - 1 = a - 1 = 2 - 1 = 1$

$v_2 = $ df for $MS_E = ab(n-1) = 2 \times 3(7) = 42$

$\mu = \frac{\sum_{m=1}^{a}\mu_m}{a} = \frac{31 + 25.75}{2} = 28.375$

$\phi = \sqrt{\frac{n'\sum_{m=1}^{a}(\mu_m - \mu)^2}{as^2}} = \sqrt{\frac{24([31 - 28.375]^2 + [25.75 - 28.375]^2)}{2(14.79)}}$

$= 3.344$

From Table A.4, the researcher enters the value that corresponds to $v_1 = 1$, $v_2 = 42$ degrees of freedom with $\phi = 3.344$, $\alpha = 0.05$, and reads the β of the test, which, in this case, is about 0.03. The power of the test is $1 - \beta \approx 1.00$. Thus, with this model, there is about a zero (0%) chance of committing a type II error (stating that H_0 is true when it really is false).

Let us now compute the same test for factor B.

3. Factor B

As before:

$$k' = b = 3$$
$$n' = an = 2 \times 8 = 16$$
$$v_1 = b - 1 = 2$$
$$v_2 = \text{df for MS}_E = 42$$

$$\mu = \frac{\sum\limits_{j=1}^{b} \mu_j}{b} = \frac{23.25 + 27.25 + 34.63}{3} = 28.377$$

$$\phi = \sqrt{\frac{n' \sum\limits_{j=1}^{b} (\mu_j - \mu)^2}{bs^2}}$$

$$= \sqrt{\frac{16([23.25 - 28.377]^2 + [27.25 - 28.377]^2 + [34.63 - 28.377]^2)}{3(14.79)}}$$

$$= 4.9027$$

In Table D, finding the $v_1 = 2$, $v_2 = 42$ value at $\alpha = 0.05$, $\phi = 4.9027$, (not even on the table) the researcher sees that, for $\beta \approx 0.000$, the power of the test is ≈ 1.00. That is, there is about zero chance of making a type II error.

H. Alternative Way of Determining Power of the Test A Priori

The power of the test computed before the ANOVA is performed is similar to what was shown in Chaps. 5 and 6. The formula for the computation is:

$$\phi = \sqrt{\frac{n'\delta^2}{2k's^2}} \tag{41}$$

where:

$$n' = an, \text{ if factor } B, \text{ or } bn, \text{ if factor } A$$
$$k' = a \text{ or } b, \text{ depending upon the factor with which one is working}$$

$s^2 = \widehat{MS_E}$ (a value that would be estimated prior to conducting the study, for this is an a priori test)

δ = specified difference to detect

1. Treatment A

$k' = a = 2$

$n' = bn = 3 \times 8 = 24$

$v_1 = a - 1 = 2 - 1 = 1$

$v_2 = $ df for $MS_E = 42$

$\delta = $ set at 5 units

$s^2 = MS_E = 14.786$, which, in practice, would have to be estimated

$$\phi = \sqrt{\frac{n'\delta^2}{2k's^2}} = \sqrt{\frac{24(5)^2}{2(2)14.786}} = 3.1851$$

Entering Table D, with $v_1 = 1$, $v_2 = 42$, $\phi = 3.1851$, and $\alpha = 0.05$, one finds the β value to be about 0.015. The power of the statistical model is $1 - \beta = 0.985$ (98.5%).

2. Treatment B

$k' = b = 3$

$n' = an = 2 \times 8 = 16$

$v_1 = b - 1 = 3 - 1 = 2$

$v_2 = $ df for $MS_E = 42$

$\delta = $ set at 5 units

$s^2 = \widehat{MS_E} = 14.786$ (Note: Again, this would be estimated; we are using the actual only for demonstration purposes.)

$$\phi = \sqrt{\frac{n'\delta^2}{2k's^2}} = \sqrt{\frac{16(5)^2}{2(3)14.786}} = 2.123$$

Looking at Table A.4, with $v_1 = 2$, $v_2 = 42$, $\phi = 2.123$, and let us set $\alpha = 0.05$, we see that the power $(1 - \beta)$ is about 0.85 (45%).

I. Tests of Power, A Posteriori

After the experiment has been run and the ANOVA has been computed, the power of the statistic can be computed for factors A and B, or, if interaction is significant, the $A \times B$ combination means:

$k' = a$ when contrasting levels of factor A, and

b when contrasting levels of factor B

After the ANOVA has been calculated, determining the actual power of the model is straightforward.

$$\phi = \sqrt{\frac{(k' - 1)(\text{factor MS} - s^2)}{k's^2}} \tag{42}$$

1. Factor A

$k' = a = 2$

$MS_A = 330.750$

$v_1 = k' - 1 = 2 - 1 = 1$

$v_2 = \text{df for } MS_E = 42$

$s^2 = MS_E = 14.786$, which is now a calculated value

$$\phi = \sqrt{\frac{(2 - 1)(330.750 - 14.786)}{2(14.786)}} = 3.269$$

The power of the test $(1-\beta)$ when $\phi = 3.269$, $v_1 = 1$, $v_2 = 42$, and $\alpha = 0.05$ (from Table A.4) is about 0.97, or 97%. That is, the probability of making a type II error, given the α level, ϕ, and s^2, is $1 - 0.97$, or 3%.

2. Factor B

$k' = b = 3$

$MS_B = 532.750$

$v_1 = k' - 1 = 3 - 1 = 2$

$v_2 = \text{df for } MS_E = 42$

$s^2 = MS_E = 14.786$

Let us set $\alpha = 0.05$.

$$\phi = \sqrt{\frac{(3-1)(532.750 - 14.786)}{3(14.786)}} = 4.833$$

The power of this test, when $\phi = 4.833$, $v_1 = 2$, $v_2 = 42$, and $\alpha = 0.05$, is about 1.00, or 100%. The probability of making a type II error is about zero, or 1%.

3. Power for Factor $A \times B$ Interaction

The power of the interaction can also be computed after the ANOVA has been completed:

$$\phi = \sqrt{\frac{(A \times B \text{ degree of freedom})(\text{MS}_{AB} - s^2)}{([A \times B \text{ degrees of freedom}] + 1)s^2}} \tag{43}$$

df $A = 2 - 1 = 1$

df $B = b - 1 = 3 - 1 = 2$

$\text{MS}_{AB} = 175.000$

$v_1 = (a-1)(b-1) = (2-1)(3-1) = 2$

$v_2 = $ df for $\text{MS}_E = 42$

$s^2 = \text{MS}_E = 14.786$

$\alpha = 0.05$

$$\phi = \sqrt{\frac{(1 \cdot 2)175 - 14.786}{(1 \cdot 2 + 1)(14.786)}} = 2.688$$

For $\alpha = 0.05$, $v_1 = 2$, $v_2 = 42$, and $\phi = 2.688$ the power of the statistic $(1 - \beta)$ is 0.97, and the probability of rejecting H_A, when true, is 0.03, or 3%.

J. Sample Size Requirements

Prior to conducting an experiment or performing a study, an experimenter will want be sure that the sample size selected is adequate at:

A specified power $(1 - \beta)$
A specified alpha (significance level, α)
A specified σ^2
A specified minimum detectable difference between means

As in the case of the one-factor ANOVA, the procedure is iterative, and generally it is based upon the most important main factor effect (A or B). If the researcher suspects greater variability in one factor than another, it would be wise to use that with the greater variability estimate, $\hat{\sigma}^2$, to be on the safe, or conservative, side.

The method is performed as in Chap. 6. Using our example in the present chapter, we will apply the formula:

$$\phi = \sqrt{\frac{n'\delta^2}{2k'S^2}} \tag{43}$$

where $n' = bn$, if factor A*; an, if factor B
$k' = a$, if A; b, if B
$v_1 = k'-1$ ($a-1$ if factor A, $b-1$ if factor B)
$v_2 =$ df for MS_E
$S^2 =$ variance estimate, or MS_E
$\alpha =$ significance level for type I error
$\beta =$ level of type II error which is experimented
$\delta =$ minimum desired detectable difference between means

In our example, let us select factor A as the effect on which to base our decision. Suppose we estimate MS_E as 14.786 (which we would not know in reality because we have not performed the experiment).

$k' = a = 2$
$v_1 = 2-1 = 2-1 = 1$

It may be easier to see what is happening if we rewrite in terms of factor A.

I find it easier to determine v_2 in this way, for one needs to know what the values of a and n are, not just their product, an.

Let us continue to use Example 1:

$v_1 = a-1 = 1$
$\delta = 5$ (as before). We are using this minimum detectable difference, as it was previously set, to show how these calculations are all interrelated.
$\alpha = 0.05$, as before
$\beta = 0.10$ (so the required power $[1-\beta] = 0.90$) (we will use $1-\beta = 0.90$ for a change)
$s^2 = 14.786$, as actually calculated

The final formula, then, is:

$$\phi = \sqrt{\frac{bn\delta^2}{2k'S^2}} \tag{44}$$

---

*an or bn constitutes the entire sample size of group A or group B categorized by level; n is the actual per cell sample size.

$$\phi = \sqrt{\frac{3(n)5^2}{2(2)14.786}}$$

Let us begin the iterative process, estimating n (the within-cell replicates) as $n = 15$.

$$\phi = \sqrt{\frac{3(15)5^2}{2(2)14.786}} = 4.361$$

$v_1 = 1$

$v_2 = ab(n-1) = 2 \times 3(15-1) = 84$

Looking in Table D, $\alpha = 0.05$, $v_1 = 1$, $v_2 = 84$, $\phi = 4.361$, $1-\beta = 0.90$. We see that the power of this sample size is greater than 0.90 (actually, it is about 99.9%), so we can lower the estimate of sample size, say, 10.

Next Iteration, with $n = 10$

$$\phi = \sqrt{\frac{3(10)5^2}{2(2)14.786}} = 3.561$$

$v_1 = 1$

$v_2 = 2 \times 3(10-1) = 54$

$\alpha = 0.05$

We find that the power is still over our required 0.90 value. We can reduce the sample size, n, again, say to 5.

$$\phi = \sqrt{\frac{3(5)5^2}{2(2)14.786}} = 2.518$$

$v_1 = 1$

$v_2 = 2 \times 3(5-1) = 24$

$\alpha = 0.05$

The power for this test is about 0.92, which the researcher decides to use because it is close to 0.90. So each cell in the experiment will use an $n = 5$. The actual experiment used $n = 8$, but 5 would have been adequate.

K. Minimum Detectable Difference

As before, the minimum detectable difference is the numerical difference between means that can be detected by the two-factor factorial design at a set α, β, sample size, and σ^2. Both treatments A and B can be tested.

The formula for this test is:

$$\delta = \sqrt{\frac{2k'S^2\phi^2}{n'}} \tag{45}$$

where $k' = a$ if measuring factor A and b if measuring factor B
$n' = bn$ if measuring factor A and an if measuring factor B
$s^2 = MS_E$
ϕ must be read from Table D, at a specified α, β, and σ^2, or can be computed in determining the power and plugged into the minimum detectable difference formula.

Example 1 (cont.):   In our data set, we are interested in knowing the smallest detectable difference for both factors A and B after we have performed the study.

1. Factor A

$k' = a = 2$

$s^2 = MS_E = 14.786$

$n' = b \times n = 3 \times 8 = 24$

$\alpha = 0.05$, as before

$\beta = 0.10$, so $1 - \beta = 0.90$, as before

$v_1 = a - 1 = 2 - 1 = 1$

$v_2 = ab(n-1) = 2 \times 3(8-1) = 42$ (to be read from Table D for ϕ; find v_2 on the table corresponding to $\alpha = 0.05$, $v_1 = 1$, and $1-\beta = 0.90$, and read ϕ)

$\phi = 2.5$

Plugging these data in Eq. (46), the researcher finds that:

$$\delta = \sqrt{\frac{2(2)14.786(2.5)^2}{3 \times 8}} = 3.925$$

Hence, given $\alpha = 0.05$, $1-\beta = 0.90$, and $\sigma^2 = 14.786$, the minimum detectable difference between means in treatment A is 3.925 points. This is good, because we stated a need for a minimum of 5 points.

Hence, the researcher is quite confident that, if a significant difference exists between means, the statistic will detect it, if it is 5 points or greater. There is a "cushion" factor in this model.

2. Factor B

$$k' = b = 3$$
$$s^2 = 14.786 = MS_E$$
$$n' = a \times n = 2 \times 8 = 16$$
$$\alpha = 0.05$$
$$\beta = 0.10$$
$$v_1 = b - 1 = 3 - 1 = 2$$
$$v_2 = ab(n - 1) = 2 \times 3(7) = 42$$

ϕ is estimated from Table D, $v_1 = 2$, $v_2 = 42$, $\alpha = 0.05$, $1 - \beta = 0.90$, as ≈ 2.15.

$$\phi = \sqrt{\frac{2(3)(14.786)(2.15)^2}{2 \times 8}} = 5.063$$

The minimum detectable difference between means in the treatment B portion is 5.063, which is about the required 5.

L. Missing Values

It is critical, in this researcher's opinion, that the replicates used per cell in two-factor factorial designs be balanced or equal. If a list of data is missing, making the cell sample size, n, unbalanced, the researcher can *randomly* remove values in the cells with greater sample sizes until all cell sample sizes are equal. However, if only one data point is missing, one can substitute an estimated value, y_{ijk}, for the missing value. For example, the missing value can be estimated from:

$$\hat{y}_{ijk} = \frac{ay_{i..} + by_{.j.} - \sum_{i=1}^{a}\sum_{j=1}^{b}\sum_{k=1}^{n} y_{ijk}}{N + 1 - a - b} \tag{46}$$

where a = number of treatment levels in treatment A
b = number of treatment levels in treatment B
$y_{i..}$ = sum of the ith row totals containing the missing value
$y_{.j.}$ = sum of the jth column totals containing the missing value
$N = a \times b \times n$, including the missing value

Once the missing value is estimated, it is inserted into the data, and the ANOVA proceeds as before. However, for each data point estimated, the researcher loses one degree of freedom in the error term. So, if one value is estimated, the degrees of freedom become:

$$\text{Degrees of freedom}_{\text{ADJ}} = (ab[n-1]) - 1$$

Example 1 (cont.): Suppose the value, y_{122} (31), is missing, producing data as appear in Table 18. In this example, we are concerned with the $y_{i..}$ (row total) with the missing value and $y_{.j.}$ (column total) with the missing value. The row total (all females) is $y_{1..}$ or 713. The column total of all product 2 ($y_{.2.}$) is 405.

The total of all individual y_{ijk} value is:

$$\sum_{i=1}^{a}\sum_{j=1}^{b}\sum_{k=1}^{n} y_{ijk} = 32 + 27 + 22 + \cdots + 30 + 32 + 29 = 1331$$

The estimate of the missing value is:

$$\hat{y}_{ijk} = \frac{2(713) + 3(405) - 1331}{48 + 1 - 2 - 3} = 29.773$$

The researcher plugs 29.773 (or 30, rounded) into the MV value spot in the $y_{12.}$ cell and computes the ANOVA as before, except that the MS_E has one less degree of freedom.

If several values are missing, the mean values of each cell containing missing values can be substituted for the missing values. For each substitution, it is important to reduce the degrees of freedom in the error term by one. Hence, if three values were estimated values (m) in a fixed-effects, two-factor factorial design, the degrees of freedom would be:

$$\text{Degrees of freedom}_{\text{adj}} = ab(n-1) - m$$

where m is the number of missing values estimated.

The experiment's validity becomes very shaky if many values are estimated. This is particularly true for applied statistical researchers, for whom assumption often does not prove valid in the actual research field.

III. CONCLUDING REMARKS

A. Model I: Fixed Effects

In cases where all levels within the two factors have been intentionally chosen, the model is said to be fixed. All of the work in this chapter has been concerned with a fixed-effects model. In fixed-effect studies, which are vastly

TABLE 18 Data (with Missing Value)

Factor A—sex	Product 1		Product 2		Product 3		
1 = Female	32	28	28	26	36	46	
	27	23	MVᵃ	33	47	39	
	22	25	24	27	42	43	
	19	21	25	25	35	40	
		$y_{11.}$ 197		$y_{12.}$ 188		$y_{13.}$ 328	$y_{1..} = 713$
2 = male	18	16	27	25	24	26	
	22	19	31	32	27	30	
	20	24	27	26	33	32	
	25	31	25	24	25	29	
		$y_{21.}$ 175		$y_{22.}$ 217		$y_{23.}$ 226	$y_{2..} = 618$
$y_{.j.}$	$y_{.1.} = 372$		$y_{.2.} = 405$		$y_{.3.} = 554$		$y_{...} = 1331$

Factor B—Moisturizers

ᵃMV, missing value.

more common than either random-effects or mixed-effects models, the hypotheses tested are:

Factor A: H_0: $\mu_1 = \mu_2 \cdots = \mu_n$

H_A: At least one μ differs

Factor B: H_0 : $\mu_1 = \mu_2 \cdots = \mu_n$

H_A: At least one μ differs

The F_C tests, as the reader will recall, are:

Factor A: $\dfrac{MS_A}{MS_E}$

Factor B: $\dfrac{MS_B}{MS_E}$

$A \times B$ interaction: $\dfrac{MS_{AB}}{MS_E}$

Note: The degrees of freedom for F_T are (numerator df; denominator df).

Conclusions drawn concerning model I are only for the levels evaluated in factors A and B. The assumptions should not be generalized to make universal statements.

B. Model II: Random Effects

In some cases, the levels of both treatments A and B are selected at random from the "universal," or all possible levels "out there." In models of this type, one does not want to make inferences concerning all "levels" of a specific factor. In a two-factor factorial model, it is all levels of two factors.

Recall that the hypothesis dealt with means (μ). In the random effects model, the question is one of equivalence of variances (σ^2).

Factor A: H_0: $\sigma_1^2 = \cdots = \sigma_a^2$

H_A: The variances are not equal

Factor B: H_0: $\sigma_1^2 = \cdots = \sigma_b^2$

H_A: The variances are not equal

$A \times B$ interaction: H_0 : $\sigma_1^2 = \cdots = \sigma_{ab}^2$

H_A: The variances are not equal

The F_C test for the random-effects model is not the same as for the fixed-effects model.

Factor A: $\dfrac{MS_A}{MS_{AB}}$

Factor B: $\dfrac{MS_B}{MS_{AB}}$

$A \times B$ interaction: $\dfrac{MS_{AB}}{MS_E}$

Note: The degrees of freedom for F_T are $F_{T\alpha}$ (numerator df; denominator df)

We have covered a great deal of material in this chapter, which certainly will be of use to the applied researcher. It is important that the researcher clearly understands the methods presented. More complex factorial designs will not be discussed because they are of little value to the applied researcher.

8

Two-Factor Factorial Completely Randomized Blocked Designs

As in the case of the complete block design in the one-factor analysis of variance, there are times when complete randomization is not the best path for the experimenter to pursue, particularly in terms of practicality. There are many times when it is not feasible, for example, in heating or temperature experiments, such as D-value computations of the lethality rate of steam heat for specific bacterial spores. It may be practical only to run all the replicate samples at one temperature, then subsequent replicates at other temperatures, and so on. In this case, temperature 1 would represent block 1; temperature 2, block 2; and on to temperature n. Another real problem for which this design is useful consists of experiments so large in size that it is not possible to run the entire study in a single time period, say, a day. It may take 2 or 3 days. In this case, the test days are blocks. Other applications include different batches of a material, different operators or technicians, or different times, blocked to enhance the statistical power.

The concept of blocking two-factor designs is a direct extension of the one-factor complete block design, so we will not spend a lot of time on its discussion, except to provide procedural or calculation requirements. Only the fixed-effects model will be discussed, for it is by far the most applicable.

The two-factor factorial, blocked design has the linear form:

$$y_{ijk} = \mu + A_i + B_j + (AB)_{ij} + C_k + \epsilon_{ijk} \qquad (1)$$

where

i	$= 1,2,\ldots a$
j	$= 1,2,\ldots b$
k	$= 1,2,\ldots n$
μ	$=$ grand mean
A_i	$=$ treatment A at ith level
B_j	$=$ treatment B at jth level
$(AB)_{ij}$	$= A \times B$ Interaction
C_k	$=$ the blocking effect of the kth block
ϵ_{ijk}	$=$ NID$(0,\sigma^2)$; the error is an aggregate of factors A and B, the $A \times B$ interaction, and the block effect

Note that, in this blocking design, one does not completely randomize all abn values but restricts randomization to within each block. We will assume that no interaction between the blocks and treatments occurs. If there is interaction, it will be added (confounded) to the error term, inflating it. Hence, the researcher will want to be observant for "strange" or unexplained increases in MS_E. In point of fact, the error term is composed of (AC), (BC), and (ABC), all of which we assume are near zero.

The analysis of variance table for the two-factor factorial, randomized complete block design is presented in Table 1.

I. EXPECTED MEAN SQUARES

Notice again that the variance components of this model will all equal an unbiased estimate of σ^2, given that no treatment/interaction blocking effects are present. Otherwise, the error term σ^2 also contains the treatment effect, interaction effect, or blocking effect embedded in it.

$$\text{Treatment } A = \underbrace{\sigma^2}_{\text{Pure error}} + \underbrace{\frac{bn \sum A_i^2}{a-1}}_{\substack{\text{Treatment } A \\ \text{effect}}}$$

$$\text{Treatment } B = \underbrace{\sigma^2}_{\text{Pure error}} + \underbrace{\frac{an \sum B_j^2}{b-1}}_{\substack{\text{Treatment } B \\ \text{effect}}}$$

TABLE 1 Analysis of Variance Table for Two-Factor Factorial, Randomized Complete Block Design

Source of variation	Sum of squares	Degrees of freedom	Mean square	F_C	F_T
Treatment A	(SS_A) $\dfrac{1}{bn}\sum_{i=1}^{a} y_{i..}^2 - \dfrac{y_{...}^2}{abn}$	$a-1$	$\dfrac{SS_A}{a-1} = MS_A$	$\dfrac{MS_A}{MS_E}$	$F_{\alpha[(a-1);(ab-1)(n-1)]}$
Treatment B	(SS_B) $\dfrac{1}{an}\sum_{j=1}^{b} y_{.j.}^2 - \dfrac{y_{...}^2}{abn}$	$b-1$	$\dfrac{SS_B}{b-1} = MS_B$	$\dfrac{MS_B}{MS_E}$	$F_{\alpha[(b-1);(ab-1)(n-1)]}$
$A \times B$ interaction	(SS_{AB}) $\dfrac{1}{n}\sum_{i=1}^{a}\sum_{j=1}^{b} y_{ij.}^2 - \dfrac{y_{...}^2}{abn} - SS_A - SS_B$	$(a-1)(b-1)$	$\dfrac{SS_{AB}}{(a-1)(b-1)} = MS_{AB}$	$\dfrac{MS_{AB}}{MS_E}$	$F_{\alpha[(a-1)(b-1);(ab-1)(n-1)]}$
Blocks	(SS_{BLOCK}) $\dfrac{1}{ab}\sum_{k=1}^{n} y_{..k}^2 - \dfrac{y_{...}^2}{abn}$	$(n-1)$	$\dfrac{SS_{BLOCK}}{(n-1)}$		No test
Error	(SS_E) $SS_T - SS_A - SS_B - SS_{AB} - SS_{BLOCKS} = SS_E$	$(ab-1)(n-1)$	$\dfrac{SS_E}{(ab-1)(n-1)} = MS_E$		
Total	(SS_T) $\sum_{i=1}^{a}\sum_{j=1}^{b}\sum_{k=1}^{n} y_{ijk}^2 - \dfrac{y_{...}^2}{abn}$	$abn-1$			

$$\text{Treatment } A \times B = \underbrace{\sigma^2}_{\text{Pure error}} + \underbrace{\frac{n \sum \sum (AB)^2_{ij}}{(a-1)(b-1)}}_{\substack{\text{Treatment } A \times B \\ \text{effect}}}$$

$$\text{Block effect} = \underbrace{\sigma^2}_{\text{Pure error}} + \underbrace{ab\sigma^2_c}_{\substack{\text{Block} \\ \text{effect}}}$$

Pure Error $= \sigma^2 =$ Random Error

Example 1. A chemist working on a pilot purification extraction procedure is interested in evaluating three different antibiotic products using two different extraction methods. This study cannot be conducted in 1 day, so the researcher decides to utilize a two-factor design with days being blocked. The study will restrict randomization to being within each of three blocks. The values collected are in percentages, which have been coded to equal whole numbers (e.g., 89% = 89). The study design is presented in Table 2.

Note that at several samplings (Table 3), the percentage recorded was over 100. This is a normal phenomenon and has to do with random error. Also, note that the researcher has designed this study as a screening study. It is merely a preliminary study to provide the basis for the researcher to expand the study into a larger, more definitive one.

The researcher would like to know whether the two extraction methods are equivalent. If so, she will use method 2, for it is cheaper and faster. The researcher would also like to know whether there is a difference in the extraction efficiency for the same glycoamino antibiotic in three separate formulas.

TABLE 2 ANOVA Table, Represented Notation

		Day (block)					
	Factor B, extraction method	1		2		3	
		1	2	1	2	1	2
Factor A, antibiotic	1	y^a_{111}	y_{121}	y_{112}	y_{122}	y_{113}	y_{123}
	2	y_{211}	y_{221}	y_{212}	y_{222}	y_{213}	y_{223}
	3	y_{311}	y_{321}	y_{312}	y_{322}	y_{313}	y_{323}

[a] y_{ijk}

TABLE 2B   ANOVA Table, Actual Values Collected

| | | Day (block) | | | | | |
| | | 1 | | 2 | | 3 | |
	Factor B, extraction method	1	2	1	2	1	2
Factor A, antibiotic	1	82	78	84	73	88	84
	2	94	79	88	72	98	82
	3	106	85	90	75	104	87

Using the six-step procedure, let us work the problem.

Step 1.   Formulate the hypothesis:

Factor A 　　　　　 H_0: $\mu_1 = \mu_2 = \mu_3$ (The proportion of extraction of glycoamino is the same for each product.)

　　　　　　　　　 H_A: The above is not true.

Factor B 　　　　　 H_0 : $\mu_1 = \mu_2$ (Extraction methods 1 and 2 provide the same results.)

　　　　　　　　　 H_A : $\mu_1 \neq \mu_2$

$A \times B$ Interaction: 　 H_0: There is no significant interaction between factors A and B.

　　　　　　　　　 H_A: The above is not true.

Step 2.   Select α and n. The researcher has determined to use the smallest sample size possible and run the study over 3 days (blocks) and also to use $\alpha = 0.05$ for the interaction but $\alpha = 0.10$ for the main effects. That is, she wants to be more protected from type I error for interaction but less so for the main effects. In point of fact, she is being less conservative for type I error, thereby to discover a possible difference if one may exist within each of the main effects.

Step 3.   The linear model to be used is

$$y_{ijk} = \mu + A_i + B_j + (AB)_{ij} + C_k + \epsilon_{ijk} \tag{1}$$

where

　　　　 A_i = the ith level of factor A
　　　　 B_j = the jth level of factor B

$(AB)_{ij} =$ the interaction of the ith level of factor A and the jth level of factor B

$C_k =$ the kth level block effect

$\epsilon_{ijk} =$ error term

$a = 3$	degrees of freedom $= a - 1 = 3 - 1 = 2$
$b = 2$	$b - 1 = 2 - 1 = 1$
$n = 3$	$n - 1 = 3 - 1 = 2$
$AB = 3 \times 2$	$(a - 1)(b - 1) = 2 \times 1 = 2$
error $= (ab - 1)(n - 1) = (3 \times 2 - 1)(3 - 1) = 10$	

Step 4.   Establish decision rule.

Factor A: $F_{\alpha[b-1; (ab-1)(n-1)]} = F_{0.10[2, 10]} = 2.92$

If $F_c > 2.92$, reject H_0 at $\alpha = 0.10$. A significant difference in products exists.

Factor B: $F_{\alpha[b-1; (ab-1)(n-1)]} = F_{0.10[1, 10]} = 3.29$

If $F_c > 3.29$, reject H_0 at $\alpha = 0.10$. A significant difference exists in the methods.

$A \times B$ interaction: $F_{\alpha[(a-1)(b-1); (ab-1)(n-1)]} = F_{0.05[2, 10]} = 4.10$

If $F_c > 4.10$, reject H_0; significant factor $A \times B$ interaction exists at $\alpha = 0.05$.

Step 5.   Conduct the experiment. Table 3 provides the data.

Components

Factor $A = y_{i..} = 489 + 513 + 547 = 1549$

Factor $B = y_{.1.} = 282 + 262 + 290 = 834$

$\qquad\qquad y_{.2.} = 242 + 220 + 253 = 715$

Factor $A \times B = y_{ij.} = y_{11.} = 82 + 84 + 88 = 254$

$\qquad\qquad\qquad y_{12.} = 78 + 73 + 84 = 235$

$\qquad\qquad\qquad y_{21.} = 94 + 88 + 98 = 280$

$\qquad\qquad\qquad y_{22.} = 79 + 72 + 82 = 233$

$\qquad\qquad\qquad y_{31.} = 106 + 90 + 104 = 300$

$\qquad\qquad\qquad y_{32.} = 85 + 75 + 87 = 247$

$$SS_A = \frac{1}{bn} \sum_{i=1}^{3} y_{i..}^2 - \frac{y_{i..}^2}{abn}$$

$$= \frac{1}{2(3)}[489^2 + 513^2 + 547^2] - \frac{1549^2}{3 \cdot 2 \cdot 3}$$

$$= 133,583.167 - 133,300.056$$

$$= 283.111$$

TABLE 3 Data

Factor B, extraction method ($y_{j.}$)	Day (block; $y_{..k}$)						
	1		2		3		
	1	2	1	2	1	2	
Factor A, Antibiotic Formulation 1	82	78	84	73	88	84	$489 = y_{1..}$
2	94	79	88	72	98	82	$513 = y_{2..}$
3	106	85	90	75	104	87	$547 = y_{3..}$
	$y_{.1} = 524$		$y_{..2} = 482$		$y_{..3} = 543$		
$y_{.j.}$	$282 = y_{.1.}$	$242 = y_{.2.}$	$262 = y_{.1.}$	$220 = y_{.2.}$	$290 = y_{.1.}$	$253 = y_{.2.}$	$1549 = y_{....}$

$$SS_B = \frac{1}{an} \sum_{j=1}^{2} y_{.j.}^2 - \frac{y_{.j.}^2}{abn}$$

$$= \frac{1}{3(3)}[834^2 + 715^2] - \frac{1549^2}{3 \cdot 2 \cdot 3}$$

$$= 134,086.770 - 133,300.056$$

$$= 786.714$$

$$SS_{\text{BLOCK}} = \frac{1}{ab} \sum_{k=1}^{3} y_{..k}^2 - \frac{y_{...}^2}{abn}$$

$$= \frac{1}{2(3)}[524^2 + 482^2 + 543^2] - \frac{1549^2}{3 \cdot 2 \cdot 3}$$

$$= 133,624.833 - 133,300.056$$

$$= 324.778$$

$$SS_{AB} = \frac{1}{n} \sum_{i=1}^{3} \sum_{j=1}^{2} y_{ij.}^2 - \frac{y_{...}^2}{abn} - SS_A - SS_B$$

$$= \frac{1}{3}\left[254^2 + 235^2 + 280^2 + 233^2 + 300^2 + 247^2\right]$$

$$- \frac{1549^2}{3 \cdot 2 \cdot 3} - SS_A - SS_B$$

$$= 134,479.667 - 133,300.056 - SS_A - SS_B$$

$$= 1,179.611 - SS_A - SS_B$$

$$= 1,179.611 - 283.111 - 786.714$$

$$= 109.786$$

$$SS_{\text{TOTAL}} = \sum_{i=1}^{a} \sum_{j=1}^{b} \sum_{k=1}^{n} y_{ijk}^2 - \frac{y_{...}^2}{abn}$$

$$= \sum_{i=1}^{a} \sum_{j=1}^{b} \sum_{k=1}^{n}[82^2 + 94^2 + 106^2 + \cdots + 84^2 + 82^2 + 87^2]$$

$$- \frac{1549^2}{3 \cdot 2 \cdot 3}$$

$$= 134,897 - 133,300.056$$

$$= 1596.944$$

TABLE 4   ANOVA Table for Two-Factor Randomized Block Design

Source of variance	Sum of squares	Degrees of freedom	Mean square	Fc	F_T	S = Significant NS = Not significant
Factor A (product formulation)	283.111	2	141.56	15.296	2.92	S; $\alpha = 0.10$
Factor B (method)	786.714	1	786.71	84.96	3.29	S; $\alpha = 0.10$
Factor A × B interaction	109.78	2	54.89	5.93	4.10	S; $\alpha = 0.05$
Block effects (days)	324.778	2	162.89			
Error	92.555	10	9.26			
Total	1596.944	17				

$$SS_E = SS_T - SS_A - SS_B - SS_{\text{BLOCK}} - SS_{AB}$$
$$= 1596.944 - 283.111 - 786.714 - 324.778 - 109.786$$
$$= 92.555$$

The next step is to construct the analysis of variance table (Table 4).

Step 6.   Immediately the researcher sees that there is significant interaction between product formulations and extraction method used. In addition, the researcher sees that the error term does not appear inflated with $A \times$ block, $B \times$ block, and $A \times B \times$ block interaction, because it is relatively small. Yet, one cannot tell for sure without relying on experience. Because the main effects interaction ($A \times B$) term is significant, the researcher plots the mean values (Fig. 1) for the $\bar{y}_{ij.}$, where:

$\bar{y}_{11.} = 84.67$
$\bar{y}_{12.} = 78.33$
$\bar{y}_{21.} = 93.33$
$\bar{y}_{22.} = 77.67$
$\bar{y}_{31.} = 100.00$
$\bar{y}_{32.} = 82.33$

Upon closer investigation, the researcher sees that method 1 provides higher extractions than method 2. The practical importance of this

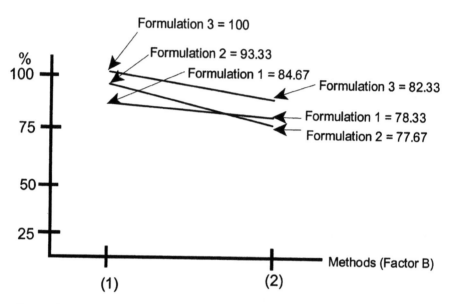

FIGURE 1   Plotted mean values.

interaction is not significant for the researcher. She feels that the sensitivity of the interaction is too great (MS_E), based on her field experience, and decides to ignore it in this pilot study. She is pleased that the block effect did reduce variability but decides, for the next study, to pool days (ignore the day effect), which will increase the error term. She sees that the main effect, A (antibiotic formulation), has varying extraction effects. And, because formulations differ, she will expand this component in the next study, carefully noting what happens. Also, she decides to use extraction method 1 because it provides consistently better extraction results. In the next study, she will omit extraction method 2.

It is important for the researcher to ground the statistics in the field of his or her expertise instead of looking at the statistical analysis as a "holy" vehicle. But this requires expertise in both statistics and one's primary field.

A computer printout of this evaluation is presented in Table 5. The generalized linear model was used on a MiniTab software package.

The means for the main effects and interaction are provided in Table 6.

TABLE 5   MiniTab Generalized Linear Model

ANALYSIS OF VARIANCE FOR EXTRACTION

Source	DF	Seq SS	Adj SS	Adj MS	F	P
C1	2	283.11	283.11	141.56	15.29	.001
C2	1	786.72	786.72	786.72	85.00	.000
C3	2	324.78	324.78	162.39	17.55	.001
C1*C2	2	109.78	109.78	54.89	5.93	.020
ERROR	10	92.56	92.56	9.26		
TOTAL	17	1596.94				

Note: C_1 = factor A, C_2 = factor B, C_3 - blocks (days), $C_4 = y_{ijk}$, $C_5 = \hat{y}_{ijk}$, $C_6 = y\epsilon_{ijk}$.

Note: The predicted value $\hat{y}_{ijk} = \hat{\mu} + \hat{A} + \hat{B} + \widehat{AB} + \hat{C}$ where:

$$\hat{\mu} = \bar{y}_{...}$$
$$A = \bar{y}_{1..} - \bar{y}_{...}$$
$$B = \bar{y}_{.j.} - \bar{y}_{...}$$
$$C = \bar{y}_{..k} - \bar{y}_{...}$$
$$AB_{ij} = \bar{y}_{ij.} - \bar{y}_{i..} - \bar{y}_{.j.} + \bar{y}_{...}$$

TABLE 6   Means for Main Effects and Interactions

(A) PRODUCT =	C_1		MEAN
	1		81.50
	2		85.50
	3		91.17
(B) METHOD =	C_2		
	1		92.67
	2		79.44
(C) DAY (BLOCK) =	C_3		
	1		87.33
	2		80.33
	3		90.50
PRODUCT × METHOD INTERACTION =	$C_1 \times C_2$		
	1	1	84.67
	1	2	78.33
	2	1	93.33
	2	2	77.67
	3	1	100.00
	3	2	82.33

TABLE 7 Input/Output Data Table

ROW	C1	C2	C3	C4	C5	C6
1	1	1	1	83	85.944	− 3.94444
2	2	1	1	96	94.6111	− 6.61111
3	3	1	1	106	101.278	4.72222
4	1	1	1	78	79.611	− 1.61111
5	2	2	1	79	78.944	0.05558
6	3	2	1	83	87.611	1.38889
7	1	1	2	84	78.944	5.05596
8	2	1	2	88	87.611	0.38889
9	3	1	2	90	94.278	− 4.27778
10	1	2	2	72	72.611	0.38889
11	2	2	2	72	71.944	0.05556
12	3	2	2	73	76.611	− 1.61111
13	1	1	3	88	89.111	− 1.11111
14	2	1	3	98	47.778	0.22222
15	3	1	3	104	104.444	− 0.44444
16	1	2	3	84	82.778	1.22222
17	2	2	3	82	82.111	− 0.11111
18	3	2	3	87	88.778	0.22222

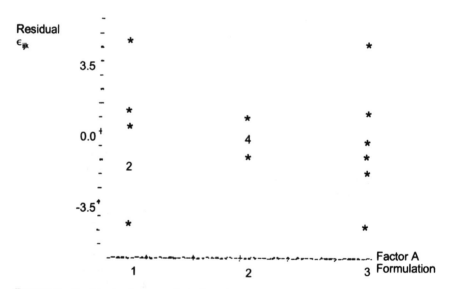

FIGURE 2 Residual values ϵ_{ijk} plotted against main effect A (formulation).

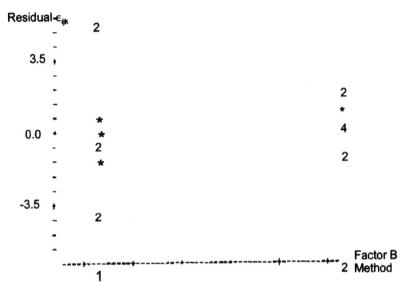

FIGURE 3   Residual values ϵ_{ijk} plotted against factor *B* (method).

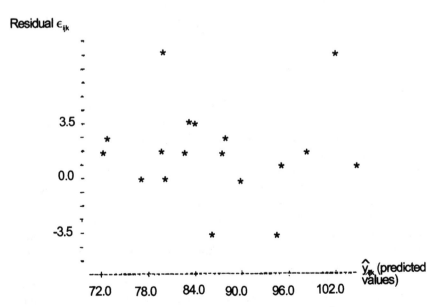

FIGURE 4   Residual values ϵ_{ijk} plotted against predicted values $\hat{y}_{ijk}$.

For example,

$$\hat{y}_{111} = \bar{y}_{...} + (\bar{y}_{1..} - \bar{y}_{...}) + (\bar{y}_{.1.} - \bar{y}_{...}) + (\bar{y}_{..1} - \bar{y}_{...}) + (\bar{y}_{11.} - \bar{y}_{1..} - \bar{y}_{.1.} + \bar{y}_{...})$$
$$= 86.06 + (81.50 - 86.06) + (92.67 - 86.06)$$
$$+ (87.33 - 86.06) + (84.67 - 81.50 - 92.67 + 86.06)$$
$$= 85.94$$

The formula for deriving $\hat{y}_{ijk}$ can be simplified with some algebraic manipulation to

$$\hat{y}_{ijk} = \bar{y}_{ij.} + \bar{y}_{..k} - \bar{y}_{...} \quad (\text{e.g.}, \hat{y}_{111} = 84.67 + 87.33 - 86.06 = 85.94)$$

Let us now look at some residual plots. Figure 2 portrays the residual values, ϵ_{ijk}, plotted against the three antibiotic formulations (main effect A). Notice that the residuals for all three formulations in factor A are uniformly distributed about zero.

Figure 3 portrays the residual values, ϵ_{ijk}, plotted against main effect B (extraction method). Notice that the values in the two levels of factor B are uniformly distributed about zero.

Figure 4 presents a plot of the residual values, ϵ_{ijk} against the predicted values $\hat{y}_{ijk}$. Again, the residuals versus fitted or predicted values seem to be centered about zero.

The researcher also should perform exploratory data analysis on the residual values, including stem-and-leaf displays, letter-value displays, and boxplots.

II. MULTIPLE CONTRASTS

Multiple contrasts can be made of the main effects (factors A and B) as well as the interaction. As discussed previously, if the interaction of the main effects is significant, the researcher will want to be careful in evaluating the main effects by themselves. Based upon Fig.1, the interaction of formulations 1 and 2 flip-flops between methods 1 and 2. Using extraction method 1, the extraction quantity of formulation 2 is slightly higher than that for formulation 1, but when using extraction method 2, the extraction of formulation 1 is slightly greater than that for formulation 2.

The researcher now has dismissed the interaction's significance to her goal, that of picking an extraction method. She has decided, also, to expand the investigation of the extraction method of choice (method 1) into a more intense future study.

However, you, as the researcher, may not want to handle the analysis as she did. You may want to explore the interaction effects as well as the main effects via multiple contrasts.

We will forgo any orthogonal (a priori) evaluation because the likelihood of the researcher knowing what contrasts are important *before* conducting the study is not high. Instead, we will focus on the a posteriori contrasts that the researcher decides to perform after a study has been completed and the H_0 hypothesis rejected.

As in the last chapter, when a main factor contains only two levels, no further contrasts are necessary because the F-test would provide only a retest of their significance. That is, the researcher already knows that there is a significant difference between methods 1 and 2 (factor B, extraction method) at the set α.

Suppose the researcher wanted to evaluate the main effects of factor A, although this will undoubtedly provide contradictory results between products 1 and 2 because results will differ depending upon the method used.

III. SCHEFFE'S METHOD

Recall that Scheffe's method is used to compare a number of different contrasts. It is useful for comparing any number of combination contrasts but not for all pairs of means.

The test can be used for both factor A ($y_i..$) and factor B ($y._j.$) as well as the $A \times B$ interaction ($y_{ij}.$). For standardization, we call the $y_i..$s the row totals, and the $y._j.$s the column totals.

The standard error of the contrast (C) is:

$$S_c = \sqrt{MS_E \sum \left(\frac{c^2}{n}\right)} \tag{2}$$

which is, for factor A:

$$S_c = \sqrt{MS_E \sum_{i=1}^{a} \left(\frac{c_i^2}{n}\right)}$$

and for factor B:

$$S_c = \sqrt{MS_E \sum_{j=1}^{b} \left(\frac{c_j^2}{n}\right)}$$

In this example, only factor A is of importance because factor B is at two levels and is known to be significant.

Factor A Contrasts (C_i)

$$C_i = C_1 \bar{y}_{1..} + C_2 \bar{y}_{2..} + \cdots + C_a \bar{y}_{a..}$$

The critical value with which C_i should be compared is $S_{\alpha_j} = S_{C_i} \sqrt{(a-1)F_{\alpha(a-1);(ab-1)(n-1)}}$.

If C_j (factor B) is evaluated, use the form $S_{\alpha_j} = S_{C_j} \sqrt{(b-1)F_{\alpha(b-1);(ab-1)(n-1)}}$.

Hypothesis: If $|C_i| > S_{\alpha_i}$, reject H_0

Recall: $y_{i..} = y_{1..} = 489;$ $\bar{y}_{1..} = \dfrac{489}{6} = 81.50$

$= y_{2..} = 513;$ $\bar{y}_{2..} = \dfrac{513}{6} = 85.50$

$= y_{3..} = 547;$ $\bar{y}_{3..} = \dfrac{547}{6} = 91.17$

Suppose the researcher wants to contrast:

$$C_1 = \mu_1 - \frac{\mu_2 + \mu_3}{2} = 0 \quad 81.5 - \frac{85.5 + 91.17}{2} = -6.84$$

The hypothesis set is written:

C_1: H_0: $\mu_1 - \dfrac{\mu_2 + \mu_3}{2} = 0$

H_A: $\mu_1 - \dfrac{\mu_2 + \mu_3}{2} \neq 0$

$C_1 = \bar{y}_{1..} - \dfrac{\bar{y}_{2..} + \bar{y}_{3..}}{2}$

$C_1 = 81.5 - \dfrac{85.5 + 91.17}{2} = -6.84$

Recall from Table 4 that $MS_E = 9.256$.

$$S_{C_1} = \sqrt{MS_E \sum_{i=1}^{3} \frac{C_i}{n_i}} = \sqrt{9.256 \left(\frac{1^2 + (-1/2)^2 - (1/2)^2}{6} \right)} \quad \text{or}$$

$$\sqrt{9.256 \left(\frac{1^2}{6} + \frac{(-1/2)^2}{6} + \frac{(-1/2)^2}{6} \right)} = 1.52$$

$$S_{\alpha_1} = S_{C_{0.05,C_1}} \sqrt{(a-1)F_{\alpha[a-1;(ab-1)(n-1)]}}$$
$$= 1.52\sqrt{(3-1)F_{0.05(2;10)}}$$
$$= 1.52\sqrt{2(4.10)}$$
$$= 4.35$$

If $|C_i| > S_{\alpha_i}$ reject H_0 at α.

$|C_1| = |-6.84| > 4.35$, so the H_0 hypothesis for contrast 1 (C_1), $(H_0: \mu_1 - (\mu_2 + \mu_3)/2 = 0)$, is rejected at $\alpha = 0.05$.

Contrast 2 is:

$$C_2: H_0: \mu_2 - \mu_3 = 0$$
$$H_A: \mu_2 - \mu_3 \neq 0$$

$$C_2 = \bar{y}_{2..} - \bar{y}_{3..} = 85.50 - 91.17 = -5.67$$

$$S_{C_2} = \sqrt{MS_E \sum_{i=1}^{2} \frac{C_i}{n_i}} = \sqrt{9.256\frac{(1^2 + (-1)^2)}{6}} = 1.76$$

$$S_{\alpha_2} = 1.76\sqrt{2(4.10)} = 5.04$$

$|C_2| = |-5.67| > 5.04$, so the H_0 hypothesis for contrast 2 (C_2), $(H_0: \mu_2 = \mu_3)$ is rejected at $\alpha = 0.05$.

Here is where the problem of interaction comes into play. One cannot contrast the main effects of factor A without taking into account factor B. For a case in point, if the researcher were to compare μ_1 with μ_2 and a difference was detected, she or he would have to be sure to note that at factor B, method 1, product 2 provides a greater extraction percentage than product 1. But at factor B, method 2, product 1 provides a greater extraction percentage than product 2. Hence, the researcher would usually contrast not main effects ($y_{i..}$ or $y_{.j.}$) but interactions (y_{ij}) to get a view of what the data reveal.

For the researcher, the Scheffe method is most useful when evaluating particularly complex contrasts, such as $C_1[\mu_1 - (\mu_2 + \mu_3)/2]$. If the researcher wants to compare all pairs of means, the LSD, Duncan's multiple range, Newman–Keuls, or Tukey's test can be used. They tend to be more sensitive to differences between mean pairs than is the Scheffe method.

IV. LEAST SIGNIFICANT DIFFERENCE (LSD)

Recall that the least significant difference procedure compares all pairs of means and can be used for both the main effects and the interaction terms.

Because factor B had only two levels, there is no need to compare them, for we already know they are significantly different.

Because the LSD procedure is used to compare mean pairs, it is important from the researcher's perspective that, in the blocked design, there be no missing values. If one block is missing a value, the other blocks should be reduced randomly one block value each to make the design balanced.

The LSD test formula for factor B is:

$$LSD = t_{\alpha/2;(ab-1)(n-1)}\sqrt{\frac{2MS_E}{an}}$$

For factor A, substitute a for b, $\sqrt{\frac{2MS_E}{bn}}$

The hypothesis test is:

$$H_0: \mu_i - \mu_j = 0$$

$$H_A: \mu_i - \mu_j \neq 0$$

If $|\bar{y}_i - \bar{y}_j| > LSD$, reject H_0 at α.

There are $[a(a-1)]/2 = (3 \times 2)/2 = 3$ possible contrasts for factor A. The Factor A means are:

$$\bar{y}_{1..} = 81.50$$

$$\bar{y}_{2..} = 85.50$$

$$\bar{y}_{3..} = 91.17$$

$$LSD = t_{\alpha/2;\ (2b-1)(n-1)}\sqrt{\frac{2MS_E}{bn}}$$

for $b = 2, a = 3, n = 3,$ and $MS_E = 9.256$

Let us set α at 0.05. $t_{\alpha/2\cdot(2b-1)(n-1)} = t_{0.05/2(3\cdot2-1)(3-1)} = t_{0.025;10}$ From the students t table (Table B), $t = 2.228$

$$LSD = 2.228\sqrt{\frac{2(9.256)}{2 \times 3}} = 3.91$$

The three contrasts are:

LSD	S = Significant NS = Not significant
$\bar{y}_{1..} - \bar{y}_{2..} = \|81.50 - 85.50\| = 4 > 3.91$	S
$\bar{y}_{1..} - \bar{y}_{3..} = \|81.50 - 91.17\| = 9.67 > 3.91$	S
$\bar{y}_{2..} - \bar{y}_{3..} = \|85.50 - 91.17\| = 5.67 < 3.91$	S

V. DUNCAN'S MULTIPLE RANGE TEST

We have used the Duncan's multiple range test over the last several chapters. It is useful for comparing all pairs of means. Again, the more advanced designs, such as the complete block two-factor factorial experiments we are using, will be used primarily for research and development. The reason is that, in the world at large, it will be more difficult for nonstatisticians to comprehend them. It is strongly recommended that sample sizes be the same to provide a balanced design. If a value is missing, however, one can estimate it with the method used in Chap. 7 and increase degrees of freedom for the error term by one. Hence, degrees of freedom would be $MS_E = (ab - 1)(n - 1) - 1$.

Both the main effects and interaction can be compared using Duncan's multiple range test. Recall that one arranges the a (or b) treatment means of each factor tested in ascending order. This is followed by computing the standard error of each factor.

For factor A, it is:

$$S_{\bar{y}_{i..}} = \sqrt{\frac{MS_E}{bn}}$$

For factor B, it is:

$$S_{\bar{y}_{.j.}} = \sqrt{\frac{MS_E}{an}}$$

Ascending order (treatment means of factor A):

$$\bar{y}_{1..} = 81.50$$

$$\bar{y}_{2..} = 85.50$$

$$\bar{y}_{3..} = 91.17$$

Computation of standard error:

$$S_{\bar{y}_{1..}} = \sqrt{\frac{MS_E}{bn}} = \sqrt{\frac{9.256}{2 \times 3}} = 1.24$$

From Duncan's multiple range table (see Table A.5), one obtains the value of $r_{\alpha(p,f)}S_{\bar{y}_{i..}}$ for $p = 2, 3 \ldots, a$. (For treatment B, this would be $r_{\alpha(p,f)}S_{\bar{y}_{.j.}}$ for $p = 2, 3, \ldots, b$).

The observed differences between the means are then compared, beginning with the largest to the smallest, which is compared with R_a (R_b if factor B). Next, the largest to the second smallest is compared with R_{a-1} (or R_{b-1} if factor B). For Factor A, the interaction process continues until all possible $[a(a-1)]/2 = (3 \times 2)/2 = 3$ comparisons have been made. If the observed pair difference, is greater than the R value, the mean pair difference is significant at α. No difference between a pair of means is considered significant if the two means involved lie between pairs of means that are not significant.

$$R_2 = r_{0.05(2,10)}S_{\bar{y}_i.} \qquad R_3 = r_{0.05(3,10)}S_{\bar{y}_i.}$$
$$R_2 = 3.15(1.24) \qquad R_3 = 3.30(1.24)$$
$$R_2 = 3.91 \qquad R_3 = 4.09$$

Contrast	S = Significant NS = Not significant
$\bar{y}_{3..} - \bar{y}_{1..} = 91.17 - 81.50 = 9.67 > 4.09$	S
$\bar{y}_{3..} - \bar{y}_{2..} = 91.17 - 85.50 = 5.67 > 3.91$	S
$\bar{y}_{2..} - \bar{y}_{1..} = 85.50 - 81.50 = 4.00 > 3.91$	S

However, by not checking out the interactions, which are significant in this case, the researcher would miss the point that formulations 1 and 2 flip-flop, depending upon whether they are evaluated using factor B method 1 or 2.

VI. NEWMAN–KEULS TEST

The application of this test is very similar to what was done in the previous chapter. Like the Duncan multiple range and LSD tests, the test is designed to compare all possible combinations of treatment level means. It can be utilized for both main effects, factors A ($\bar{y}_{i.}$) and B ($\bar{y}_{.j}$), and the interaction means ($\bar{y}_{.j}$).

As before, the researcher calculates a set of k_p values for each factor:

$$k_p = q_{\alpha(p,f)}S_{\bar{y}} \tag{3}$$

For main effect factor A, the form is:
$$k_p = q_{\alpha(p,f)}S_{\bar{y}_{i..}} \qquad \text{where } p = 2, 3 \ldots, a \text{ and } f = \text{degrees of freedom MS}_E$$
For main effect B, the form is:
$$k_p = q_{\alpha(p,f)}S_{\bar{y}_{.j}} \qquad \text{where } p = 2, 3 \ldots, b \text{ and } f = \text{degrees of freedom MS}_E$$
Recall that factor B had only two levels, so the evaluation need not go further.

As with Duncan's multiple range test, the investigator first computes the k_p value for factor A:

$$k_p = q_{\alpha(p,f)}S_{\bar{y}_{i..}}$$

$$S_{\bar{y}_{i..}} = \sqrt{\frac{MS_E}{bn}} = \sqrt{\frac{9.256}{6}} = 1.24$$

Then, calculate k_p, where $p = 2, 3$, letting $\alpha = 0.05$.
    Find q_α in the Studentized range table (see Table A.1).

$$q_{0.05(2,10)} = 3.15$$

$$q_{0.05(3,10)} = 3.88$$

$$k_p = q_{\alpha(p,f)} S_{\bar{y}_{i..}}$$

$$k_2 = 3.15(1.24) = 3.91$$

$$k_3 = 3.88(1.24) = 4.81$$

Next, we arrange the $\bar{y}_{i..}$ values in ascending order:

$$\bar{y}_{1..} = 81.50$$

$$\bar{y}_{2..} = 85.50$$

$$\bar{y}_{3..} = 91.17$$

Compute contrasts as in the Duncan method:

Contrast	S = Significant NS = Not significant
$\bar{y}_{3..} - \bar{y}_{1..} = 91.17 - 81.50 = 9.67 > 4.81$	S
$\bar{y}_{3..} - \bar{y}_{2..} = 91.17 - 85.50 = 5.67 > 3.91$	S
$\bar{y}_{2..} - \bar{y}_{1..} = 85.50 - 81.50 = 4.00 > 3.91$	S

As stated previously, it is not a good idea to compare main effects without being extremely careful when interaction is present.

VII. TUKEY TEST

The Tukey test procedure is straightforward. Both main effects factors A and B, and the interaction effects can be contrasted. As before, the Tukey test considers any pair difference (absolute) that is greater than T_α significant at α.

For main effect factor A, the form is: $T_\alpha = q_{\alpha(a,f)}S_{\bar{y}_{i..}}$

For main effect factor B, the form is: $T_\alpha = q_{\alpha(b,f)}S_{\bar{y}_{.j.}}$

All $[a(a-1)]/2$ or $[b(b-1)]/2$ mean pairs for main effect factors A and B, respectively, are computed. And, as before, because $b=2$, only factor A will be contrasted.

Factor A

$$T_\alpha = q_{\alpha(a,f)}S_{\bar{y}_{i..}}$$

$$S_{\bar{y}_{i..}} = \sqrt{\frac{MS_E}{bn}} = \sqrt{\frac{9.256}{2 \cdot 3}}$$

$$S_{\bar{y}_{i..}} = 1.24$$

For factor B:

$$S\bar{y}_{.j.} = \sqrt{\frac{MS_E}{an}}$$

$$T_{0.05} = q_{0.05(3,10)}1.24 = 3.88(1.24) = 4.81$$

Where $f=$ degrees of freedom for $MS_E = (ab-1)(n-1) = 10$

$\alpha = 0.05$, and $a = 3$

Decision rule:

$$H_0: \mu_i = \mu_j$$
$$H_A: \mu \neq \mu_j$$

If $|\bar{y}_{i..} - \bar{y}_{j..}| > T_\alpha$ reject H_0 (there is no difference between mean pairs) at α.

Contrast	S = Significant NS = Not significant
$\bar{y}_{3..} - \bar{y}_{1..} = 91.17 - 81.50 = 9.67 > 4.81$	S
$\bar{y}_{3..} - \bar{y}_{2..} = 91.17 - 85.50 = 5.67 > 4.81$	S
$\bar{y}_{2..} - \bar{y}_{1..} = 85.50 - 81.50 = 4.00 < 4.81$	NS

As before, the same warnings apply. It is very risky determining main effects factors A and/or B when $A \times B$ interaction is significant. Formulations 1 and 2 flip-flop in the proportion of extraction, depending upon the method.

VIII. COMPARING BOTH FACTORS *A* AND *B*

When interaction is significant, as it is in this case, it is often not useful to contrast main effects. It is, however, useful to compare combinations of factors *A* and *B*.

As in Chap. 7, instead of comparing column or row means (main effects), we now compare cell means or main effects factor combinations $A \times B$.

As stated in the main effects contrast portion of this chapter, the probability of knowing what contrasts one wants to test *prior to* conducting the study is essentially zero. Hence, we will not discuss *a priori* orthogonal contrasts. Let us instead go back through the contrasts we employed for the main effects and employ them for cell combinations. The cell means for the main effect combinations averaged over the blocks or days are:

$$A_1 B_1 = \bar{y}_{11.} = 84.67 \qquad A_1 B_2 = \bar{y}_{12.} = 78.33$$

$$A_2 B_1 = \bar{y}_{21.} = 93.33 \qquad A_2 B_2 = \bar{y}_{22.} = 77.67$$

$$A_3 B_1 = \bar{y}_{31.} = 100.00 \qquad A_3 B_2 = \bar{y}_{32.} = 82.33$$

These values are those of interest for the $A \times B$ factor contrast methods discussed. Let us begin with Scheffe's method.

IX. SCHEFFE'S METHOD

Recall that Scheffe's method is used mainly to compare several combinations of contrasts. It is not as efficient for comparing all pairwise contrasts as the LSD, Duncan's multiple range test, Newman–Keuls, or Tukey's method. And recall that type I error (α) will be, at most, α for the combined contrasts.

Suppose the researcher wants to perform the following two contrasts:

C_1: H_0: $\mu_{11.} = \mu_{32.}$

$\qquad H_A$: $\mu_{11.} \neq \mu_{32.}$

C_2: H_0: $\mu_{11.} + \mu_{21.} + \mu_{31.} = \mu_{12.} + \mu_{22.} + \mu_{32.}$

$\qquad H_A$: $\mu_{11.} + \mu_{21.} + \mu_{31.} \neq \mu_{12.} + \mu_{22.} + \mu_{32.}$

Recall that the critical value the C_i values are compared with is:

$$S_{\alpha_i} = S_{c_i}\sqrt{(a-1)(b-1)F_{\alpha[(a-1)(b-1);(ab-1)(n-1)]}}$$

where

$$S_{c_i} = \sqrt{MS_E \sum\left(\frac{c_{ij}^2}{n}\right)} \quad \text{and} \quad MS_E = 9.256.$$

The decision rule is:

If $|C_i| > S_{\alpha_i}$ reject H_0 at α.

$C_1 = \bar{y}_{11.} - \bar{y}_{32.}$

$\quad = |84.67 - 82.33| = 2.34$

$C_2 = \bar{y}_{11.} + \bar{y}_{21.} + \bar{y}_{31.} - \bar{y}_{12.} - \bar{y}_{22.} - \bar{y}_{32.}$

$\quad = |84.67 + 93.33 + 100.00 - 78.33 - 77.67 - 82.33| = 39.67$

$$S_{c_1} = \sqrt{MS_E\left(\frac{1^2 + (-1^2)}{3}\right)} = \sqrt{9.256\left(\frac{1^2 + (-1^2)}{3}\right)} = 2.48$$

$$S_{c_2} = \sqrt{9.256\left(\frac{1^2 + 1^2 + 1^2 + (-1^2) + (-1^2) + (-1^2)}{3}\right)} = 4.30$$

For contrast 1 (C_1), the test hypothesis is:

$C_1 = H_0: \mu_{11.} = \mu_{22.}$

$\quad\quad H_A: \mu_{11.} \neq \mu_{32.}$

Let $\alpha = 0.05$

$S_{\alpha_1} = S_{c_1}\sqrt{(a-1)(b-1)F_{\alpha[(a-1)(b-1);(ab-1)(n-1)]}}$

$S_{\alpha_1} = S_{c_1}\sqrt{(3-1)(2-1)(4.10)} = 2.48\sqrt{2(4.10)} = 7.10$

Because $C_1 = 2.34 < 7.10$, one cannot reject H_0 at $\alpha = 0.05$.
    For contrast 2 (C_2), the test hypothesis is:

$C_2 = H_0: \mu_{11.} + \mu_{21.} + \mu_{31.} = \mu_{12.} + \mu_{22.} + \mu_{32.}$

$\quad\quad H_A$: The above is not true.

Let $\alpha = 0.05$.

$$S_{\alpha_2} = S_{C_2}\sqrt{(3-1)(2-1)(4.10)} = 4.30\sqrt{2(4.10)} = 12.31$$

Because $C_2 = 39.67 > 12.31$, reject H_0 at $\alpha = 0.05$.

X. LEAST SIGNIFICANT DIFFERENCE (LSD)

We have now arrived at one of the most useful procedures for comparison of treatment means when interaction exists. Because the researcher can compare all possible pairs of $A \times B$ means, he or she will have a much better idea of where differences exist relative to the effects of main factor $A \times B$. There are six mean values corresponding to the three levels of factor A and the two levels of factor B, so the number of contrasts possible for the cell means ($\bar{y}_{ij.}$) is:

$$\frac{ab(ab-1)}{2} = \frac{3 \cdot 2(3 \cdot 2 - 1)}{2} = 15$$

The least significant difference value, (LSD), is

$$t_{\frac{\alpha}{2},(ab-1)(n-1)}\sqrt{\frac{2MS_E}{n}}$$

This is for a balanced design where the replicate n values are the same, which is important in blocked studies. We have already discussed appropriate ways to handle missing values.

The test hypotheses are:

$$H_0: \mu_{ij.} - \mu_{ji.} = 0$$

$$H_A: \mu_{ij.} - \mu_{ji.} \neq 0$$

The decision rule is:

If $|\bar{y}_{ij.} - \bar{y}_{ji.}| > t_{\frac{\alpha}{2},(ab-1)(n-1)}\sqrt{\frac{2MS_E}{n}}$, reject H_0 at α.

In our example:

$$\sqrt{\frac{2MS_E}{n}} = \sqrt{\frac{2(9.256)}{3}} = 2.48$$

Let $\alpha = 0.05$ and $\alpha/2 = 0.025$; for $df = 10$, $t_{(0.025,\ 10)} = 2.228$. So, putting this all together, LSD $= 2.228(2.48) = 5.53$. If $|\bar{y}_{ij.} - \bar{y}_{ji.}| > 5.53$, reject H_0 at α.

Contrasts	S = Significant NS = Not significant
$\bar{y}_{21.}$ VS. $\bar{y}_{11.} = |93.33 - 84.67| = 8.66 > 5.53$	S
$\bar{y}_{31.}$ VS. $\bar{y}_{11.} = |100.0 - 84.67| = 15.33 > 5.53$	S
$\bar{y}_{12.}$ VS. $\bar{y}_{11.} = |78.33 - 84.67| = 6.34 > 5.53$	S
$\bar{y}_{22.}$ VS. $\bar{y}_{11.} = |77.67 - 84.67| = 7.00 > 5.53$	S
$\bar{y}_{32.}$ VS. $\bar{y}_{11.} = |82.33 - 84.67| = 2.34 < 5.53$	S
$\bar{y}_{31.}$ VS. $\bar{y}_{21.} = |100.00 - 93.33| = 6.67 > 5.53$	NS
$\bar{y}_{12.}$ VS. $\bar{y}_{21.} = |78.33 - 93.33| = 15.00 > 5.53$	S
$\bar{y}_{22.}$ VS. $\bar{y}_{21.} = |77.67 - 93.33| = 15.66 > 5.53$	S
$\bar{y}_{32.}$ VS. $\bar{y}_{21.} = |82.33 - 93.33| = 11.00 > 5.53$	S
$\bar{y}_{12.}$ VS. $\bar{y}_{31.} = |78.33 - 100.00| = 21.67 > 5.53$	S
$\bar{y}_{22.}$ VS. $\bar{y}_{31.} = |77.67 - 100.00| = 22.33 > 5.53$	S
$\bar{y}_{32.}$ VS. $\bar{y}_{31.} = |82.33 - 100.00| = 17.67 > 5.53$	S
$\bar{y}_{12.}$ VS. $\bar{y}_{32.} = |78.33 - 82.33| = 4.00 < 5.53$	NS
$\bar{y}_{22.}$ VS. $\bar{y}_{32.} = |77.67 - 82.33| = 4.66 < 5.53$	NS
$\bar{y}_{12.}$ VS. $\bar{y}_{22.} = |78.33 - 77.67| = 0.66 < 5.53$	NS

It would be helpful to consult Fig. 1 to see where the differences are.

Therefore, using method 2, none of the three formulations differ from each other in extraction percentage. Also, formulation 1, method 1 is equivalent to them. All other combination pairs are significantly different from each other at $\alpha = 0.05$.

XI. DUNCAN'S MULTIPLE RANGE TEST

As noted earlier, Duncan's multiple range test can also be used to compare all possible $A \times B$ mean pair ($\bar{y}_{ij.}$) combinations. Again, we will consider only the balanced experimental design contrasts. The cell means ($\bar{y}_{ij.}$) are, as usual, ranked in ascending order.

The test hypothesis is:

H_0: $\mu_{ij.} - \mu_{ji.} = 0$

H_A: $\mu_{ij.} - \mu_{ji.} \neq 0$

Decision rule:

If $\bar{y}_{ij.} - \bar{y}_{ji.} > r_{\alpha(p,f)}S_{\bar{y}_{ij.}}$, reject H_0 at α.

The cell means $(\bar{y}_{ij.})$ are arranged in ascending order:

$\bar{y}_{22.} = 77.67$

$\bar{y}_{12.} = 78.33$

$\bar{y}_{32.} = 82.33$

$\bar{y}_{11.} = 84.67$

$\bar{y}_{21.} = 93.33$

$\bar{y}_{31.} = 100.00$

The standard error of the mean is calculated as:

$$S_{\bar{y}_{ij.}} = \sqrt{\frac{MS_E}{n}} = \sqrt{\frac{9.256}{3}} = 1.76$$

The r value is found in Table A.5.

Let $\alpha = 0.05$

$$R_p = r_{\alpha(p,f)}S_{\bar{y}_{ij.}}$$

$p = 2, 3 \cdots a \cdot b = 2, 3 \cdots 6$

$f = ab(n-1)(n-1) = (3 \cdot 2 - 1)(3-1) = 10$

$R_2 = r_{0.05(2,10)}S_{\bar{y}_{ij.}} = 3.15(1.76) = 5.54$

$R_3 = r_{0.05(3,10)}S_{\bar{y}_{ij.}} = 3.30(1.76) = 5.81$

$R_4 = r_{0.05(4,10)}S_{\bar{y}_{ij.}} = 3.37(1.76) = 5.93$

$R_5 = r_{0.05(5,10)}S_{\bar{y}_{ij.}} = 3.43(1.76) = 6.04$

$R_6 = r_{0.05(6,10)}S_{\bar{y}_{ij.}} = 3.46(1.76) = 6.09$

The number of possible contrasts: $[ab(ab - 1)]/2 = [3 \cdot 2(3 \cdot 2 - 1)]/2 =$ 15 total contrasts.

	S = Significant NS = Not significant
$\bar{y}_{31.} - \bar{y}_{22.} = 100.00 - 77.67 = 22.33 > 6.09 = (R_6)$	S
$\bar{y}_{31.} - \bar{y}_{12.} = 100.00 - 78.33 = 21.67 > 6.04 = (R_5)$	S
$\bar{y}_{31.} - \bar{y}_{32.} = 100.00 - 82.33 = 17.67 > 5.93 = (R_4)$	S
$\bar{y}_{31.} - \bar{y}_{11.} = 100.00 - 84.67 = 15.33 > 5.81 = (R_3)$	S
$\bar{y}_{31.} - \bar{y}_{21.} = 100.00 - 93.33 = 6.67 > 5.54 = (R_2)$	S
$\bar{y}_{21.} - \bar{y}_{22.} = 93.33 - 77.67 = 15.66 > 6.04 = (R_5)$	S
$\bar{y}_{21.} - \bar{y}_{12.} = 93.33 - 78.33 = 15.00 > 5.93 = (R_4)$	S
$\bar{y}_{21.} - \bar{y}_{32.} = 93.33 - 82.33 = 11.00 > 5.81 = (R_3)$	S
$\bar{y}_{21.} - \bar{y}_{11.} = 93.33 - 84.67 = 8.66 > 5.54 = (R_2)$	S
$\bar{y}_{11.} - \bar{y}_{22.} = 84.67 - 77.67 = 7.00 > 5.93 = (R_4)$	S
$\bar{y}_{11.} - \bar{y}_{12.} = 84.67 - 78.33 = 6.34 > 5.81 = (R_3)$	S
$\bar{y}_{11.} - \bar{y}_{32.} = 84.67 - 82.33 = 2.34 < 5.54 = (R_2)$	NS
$\bar{y}_{32.} - \bar{y}_{22.} = 82.33 - 77.67 = 4.66 < 5.81 = (R_3)$	NS
$\bar{y}_{32.} - \bar{y}_{12.} = 82.33 - 78.33 = 4.00 < 5.54 = (R_2)$	NS
$\bar{y}_{12.} - \bar{y}_{22.} = 78.33 - 77.67 = 0.66 < 5.54 = (R_2)$	NS

XII. NEWMAN–KEULS TEST

The Newman–Keuls test can also used to compare all possible pairs of $A \times B$ cell means $(\bar{y}_{ij.})$. Recall that in performing this test, a set of critical values is computed using the formula:

$$K_p = q_{\alpha(p,f)}S_{\bar{y}_{ij.}} \qquad p = 2, 3 \ldots ab$$

Note also that the standard error of the mean represents the cell means $(\bar{y}_{ij.})$. The MS_E value is still used, but the divisor is n, not an or bn, as for the treatment standard error computation.

For our present example, $ab = 3 \times 2 = 6$, $p = 2, 3, 4, 5, 6$; $f = df$ for MS_E, or $(ab - 1)(n - 1) = 10$. Let $\alpha = 0.05$

$$S_{\bar{y}_{ij.}} = \sqrt{\frac{MS_E}{3}} = \sqrt{\frac{9.256}{3}} = 1.76$$

The test hypothesis for each mean compared is:

$H_0: \mu_{ij.} - \mu_{ji.} = 0$

$H_A: \mu_{ij.} - \mu_{ji.} \neq 0$

Decision rule:

    Reject H_0 if $\bar{y}_{ij.} - \bar{y}_{ji.} > k_p$

    Compute the k_p values, using the Studentized range statistic table (see Table A.12) for $q_{\alpha(p,f)}$:

$$k_P = q_{\alpha(p,f)} S_{\bar{y}_{ij.}}$$

$$k_2 = q_{0.05(2,10)} 1.76$$
$$k_2 = 3.15(1.76)$$
$$k_2 = 5.54$$

$$k_3 = q_{0.05(3,10)} 1.76$$
$$k_3 = 3.88(1.76)$$
$$k_3 = 6.83$$

$$k_4 = q_{0.05(4,10)} 1.76$$
$$k_4 = 4.33(1.76)$$
$$k_4 = 7.62$$

$$k_5 = q_{0.05(5,10)} 1.76$$
$$k_5 = 4.66(1.76)$$
$$k_5 = 8.20$$

$$k_6 = q_{0.05(6,10)} 1.76$$
$$k_6 = 4.91(1.76)$$
$$k_6 = 8.64$$

The cell means are arranged in ascending order:

$$\bar{y}_{22.} = 77.67$$
$$\bar{y}_{12.} = 78.33$$
$$\bar{y}_{32.} = 82.33$$

$$\bar{y}_{11.} = 84.67$$
$$\bar{y}_{21.} = 93.33$$
$$\bar{y}_{31.} = 100.00$$

As before, the $[ab(ab-1)]/2 = [3 \cdot 2(3 \cdot 2 - 1)]/2 = 30/2 = 15$ contrasts are:

	S = Significant NS = Not significant
$\bar{y}_{31.} - \bar{y}_{22.} = 100.00 - 77.67 = 22.33 > 8.64 = (K_6)$	S
$\bar{y}_{31.} - \bar{y}_{12.} = 100.00 - 78.33 = 21.67 > 8.20 = (K_5)$	S
$\bar{y}_{31.} - \bar{y}_{32.} = 100.00 - 82.33 = 17.67 > 7.62 = (K_4)$	S
$\bar{y}_{31.} - \bar{y}_{11.} = 100.00 - 84.67 = 15.33 > 6.83 = (K_3)$	S
$\bar{y}_{31.} - \bar{y}_{21.} = 100.00 - 93.33 = 6.67 > 5.54 = (K_2)$	S
$\bar{y}_{21.} - \bar{y}_{22.} = 93.33 - 77.67 = 15.66 > 8.20 = (K_5)$	S
$\bar{y}_{21.} - \bar{y}_{12.} = 93.33 - 78.33 = 15.00 > 7.62 = (K_4)$	S
$\bar{y}_{21.} - \bar{y}_{32.} = 93.33 - 82.33 = 11.00 > 6.83 = (K_3)$	S
$\bar{y}_{21.} - \bar{y}_{11.} = 93.33 - 84.67 = 8.66 > 5.54 = (K_2)$	S
$\bar{y}_{11.} - \bar{y}_{22.} = 84.67 - 77.67 = 7.00 < 7.62 = (K_4)$	NS
$\bar{y}_{11.} - \bar{y}_{12.} = 84.67 - 78.33 = 6.34 < 6.83 = (K_3)$	NS
$\bar{y}_{11.} - \bar{y}_{32.} = 84.67 - 82.33 = 2.34 < 5.54 = (K_2)$	NS
$\bar{y}_{32.} - \bar{y}_{22.} = 82.33 - 77.67 = 4.60 < 6.83 = (K_3)$	NS
$\bar{y}_{32.} - \bar{y}_{12.} = 82.33 - 78.33 = 4.00 < 5.54 = (K_2)$	NS
$\bar{y}_{12.} - \bar{y}_{22.} = 78.33 - 77.67 = 0.66 < 5.54 = (K_2)$	NS

It will be helpful to review Fig. 1 to see where the mean pair differences are. These results differ from those of the LSD and Duncan's multiple range test in that $\bar{y}_{11.} = \bar{y}_{12.}$ and $\bar{y}_{11.} = \bar{y}_{22.}$.

XIII. TUKEY TEST

This test, as we have seen, is also one to compare all possible mean pairs. The test is straightforward for comparing cell $(A \times B)$ means $(\bar{y}_{ij.})$.

The test hypothesis is:

H_0: $\mu_{ij.} - \mu_{ji.} = 0$

H_A: $\mu_{ij.} - \mu_{ji.} \neq 0$

Reject H_0 if $|\bar{y}_{ij.} - \bar{y}_{ji.}| > t_\alpha$, where $t_\alpha = q_{[\alpha(ab-1)(n-1)]}S_{\bar{y}_{ij.}}$. The Studentized range (Table L) is used to determine q_α.

Again, the number of pairs of contrasts is

$$\frac{ab(ab-1)}{2} = \frac{(3 \times 2)(3 \times 2 - 1)}{2} = \frac{30}{2} = 15$$

Let $\alpha = 0.05$.

$$S_{\bar{y}_{ij\cdot}} = \sqrt{\frac{MS_E}{n}} = \sqrt{\frac{9.256}{3}} = 1.76$$

$$t_\alpha = q_{\alpha[ab;(ab-1)(n-1)]}S_{\bar{y}_{ij\cdot}}$$

$$t_{0.05} = q_{\alpha[3\cdot2;(3\cdot2-1)(3-1)]}1.76$$

$$t_{0.05} = q_{\alpha[6;10]}1.76$$

$$t_{0.05} = 4.91(1.76) = 8.64$$

	S = Significant NS = Not significant
$\bar{y}_{21\cdot} - \bar{y}_{11\cdot} = \|93.33 - 84.67\| = 8.66 > 8.64$	S
$\bar{y}_{31\cdot} - \bar{y}_{11\cdot} = \|100.00 - 84.67\| = 15.33 > 8.64$	S
$\bar{y}_{12\cdot} - \bar{y}_{11\cdot} = \|78.33 - 84.67\| = 6.34 < 8.64$	NS
$\bar{y}_{22\cdot} - \bar{y}_{11\cdot} = \|77.67 - 84.67\| = 7.00 < 8.64$	NS
$\bar{y}_{32\cdot} - \bar{y}_{11\cdot} = \|82.33 - 84.67\| = 2.34 < 8.64$	NS
$\bar{y}_{31\cdot} - \bar{y}_{21\cdot} = \|100.00 - 93.33\| = 6.67 < 8.64$	NS
$\bar{y}_{12\cdot} - \bar{y}_{21\cdot} = \|78.33 - 93.33\| = 15.00 > 8.64$	S
$\bar{y}_{22\cdot} - \bar{y}_{21\cdot} = \|77.67 - 93.33\| = 15.66 > 8.64$	S
$\bar{y}_{32\cdot} - \bar{y}_{21\cdot} = \|82.33 - 93.33\| = 11.00 > 8.64$	S
$\bar{y}_{12\cdot} - \bar{y}_{31\cdot} = \|78.33 - 100.00\| = 21.67 > 8.64$	S
$\bar{y}_{22\cdot} - \bar{y}_{31\cdot} = \|77.67 - 100.00\| = 22.33 > 8.64$	S
$\bar{y}_{32\cdot} - \bar{y}_{31\cdot} = \|82.33 - 100.00\| = 17.67 > 8.64$	S
$\bar{y}_{22\cdot} - \bar{y}_{12\cdot} = \|77.67 - 78.33\| = 0.66 < 8.64$	NS
$\bar{y}_{32\cdot} - \bar{y}_{12\cdot} = \|82.33 - 78.33\| = 4.00 < 8.64$	NS
$\bar{y}_{22\cdot} - \bar{y}_{32\cdot} = \|77.67 - 82.33\| = 4.66 < 8.64$	NS

Note that this statistic is more conservative in detecting differences than those we used earlier, i.e., LSD, Duncan's, and Newman–Keuls.

XIV. POWER OF THE TEST (FIXED-EFFECTS MODEL)

A. Power Computation Before Conducting the Experiment

As statistical designs become more complex, the computation of the power before running the test becomes more tricky, particularly when the two-factor factorial experiment has been blocked concerning replicates, as in this case. But the computation is still useful, particularly in that it creates a "useful ballpark." Unfortunately, replication-over-time (blocked) designs are more difficult, in practice, to control than a completely randomized design. It is important to compute the power after the test has been conducted, particularly if the H_0 hypothesis is chosen. This will ensure that the differences one expects to detect will be detected.

As in Chap. 7, the main effects, A and B, are computed separately as:

$$\phi = \sqrt{\frac{n' \sum_{n=1}^{k'} (\mu_m - \mu_j)^2}{k' S^2}}$$

where $k' = a$ or b, depending upon which factor
$n' = bn$, if factor A and an, if factor B
$S^2 = MS_E$

$\mu = \frac{\sum_{i=1}^{k'}}{k'} \mu_m =$ population mean for each level within each factor.

$\mu_{m_a} = \frac{\sum^{\mu_a} \mu_i}{a}$ for factor A or $\mu_{m_b} = \frac{\sum^{\mu_b} \mu_i}{b}$ for factor $B =$ mean of the means or grand mean.

Determining the power of a two-factor factorial completely randomized block design is straightforward. I have found this procedure to be useful in trying to gauge the actual value of a specific test design, in the real world, in being able to detect a true difference in treatments.

As before, factors A and B (main effects) are computed separately. In this example, we will perform the test for both factors.

1. Factor A

Let $\alpha = 0.05$

$k' = a = 3$

$n' = bn = 2 \times 3 = 6$

$v_1 = k' - 1 = a - 1 = 3 - 1 = 2$

$v_2 = \text{df } MS_E = (ab - 1)(n - 1) = 10$

$S^2 = MS_E = 9.256$

$\bar{y}_{i..} = \dfrac{y_{i..}}{bn}$

$\bar{y}_{1..} = \dfrac{y_{1..}}{bn} = \dfrac{489}{2 \cdot 3} = 81.50$

$\bar{y}_{2..} = \dfrac{y_{2..}}{bn} = \dfrac{513}{2 \cdot 3} = 85.50$

$\bar{y}_{3..} = \dfrac{y_{3..}}{bn} = \dfrac{547}{2 \cdot 3} = 91.17$

$$\mu_{m_a} = \frac{\sum\limits_{m=1}^{a} \mu_i}{a} = \frac{81.50 + 85.50 + 91.17}{3} = 86.06$$

$$\phi = \sqrt{\frac{bn\sum\limits_{i=1}^{a}(\mu_i - \mu_{m_a})^2}{aS^2}}$$

$$= \sqrt{\frac{6[(81.50 - 86.06)^2 + (85.50 - 86.06)^2 + (91.17 - 86.06)^2]}{3(9.256)}} = 3.19$$

From the power determination table (Table A.4), the researcher enters the table with $v_1 = 2$, $v_2 = 10$, $\alpha = 0.05$, and $\phi = 3.19$. Reading the operating characteristics of the curve, one sees is $1 - \beta = 0.98$ is 98%, hence, the power of the test. There is a 2% chance that the researcher will say that no difference exists between treatments in factor A when a difference does exist.

2. Factor B

The procedure is very similar to that of factor A.
Let $\alpha = 0.05$

$$k' = b = 2$$

$$n' = an = 3 \times 3 = 9$$

$$v_1 = b - 1 = 2 - 1 = 1$$

$$v_2 = df\ MS_E = (ab - 1)(n - 1) = 10$$

$$S^2 = MS_E = 9.256$$

$$\bar{y}_{j.} = \frac{y_{j.}}{an}$$

$$\bar{y}_{.1.} = \frac{y_{.1.}}{an} = \frac{834}{3.3} = 92.67$$

$$\bar{y}_{.2.} = \frac{y_{.2.}}{an} = \frac{715}{3.3} = 79.44$$

$$\mu_{m_b} = \frac{\sum\limits_{m=1}^{b} \mu_m}{b} = \frac{92.67 + 79.44}{2} = 86.06$$

$$\phi = \sqrt{\frac{an \sum_{i=1}^{b}(\mu_j - \mu_b)^2}{b\,S^2}}$$

$$= \sqrt{\frac{9(92.67 - 86.06)^2 + (79.33 - 86.06)^2}{2(9.256)}} = 6.58$$

From Table A.4, the researcher enters the table with $v_1 = 1$, $v_2 = 10$, $\alpha = 0.05$, and $\phi = 6.58$ and finds that $1 - \beta = 0.99$. Hence, the probability of β error is less than 1%.

XV. POWER DETERMINATION AFTER THE EXPERIMENT HAS BEEN CONDUCTED

This is very important as the researcher conducts an experiment and, for example, a difference in factor A cannot be found. The researcher then will want to know the power of the statistic. That is, would the design actually detect a difference if one exists?

As before, the power of the test can be computed for both main effects, but separately.

Recall, $k' = a$ if factor A and b if factor B.

$$\phi = \sqrt{\frac{(k' - 1)(\text{factor MS} - S^2)}{k'S^2}}$$

Example for factor A
Let $\alpha = 0.05$

$$k' = a = 3$$

$$\text{MS}_A = 141.556$$

$$v_1 = k' - 1 = a - 1 = 3 - 1 = 2$$

$$v_2 = \text{df MS}_E = (ab - 1)(n - 1) = (3 \cdot 2 - 1)(3 - 1) = 10$$

$$S^2 = \text{MS}_E = 9.256$$

$$\phi = \sqrt{\frac{(3 - 1)(141.556 - 9.256)}{3(9.256)}} = 3.09$$

From Table A.4, with $v_1 = 2$, $v_2 = 10$, $\alpha = 0.05$, and $\phi = 3.09$, which is too extreme for the Table A.4 value, $\beta = 0.02$, $1 - \beta = 0.98$. Given that a true difference exists with factor A's levels, one is more than 98% confident that the statistic will pick it up.

There are occasions when the researcher may want to check the power of the interaction effect. For example, if the researcher has performed an experiment and does not witness an interaction effect, even though the two-factor experiment was run as a randomized complete block design, she or he may want to compute the power to be sure the study was capable of detecting interaction, given that it was there.

The power computation for $A \times B$ interaction is:

$$\phi = \sqrt{\frac{(A \times B \text{ degrees of freedom})(MS_{AB} - S^2)}{[(A \times B \text{ degrees of freedom}) + 1]S^2}} \tag{4}$$

df for $A = a - 1 = 3 - 1 = 2$

df for $B = b - 1 = 2 - 1 = 1$

$MS_{AB} = 54.89$

$v_1 = (a - 1)(b - 1) = (3 - 1)(2 - 1) = 2$

$v_2 = $ df for $MS_E = 10$

$S^2 = MS_E = 9.256$

Let $\alpha = 0.05$

$$\phi = \sqrt{\frac{(2 \cdot 1)(54.89 - 9.256)}{(2 \cdot 1 + 1)(9.256)}} = 1.81$$

For $v_1 = 2, v_2 = 10, \alpha = 0.05,$ and $\phi = 1.81, 1 - \beta \approx 0.68.$ The power of the test is $\approx 0.68,$ which means there is a 32% probability of concluding that an interaction is not significant when it is.

XVI. SAMPLE SIZE REQUIREMENTS

Although the power, sample size, and detection limits are all related, there are many times a researcher wants to determine the sample size with a set β prior to conducting the study.

The attributes that the researcher must specify ahead of time are:

The power $(1 - \beta)$
The value of alpha (significance level, α)
The σ^2
The minimum detectable difference between means

As in the case of the two-factor factorial experiment and the one-factor ANOVA, the procedure is accomplished by iteration. Generally, the sample

---

size of the experiment is determined on the basis of the more critical main effect (A or B).

The method is performed, as in Chap. 7, using the formula:

$$\phi = \sqrt{\frac{n'\delta^2}{2k'S^2}}$$

where $n' = bn$ if factor A and an if factor B
$k' = a$ if A and b if B
df for $v_1 = k' - 1$ ($a - 1$ if A, $b - 1$ if B)
df for $v_2 = $ df $MS_E = (ab - 1)(n - 1)$, which is unknown
$S^2 = $ variance estimate ($\hat{\sigma}^2$) of MSE
$\delta = $ minimum desired detectable difference between means

In our example, let us use factor A.

$S^2 = 10$ (by estimate)

$\alpha = 0.05$, in this case

$\beta = 0.20$

$\delta = 5$

df for $v_1 = k' - 1 = a - 1 = 3 - 1 = 2$

$$\phi = \sqrt{\frac{n'\delta^2}{2k'S^2}} \quad \text{or} \quad \sqrt{\frac{n'\delta^2}{2aS^2}} = \sqrt{\frac{(2 \times n)5^2}{2(3)10}}$$

It is easier to rewrite n' as "bn" (or "an" for factor B) in determining the sample size, where $n_{bl} = $ the number of blocks. The sample size in this case is directly related to the number of blocks.

Suppose we estimate $n_{bl} = 4$ for the first iteration. That means we would have to replicate the study in its entirety over 4 days or replicated days.

$n = 4$

$$\phi = \sqrt{\frac{2(4)5^2}{2(3)10}} = 1.83$$

Let $\alpha = 0.05$

$v_1 = 2$
$v_2 = (ab - 1)(n - 1) = (3 \cdot 2 - 1)(4 - 1) = 15$

From Table A.4, with $v_1 = 2$, $v_2 = 15$, $\alpha = 0.01$, and $\phi = 1.83$, we see $1 - \beta \approx 0.74$, which $\beta \approx 0.26$ is larger than our specified β, which is set at 0.20. Let us take the next iteration to be $n = 5$, or five blocks.

$$\phi = \sqrt{\frac{2 \cdot (5)5^2}{2(3)10}} = 2.04$$

df for $v_1 = 2$

df for $v_2 = (ab - 1)(n - 1) = (3 \times 2 - 1)(5 - 1) = 20$

From Table A.4, we see that $1 - \beta \approx 0.82$, which is about right. Hence, the experiment should have five replicate blocks.

XVII. MINIMUM DETECTABLE DIFFERENCE

There are a number of occasions when one is interested in approaching the experiment from a detectable difference between means perspective.

The procedure is as we saw in Chap. 7. The researcher states a numerical value that is the minimum value or difference she or he will accept in detecting a difference in means. The α value, the β value, n (number of replicates), and σ^2 are set.

The formula for this determination is:

$$\delta = \sqrt{\frac{2k'S^2\phi^2}{n'}}$$

where $k' = a$ if factor A and b if factor B

$n' = bn$, if factor A and an, if factor B

$S^2 = \text{MS}_E$

ϕ is read from Table A.4 at a specified $1 - \beta$, v_1, v_2, and α level.

Using the example in this chapter, the researcher will usually be more concerned with one factor than the other, if done before the experiment, or may compute both factor δs after the study has been conducted.

1. Factor A (After the Study Has Been Completed)

$k' = a = 3$

$S^2 = \text{MS}_E = 9.256$

df for $v_1 = a - 1 = 3 - 1 = 2$

df for $v_2 = (ab - 1)(n - 1) = (3.2 - 1)(3 - 1) = (5)(2) = 10$

$n' = bn = 2 \times 3 = 6$ This is an n of 6 blocks, or days.

Let $\alpha = 0.01$

$\beta = 0.20$

ϕ is read from Table D. At $1 - \beta = 0.80$, $\alpha = 0.01$, $v_1 = 2$, and $v_2 = 10$, $\phi \approx 2.8$.

$$\delta = \sqrt{\frac{2(3)(9.256)(2.8)^2}{6}} = 8.52$$

So at $\alpha = 0.01$, $\beta = 0.20$, $S^2 = 9.256$, the minimum detectable difference between means in factor A is 8.52 points.

2. Factor B

$k' = b = 2$

$S^2 = 9.256$

df for $v_1 = b - 1 = 2 - 1 = 1$

df for $v_2 = (ab - 1)(n - 1) = 5 \times 2 = 10$

$n' = an = 3 \times 3 = 9$

Let $\alpha = 0.01$

$\beta = 0.20$

Read directly from Table D, at $\alpha = 0.01$, $1 - \beta = 0.80$, $v_1 = 1$, and $v_2 = 10$, $\phi = 2.9$.

$$\delta = \sqrt{\frac{2(2)(9.256)(2.9)^2}{9}} = 5.88$$

The minimum detectable difference between means in factor B is 5.88 at $\alpha = 0.01$ and $\beta = 0.20$.

XVIII. CONCLUSION

Although no researcher will depend on any one experimental design, the applied researcher now has added and greater flexibility in a two-factor ANOVA design. This is particularly valuable when a study or experiment cannot be replicated in 1 day or test period.

9

Useful Small-Scale Pilot Designs: 2^k Designs

A very useful factorial design for researchers is a 2^k factorial design. The 2^k factorial has two levels, with k factors, and is used when the researcher desires to measure joint effects. The two levels are usually qualitative in that they represent high/low, strong/soft, with/without combinations. However, quantitative levels are often used (e.g., 250°F/210°F, 15 PSI/30 PSI). This design is particularly useful in screening or pilot studies.

The assumptions in this chapter concerning the 2^k design are as follows:

1. The factors are fixed.
2. The design is completely randomized.
3. The distribution underlying the data is *normal.*

These are the usual ones met, particularly in the early stages of product development when a number of factors are evaluated. This design provides the smallest number of runs with k factors in a complete factorial design and, hence, is common in pilot or screening studies. Also, because there are only two levels for each factor evaluated by the design, it is not outrageous to assume the responses are linear or can be linearized by a transformation (e.g., $\log_{10}$) over the range of the factor levels evaluated. I have used this type of design extensively over the years and find, in practice (industrial microbiology), that this is a reasonable assumption. Yet, checking the model is still important.

Finally, the computation of this type of design is straightforward. I especially like to perform these by hand (calculator and pencil) because the process *forces* me to look at the data, the factors, and the levels from a microbiological perspective, a research perspective, and a statistical perspective. This enables me to see things (interactions, etc.) that provide guidance for the next experimental iteration. Just getting the end results in a computer printout does not allow me to *know* the data or to bring to bear my insight as a research microbiologist.

I. THE 2^2 FACTORIAL DESIGN

We will concentrate on a 2^2 design, also known as the 2×2 (2 by 2) design, which has two factors, A and B, at two levels each, often extremes of one another (e.g., high/low, strong/weak, full strength/half strength).

The linear model for this design is:

$$y_{ij} = \mu + A_i + B_j + (AB)_{ij} + \epsilon_{ijk} \tag{1}$$

where $\mu =$ common average
$A_i =$ factor A; $i = 1, 2$
$B_j =$ factor B; $j = 1, 2$
$n = 1, \ldots, k$ (replicates)

Suppose a researcher wants to evaluate the antimicrobial activity of a compound at two different concentrations, in two different vehicles, and at two dilution levels—2% chlorhexidine gluconate (CHG) with enhancers and 4% chlorhexidine gluconate at water dilution levels of use strength (10%) and full strength (100%). The researcher wants to develop a 2% CHG product with an alcohol enhancer that is more effective (greater bacterial kill) immediately after application than the 4% CHG.

Most researchers assign the levels to nominal categories. Let us call factor A product concentration, where 4% = the high level and 2% = the low level. Let us also designate the dilution levels, full and 10% strength, as high and low factor B, respectively. Notice that both factors in this design will be evaluated in combination with one another. There is no situation in this design where one tests only factor A or only factor B.

II. EFFECT OF EACH FACTOR

The effect of each factor is defined as the change in response produced by a change in the level of that factor. Figure 1 illustrates the 2^2 design as it is conventionally presented.

At a low level of B (10% strength), the observed effect of A is the level minus the low level, or $a - (1)$. The observed effect of A at a high level of B is $ab - b$. The average effect of moving from a low level of A to a high level is:

$$A = \tfrac{1}{2}[a - (1) + ab - b]$$

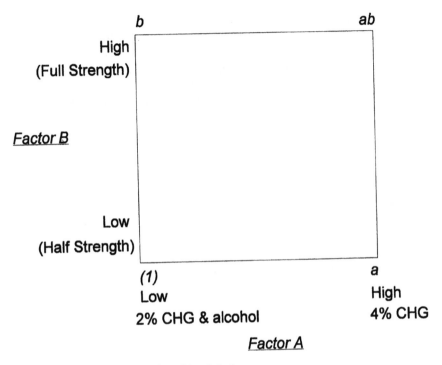

FIGURE 1   Graphic presentation of 2 × 2 design.

or

$$A_{\text{effect}} = \tfrac{1}{2}[ab + a - b - (1)]^*$$

The observed effect of B at a high level of A is $ab - a$. The observed effect of B at a low level of A is $b - (1)$. The average B effect is:

$$B = \tfrac{1}{2}[ab - a + b - (1)]$$

or

$$B_{\text{effect}} = \tfrac{1}{2}[ab + b - a - (1)]^\dagger$$

When factor A is high and factor B is low, the combination may be seen listed in various texts as $a'b^\circ$ or a^+b^- or just "a," and when factor A is low and factor B is high, the combination may be portrayed as $a^\circ b'$ or $a^- b^+$ or

---

*When replications of the test are used, the A effect is $\frac{1}{2n}[ab + a - b - (1)]$, where $n =$ number of replicates.
†When the experiment is replicated, the B effect is $(1/2n)[ab + b - a - (1)]$, where $n =$ number of replicates.

just "b." When factor A is high and factor B is high, the combination may be written as $a'b'$, or a^+b^+ or just "ab," and when factor A is low and factor B is low, the combination may be written as $a°b°$ or a^-b^- or (1).

The interaction effect in this model is represented by the difference between the A effect at a high level of B and the A effect at a low level of B, or the B effect at a high level of A and the B effect at a low level of A. Either way provides the AB effect:

$$AB = \tfrac{1}{2}[ab - b - a + (1)]$$

or

$$AB_{\text{effect}} = \tfrac{1}{2}[ab + (1) - a - b]^*$$

Some authors present the formulas for determining A, B, and AB in terms of mean differences, where the high level is depicted by a " $+$ " and the low level by a " $-$."

1. A factor
$$A = \bar{y}_{a+} - \bar{y}_{a-}$$
$$= \frac{ab + a}{2} - \frac{b + (1)}{2}$$
$$= \tfrac{1}{2}[ab + a - b - (1)]$$

This, by the way, is the same formula presented previously for the main effect of A.

2. B factor
$$B = \bar{y}_{b+} - \bar{y}_{b-}$$
$$= \frac{ab + b}{2} - \frac{a + (1)}{2}$$
$$= \tfrac{1}{2}[ab + b - a - (1)]$$

3. AB interaction effect
$$AB = \frac{ab + (1)}{2} - \frac{a + b}{2}$$
$$= \tfrac{1}{2}[ab + (1) - a - b]$$

---

*If replicates are performed, the AB effect is $(1/2n)[ab + (1) - a - b]$, where $n =$ number of replicates.

Hence, when A or B is negative, the increase from low (e.g., A^-) to high (A^+) decreases the net effect. When the value of A or B is positive, the result of moving from low (e.g., A^-) to high (A^+) is an increase in the net effect.

The 2^2 experiment uses a direct contrast method to determine the main factor effects and interaction effects of factors A and B. The two main effects (factors A and B) and the interaction effect ($A \times B$) make up the three possible contrasts. Because the design is orthogonal, the entire test sequence is based upon orthogonal contrast procedures, which have the form:

$$SS_{CONTRAST} = \frac{(\sum Cy)^2}{\sum C^2} \qquad (2)$$

and, when replicated,

$$SS_{CONTRAST} = \frac{(\sum Cy)^2}{n \sum C^2}$$

We have used this formula modified for orthogonal contrasts of main effect factors and interactions in the previous chapters, so it is nothing new.

The 2^2 design is an orthogonal design (Table 1). The numerator portion of the contrast [Eq. (2)] is derived as shown in the following.

The factor A main effect coefficient order is (reading down column A) $A = [ab + a - b - (1)]^2$.
The factor B main effect is $B = [ab + b - a - (1)]^2$.
The interaction of $A \times B$ effect is $A \times B = [ab - a - b + (1)]^2$.

The denominator portion of the contrast [Eq. (2)] is:

$$\sum C^2 = \sum (-1)^2 + 1^2 + (-1)^2 + 1^2 = 4$$

Hence, the denominator for each contrast is always 4, and when $n = 1$ (no replications) the final formulas are:

$$SS_A = \frac{[ab + a - b - (1)]^2}{4} \qquad (3)$$

TABLE 1 Linear Contrast Coefficients for A, B, and AB

Treatment portions	A	B	AB
(1)	−1	−1	+1
a	+1	−1	−1
b	−1	+1	−1
ab	+1	+1	+1

$$SS_B = \frac{[ab + b - a - (1)]^2}{4} \tag{4}$$

$$SS_{AB} = \frac{[ab + (1) - a - b]^2}{4} \tag{5}$$

With n replicates, the formulas are:

$$SS_A = \frac{[ab + a - b - (1)]^2}{4n} \tag{6}$$

$$SS_B = \frac{[ab + b - a - (1)]^2}{4n} \tag{7}$$

$$SS_{AB} = \frac{[ab + (1) - a - b]^2}{4n} \tag{8}$$

If the effect (A or B) is negative, then going from a low to a high level of either factor reduces the output, as the level of A or B is increased. If the effect is positive, increasing the level increases the output. If the interaction effect is large, one cannot talk about the main effects by themselves.

The formulas for $\bar{A}$, $\bar{B}$, and $\overline{AB}$ are:

$$\bar{A} = \frac{1}{2n}[ab + a - b - (1)]$$

$$\bar{B} = \frac{1}{2n}[ab + b - a - (1)]$$

$$\overline{AB} = \frac{1}{2n}[ab + (1) - a - b]$$

where n = number of replicates.

Graphing of data, as before, is also useful. I find that replicating this type of study three times ($n = 3$) will generally provide valid data at cost-effective levels.

Example 1: A research scientist has two factors, A and B. She would like to evaluate two concentrations of an antibiotic with two binder levels. The goal is to find dissolution rates in an acid medium (pH 5.5).

The concentration levels of antibiotic the researcher has designated factor A. The a^+ level is 0.15%, and the a^- level is 0.08%. She assigns the binder levels to factor B: the high binder level (b^+) is 50 mg, and the low binder level (b^-) is 25 mg. The researcher replicates the experiment in its entirety three times. The following data are dissolution rates, in seconds.

	REPLICATES	Total
$(1) = a^- b^-$	69, 72, 74	215
$a = a^+ b^-$	64, 67, 65	196
$b = a^- b^+$	63, 65, 65	193
$ab = a^+ b^+$	69, 71, 67	207

Before continuing, let us calculate the terms in the ANOVA table for the 2^2 design (Table 2), using the six-step procedure:

Step 1. Formulate the hypotheses (These are three):

Factor A: H_0: The 0.15% antimicrobial is equivalent to 0.08% in dissolution rates.

H_A: The above is not true.

Factor B: H_0: The 50-mg binder and the 25-mg binder are equivalent in dissolution rates.

H_A: The above is not true.

AB interaction: H_0: There is no interaction between main factor effects A and B.

H_A: There is significant interaction between main factor effects A and B.

Step 2. Let us set $\alpha = 0.10$ because this is an exploratory study. The researcher is willing to reduce α in order to prevent excessive β error (recall that α error is the probability of rejecting H_0 when it is actually

TABLE 2 ANOVA Table

Source of variation	Sum of squares	Degrees of freedom	Mean square	F_C	F_T
Factor A	$\frac{[ab+a-b-(1)]^2}{4n} = SS_A$	$a - 1$ (which is always 1)	$\frac{SS_A}{1} = MS_A$	$\frac{MS_A}{MS_E}$	$F_{\alpha[1;ab(n-1)]}$
Factor B	$\frac{[ab+b-a-(1)]^2}{4n} = SS_B$	$b - 1$ (which is always 1)	$\frac{SS_B}{1} = MS_B$	$\frac{MS_B}{MS_E}$	$F_{\alpha[1;ab(n-1)]}$
$A \times B$ interaction	$\frac{[ab+(1)-a-b]^2}{4n} = SS_{AB}$	$(a-1)(b-1)$ (which is always 1)	$\frac{SS_{AB}}{1} = MS_{AB}$	$\frac{MS_{AB}}{MS_E}$	$F_{\alpha[1;ab(n-1)]}$
Error	$SSE = SS_T - SS_A - SS_B - SS_{AB}$	$ab(n-1)$	$\frac{SS_E}{ab(n-1)} = MS_E$		
Total	$\sum_{i=1}^{2}\sum_{j=1}^{2}\sum_{k=1}^{n} y_{ijk} - \frac{y^2 \cdots}{4n}$ $= SS_T$	$abn - 1$			

true, and β error is the probability of failing to reject H_0 when it is actually false). The entire study will be replicated three times ($n = 3$).

Step 3. The ANOVA test for a completely randomized 2^2 design, of course, will be used in this evaluation.

Step 4. Decision rules:

Factor A: If F_C calculated for factor $A > F_T$, reject H_0 at $\alpha = 0.10$.
$F_T = F_{0.10\ (1,\ ab(n-1))} = F_{0.10\ (1,\ 8)} = 3.46$ (from Table 3 the F distribution)

Factor B: If F_C calculated for factor $B > F_T$, reject H_0 at $\alpha = 0.10$.
$F_T = F_{0.10\ (1,\ ab(n-1))} = F_{0.10\ (1,\ 8)} = 3.46$ (from Table 3 the F distribution)

Factor AB: If F_C calculated for the interaction term $> F_T$, reject H_0 at $\alpha = 0.10$.
$F_T = F_{0.10\ (1,\ ab(n-1))} = F_{0.10\ (1,\ 8)} = 3.46$ (from Table 3 the F distribution)

Step 5. Perform ANOVA. A schema (Fig. 2) is a very useful map, prior to performing the test.

$$SS_A = \frac{[ab + a - b - (1)]^2}{4n} = \frac{[207 + 196 - 193 - 215]^2}{4(3)} = 2.08$$

$$SS_B = \frac{[ab + b - a - (1)]^2}{4n} = \frac{[207 + 193 - 196 - 215]^2}{4(3)} = 10.08$$

$$SS_{AB} = \frac{[ab + (1) - a - b]^2}{4n} = \frac{[207 + 215 - 196 - 193]^2}{4(3)} = 90.75$$

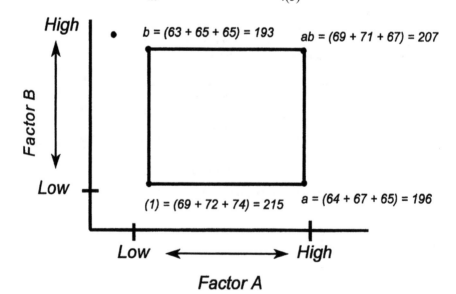

FIGURE 2 ANOVA schema.

$$SS_T = \sum_{i=1}^{2} \sum_{j-1}^{2} \sum_{k=1}^{3} \frac{y_{ijk}^2 - y_{...}^2}{4n}$$

where $y_{...} = \sum y_{ijk} = 811.00$

$$SS_T = 69^2 + 72^2 + \cdots + 71^2 + 67^2 - \frac{811^2}{12}$$

$$SS_T = 54941.00 - \frac{811^2}{12} = 130.92$$

$$SS_E = SS_T - SS_A - SS_B - SS_{AB} = 130.92 - 2.08 - 10.08 - 90.75 = 28.01$$

The next step is to construct an ANOVA table (Table 3).

Step 6. Discussion. The researcher clearly sees that the interaction of factors A and B is statistically significant at $\alpha = 0.10$. Because the interaction term is significant, it is not a good idea to test the main effects directly, for they interact. This discovery moves the researcher to look at the interaction more carefully. By the way, the average effects of A, B, and AB are:

$$\bar{A} = \frac{1}{2(n)}[ab + a - b - (1)]$$

$$= \frac{1}{2(3)}[207 + 196 - 193 - 215] = -0.83$$

$$\bar{B} = \frac{1}{2(n)}[ab + b - a - (1)]$$

$$= \frac{1}{2(3)}[207 + 193 - 196 - 215] = -1.83$$

TABLE 3 ANOVA Table

Source of variation	Sum of squares	Degrees of freedom	Mean square	F_C	F_T	S = Significant NS = Not significant
Factor A	2.08	1	2.08	0.59	3.46	–
Factor B	10.08	1	10.08	2.88	3.46	–
AB interaction	90.75	1	90.75	25.93	3.46	S
SS_E	28.01	8	3.50			
SS_{TOTAL}	130.92	11				

$$\overline{AB} = \frac{1}{2(n)}[ab + (1) - a - b]$$

$$= \frac{1}{2(3)}[207 + 215 - 196 - 193] = 5.50$$

Because the interaction of A and B was significant, the researcher knows she cannot discuss the main effects independently. That is, if one discusses factor A, it must be relative to factor B. As a visual aid to interpretation, it is useful to graph the data (Fig. 3).

$$A^- B^+ = B = 193; \quad \bar{y}_B = \frac{193}{3} = 64.63$$

B high

$$A^+ B^+ = ab = 207; \quad \bar{y}_{AB} = \frac{207}{3} = 69.00$$

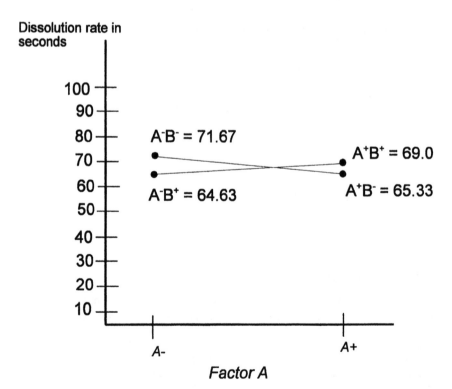

FIGURE 3   Data graph.

$$A^-B^- = (1) = 215; \quad \bar{y}_{(1)} = \tfrac{215}{3} = 71.67$$

B low

$$A^+B^- = a = 196; \quad \bar{y}_A = \tfrac{196}{3} = 65.33$$

When factor A is low, B high has a faster reaction time than B low. However, when factor A is high, B low is faster than B high in dissolution rate time. The investigator suspects that some unknown component, C, or several, C, D, and E, are influencing the dissolution rate. So, she decides to explore several other compounds in experiments we will not examine here.

III. MODEL ADEQUACY

The linear model, $\hat{y} = b_0 + b_1(a) + b_2(b) + b_3(ab)$, can be used to ensure the validity of the model.

$$b_0 = \frac{y_{...}}{abn} \qquad\qquad (9)$$

where $a = 2$, $b = 2$, n = number of replicates, and where

$$b_1 = \text{factor } A = \frac{1}{4(n)}[ab + a - b - (1)] \qquad\qquad (10)$$

$$b_2 = \text{factor } B = \frac{1}{4(n)}[ab + b - a - (1)] \qquad\qquad (11)$$

$$b_3 = \text{factor } AB \text{ interaction} = \frac{1}{4(n)}[ab + (1) - a - b] \qquad\qquad (12)$$

$a = 1$, if A^+, or -1, if A^-, and $b = 1$, if B^+, or -1, if B^-.
   Using Example 1,

$$b_0 = \frac{y_{...}}{abn} = \frac{811}{2(2)(3)} = 67.58*$$

$$b_1 = A \text{ factor} = \frac{1}{4(n)}[ab + a - b - (1)]$$

$$= \frac{1}{4(3)}[207 + 196 - 193 - 215] = -0.42$$

---

*Note: b_0 happens to be $\bar{y}_{...}$

$$b_2 = B \text{ factor} = \frac{1}{4(n)}[ab + b - a - (1)]$$

$$= \frac{1}{4(3)}[207 + 193 - 196 - 215] = -0.92$$

$$b_3 = AB \text{ interaction factor} = \frac{1}{4(n)}[ab + (1) - a - b]$$

$$= \frac{1}{4(3)}[207 + 215 - 196 - 193] = 2.75$$

The linear regression model to use to check the model's adequacy is then:

$$\hat{y} = 67.58 - 0.42(a) - 0.92(b) + 2.75(ab) \tag{13}$$

The $\hat{y}$ values will be used to compute estimates for each of the four combinations.

For (1), where both a and b are at low levels ($a^- b^-$), hence $a = -1$, and $b = -1$:

$$\hat{y}_{a\text{-}b\text{-}} = 67.58 - 0.42(-1) - 0.92(-1) + 2.75[(-1)(-1)]$$

$$\hat{y}_{a\text{-}b\text{-}} = 67.58 + 0.42 + 0.92 + 2.75$$

$$\hat{y}_{a\text{-}b\text{-}} = 71.67$$

The residual can be computed for this group in the usual way, $\epsilon = y - \hat{y}$, where $y =$ the actual value and $\hat{y}$ the predicted value, for $y - \hat{y}$.

$$e_1 = 69 - 71.67 = -2.67$$

$$e_2 = 72 - 71.67 = 0.33$$

$$e_3 = 74 - 71.67 = 2.33$$

For $a^+ b^-$, where a is at the high level and b at the low, $a = 1$, and $b = -1$:

$$\hat{y}_{a\text{+}b\text{-}} = 67.58 - 0.42(1) - 0.92(-1) + 2.75[(1)(-1)] = 65.33$$

$$e_1 = 64 - 65.33 = -1.33$$

$$e_2 = 67 - 65.33 = 1.67$$

$$e_3 = 65 - 65.33 = -0.33$$

For a^-b^+, where a is low and b is high, $a = -1$, and $b = 1$:

$$\hat{y}_{a^-b^+} = 67.58 - 0.42(-1) - 0.92(1) + 2.75[(-1)(1)] = 64.33$$
$$e_1 = 63 - 64.33 = -1.33$$
$$e_2 = 65 - 64.33 = 0.67$$
$$e_3 = 65 - 64.33 = 0.67$$

For a^+b^+, where both a and b are high, $a = 1$, and $b = 1$:

$$\hat{y}_{a^+b^+} = 67.58 - 0.42(1) - 0.92(1) + 2.75[(1)(1)] = 68.99$$
$$e_1 = 69 - 68.99 = 0.01$$
$$e_2 = 71 - 68.99 = 2.01$$
$$e_3 = 67 - 68.99 = -1.99$$

IV. 2^2 FACTORIAL DESIGNS CALCULATED WITH STATISTICAL SOFTWARE

Many software packages can be used to compute this 2^2 design, including SPSSX, SAS, and MiniTab. Because MiniTab is exceptionally popular and user-friendly, its structure will be demonstrated using the general linear model.

The key point to keep in mind is that no factor is strictly A or strictly B, so one cannot code for just A or just B. Fortunately, one has to code with only -1 or $+1$, depending upon whether A is high or low or B is high or low.

The data are keyed in as presented in Table 4.

TABLE 4 Data

Row	C1	C2	C3
n	a	b	y
1	-1	-1	69
2	-1	-1	72
3	-1	-1	74
4	1	-1	64
5	1	-1	67
6	1	-1	65
7	-1	1	63
8	-1	1	65
9	-1	1	65
10	1	1	69
11	1	1	71
12	1	1	67

TABLE 5   ANOVA Table

		ANALYSIS OF VARIANCE				
Source	DF	Seq SS	Adj SS	Adj MS	F	P
C1	1	2.083	2.083	2.083	0.60	.463
C2	1	10.083	10.083	10.083	2.88	.128
C1*C2	1	90.750	90.750	90.750	25.93	.000
ERROR	8	28.000	28.000	3.500		
TOTAL	11	130.917				

The general linear command is GLM C3 = C1 C2 C2*C3 where C3 = y, C1 = A factor, C2 = B factor, and C2 * C3 = interaction of A and B.

The fits or predictions can be computed, as can the residuals and means. The entire command structure is:

MTB > GLM C3 = C1 C2 C1*C2
SUBC > FITS C4;
SUBC > RESIDS C5;
SUBC. MEANS C1 C2.

The ANOVA for the data is presented in Table 5.

Notice that the content matches that of Table 3, constructed from the data computed by hand. Computations of the model diagnostics are presented in Table 6.

The model adequacy is checked first by means of a plot of the residuals versus the fitted or predicted values (Fig. 4).

The residual data appear to be randomly distributed, with greater spread, however, as the predicted values increase. This is probably not a concern.

The researcher also prints a plot of the residuals versus the actual values to get a feeling for their relative proximities.

On examining Fig. 5, the researcher is puzzled by the plot but not overly concerned. Because she has not worked with this antibiotic compound previously, she has no "background data" with which to compare. So, she continues digging deeper, looking for clues to explain the data phenomena.

She first prints a stem–leaf display (Fig. 6) and sees that the residual data are spread fairly uniformly about the median but also notices the "gappiness" of the data. She considers this to be a result of using only three replicates and is not overly concerned.

She next generates a letter-value display (Table 7) and concludes that the data are too few and too dispersed to see anything of use. She does notice

TABLE 6   Model Diagnostics

Row	C1 a	C2 b	C3 y	C4 y [a]	C5 e [b]
1	−1	−1	69	71.6667	−2.66666
2	−1	−1	72	71.6667	0.33334
3	−1	−1	74	71.6667	2.33334
4	1	−1	64	65.3333	−1.33334
5	1	−1	69	65.3333	1.66666
6	1	−1	65	65.3333	−0.33334
7	−1	1	63	64.3333	−1.33334
8	−1	1	65	64.3333	0.66666
9	−1	1	65	64.3333	0.66666
10	1	1	69	69.0000	0.00000
11	1	1	71	69.0000	2.00000
12	1	1	67	69.0000	−2.00000

[a] The predicted values (C4) were previously calculated by hand, using the formula $\hat{y} = b_0 + b_1(a) + b_2(b) + b_3(ab)$.
[b] $e = y - \hat{y}$.

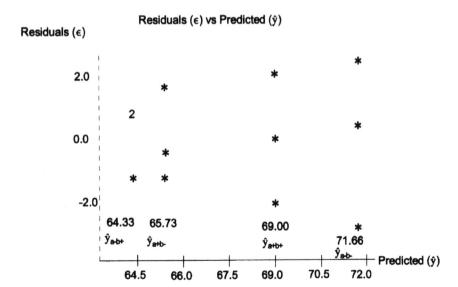

FIGURE 4   Plot of residual versus predicted values.

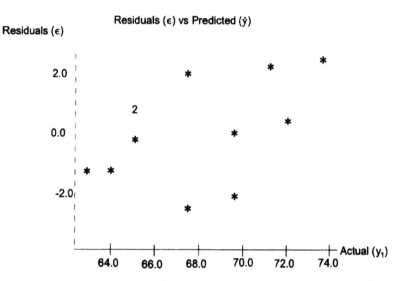

FIGURE 5   Plot of residual versus actual values.

	Stem	Leaf
1	-2	6
2	-2	0
2	-1	
4	-1	33
4	-0	
5	-0	3
(2)	0	03
5	0	66
3	1	
3	1	6
2	2	03

FIGURE 6   Stem-and-leaf display of residuals.

TABLE 7   Letter-Value Display of Residuals

	Depth	Lower	Upper	Mid	Spread
N	12				
M	6.5		0.167	0.167	
H	3.5	− 1.333	1.167	− 0.083	2.500
E	2.0	− 2.000	2.000	0.000	4.000
	1	− 2.667	2.333	− 0.167	5.000

that the midrange values are not really increasing or decreasing as a trend, so the residual data are not skewed.

Finally, she computes a boxplot (Fig. 7) with notches and, again, this reveals nothing out of the ordinary.

She then looks at all the data, trying to see some pattern, not only from a statistical perspective but also from an experimental one, based on knowledge of her major field speciality of chemistry. Nothing is apparent, so she conducts another series of studies and critically observes the results to learn more about what the phenomena reveal. At this time, she is satisfied with the model's adequacy but remains puzzled about the characteristics of the main effects and interaction. She decides to hold a meeting with her project team members to "bounce the data results" off them.

Although this approach is not often seen in statistical testing, it is the overriding process in one's field. What is going on is just not known—yet.

V.   BLOCKING A 2^2 DESIGN

There are times when it is not possible to run all n replicates on the same day with the same technicians or even under the same conditions (different batch ingredients, different equipment, etc.). At other times, it is desirable to vary conditions such as technicians, material brands, or lots to ensure robustness. This is particularly true in evaluating antibiotics, disinfectants,

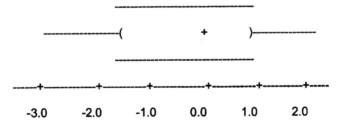

FIGURE 7   Boxplot of residuals.

bioengineering products, and biotechnology processes. In methods development, a researcher may purposely vary raw materials, for example, to find the combination that provides favorable end results.

Blocking an n-replicated design, then, is the obvious next step in a 2^2 design. Fortunately, the 2^2 design we have just explored can be used in the blocked design, with a difference, although slight, that is critical to understanding the procedure. Instead of replicating the study n times, the study is blocked B times. The blocks comprise the different conditions under which the experiment is conducted, not homogeneous ones, as in the case of the completely randomized 2^2 factorial design. Each set of nonhomogeneous conditions defines a block, and each replicate is run in one block. The run order [(1), a, b, ab], however, within each block is randomly assigned.

For demonstration purposes, let us use Example 1 as our example for this section. The only difference will be that, instead of the three n replicates being conducted under homogeneous conditions, let us assume they were conducted using different technicians, and each replicate constitutes a block, or B. The experimenter, while not interested in technician-to-technician error, did not want the effect to confound the study. The study results, then, are presented in Table 8.

The ANOVA table for a complete blocked 2^2 factorial design is presented in Table 9.

Let us now perform the six-step procedure using the data from Example 1.

Step 1. Formulate the test hypothesis:
Factor A: H_0: The 0.15% antimicrobial is equivalent to the 0.08% antimicrobial in dissolution rate.
$\quad\quad H_A$: The above is not true.
Factor B: H_0: The 50-mg binder and the 25-mg binder are equivalent in dissolution rates.
$\quad\quad H_A$: The above is not true.

TABLE 8   Blocks

	Blocks			Total treatment combination
	1	2	3	
$(1) = a^- b^-$	69	72	74	215
$a = a^+ b^-$	64	67	65	196
$b = a^- b^+$	63	65	65	193
$ab = a^+ b^+$	69	71	67	207
Total blocks	265	275	271	

TABLE 9 ANOVA Table for Complete 2^2 Factorial Design

Source of variation	Sum of squares	Degrees of freedom	Mean square	F_C	F_T
Factor A	$\frac{[ab+a-b-(1)]^2}{4B} = SS_A$	1	$\frac{SS_A}{1}$	$\frac{MS_A}{MS_E}$	$F_{\alpha[1;ab(B-1)]}$
Factor B	$\frac{[ab+b-a-(1)]^2}{4B} = SS_B$	1	$\frac{SS_B}{1}$	$\frac{MS_B}{MS_E}$	$F_{\alpha[1;ab(B-1)]}$
AB interaction	$\frac{[ab+(1)-a-b]^2}{4B} = SS_{AB}$	1	$\frac{SS_{AB}}{1}$	$\frac{MS_{AB}}{MS_E}$	$F_{\alpha[1;ab(B-1)]}$
Block effect	$\frac{\sum (B_k)^2}{4} - \frac{y^2_{...}}{4B} = SS_{BL}$	$B-1$	$\frac{SS_{BL}}{B-1}$	Generally not tested	
Error	$SSE = SS_T - SS_A$ $\quad - SS_B - SS_{AB}$ $\quad - SS_{BL}$	$(ab-1)$ $(B-1)$	$\frac{SS_E}{ab(B-1)}$		
Total	$\sum\limits_{i=1}^{2}\sum\limits_{j=1}^{2}\sum\limits_{k=1}^{B} y_{ijk} - \frac{y^2_{...}}{4B} = SS_T$	$abB-1$			

Note: B = total number of blocks.

AB interaction: H_0: There is no interaction between main effects A and B.

$\quad\quad\quad\quad H_A$: The above is not true.

Step 2. Again, we will set $\alpha = 0.10$ and B = number of blocks = 3.

Step 3. The randomized block 2^2 factor design will be used.

Step 4. Decision rule:

Factor A: If F_C calculated for factor $A > F_T$, reject H_0 at $\alpha = 0.10$.

$\quad\quad\quad F_T = F_{0.10\,(1,\,ab(B-1))} = F_{0.10\,(1,\,8)} = 3.46$ (from Table C (F table))

Factor B: If F_C calculated for factor $B > F_T$, reject H_0 at $\alpha = 0.10$.

$\quad\quad\quad F_T = F_{0.10\,(1,\,ab(B-1))} = F_{0.10\,(1,\,8)} = 3.46$ (from Table C (F table))

Factor $A \times B$: If F_C calculated for the interaction term $> F_T$, reject H_0 at $\alpha = 0.10$.

$\quad\quad\quad F_T = F_{0.10\,(1,\,ab(B-1))} = F_{0.10\,(1,\,8)} = 3.46$ (from Table C (F table))

Step 5. Compute the statistic. From Table 8:

	$B_k =$
(1) = 215	Block 1 = B_1 = 265
$a = 196$	Block 2 = B_2 = 275
$b = 193$	Block 3 = B_3 = 271
$ab = 207$	B = number of blocks = 3

The sum of

$$SS_A = \frac{[ab+a-b-(1)]^2}{4B} = \frac{[207+196-193-215]^2}{4(3)} = 2.08$$

$$SS_B = \frac{[ab+b-a-(1)]^2}{4B} = \frac{[207+193-196-215]^2}{4(3)} = 10.08$$

$$SS_{AB} = \frac{[ab+(1)-a-b]^2}{4B} = \frac{[207+215-196-193]^2}{4(3)} = 90.75$$

$$SS_{Block} = \frac{\sum B_k^2}{4} - \frac{y_{...}^2}{4B} = \frac{265^2 + 275^2 + 271^2}{4} - \frac{811^2}{4(3)}$$

$$= 54,822.75 - 54,810.08 = 12.67$$

$$SS_T = \sum_{i=1}^{2} \sum_{j=1}^{2} \sum_{k=1}^{B} y_{ijk}^2 - \frac{y_{...}^2}{4B}$$

$$SS_T = 69^2 + 72^2 + \cdots + 71^2 + 67^2 - \frac{811^2}{12} = 54,941.00 - \frac{811^2}{12} = 130.92$$

$$SS_E = SS_T - SS_A - SS_B - SS_{AB} - SS_{Block}$$

$$= 130.92 - 2.08 - 10.08 - 90.75 - 12.67 = 15.34$$

The ANOVA table (Table 10) is then constructed for these data.

Step 6. Discussion. The comparison of main effects A and B makes little sense because the interaction between them is so high. The researcher decides to meet with her team in an attempt to determine what phenomena are operative in this kinetic chemical process.

TABLE 10   ANOVA Table

Source of variation	Sum of squares	Degrees of freedom	Mean square	F_C	F_T	S = Significant NS = Not significant
Factor A	2.08	1	2.08	0.81	3.46	a
Factor B	10.08	1	10.08	3.94	3.46	a
AB interaction	90.75	1	90.75	35.45	3.46	S
Block effect	12.67	2	6.34	—		
SS_E	15.34	6	2.56			
SS_{TOTAL}	130.92	11				

[a]Because the interaction term is significant, any significant outcomes for an individual factor must be clearly framed in terms of the other main factor.

The average effects of A, B, and AB are the same as calculated earlier, except that n is replaced by B.

$$\bar{A} = \frac{1}{2(B)}[ab + a - b - (1)]$$

$$= \frac{1}{2(3)}[207 + 196 - 193 - 215] = -0.83$$

$$\bar{B} = \frac{1}{2(B)}[ab + b - a - (1)]$$

$$= \frac{1}{2(3)}[207 + 193 - 196 - 215] = -1.83$$

$$\overline{AB} = \frac{1}{2(B)}[ab + (1) - a - b]$$

$$= \frac{1}{2(3)}[207 + 215 - 196 - 193] = 5.50$$

The meaning of these data, then, remains the same. Because of the factor AB interaction, the main effects cannot be discussed independently.

VI. MODEL ADEQUACY

The linear model for this blocked 2^2 factorial design is:

$$y_{ijk} = \mu + A_i + B_j + (AB)_{ij} + B_k + \epsilon_{ijk}$$

where A = factor A, B = factor B, AB = factor $A \times B$ interaction, and B_k = blocks.

Rewriting the model for predictive purposes:

$$\hat{y} = b_0 + b_1a + b_2b + b_3(ab) + B + \epsilon$$

where:

$$b_0 = \frac{y_{...}}{abn}$$

$$a = 2, \qquad b = 2, \qquad B = \text{number of blocks} = 3$$

$$b_1 = \text{factor } A = \frac{1}{4(B)}[ab + a - b - (1)]$$

$$b_2 = \text{factor } B = \frac{1}{4(B)}[ab + b - a - (1)]$$

$$b_3 = \text{factor } AB = \frac{1}{4(B)}[ab + (1) - a - b]$$

and $a = 1$, if a^+, or -1, if a^-, $b = 1$, if b^+, or -1, if b^-.

The researcher will need to perform a contrast-type operation and compute B_k contrasts. It does not matter how one labels the constants.

Let us call $B_1 = 1$ for block 1, $B_2 = 2$ for block 2, and $B_3 = 3$ for block 3.

The block sum total for block 1 is 265, block 2 is 275, and block 3 is 271 (Table 8).

$$\hat{B}_1 = \frac{1}{2}\left(\frac{\sum B_1}{\text{number of blocks}} - \frac{\sum B_2 + \sum B_3}{\text{number of blocks} \times \text{number of } B_k \text{ in numerator}}\right)$$

$$= \frac{1}{2}\left[\frac{265}{3} - \frac{275 + 271}{3(2)}\right] = \frac{88.33 - 91.00}{2} = \frac{-2.67}{2} = -1.33$$

$\hat{B}_2$

$$= \frac{1}{2}\left(\frac{\sum B_2}{\text{number of blocks}} - \frac{\sum B_1 + \sum B_3}{\text{number of blocks} \times \text{number of blocks in numerator}}\right)$$

$$= \frac{1}{2}\left[\frac{275}{3} - \frac{265 + 271}{3(2)}\right] = \frac{91.67 - 89.33}{2} = \frac{2.33}{2} = 1.17$$

$\hat{B}_3$

$$= \frac{1}{2}\left(\frac{\sum B_3}{\text{number of blocks}} - \frac{\sum B_1 + \sum B_2}{\text{number of blocks} \times \text{number of blocks in numerator}}\right)$$

$$= \frac{1}{2}\left[\frac{271}{3} - \frac{265 + 275}{3(2)}\right] = \frac{90.33 - 90.00}{2} = \frac{0.33}{2} = 0.17$$

So $B_k =$

If block 1, $\hat{B}_1 = -1.33$
If block 2, $\hat{B}_2 = 1.17$
If block 3, $\hat{B}_3 = 0.17$

The linear model is then:

$$\hat{y} = b_0 + b_1(a) + b_2(b) + b_3(ab) + B_k = 67.58 - 0.42a - 0.92b + 2.75(ab) + B_k$$

where: $k = 1, 2, 3$
$B_1 = -1.33$
$B_2 = 1.17$
$B_3 = 0.17$

For $(1) = a^- b^-$, block 1: $a = -1, b = -1$, and $B_1 = -1.34$

$\hat{y}_{a^- b^-} = 67.58 - 0.42(-1) - 0.92(-1) + 2.75[(-1)(-1)] + (-1.33) = 70.34$

For $(1) = a^- b^-$, block 2: $a = -1, b = -1$, and $B_2 = 1.17$

$\hat{y}_{a^- b^-} = 67.58 - 0.42(-1) - 0.92(-1) + 2.75[(-1)(-1)] + (1.17) = 72.84$

For $(1) = a^- b^-$, block 3: $a = -1, b = -1$, and $B_3 = 0.17$

$\hat{y}_{a^- b^-} = 67.58 - 0.42(-1) - 0.92(-1) + 2.75[(-1)(-1)] + (0.17) = 71.84$

For $a = a^+ b^-$, block 1: $a = 1, b = -1$, and $B_1 = -1.33$

$\hat{y}_{a^+ b^-} = 67.58 - 0.42(1) - 0.92(-1) + 2.75[(1)(-1)] - 1.33 = 64.00$

For $a = a^+ b^-$, block 2: $a = 1, b = -1$, and $B_2 = 1.17$

$\hat{y}_{a^+ b^-} = 67.58 - 0.42(1) - 0.92(-1) + 2.75[(1)(-1)] + 1.17 = 66.50$

For $a = a^+ b^-$, block 3: $a = 1, b = -1$, and $B_3 = 0.17$

$\hat{y}_{a^+ b^-} = 67.58 - 0.42(1) - 0.92(-1) + 2.75[(1)(-1)] + 0.17 = 65.50$

For $b = a^- b^+$, block 1: $a = -1, b = 1$, and $B_1 = -1.33$

$\hat{y}_{a^- b^+} = 67.58 - 0.42(-1) - 0.92(1) + 2.75[(-1)(1)] - 1.33 = 63.00$

For $b = a^- b^+$, block 2: $a = -1, b = 1$, and $B_2 = 1.17$

$\hat{y}_{a^- b^+} = 67.58 - 0.42(-1) - 0.92(1) + 2.75[(-1)(1)] + 1.17 = 65.50$

For $b = a^- b^+$, block 3: $a = -1, b = 1$, and $B_3 = 0.17$

$\hat{y}_{a^- b^+} = 67.58 - 0.42(-1) - 0.92(1) + 2.75[(-1)(1)] + 0.17 = 64.50$

For $ab = a^+ b^+$, block 1: $a = 1, b = 1$, and $B_1 = -1.34$

$\hat{y}_{a^+ b^+} = 67.58 - 0.42(1) - 0.92(1) + 2.75[(1)(1)] - 1.33 = 67.66$

For $ab = a^+ b^+$, block 2: $a = 1, b = 1$, and $B_2 = 1.17$

$\hat{y}_{a^+ b^+} = 67.58 - 0.42(1) - 0.92(1) + 2.75[(1)(1)] + 1.17 = 70.16$

For $ab = a^+ b^+$, block 3: $a = 1, b = 1$, and $B_3 = 0.17$

$\hat{y}_{a^+ b^+} = 67.58 - 0.42(1) - 0.92(1) + 2.75[(1)(1)] + 0.17 = 69.16$

VII. COMPUTER-GENERATED DATA (COMPLETE BLOCK 2^2 DESIGN)

Using the general linear model routine in computer software, the complete block 2^2 factorial design study can be generated. The same commands as those for the randomized 2^2 factorial design can be used, but the variable list must be increased by one to accommodate the block effect. Table 11 portrays the input data. $C_1 =$ factor $A = -1$ if a^-, 1 if a^+. $C_2 =$ factor $B = -1$ if b^-, 1 if b^+. C_3 and C_4 are different ways of coding the block effect for MiniTab. The data can be entered sequentially (1, 2, 3) or orthogonally ($-1, 0, 1$). One does not need both. In this example, the block data were used in C_3. $C_5 =$ Dissolution rate in seconds

Using MiniTab, the command structure is:
MTB > GLM C5 = C1 C2 C3 C1*C2;
SUBC > FITS C6;
SUBC > RESIDS C7;
SUBC > MEANS C1 C2.
$C_6 = \hat{y}$, or the predicted value
$C_7 = y - \hat{y} = e$, or the residual values.

The ANOVA table for these data appears in Table 12.

Notice that Table 12 shows the same outcomes as the table generated earlier using pencil and paper (Table 10) in step 5. Table 13 presents the input data, as before (Table 11), with the addition of both the fits ($\hat{y}$) and the residuals (e) in fields C_6 and C_7, respectively.

TABLE 11 Input Data, Complete Block 2^2 Design

Row	C1	C2	C3	C4	C5
1	-1	-1	1	-1	69
2	-1	-1	2	0	72
3	-1	-1	3	1	74
4	1	-1	1	-1	64
5	1	-1	2	0	67
6	1	-1	3	1	65
7	-1	1	1	-1	63
8	-1	1	2	0	65
9	-1	1	3	1	65
10	1	1	1	-1	69
11	1	1	2	0	71
12	1	1	3	1	67

TABLE 12   Analysis of Variance for Complete Block 2^2 Factorial

Source	DF	$S_{eq}SS$	Adj_jSS	Adj_jMS	F	P
C1	1	2.083	2.083	2.083	0.82	0.401
C2	1	10.083	10.083	10.083	3.95	0.094
C3	2	12.667	12.667	6.333	2.48	0.164
C1*C2	1	90.750	90.750	90.750	35.51	0.001
ERROR	6	15.333	15.333	2.556		
TOTAL	11	130.917				

The experimenter would carry this analysis further, as we did in Sec. IV, performing stem–leaf displays, letter-value displays, and boxplots of the residuals, as well as plotting the residuals against the predicted values ($\hat{y}$).

VIII. CONFOUNDING THE 2^2 DESIGN

In many pilot type studies using a 2^2 design, the researcher may not be able to conduct the study in one full block [(1) $a\,b\,ab$] at one time due to time or material constraints, for example. In addition, one technician or team may conduct part of the experiment and others, another portion. In this situation, the "actual block size" is "incomplete," or smaller than the number of treatment combinations that make up one replicate.

Suppose that in Example 1, a researcher has one team conduct the experiment portion where factor A is low and factor B is low [(1)] as well as

TABLE 13   Computer Input Data

Row	C1	C2	C3	C5	C6	C7
1	−1	−1	1	69	71.6667	−2.66666
2	−1	−1	2	72	71.6667	0.33334
3	−1	−1	3	74	71.6667	2.33334
4	1	−1	1	64	65.3333	−1.33334
5	1	−1	2	67	65.3333	1.66666
6	1	−1	3	65	65.3333	−0.33334
7	−1	1	1	63	64.3333	−1.33334
8	−1	1	2	65	64.3333	0.66666
9	−1	1	3	65	64.3333	0.66666
10	1	1	1	69	69.0000	0.00000
11	1	1	2	71	69.0000	2.00000
12	1	1	3	67	69.0000	−2.00000

the portion where factor A is high and factor B is high (ab). A second group is assigned to conduct the components where factor A is high and factor B is low (a) and where factor A is low and factor B is high (b). Team 1, then, conducts block (1) and ab ($\begin{smallmatrix}1\\ab\end{smallmatrix}$), and team 2 conducts the block a and b ($\begin{smallmatrix}a\\b\end{smallmatrix}$).

Here, the experiment whole— (1), a, b, ab— is said to be "confounded." Generally, confounding is designed such that the interaction effect is confounded (mixed with) the block effect so that the main effects can be seen clearly. This can be a real problem to an experimenter, but modifying the design structure sometimes is all one can do, particularly in research and development. The 2^2 factorial design, when confounded, requires replicates for the data to make any sense. Often, it is wiser to confound these designs partially instead of confounding them completely. The experimenter would randomize which of the two partial blocks is assigned to team 1 or team 2 as well as the order of performing the experiment within each of these blocks, if they are conducted sequentially.

But what does one confound with blocks? The standard statistical answer is the interaction term. But this is not always the best. To see how it is done, let us look at Table 14.

Table 14 portrays the linear combination of each effect in terms of its sign, for example, $A = ab + a - b - (1)$ or, more appropriately, $A = 1/2$ $[ab + a - b - (1)]$ and $B = [ab - a + b - (1)]$ or, more appropriately, $B = 1/2[ab - a + b - (1)]$.

Now to confound AB with blocks, one merely finds the pluses and minuses in the AB column and puts them in different blocks: (1) and ab are positive and go in one block, and a and b are negative, so they go into another (Fig. 8).

There are times when one does not want to confound the AB interaction effect with the block effect. Suppose one wants to confound the A effect with blocks, because one wants to measure the AB interaction. The same procedure is used. Consulting the A column of Table 14, one assigns treatment

TABLE 14 Factor Effects

Treatment combination	Main factor effects		
	A	**B**	**AB**
(1)	−	−	+
a	+	−	−
b	−	+	−
ab	+	+	+

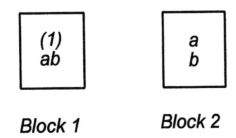

Block 1 **Block 2**

FIGURE 8   *AB* interaction confounded with blocks.

combinations with the + sign to one block and the − treatment combinations to the other (Fig. 9).

This, of course, results in the *A* effect being confounded with blocks, so one will not be able to determine the *A* effect. Conversely, if the researcher chooses to confound the *B* effect with blocks, she consults Table 14, finds the *B* column, and places the treatment combinations with a + sign in one block and a − sign in the other (Fig. 10).

It is often useful to measure the replication variability by computing the replication effect. If the contribution to replication variability is not large, it can be pooled with the error term to increase the error term's degrees of freedom while reducing MS_E.

The analysis of variance table for this design is presented in Table 15.

To be sure the reader understands this procedure, let us rework Example 1, as if it were run in two blocks of three replicates. Generally, it is wise to replicate experiments anyway to estimate the random error component. The entire study is then repeated *n* times. Although this study is blocked in the way it is, and it is termed confounded, one can confound the study by blocking it differently in ways previously discussed.

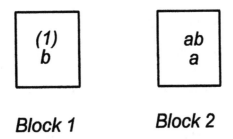

Block 1 **Block 2**

FIGURE 9   *A* factor confounded with blocks.

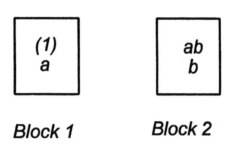

Block 1   **Block 2**

FIGURE 10   *B* factor confounded with blocks.

IX. COMPLETELY CONFOUNDED DESIGN

Completely confounded designs are ones in which the same variables are confounded throughout the entire experimental sequence.

For this example, then, the experimental data are represented in Table 16 and Fig. 11. Research team 1 conducts the portion of the study where factors *A* and *B* are both high and low. Research team 2 conducts the portion of the study where factor *A* and factor *B* are high.

Let us then perform the experiment, beginning with the six-step procedure.

Step 1.   Formulate the test hypothesis:

Factor *A*: H_0: The 0.15% antimicrobial is equivalent to the 0.08% in dissolution rates.
H_A: The above is not true.

Factor *B*: H_0: The 50-mg binder and the 25-mg binder are equivalent in dissolution rates.
H_A: The above is not true.

Replicate variability: H_0: The replicates are not significantly different.
H_A: The above is not true.

AB interaction/blocks: H_0: Because the interaction (*AB*) and blocks are confounded, one does not know whether the effect is due to blocking or to *AB* interaction or to a combination of these.

From Table 14, we know the blocks will have the form in Fig. 12.

Step 2.   Let $\alpha = 0.05$. $R = 3$, because the design is replicated three times.

Step 3.   The ANOVA model to be used is a confounded 2^2 factorial design. The confounding will occur between blocks and the *AB* interaction.

TABLE 15 ANOVA Table

Source of variation	Sum of squares	Degrees of freedom	Mean square	F_C	F_T
Factor A	$\dfrac{[ab+a-b-(1)]^2}{4R^a} = SS_A$	1	$\dfrac{SS_A}{1} = MS_A$	$\dfrac{MS_A}{MS_E}$	$F_{\alpha[1;\,\text{df MSE}]}$
Factor B	$\dfrac{[ab-a+b-(1)]^2}{4R} = SS_B$	1	$\dfrac{SS_B}{1} = MS_B$	$\dfrac{MS_B}{MS_E}$	$F_{\alpha[1;\,\text{df MSE}]}$
Replicate	$\sum_{i=1}^{I}\dfrac{R_i^2}{4} - \dfrac{Y_{\ldots}^2}{4R} = SS_{Rep}$	$R-1$	$\dfrac{SS_{Rep}}{R-1} = MS_{Rep}$	$\dfrac{MS_{Rep}}{MS_E}$	$F_{\alpha[R-1;\,\text{df MSE}]}$
AB interaction and block effect b	$\dfrac{[ab+(1)-a-b]^2}{4R} = SS_{AB/B}$	1	$\dfrac{SS_{AB/B}}{1} = MS_{AB/B}^{\,c}$		
Error (replicate effect)	$SS_E = SS_T - SS_A - SS_B$ $- SS_{AB/B} SS_{Rep}$	$(ab-1)(R-1)$	$\dfrac{SS_E}{((ab-1)(R-1))} = MS_E$		
Total	$\sum_{i=1}^{3}\sum_{j=1}^{2}\sum_{k=1}^{B} Y_{ijk}^2 - \dfrac{Y_{\ldots}^2}{4R} = SS_T$	$ab(R-1)$			

[a] R = number of replicates [if the replicate effect is insignificant, add it (SS_R) to the SS_E term, as well as its $R-1$ degrees of freedom, for increased power.]
$\dfrac{[ab+(1)-a-b]^2}{4R} = \dfrac{\sum(\text{blocks})^2}{(\text{number of observations per block})R} - \dfrac{Y_{\ldots}^2}{4R} = SS_{AB}/\text{block effect}$
SS_E is actually composed of the Block × Treatment A and B interaction, as well as error. The researcher assumes they are 0, leaving only the actual error term.
[c] It is not useful to compute F_c due to confounding the block effect with interaction. However, if the researcher wants to measure the combination; $F_c = MS_{AB/B}/MS_E$ and $F_T = F_\alpha[1;\,\text{df } MSE]$.

TABLE 16 Completely Confounded Design Data

	Replicates					Replicates			
Team 1	1	2	3	Total	Team 2	1	2	3	Total
$(1) = a^-b^-$	69	72	74	215	$a = a^+b^-$	64	67	65	196
$ab = a^+b^+$	69	71	67	207	$b = a^-b^+$	63	65	65	193
	138	143	141	422		127	132	130	389

Step 4. Decision rule:

Factor A: If $F_{calculated} > F_{tabled}$, reject H_0 at $\alpha = 0.05$.
$$F_T = [0.05(1; (ab - 1)(R - 1))]$$

$$= F_{0.05[1,(2 \times 2 - 1)(3-1)]} = F_{0.05[1,6]} = 5.99 \text{ (Table A.3)}$$

Factor B: If $F_{calculated} > F_{tabled}$, reject H_0 at $\alpha = 0.05$.
$$F_T = [0.05(1; (ab - 1)(R - 1))] = F_{0.05[1,(2 \times 2 - 1)(3-1)]} = F_{0.05[1,6]} = 5.99$$

Replicates: If $F_{calculated} > F_{tabled}$, reject H_0 at $\alpha = 0.05$.

$$F_T = [0.05((R - 1); (ab - 1)(R - 1))] = F_{0.05[(2,6)]} = 5.14$$

Step 5. Compute the statistic.
$$SS_A = \frac{[ab + a - b - (1)]^2}{4R} = \frac{(207 + 196 - 193 - 215)^2}{4(3)} = 2.08$$

$$SS_B = \frac{[ab + b - a - (1)]^2}{4R} = \frac{(207 + 193 - 196 - 215)^2}{12} = 10.08$$

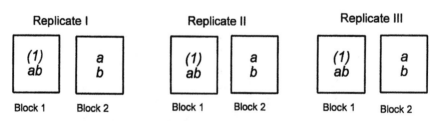

Replicate I   Replicate II   Replicate III

| (1) | a |
| ab | b |

Block 1   Block 2

| (1) | a |
| ab | b |

Block 1   Block 2

| (1) | a |
| ab | b |

Block 1   Block 2

FIGURE 11 Completely confounded design data.

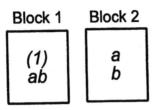

FIGURE 12 *AB* interaction blocks.

$$SS^*_{AB \text{ Blocks}} = \frac{[ab + (1) - a - b]^2}{4R} = \frac{(207 + 215 - 196 - 193)^2}{4(3)} = 90.75$$

$$SS_{\text{Block}} = \frac{\sum(\text{Blocks})^2}{\text{number of observations per block}_{(R)}} - \frac{y^2_{...}}{4R}$$

$$= \frac{422^2 + 389^2}{3(2)} - \frac{811^2}{12} = 90.75$$

$$SS_{\text{Replicates}} = \frac{\sum\limits_{i=1}^{3} R_i^2}{4} - \frac{y^2_{...}}{4R} = \frac{265^2 + 275^2 + 271^2}{4} - \frac{811^2}{12} = 12.67$$

where $R_1 = 138 + 127$, $R_2 = 143 + 132$, and $R_3 = 141 + 130$,

$$SS_T = \sum_1^3 \sum_1^2 \sum_1^2 y^2_{ijk} - \frac{y^2_{...}}{4R} = 69^2 + 72^2 + \cdots + 71^2 + 67^2 - \frac{811^2}{4(3)} = 130.92$$

$$SS_E = SS_T - SS_A - SS_B - SS_{AB/B}$$
$$= 130.92 - 2.08 - 10.08 - 90.75 - 12.67 = 15.34$$

Step 6. Discussion (see Table 17).

There is a problem with this design, however. We saw from Example 1 that there was significant interaction. We used the same data as before, so we know interaction is significant, but with this completely confounded design (*AB* interaction with blocks) we cannot know for sure what is happening. Is the block effect the culprit in the high value (90.75), or is it the interaction of factors *A* and *B*, or both? We cannot know by this design but could probably have a very grounded hunch. But the hunch could be wrong. This is a danger of using a completely confounded design. The researcher, upon seeing these data, would no doubt be puzzled and perhaps run the study again.

Finally, the researcher does not have to compute $SS_{\text{Replicates}}$ in this design. When it is not computed, (its effect) becomes a part of SS_E. The

---

* The block calculation will also result in the SS_{AB} value, for they are confounded.

TABLE 17   ANOVA Table

Source of variation	Sum of squares	Degrees of freedom	Mean square	F_c	F_T	S = Significant NS = Not significant
Factor A	2.08	1	2.08	0.81	5.99	NS
Factor B	10.08	1	10.08	3.94	5.99	NS
AB interaction with blocks	90.75	1	90.75[a]	35.45	5.99	S
$SS_{Replicates}$	12.67	2	6.33	2.47[b]	5.14	
SS_{ERROR}	15.34	6	2.56			
SS_{TOTAL}	130.92	11				

[a]Researcher asks why this ($MS_{AB/B}$) is so high. Block effect, interaction, or both.
[b]Researcher sees that the replicate is not significant. So, instead of going on, the researcher decides to pool the $SS_{Replicates}$ effect with SS_{Error} to gain two degrees of freedom.

degrees of freedom, then, are $ab(R-1)$ in the error term instead of $(ab-1)(R-1)$ (see Table 18).

X. DIAGNOSTIC CHECKING

For the confounded 2^2 factorial design, this researcher rarely checks the model adequacy, simply because there are too many "holes" in the confounded design. In my opinion, the confounded study design is very useful for "quick and dirty" explorations, but conclusive understanding must be ruled out.

TABLE 18   Revised ANOVA Table ($SS_{Replicate}$ Pooled with SS_{Error})

Source of variation	Sum of squares	Degrees of freedom	Mean square	F_c	F_T	S = Significant NS = Not significant
Factor A	2.08	1	2.08	0.59	5.32[a]	NS
Factor B	10.08	1	10.08	2.88	5.32	NS
AB interaction with blocks	90.75	1	90.75	—		
SS_{Error}[b]	$12.67 + 15.34 = 28.0$	$2 + 6 = 8$	3.50			
SS_{TOTAL}	130.92	11				

[a]F_T for factor A and $B = F_{0.05}(1, 8) = 5.32$.
[b]SS_E is now composed of SS_E plus $SS_{REPLICATES}$.

If one does want to see how well the model fits the data, however, the following is the procedure. It is suggested that evaluation be of the main effects A and B as well as the AB interaction/block effect, leaving the replicate effect alone.

XI. MODEL ADEQUACY

The linear model is:

$$y = b_0 + b_1(a) + b_2(b) + b_3(ab) \tag{14}$$

is sufficient.

$$b_0 = \frac{y_{...}^2}{abR}$$

$a = 2$ $a = 1$ if a^+, or -1 if a^-

$b = 2$ $b = 1$ if b^+, or -1 if b^-

$R =$ number of replicates (not blocks) $= 3$

From Example 1, recall that $ab = 207$, $b = 193$, $a = 196$, and $(1) = 215$.

$$b_1 = \text{factor } A = \frac{1}{4R}[ab + a - b - (1)]$$

$$b_2 = \text{factor } B = \frac{1}{4R}[ab + b - a - (1)]$$

$$b_3 = \text{factor } AB = \frac{1}{4R}[ab + (1) - a - b]$$

Using the data from Example 1,

$$b_0 = \frac{y_{...}^2}{abR} = \frac{811}{2(2)(3)} = 67.58 = \bar{y}$$

$$b_1 = a \text{ factor } = \frac{1}{4R}[ab + a - b - (1)]$$

$$= \frac{1}{4(3)}[207 + 196 - 193 - 215] = -0.42$$

$$b_2 = b \text{ factor } = \frac{1}{4R}[ab + b - a - (1)]$$

$$= \frac{1}{4(3)}[207 + 193 - 196 - 215] = -0.92$$

$b_3 = ab$ interaction/block effect

$$= \frac{1}{4R}[ab + (1) - a - b] = \frac{1}{4(3)}[207 + 215 - 196 - 193] = 2.75$$

The linear model to check the model's adequacy, then, is:

$$\hat{y} = 67.58 - 0.42(a) - 0.92(b) + 2.75(ab)$$

Notice that these are precisely the formula and values calculated in Eq. (13). The actual calculations will not be redone as the outcome is exactly the same. The only difference is that the $b_3(ab)$ is no longer only the AB interaction effect but is the AB interaction and the block effect.

XII. COMPUTER-GENERATED RESULTS

Let us now review how the exercise is computed with a general linear model. Suppose initially the researcher used the model that was in the form:

$$\hat{y} = \beta_0 + \beta_1(a) + \beta_2(b) + \beta_3(ab) + \beta_4(R)$$

where $\hat{y}$ = predicted value of dissolution rate
$b_0 = \mu$
a = factor A = 1 if a^+, or -1 if a^-
b = factor B = 1 if b^+, or -1 if b^-
ab = both the AB interaction and the block effect in this confounded design
R = replicates

The data are keyed in as presented in Table 19.
The MiniTab computer program command is:

GLM C4 = C1 C2 C1*C2 C3.

The computer printout is presented in Table 20. It is the same as calculated in Table 17.

Because the replicate effect (C_3) was not significant, the investigator chose to pool it with the error term. The investigator could just add the degrees of freedom terms as well as the sum-of-squares terms ($SS_{rep} + SS_E$) and recompute the F values or redo the computer calculation.

To redo the computation, the GLM key strokes are:

GLM C4 =   C1 C2 C1* C2.

The modified ANOVA Table appears as Table 21. This is the same ANOVA that was computed in Table 18. The actual values (y), the predicted values ($\hat{y}$), and the error ($y - \hat{y}$) are presented in Table 22.

XIII. PARTIAL CONFOUNDING

In the last section, we discussed complete confounding, where the same variable effect (ab) is confounded continually through the entire sequence of

TABLE 19 Data Table

Row	C1	C2	C3	C4
1	−1	−1	1	69
2	−1	−1	2	72
3	−1	−1	3	74
4	1	1	1	69
5	1	1	2	71
6	1	1	3	67
7	1	−1	1	64
8	1	−1	2	67
9	1	−1	3	65
10	−1	1	1	63
11	−1	1	2	65
12	−1	1	3	65

C1 $= a =$ 1 if a^+; $-$ 1 if a^-.
C2 $= b =$ 1 if b^+; $-$ 1 if b^-.
C3 $=$ replicate $=$ 1, if replicate 1; 2, if replicate 2; 3, if replicate 3.
C4 $=$ dissolution rate value.

replicates. By designing the study in this way, one loses the ability to measure the AB interaction effect because it is confounded with the block effect.

A different way of designing the study is to confound certain variable effects "partially," that is, not to confound the same effect continually. A design I find particularly useful is one where three replicates of two experimental blocks are performed, confounding A, B, and AB effects with blocks one time each. This does not have to remain constant, for in the 2^2 design one can do a combination of, say, ab and a, ab and b, a and b, or a and b and ab. The effect for A, B, or AB is lost, however, when confounded with the block effect.

TABLE 20 2 × 2 Analysis of Variance

Source	Df	Seq SS	Adj SS	Adj MS	F	P
C1	1	2.083	2.083	2.083	0.82	.401
C2	1	10.083	10.083	10.083	3.95	.094
C1*C2	1	90.750	90.750	90.750	35.51	.001
C3	2	12.667	12.667	6.333	2.48	.164
Error	6	15.333	15.333	2.556		
Total	11	130.917				

TABLE 21   Analysis of Variance

Source	Df	Seq SS	Adj SS	Adj MS	F	P
C1	1	2.083	2.083	2.083	0.60	.463
C2	1	10.083	10.083	10.083	2.88	.128
C1*C2	1	90.750	90.750	90.750	25.93	.000
Error	8	28.000	28.000	3.500		
Total	11	130.917				

Hence, our example using three replicates confounds A, B, and AB one time each; the actual main effects (A and B) and the interaction of A and B have been replicated twice.

The procedure for partial confounding is fairly straightforward. First, Table 14 is reconstructed. This is simply a table of pluses and minuses based on the factor effect (Table 23).

Recall that factor A is $ab + a - b - (1)$, read directly, row by row, on column A. Recall also that to confound A, B, or AB with blocks, one blocks the + treatments and the − treatments separately. Hence, to confound factor A with blocks, the blocks would be as shown in Fig. 13.

This process is conducted for each of the three replicates, using Table 23 to confound AB, A, and B with blocks one time each (Fig. 14).

In conducting the study, both the blocks are randomized, as are the treatments within the blocks, in terms of run order. Block assignment 1 or 2

TABLE 22   Actual Values

y	$\hat{y}$	$y - \hat{y} = \epsilon$
69	71.6667	− 2.66666
72	71.6667	0.33334
74	71.6667	2.33334
69	69.0000	0.00000
71	69.0000	2.00000
67	69.0000	− 2.00000
64	65.3333	− 1.33334
67	65.3333	1.66666
65	65.3333	− 0.33334
63	64.3333	− 1.33334
65	64.3333	0.66666
65	64.3333	0.66666

Useful Small-Scale Pilot Designs

383

TABLE 23   Factor Effects

Treatment combination	Main factor effects		
	A	**B**	**AB**
(1)	−	−	+
a	+	−	−
b	−	+	−
ab	+	+	+

does not matter. In other words, for replicate II, block 1 could be depicted as shown in Fig. 15, or it could be as presented in Fig. 16.

The main effects (A, B) and the interaction effects are computed with two values per treatment, instead of three, as before. This is because, in one of the three replicates, the A, B, and AB effects are confounded with the block effect.

$$SS_A = \frac{[ab + a - b - (1)]^2}{4n}$$

where n is the number of times the A effect is measured (which is 2, in this situation).

$$SS_B = \frac{[ab + b - a - (1)]^2}{4n} \quad \text{and } n = \text{ number of } B \text{ measurements}$$

$$SS_{AB} = \frac{[ab + (1) - a - b]^2}{4n} \quad \text{and } n = \text{ number of } AB \text{ measurements}$$

$$SS_{\text{replicates}} = \frac{\sum R^2}{4} - \frac{y_{...}^2}{N}, \quad \text{where } N = abR$$

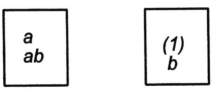

FIGURE 13   Factor A confounded with blocks.

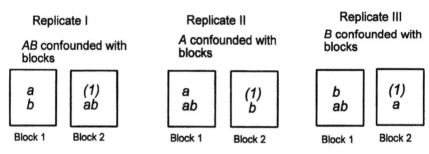

FIGURE 14   *AB, A,* and *B* confounded with blocks in three replicates.

$$SS_{\text{blocks (with replicates)}} = SS_A(\text{for confounded replicate})$$
$$= SS_B(\text{for confounded replicate})$$
$$= SS_{AB}(\text{for confounded replicate})$$

$$SS_{\text{TOTAL}} = \sum_{i=1}^{a}\sum_{j=1}^{b}\sum_{k=1}^{R} Y_{ijk}^2 - \frac{y_{...}^2}{N}$$

$$SS_E = SS_{\text{TOTAL}} - SS_A - SS_B - SS_{AB}$$
$$- SS_{\text{blocks within replicates}} - SS^*_{\text{number of replicates}}$$

Table 24 presents the ANOVA table for partially confounded designs.

Let us perform an example to clarify how the study is performed, using our original data from Example 1, reconstructed below:

	REPLICATES		
Treatment	1	2	3
ab =	69	71	67
a =	64	67	65
b =	63	65	65
(1) =	69	72	74
Replicate totals	265	275	271

---

*As before, if SS_{Reps} is not significant, it is often useful to add it to SS_E to obtain a larger number of degrees of freedom for the error term.

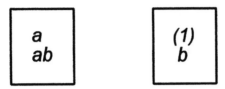

FIGURE 15   Block assignment.

It is also useful to review Table 23.

    This study is composed of three replicates. The researcher wants to retrieve information on the main effects A and B as well as AB interaction. Hence, the researcher will partially confound this study with each of these treatment effects in one replicate each. Using the factor effects schematic (Fig. 14) and finding column AB, the researcher makes sure that the two treatments with negative ($-$) signs are in one block, and the positive ($+$) signs in the other and then repeats the procedure for the A and B treatments.

    Hence, the researcher now has the partially confounded 2^2 factorial design in place. The next task is to perform the six-step procedure.

    Step 1.   Formulate the hypothesis.

    Factor A: H_0: The 0.15% antimicrobial is equivalent to the 0.08% in dissolution rate.

                  H_A: The above is not true.

    Factor B: H_0: The 50-mg binder and the 25-mg binder are equivalent in dissolution rates.

                  H_A: The above is not true.

    AB interaction: H_0: Factors A and B are independent of each other.

                       H_A: The above is not true.

    Step 2.   The researcher sets α at 0.10. Because the study design is small scale, one is looking for "potential" difference to explore in greater detail later. If one wants to screen products, accepting only those that are markedly better, $\alpha = 0.05$ may be preferred.

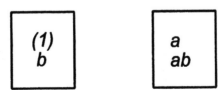

FIGURE 16   Alternative block assignment.

TABLE 24 Partial Confounding

Source of variation	Sum of squares	Degrees of freedom	Mean square	F_C	F_T
Factor A	$SS_A = \dfrac{[ab+a-b-(1)]^2}{4n^a}$	1	$\dfrac{SS_A}{1} = MS_A$	$\dfrac{MS_A}{MS_E}$	$F_{\alpha[1:df MSE]}$
Factor B	$SS_B = \dfrac{[ab+b-a-(1)]^2}{4n}$	1	$\dfrac{SS_B}{1} = MS_B$	$\dfrac{MS_B}{MS_E}$	$F_{\alpha[1:df MSE]}$
AB interaction	$SS_{AB} = \dfrac{[ab+(1)-a-b]^2}{4n}$	1	$\dfrac{SS_{AB}}{1} = MS_{AB}$	$\dfrac{MS_{AB}}{MS_E}$	$F_{\alpha[1:df MSE]}$
SS_{Blocks} with Replicates	$(SS_A + \text{confounded block}) +$ $(SS_B + \text{confounded block}) +$ $(SS_{AB} + \text{confounded block})$	3	$\dfrac{SS_{Blocks}}{3} = MS_{Blocks}$	$\dfrac{MS_{Blocks}}{MS_E}$	
SS_{REPS}^{b}	$SS_{REPS} = \dfrac{\sum R^2}{4} - \dfrac{y_{...}^{2c}}{N}$	$R-1$	$\dfrac{SS_{Reps}}{R-1} = MS_{Reps}$	$\dfrac{MS_{Reps}}{MS_E}$	
SS_{Error}	$SS_E = SS_T - SS_A - SS_B - SS_{AB}$ $-SS_{Blocks} - SS_{Reps}$	df SS_T − df SS_A − df SS_B −df SS_{AB} − df SS_{BLOCKS} −df SS_{REPS}	$\dfrac{SS_E}{df\,SS_E} = MS_E$	MS_E	
Total	$\displaystyle\sum_{i=1}^{2}\sum_{j=1}^{2}\sum_{k=1}^{N} y_{ijk}^2 - \dfrac{y_{...}^2}{N}$	$N-1$			

[a] n = number of replicates. The effect is *not confounded with blocks.*
[b] If $F_{calculated}$ for replicates is not significant, one can pool $SS_E + SS_{Reps}$, as well as $df_{Reps} + df_{Error}$. If researcher does not want to measure $SS_{replicates}$, do not subtract the effect from SS_{Total} in the calculation of SS_{Error}.
[c] $abR = N$.

The study will be replicated three times, confounding treatment factors A, B, and AB once each.

Step 3. The ANOVA model to be used is a partially confounded design (Table 24).

Step 4. Decision rule:

Factor A: If $F_{calculated} > F_{tabled}$, reject H_0 at $\alpha = 0.10$.

$F_{Tabled} = F_{0.10[1,df\ SSE3]} = F_{0.10\ [1,\ 3]} = 5.54$ (Table C),

Factor B: If $F_{calculated} > F_{tabled}$, reject H_0 at $\alpha = 0.10$.

$F_{Tabled} = F_{0.10[1,\ 3]} = 5.54$

Factor AB: If $F_{calculated} > F_{tabled}$, reject H_0 at $\alpha = 0.10$.

$F_{Tabled} = F_{0.10\ [1,\ 3]} = 5.54$

Step 5. Perform the calculations.

$$SS_A = \frac{[ab + a - b - (1)]^2}{4n}$$

Note that one does not use the data in replicate 2, for it is confounded with block effect. Hence, $n =$ number of replicates A not confounded $= 2$.

$$SS_A = \frac{[(69 + 67) + (64 + 65) - (63 + 65) - (69 + 74)]^2}{4(2)} = 4.50$$

$$SS_B = \frac{[ab + b - a - (1)]^2}{4(2)}$$

Replicate 3 is the one where B is confounded with block effects, so only replicates 1 and 2 are used.

$$\frac{[(69 + 71) + (63 + 65) - (64 + 67) - (69 + 72)]^2}{4(2)} = 2.00$$

$$SS_{AB} = \frac{[ab + (1) - a - b]^2}{4(2)}$$

Again, using only the replicates where AB is not confounded, replicates 2 and 3 are calculated.

$$SS_{AB} = \frac{[(71 + 67) + (72 + 74) - (67 + 65) - (65 + 65)]^2}{4(2)} = 60.50$$

where $k = 1$ levels per factor $= 2$

$$SS_{REPS} = \frac{\sum R^2}{2^k} - \frac{y_{...}^2}{N} = \frac{265^2 + 275^2 + 271^2}{4} - \frac{811^2}{12} = 12.67$$

$SS_{blocks+A+B+AB(\text{blocks within reps})}$

$= SS_A$ for replicates confounded

$+ SS_B$ for replicates confounded

$+ SS_{AB}$ for replicates confounded

$$SS_{A/\text{block }2} = \frac{[ab + a - b - (1)^2}{4n} = \frac{(71 + 67 - 65 - 72)^2}{4} = 0.25$$

$$SS_{B/\text{block }3} = \frac{[ab + b - a - (1)]^2}{4n} = \frac{(67 + 65 - 65 - 74)^2}{4} = 12.25$$

$$SS_{AB/\text{block }1} = \frac{[ab + (1) - a - b]^2}{4n} = \frac{(69 + 69 - 64 - 63)^2}{4} = 30.25$$

$$SS_{blocks/A+B+AB} = 0.25 + 12.25 + 30.25 = 42.75$$

$$SS_T = \sum\sum\sum y_{ijk}^2 - \frac{y_{...}^2}{4R} = 69^2 + 71^2 + \cdots + 72^2 + 74^2 - \frac{811^2}{4(3)} = 130.92$$

$$SS_E = SS_{TOTAL} - SS_A - SS_B - SS_{AB} - SS_{REPS}$$

$$- SS_{BLOCKS\ WITHIN\ REPS}$$

$$SS_E = 130.92 - 4.50 - 2.00 - 60.56 - 12.67 - 42.75 = 8.44$$

Step 6. Discussion. Construct the ANOVA Table (Table 25).

Based on this analysis, neither of the main effects A or B is significant, but the interaction is. This is a critical finding, for the researcher is in a much better position having measured A, B, and the AB interaction. In practice, it is a good idea to go immediately to the interaction and evaluate it. If it is significant, it is not really necessary to compute the main effects A and B because they must be evaluated jointly and not independently.

The researcher could perform a simple adjustment to increase the degrees of freedom in SS_E, hoping to decrease the size of MS_E, by merely adding SS_{REPS} to SS_E and their respective degrees of freedom (df).

$$SS'_E = SS_E + SS_{REPS} = 8.44 + 12.67 = 21.11$$

$$df\ SS'_E = df\ SS_E + df\ SS_{REPS} = 3 + 2 = 5$$

TABLE 25   ANOVA Table

Source of variation	Sum of squares	Degrees of freedom	Mean square	F_C	F_T	S = Significant NS = Not significant
Factor A (reps I, III)	4.50	1	4.50	1.60	5.54	NS
Factor B (reps I, II)	2.00	1	2.00	0.71	5.54	NS
AB(reps II, III)	60.50	1	60.56	21.55	5.54	S
SS$_{Blocks with reps (SS_A/}$	42.75	3	14.25			
REP 2 + SSB/REP 3						
+ SSAB/REP 1)						
SS$_{REPS}$	12.67	2	6.34			
SS$_E$	8.44	3	2.81			
SS$_T$	130.92	11				

$$MS'_E = \frac{SS'_E}{df\ SS'_E} = \frac{21.11}{5} = 4.22$$

At this point, it is plain that a new MS'_E of 4.22 will not change any of our conclusions. However, in other cases it will, particularly because the F_{tabled} value will change. For example:

$$F_{0.10[1,3]} = 5.54$$

But with the pooling of SS_E and SS_{REPS}, the new F_{tabled} value is:

$$F_{0.10[1,5]} = 4.06$$

The lower F_T in many cases will make a difference.

The procedure for partially confounded 2^2 designs when the researcher does not want to compute SS_{REPS} is shown in Table 26. Let us compute the ANOVA table (Table 27).

This type of factorial is just as easy to perform by paper-and-pencil techniques as by computer. In fact, I find it much more useful, for it makes me stay close to the data. In both computations, however, we see that the interaction of factors A and B is significant, so there is no reason to compute the main effects A and B. It would also be wise for the investigator to plot the main effects (not confounded with blocks) averages to see the interaction effect.

Finally, the researcher must realize that partially confounded study designs are very sensitive to replicate variability. In fact, one is essentially making predictions based on a replicate size of two, which can be very dangerous because there are so few data points. This researcher recommends that

TABLE 26 Partial Confounding of 2^2 Design with Replication Effect Measured

Source of variation	Sum of squares	Degrees of freedom	Mean square	F_C	F_T
Factor A	$\dfrac{[ab+a-b-(1)]^2}{4n} = SS_A$	1	$\dfrac{SS_A}{1}$	$\dfrac{MS_A}{df/SS_E}$	$F_{\alpha[1;\,df\,SS_E]}$
Factor B	$\dfrac{[ab+b-a-(1)]^2}{4n} = SS_B$	1	$\dfrac{SS_B}{1}$	$\dfrac{MS_B}{df/SS_E}$	$F_{\alpha[1;\,df\,SS_E]}$
AB interaction	$\dfrac{[ab+(1)-a-b]^2}{4n} = SS_{AB}/B$	1	$\dfrac{SS_{AB}}{1}$	$\dfrac{MS_{AB}}{df/SS_E}$	$F_{\alpha[1;\,df\,SS_E]}$
Blocks effect	(SS$_A$ for confounded block) + (SS$_B$ for confounded block) + (SS$_{AB}$ for confounded block)	3	$\dfrac{SS_{Blocks/REP}}{3}$		
SS$_E$(replicate effect)	$SS_T - SS_A - SS_B - SS_{AB} - SS_{Blocks/REPS}$	$df/SST - df/SS_A$ $-df/SS_B - df/SS_{AB}$ $-df/SS_{BLOCKS/Reps} = df/SS_E$ (by subtraction)	$\dfrac{SS_E}{df/SS_E}$	$\dfrac{SS_E}{df/SS_E}$	
Total	$\displaystyle\sum_{i=1}^{2}\sum_{j=1}^{2}\sum_{k=1}^{R} y_{ijk}^2 - \dfrac{y_{...}^2}{N}$	$N-1$			

[a] $abR = N$.

TABLE 27 ANOVA Table

Source of variation	Sum of squares	Degrees of freedom	Mean square	F_C	F_T	S = Significant NS = Not significant
Factor A	4.50	1	4.50	1.07	3.59	—
Factor B	2.00	1	2.00	0.47	3.59	—
AB interaction	60.56	1	60.56	14.35	3.59	S
Block effect	42.75	3	14.25			
SS_{Error}	130.92 − 4.50	11 −1 −1	4.22			
	− 2.00 − 60.56	−1 −3 = 5				
	− 42.75 = 21.11					
SS_{TOTAL}	130.92	11				

such designs be used only in preliminary screening studies. In addition, I would not recommend an α value less than 0.10. Using $\alpha = 0.05$, the difference required for significance would be obvious without the use of statistical analyses.

The researcher now has one more series of powerful tests at his or her disposal.

10

Nested Statistical Designs

Hierarchical or nested statistical designs can be very useful for researchers. For example, if one has, three groups of individuals (blacks, Hispanics, Caucasians) and they are treated with a drug for several different diseases, is there a difference between the groups in treatment effectiveness? Or suppose one outsources the same kinds of testing, tests A, B, and C, to three different laboratory facilities. How equivalent are the results from one laboratory to another in these tests?

What differentiates the hierarchical or nested design from a factorial design is the following. Test A in a factorial design would always be considered the constant factor in terms of method interpretation, microbiological techniques, and reagents used. But in reality, because test A was performed in different facilities, it may not be just a factor but also a variable. Test A in one laboratory would be standardized to a degree, but not entirely. There would be laboratory-to-laboratory variability [32]. The same is true for tests B and C. Because the tests are similar among laboratories, but not identical, a comparative analysis necessitates a nested or hierarchical design, as depicted in Fig. 1.

Because test A is not identical in each laboratory, it is said to be "nested," or a subset in each laboratory, and, in very real ways, is unique to each. An important question for the researcher to address then is, are the laboratories different from each other in how they perform the same tests?

A nested design is also valuable for evaluating work teams. Suppose there are three work teams, A, B, and C, each performing four different tests. Nested designs can be used to determine whether any of the teams differ in performance of any of the tests, as depicted in Fig. 2.

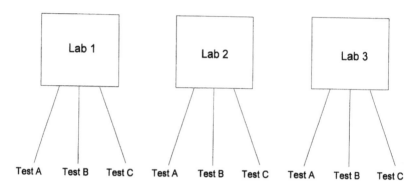

FIGURE 1 Testing among laboratories.

Some researchers, however, would not design these studies hierarchically. The determining factor for whether a design is a *factorial* or a *nested* one is whether it is more appropriately written in *factorial* or *nested* form. If the design makes more sense depicted as in Fig. 3, it is factorial. That is, the assumption must be that tests 1, 2, and 3 are identical in factors *A*, *B*, and *C*. The structure illustrated in Fig. 4 is a nested one in which tests are assumed not identical in groups *A*, *B*, and *C*, and, hence, it makes more sense to identify them numerically, 1 through 9.

Some critical thinking is often required to make this determination. But as with everything in statistics, it is important that one communicate clearly what one decided to do and, then, how it was done. *Context* is as important as *content*. Context gives the researcher and the reader a specific perspective from which to interpret the data. An argument can always be presented that a different perspective should have been applied, and such disputes are not uncommon in statistical processes [5].

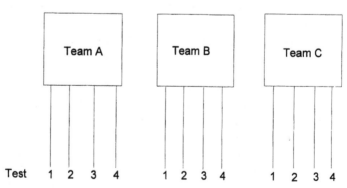

FIGURE 2 Nested design.

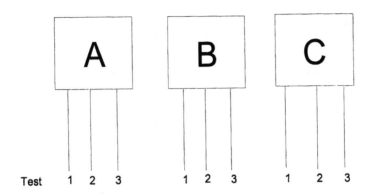

FIGURE 3 Factorial design.

When appropriate, a nested design will provide greater statistical power than a nonnested design [27]. The model is straightforward.

$$y_{ijk} = \mu + A_i + B_{j(i)} + \epsilon_{(ij)k} \tag{1}$$

where $i = 1, 2, \ldots a$, factor A
$\quad j = 1, 2, \ldots b$, factor B
$\quad k = 1, 2, \ldots n$, replicate

Note that for factor B, the value j is nested within the ith level of factor A. This design is commonly referred to as a two-stage nested design. The entire model can be expressed as:

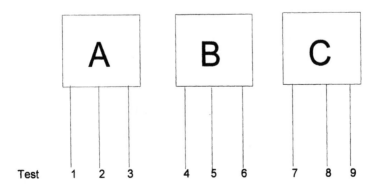

FIGURE 4 Nested design.

$$\sum_{i=j}^{a}\sum_{j=1}^{b}\sum_{k=1}^{n}(y_{ijk}-\bar{y}...)^2 = \sum_{i=1}^{a}\sum_{j=1}^{b}\sum_{k=1}^{n}[(\bar{y}_i..-\bar{y}...)+(\bar{y}_{ij}.-\bar{y}_i..)+(y_{ijk}-\bar{y}_{ij}.)]^2 \tag{2}$$

$$\underbrace{\qquad\qquad}_{\text{Total effect}} \qquad \underbrace{\qquad}_{\text{Factor } A} \quad \underbrace{\qquad}_{\text{Factor } B} \quad \underbrace{\qquad}_{\text{Error}}$$

or, in sum-of-squares totals:

$$SS_{\text{TOTAL}} = SS_A + SS_{B(A)} + SS_{\text{ERROR}} \tag{3}$$

where the error term is assumed to be normally and independently distributed with a mean of zero and a variance of σ^2 [NID $(0, \sigma^2)$].

This design is a little different from those we have encountered before in that the expected mean square values (MS_{Factors}) have, in the past, always been divided by the MS_{ERROR} term. This is not the case for this design. Generally, much procedural knowledge is required for constructing an expected mean square ($E[MS]$) table to determine which MS values are divided by which MS values, but we will simplify it and provide easy-to-use instructions (Table 1).

To determine the F calculated value, for example, for each factor other than the MS_E, one must first divide the MS factor A term by the factor $MS_{B(A)}$ or by the factor MS_E term. The MS term with one variable component fewer than the MS_A term is the one to use. Then divide the $MS_{B(A)}$ factor by the MS term that has one variable component fewer than it does.

For example, in the case where MS_A and $MS_{B(A)}$ are both fixed:

$$(MS_A) = \underbrace{\sigma^2}_{} + \underbrace{\frac{bn\sum A_i^2}{a-1}}_{} \tag{4}$$

variable component   1   2

TABLE 1   Expected Mean Square Values

Expected mean square	Factors		
	A fixed B fixed	A fixed B random	A random B random
MS_A	$\sigma^2 + \frac{bn\sum A_i^2}{a-1}$	$\sigma^2 + n\sigma_b^2 + \frac{bn\sum A_i^2}{a-1}$	$\sigma^2 + n\sigma_B^2 + bn\sigma_A^2$
$MS_{B(A)}$	$\sigma^2 + \frac{n\sum\sum B_{i(j)}^2}{a(b-1)}$	$\sigma^2 + n\sigma_B^2$	$\sigma^2 + n\sigma_B^2$
MS_{ERROR}	σ^2	σ^2	σ^2

$$MS_{B(A)} = \underbrace{\sigma^2}_{} + \underbrace{\dfrac{n \sum \sum B_{j(i)}^2}{a(b-1)}}_{}$$

variable component   1   2   (5)

$$MS_E = \underbrace{\sigma^2}_{}$$

variable component   1   (6)

Because both MS_A and $MS_{B(A)}$ have two variable components and MS_E has one, both MS_A and $MS_{B(A)}$ are divided by MS_E to determine F-calculated (F_C).

When factor A and factor B are both random, the following applies:

$$MS_A = \underbrace{\sigma^2}_{} + \underbrace{n\sigma_B^2}_{} + \underbrace{bn\sigma_A^2}_{}$$

variable components   1   2   3   (7)

$$MS_{B(A)} = \underbrace{\sigma^2}_{} + \underbrace{n\sigma_B^2}_{}$$

variable components   1   2   (8)

$$MS_E = \underbrace{\sigma^2}_{}$$

variable component   1   (9)

Because MS_A has three variable components and $MS_{B(A)}$ has two, F-calculated (F_C) for factor A is $MS_A/MS_{B(A)}$. The F_T value is found using the numerator degrees of freedom for MS_A and the denominator degrees of freedom for $MS_{B(A)}$. $F_T = F_{\alpha(df\ MS_A;df\ MS_{B(A)})}$, and using Table C to find the F_T value.

Because factor $MS_{B(A)}$ has two components and MS_E has one, the F_C value is $MS_{B(A)}/MS_E$. The F_T value is $F_{\alpha(df\ MS_{B(A)};df\ MS_E)}$. The degrees of freedom for the F_T values are simply the degrees of freedom for the main effects A and B and MS_E degrees of freedom.

When factor A is fixed and factor B is random, the following approach is applied:

$$MS_A = \underbrace{\sigma^2}_{} + \underbrace{n\sigma_B^2}_{} + \underbrace{\dfrac{bn \sum A_i^2}{a-1}}_{}$$

variable components   1   2   3   (10)

$$MS_{B(A)} = \underbrace{\sigma^2}_{1} + \underbrace{n\sigma_B^2}_{2}$$

(11)

variable components   1   2

$$MS_E = \underbrace{\sigma^2}_{1}$$

(12)

variable component   1

Because $E(MS_A)$ has three variable components and $E(MS_{B(A)})$ has two, F_C for factor A is $MS_A/MS_{B(A)}$. The F_T value, as before, is found using the numerator degrees of freedom for MS_A and the denominator degrees of freedom for $MS_{B(A)}$. $F_T = F_{\alpha(df\ MS_A;\ df\ MS_{B(A)})}$ in Table C.

Because $MS_{B(A)}$ has two variable components and MS_E has one, F_C for $MS_{B(A)}$ is $MS_{B(A)}/MS_E$. The F_T value is found using the numerator degrees of freedom for $MS_{B(A)}$ and the denominator degrees of freedom for MS_E. $F_T = F_{\alpha(df\ MS_{B(A)};df\ MS_E)}$ in Table C.

Table 2 provides a schematic of these various states of random versus fixed components, and Table 3 provides the actual ANOVA computations.

When a factor is fixed, the levels of that factor have been intentionally set, not selected randomly from the population set of all possible levels. When a factor is random, it has been selected at random from the set of all possible levels of the population. Generally, in industrial research, the models are either fixed (both factors) or mixed (A fixed, B random).

Example 1: Many times in pharmaceutical science, microbiology, biotechnology, and engineering, product-effectiveness testing is performed. In this example, a laboratory has performed time-kill kinetics studies on their various consumer antimicrobial products, using standard American Society for Testing and Materials/Food and Drug Administration

TABLE 2 Numerator and Denominator Degrees of Freedom Table

	A fixed B fixed	A fixed B random	A random B random
Factor A	$H_0: A_i = 0$ $H_A: A_i \neq 0$ $F_C = \frac{MS_A}{MS_E}$ $F_T = F_{\alpha(dfMS_A;dfMS_E)}$	$H_0: A_i = 0$ $H_A: A_i \neq 0$ $F_C = \frac{MS_A}{MS_{B(A)}}$ $F_T = F_{\alpha(dfMS_A;dfMS_{B(A)})}$	$H_0: \sigma_A^2 = 0$ $H_A: \sigma_A^2 \neq 0$ $F_C = \frac{MS_A}{MS_{B(A)}}$ $F_T = F_{\alpha(dfMS_A;dfMS_{B(A)})}$
Factor B	$H_0: B_{j(i)} = 0$ $H_A: B_{j(i)} \neq 0$ $F_C = \frac{MS_{B(A)}}{MS_E}$ $F_T = F_{\alpha(dfMS_{B(A)};dfMS_E)}$	$H_0: \sigma_B^2 = 0$ $H_A: \sigma_B^2 \neq 0$ $F_C = \frac{MS_{B(A)}}{MS_E}$ $F_T = F_{\alpha(dfMS_{B(A)};dfMS_E)}$	$H_0: \sigma_B^2 = 0$ $H_A: \sigma_B^2 \neq 0$ $F_C = \frac{MS_{B(A)}}{MS_E}$ $F_T = F_{\alpha(dfMS_{B(A)};dfMS_E)}$

TABLE 3 ANOVA Computations

Source	Sum of squares	Degrees of freedom	MS	F_C	F_T
Factor A	$\frac{1}{bn}\sum\limits_{i=1}^{a} y_{i\cdots}^2 - \frac{y_{\cdots}^2}{abn}$	$a-1$	$\frac{SS_A}{(a-1)} = MS_A$		
Factor B within A	$SS_{B(A)} = \frac{1}{n}\sum\limits_{i=1}^{a}\sum\limits_{j=1}^{b} y_{ij\cdot}^2$ $-\frac{1}{bn}\sum\limits_{i=1}^{a} y_{i\cdots}^2$	$a(b-1)$	$\frac{SS_{B(A)}}{a(b-1)} = MS_{B(A)}$	See Table 2	
Error	$\sum\limits_{i=1}^{a}\sum\limits_{j=1}^{b}\sum\limits_{k=1}^{n} y_{ijk}^2$ $-\frac{1}{n}\sum\limits_{i=1}^{a}\sum\limits_{j=1}^{b} y_{ij\cdot}^2$	$ab(n-1)$	$\frac{SS_E}{ab(n-1)} = MS_E$		
Total	$\sum\limits_{i=1}^{a}\sum\limits_{j=1}^{b}\sum\limits_{k=1}^{n} y_{ijk}^2 - \frac{y_{\cdots}^2}{abn}$	$abn-1$			

(ASTM/FDA) Tentative Final Monograph procedures. There has been a major price increase by its supplier of tryptic soy agar. The quality assurance group is disturbed about this situation in that the growth characteristics of challenge microorganisms may vary between media from different suppliers. They have issued a warning that microbiology research and development must assure the quality assurance group that substitute tryptic soy agar products are not different from the standard tryptic soy agar in terms of microbial growth characteristics. The microbiology department has found two other potential tryptic soy agar suppliers, but upon evaluation they determined that lot-to-lot variation may be excessive. That is, one lot may be acceptable and the next unacceptable.

The microbiology laboratory decides to evaluate the media from the regular supplier and the two others (fixed effect, in that the suppliers were selected on the basis of economic and availability characteristics, not at random). However, from each of the three suppliers, three lots will be selected at random (random effect). Five samples from each of the individual lots will be evaluated for microbial growth and the colony counts from each compared. The data from the study are presented in Table 4.

Let us perform the six-step procedure in evaluating this problem.

Step 1. Formulate the test hypothesis.
Company's suppliers (factor A, fixed effect)
H_0: Company A = company B = company C in terms of microbial population numbers on the agar plates.
H_A: At least one company is different from the other two in terms of microbial population numbers.

TABLE 4   Nested Design

Product suppliers (fixed)		A			B			C		
Lots selected at random		1	2	3	4	5	6	7	8	9[a]
	n									
	1	5.69[b]	4.38	4.44	5.82	5.32	5.73	5.36	5.38	6.01
	2	4.79	6.21	4.15	5.97	6.21	5.81	5.32	4.29	6.23
Replicates	3	5.23	5.48	5.39	5.81	5.73	6.13	4.79	5.71	5.82
	4	5.51	5.92	5.29	5.32	4.91	5.13	5.15	5.62	5.89
	5	5.72	4.79	4.72	5.43	5.59	5.56	5.92	5.15	5.69
Lot totals ($y_{ij.}$)		26.94	26.78	23.99	28.35	27.76	28.36	26.54	26.15	29.64
Supplier totals ($y_{i..}$)			77.71			84.47			82.33	
								$244.51 = y_{...}$		

[a]This design is nested instead of factorial because the lots can be numbered one through nine and still make sense.
[b]Actual colony count values, $\log_{10}$ scale.

Lot-to-lot effect [factor B, nested within suppliers (random)]
H_0: $\sigma^2 = \sigma^2 = \sigma^2$, or the variances of the three lots are the same.
H_A: The variances between the lots are not the same.
Step 2. Select α level and n.
The microbiology group selects $\alpha = 0.05$ because it is a standard operating procedure (SOP) decree, as is the minimum sample size of $n = 5$.
Step 3. Select method.
The two-stage nested design was used.
$y_{ijk} = \mu + A_i + B_{j(i)} + \epsilon_{(ij)k}$
where μ = grand mean
A_i = supplier effect
$B_{j(i)}$ = lot effect
$\epsilon_{(ij)k}$ is distributed as NID(0, σ^2)

Step 4. Decision rule.
Suppliers (factor A):
H_0: Company A = company B = company C.
H_A: The above is not true.
F_C (fixed) (from Table 2) $= \dfrac{\text{MS}_A}{\text{MS}_{B(A)}}$

Suppliers $= a = 3$, lots $= b = 3$, and replicates $= n = 5$.
$F_T = F_{\alpha(\text{df MS}_A; \text{ df MS}_{B(A)})} = F_{T, 0.05(a-1; a[b-1])} = F_{0.05(3-1; 3[3-1])}$
$F_{T, 0.05(2, 6)} = 5.14$ (Table A.3).
So, if $F_C > 5.14$, reject H_0 at $\alpha = 0.05$; suppliers are different.

Lot-to-lot (factor $B_{(A)}$) random effects
  H_0: The variance (σ^2) is the same between lots
  H_A: The variance (σ^2) is different between lots
  F_C (random effects) (from Table 2) $= \frac{\text{MS}_{B(A)}}{\text{MS}_E}$
  $F_T = F_{\alpha(a[b-1]; ab[n-1])} = F_{0.05(3[3-1]; 3 \times 3[5-1])} = F_{0.05(6; 36)} = 2.42$
  So, if $F_C > 2.42$, reject H_0 at $\alpha = 0.05$; there is significant lot-to-lot variability.

Step 5. Computation.

$$SS_A = SS_{\text{SUPPLIERS}} = \frac{1}{bn}\sum_{i=1}^{a} y_{i\cdot\cdot}^2 - \frac{y_{\cdot\cdot\cdot}^2}{abn}$$

$$= \frac{1}{3(5)}[77.71^2 + 84.47^2 + 82.33^2] - \frac{244.51^2}{3 \cdot 3 \cdot 5}$$

$$= 1330.15 - 1328.56$$

$$SS_A = 1.59$$

$$SS_{B(A)} = SS_{\text{LOTS WITHIN SUPPLIERS}} = \frac{1}{n}\sum_{i=1}^{a}\sum_{j=1}^{b} y_{ij\cdot}^2 - \frac{1}{bn}\sum_{i=1}^{a} y_{i\cdot\cdot}^2$$

$$= \frac{1}{5}[26.94^2 + 26.78^2 + 23.99^2 + 28.35^2 + 27.76^2 + 28.36^2$$
$$+ 26.54^2 + 26.15^2 + 29.64^2] - 1330.15$$

$$= 1332.76 - 1330.15$$

$$SS_{B(A)} = 2.61$$

$$SS_E = \sum_{i=1}^{a}\sum_{j=1}^{b}\sum_{k=1}^{n} y_{ijk}^2 - \frac{1}{n}\sum_{i=1}^{a}\sum_{j=1}^{b} y_{ij\cdot}^2$$

$$= [5.69^2 + 4.79^2 + 5.23^2 + \cdots + 5.82^2 + 5.89^2 + 5.69^2] - 1332.76$$

$$= 1340.76 - 1332.76$$

$$SS_E = 8.00$$

$$SS_{\text{TOTAL}} = \sum_{i=1}^{a}\sum_{j=1}^{b}\sum_{k=1}^{n} y_{ijk}^2 - \frac{y_{\cdot\cdot\cdot}^2}{abn} = 1340.76 - 1328.56$$

$$SS_{\text{TOTAL}} = 12.20$$

Step 6:   Construct the ANOVA Table (Table 5).
Factor *A*   (suppliers): Suppliers cannot be determined to be significantly different from one another at the $\alpha = 0.05$ level of significance.
Factor *B*   (lots within suppliers): There is no significant difference
between the lots within the suppliers in terms of variability at
$\alpha = 0.05$. Hence, we can conclude that they came from the same
population at the $\alpha = 0.05$ level of significance.

Note: Technically, in significance testing, a researcher must say "one
cannot reject the null hypothesis" at a specific α level. But in industry this is
a consistent problem because management frequently does not know how to
interpret that statement. Hence, it is easier to form the conclusion in business terms.

I. MULTIPLE COMPARISONS

In Example 1, the researcher could not reject the H_0 hypothesis, that suppliers were not different, at $\alpha = 0.05$. In addition, lot variabilities within the
three suppliers were not significantly different at $\alpha = 0.05$. But, if the H_0
hypothesis in either case had been rejected, the same multiple comparison
procedures discussed in earlier chapters could be used, with minor adjust-

TABLE 5   ANOVA Table

Factor	Sum of squares	Degrees of freedom	Mean square	F_C	F_T	Significant / not significant
Factor *A* (suppliers)	1.59	$a-1$ $3-1=2$	$0.80 = MS_A$	$\frac{MS_A}{MS_{B(A)}} = 1.82$	5.14	Not significant
Factor B_A (lots within suppliers)	2.61	$a(b-1)$ $3(3-1)$ $=6$	$0.44 = MS_{B(A)}$	$\frac{MS_{B(A)}}{MS_E} = 2.00$	2.42	Not significant
Error	8.00	$ab(n-1)$ $3 \cdot 3(5-1)$ $=36$	$0.22 = MS_E$			
Total	12.20	$abn-1$ $3 \cdot 3 \cdot 5 - 1$ $=44$				

ments. Any contrasts should be performed on the fixed-effects portions of the method rather than the random effects.

II. BONFERRONI METHOD

The Bonferroni method can be used for pairwise mean comparisons if the desired comparisons are selected *prior to* conducting the study.

A. Factor A (Suppliers; Fixed Effect)

In comparing factor A groups (suppliers), let us suppose the researchers wanted to make three comparisons and these were defined prior to conducting the study.

$$H_0: \mu_1 = \mu_2$$
$$H_0: \mu_1 = \mu_3$$
$$H_0: \mu_2 = \mu_3$$

As before, the test statistic is:

$$t' = \frac{D}{S_D} \qquad \text{where } D = |\bar{y}_{i..} - \bar{y}_{j..}|$$

$$S_D = \sqrt{\frac{2(\text{denominator MS in } F \text{ ratio})}{bn}} \qquad (13)$$

Recall that the denominator was $MS_{B(A)}$, so $S_D = \sqrt{2(MS_{B(A)})/bn}$.

B. Decision Rule

If $t' > t_{\alpha/2g;\ \text{df denominator for } F \text{ ratio}}$, a significant difference exists between the suppliers at α, where $g =$ number of contrasts.
We will compute the average values $\bar{y}_{i..}$ for the three suppliers:

$$\bar{y}_{1..} = \frac{77.71}{bn} = \frac{77.71}{15} = 5.18$$

$$\bar{y}_{2..} = \frac{84.47}{bn} = \frac{84.47}{15} = 5.63$$

$$\bar{y}_{3..} = \frac{82.33}{bn} = \frac{82.33}{15} = 5.49$$

Hence

$$D_1 = |\bar{y}_{1..} - \bar{y}_{2..}| = |5.18 - 5.63| = 0.45$$

$$D_2 = |\bar{y}_{1..} - \bar{y}_{3..}| = |5.18 - 5.49| = 0.31$$

$$D_3 = |\bar{y}_{2..} - \bar{y}_{3..}| = |5.63 - 5.49| = 0.14$$

$$S_D = \sqrt{\frac{2(MS_{B(A)})}{bn}} = \sqrt{\frac{2(0.44)}{15}} = 0.24$$

where $g = 3$ and $\alpha = 0.05$

$t_{(\alpha/2g;a[b-1])} = t_{(0.05/6;6)} = t_{(0.01,6)} = 3.14$. From the student's T table (Table A.2).

$$t_1' = \frac{D_1}{S_D} = \frac{0.45}{0.24} = 1.88$$

Because $1.88 < 3.14$, one cannot reject H_0 (as expected) at $\alpha = 0.05$.

$$t_2' = \frac{D_2}{S_D} = \frac{0.31}{0.24} = 1.29$$

Because $1.29 < 3.14$, one cannot reject H_0 (as expected) at $\alpha = 0.05$.

$$t_3' = \frac{D_3}{S_D} = \frac{0.14}{0.24} = 0.58$$

Because $0.58 < 3.14$, one cannot reject H_0 (as expected) at $\alpha = 0.05$.

It is important that the researcher not perform too many pairwise contrasts (g) with the Bonferroni procedure because more than a few make the t-table value huge, significantly reducing its power. Also, those contrasts must be selected prior to conducting the test.

When a fixed factor A component and a random factor B component are used, as in Example 1, $MS_{B(A)}$ will be used in place of MS_E for the error term denominator as well as for the degrees of freedom for the t-table value. If A and B factors are both fixed, MS_E is used as the denominator in calculating F_C.

C. Factor B

This factor is generally not evaluated when it is a random effect. However, this author has found it useful in quality assurance situations to use the hypothesis H_0: $\sigma_1^2 = \sigma_2^2 = \cdots = \sigma_k^2$ versus H_A: "at least one group does not have the same variance." Variance and ranges tend to increase, to become rather large (larger than normal), if the process is out of control. One way of assessing, not the mean value, but the variability (σ^2) is to compare the group ranges intuitively. The range is merely the largest − smallest value. For example,

	SUPPLIERS	
A	**B**	**C**
Lowest – highest	Lowest – highest	Lowest – highest
4.15 – 6.21	4.91 – 6.21	4.29 – 6.23
Range	*Range*	*Range*
2.06	1.30	1.94

Because there was no significant difference between the lots within each supplier, such evaluation is a moot process. Yet, if there had been a significant difference, the range of values might have helped isolate the supplier(s) for which lot-to-lot variability is excessive.

The Bonferroni method is not generally useful for evaluating factor B within A, particularly when the contrasts must be conceived prior to conducting the experiment [33]. *A posteriori* contrasts (conceived after the experiment has been completed) are more applicable. Let us begin with factor B within A.

D. Factor $B_{(A)}$

This factor is usually evaluated only if it is *fixed*. So, let us construct Table 6, assuming that both factor A and $B_{(A)}$ are fixed.

Let us suppose, also, that factor $B_{(A)}$ was significantly different between suppliers. We would then calculate a sum-of-squares B within A, or lots within each supplier.

Suppliers A: Lot variance

$$SS_{B(A)} = \frac{1}{n}\sum y_{ij.}^2 - \frac{y_{...}^2}{bn}$$

TABLE 6 ANOVA Table with both Factor A and $B_{(A)}$ Fixed.

Factor	Sum of squares	Degrees of freedom	Mean square	F_C
Factor A (suppliers)	1.59	2	$0.80 = MS_A$	$\frac{MS_A}{MS_E} = \frac{0.80}{0.22} = 3.64$
Factor $B_{(A)}$ (lots within suppliers)	2.61	6	$0.44 = MS_{B(A)}$	$\frac{MS_{B(A)}}{MS_E} = \frac{0.44}{0.22} = 2.00$
Error	8.00	36	$0.22 = MS_E$	
Total	12.20	44		

First supplier:

$$SS_{B(A1)} = \frac{1}{5}(26.94^2 + 26.78^2 + 23.99^2) - \frac{77.71^2}{3(5)}$$
$$= 403.69 - 402.59$$
$$= 1.10$$

Second supplier:

$$SS_{B(A2)} = \frac{1}{5}(28.35^2 + 27.76^2 + 28.36^2) - \frac{84.47^2}{3(5)}$$
$$= 475.73 - 475.68$$
$$= 0.05$$

Third supplier:

$$SS_{B(A3)} = \frac{1}{5}(26.54^2 + 26.15^2 + 29.64^2) - \frac{82.33^2}{3(5)}$$
$$= 453.34 - 451.88$$
$$= 1.46$$

The ANOVA table (Table 6) is revised accordingly (Table 7).

The researcher can now perform the three contrasts to determine which ones are significantly different, e.g.,

$$F_T = F_{\alpha(b-1); ab(n-1)} \text{ and}$$

$$F_C \text{ for } B_{(A1)} = \frac{MS_{B(A1)}}{MS_E}$$

TABLE 7 Revised ANOVA Table

Factor	Sum of squares	Degrees of freedom	Mean square	F_C
Factor A (suppliers)	1.59	2	$0.80 = MS_A$	$\frac{MS_A}{MS_E} = \frac{0.80}{0.22}$ $= 3.64$
Factor B_A	2.61	6	$0.44 = MS_{B(A)}$	$\frac{MS_{B(A)}}{MS_E} = \frac{0.44}{0.22}$ $= 2.00$
Factor $B_{(A1)}$	1.10	$(b-1)$ each $= 2$	0.55	
Factor $B_{(A2)}$	0.05	2	0.03	
Factor $B_{(A3)}$	1.46	2	0.73	
Error	8.00	36	0.22	
Total	12.20	44		

$$F_C \text{ for } B_{(A2)} = \frac{\text{MS}_{B(A2)}}{\text{MS}_E}$$

$$F_C \text{ for } B_{(A3)} = \frac{\text{MS}_{B(A3)}}{\text{MS}_E}$$

If one F_C for $B_{(Ai)}$ was significantly different from F_T, one could state that it was significantly different from the other lots. If two or all three were significantly different, one could use the LSD or Scheffe method to compare those lot groups with each other, but only if $B_{(A)}$ is *fixed*. This will be done for each contrast section.

III. SCHEFFE'S METHOD

Recall that Scheffe's method is used to compare a number of different contrasts. Scheffe's method is useful for a few of any possible contrasts but not as a contrast to compare all mean pairs. This is because, as the number of comparisons increases, the power decreases due to type I (alpha) error being, at most for all of the simultaneous comparisons, α. If only pairwise contrasts are made, the Tukey procedure gives narrower confidence limits.

A. Factor A

The $\bar{y}_{i..}$ values are evaluated in any possible combination. The standard error of the contrast is:

$$S_C = \sqrt{(\text{MS denominator})^* \sum_{i=1}^{a} \left(\frac{c_i^2}{n_i} \right)}$$

Recall that the number of contrasts is written as:

$$c_1 \mu_1 + c_2 \mu_2 + \cdots + c_m \mu_m$$

$$c_i = c_1 \bar{y}_{1..} + c_2 \bar{y}_{2..} + \cdots + c_a \bar{y}_{a..}$$

The critical value (S_{α_i}) with which the calculated c_i is compared is:

$$S_{\alpha_i} = S_{c_i} \sqrt{(a-1) F_{\alpha(a-1); \text{ degrees of freedom denominator}}}$$

Decision:
If $|C_i| > S_{\alpha_i}$, reject H_0.

---

[*]Refer to Table 2 of this chapter for selecting the appropriate denominator. In a fixed-effects model, the appropriate denominator for factor A is MS_E. In a random-effects model for factor $B_{(A)}$, with A fixed, it is $\text{MS}_{B(A)}$.

Example Cont. Recall that factor A is fixed and factor $B_{(A)}$ is random in our example. Also, one would not perform comparisons if the F_C value was not significant. In this example, it is not significant, so the computation is for demonstration purposes only.

Suppose the researcher wants to compare the lot means for all three suppliers with one another.

1. $H_0: \mu_1 = \mu_2; c_1 = |\bar{y}_{1..} - \bar{y}_{2..}| = 5.18 - 5.63 = 0.45$
2. $H_0: \mu_1 = \mu_3; c_2 = |\bar{y}_{1..} - \bar{y}_{3..}| = 5.18 - 5.49 = 0.31$
3. $H_0: \mu_2 = \mu_3; c_3 = |\bar{y}_{2..} - \bar{y}_{3..}| = 5.63 - 5.49 = 0.14$

$$S_{c_i} = \sqrt{MS_{\text{denominator}}\left(\sum \frac{c^2}{n}\right)}$$

The denominator in this example is $MS_{B(A)}$ because factor A is fixed and factor $B_{(A)}$ is random.

$$S_{c_i} = \sqrt{MS_{B(A)}\left(\sum \frac{c^2}{n}\right)}$$

$$S_{c_1} = \sqrt{0.44\left(\frac{1^2 + (-1)^2}{16}\right)} = 0.23$$

$$S_{c_2} = \sqrt{0.44\left(\frac{1^2 + (-1)^2}{16}\right)} = 0.23$$

$$S_{c_3} = \sqrt{0.44\left(\frac{1^2 + (-1)^2}{16}\right)} = 0.23$$

Letting $\alpha = 0.05$ and using Table A.3 (F distribution):

$$S_{\alpha_i} = S_{c_i}\sqrt{(a-1)F_{0.05(a-1;MS_{\text{denominator}})}} = S_{c_i}\sqrt{(a-1)F_{0.05(a-1;a(b-1))}}$$

$$S_{\alpha_1} = 0.23\sqrt{(3-1)F_{0.05(2;6)}} = 0.23\sqrt{2(5.14)} = 0.74$$

In this case, $S_{\alpha_1} = S_{\alpha_2} = S_{\alpha_3} = 0.74$.
Decision rule:
If $|C_i| > S_{\alpha_i}$, the H_0 hypothesis is rejected at α.

$|C_1| = 0.45 < 0.74$; can not reject H_0 : ($\mu_1 = \mu_2$) at $\alpha = 0.05$

$|C_2| = 0.31 < 0.74$; can not reject H_0 : ($\mu_1 = \mu_3$) at $\alpha = 0.05$

$|C_3| = 0.14 < 0.74$; can not reject H_0 : ($\mu_2 = \mu_3$) at $\alpha = 0.05$

B. Factor $B_{(A)}$

When factor $B_{(A)}$ is random, the multiple contrast procedures are generally not used, for they are meaningless. However, evaluating the ranges, as done in the Bonferroni example, is often useful [26]. But suppose $B_{(A)}$ is fixed. The hypothesis tests of B groups within factor A can be used for determining the groups contributing to the greatest variability. For example, looking at Table 7, we saw that the factor B group lots within suppliers were not significantly different in growth support when decomposed into individual lots within each supplier. The $B_{(A3)}$ was the largest mean square value, however (Table 7). Suppose $B_{(A3)}$ was significant (i.e., F_C for $B_{A_3} > F_{T(B_{A_3})}$). Then the question would be: Which lot means were significantly different from one another within that supplier (supplier C)?

If the variability within the lots of supplier C is excessive, which lots are they? Which lots significantly vary from one another? If it is variability that is key, then the range evaluation used in the Bonferroni discussion could be performed. However, if *mean* variability has any meaning, that is, lot-to-lot mean values, the following comparison can be performed.

Supplier C had the following total colony counts (from Example 1): 26.54, 26.15, and 29.64 for lots 1 through 3. The means for these lots (division by 5) are 5.31, 5.23, and 5.93, respectively. The researcher then can proceed to compare lots 1, 2, and 3, or L1 vs. L2, L2 vs. L3, and L1 vs. L3.

$$H_0: \mu_{L1} = \mu_{L2}; \qquad \bar{y}_{3(1)} - \bar{y}_{3(2)} = C_1$$

$$H_0: \mu_{L2} = \mu_{L3}; \qquad \bar{y}_{3(2)} - \bar{y}_{3(3)} = C_2$$

$$H_0: \mu_{L1} = \mu_{L3}; \qquad \bar{y}_{3(1)} - \bar{y}_{3(3)} = C_3$$

$$S_{\alpha_{(j)}} = S_{c_j}\sqrt{(b-1)}; \; F_{\alpha(b-1;ab(n-1))}$$

$$S_{c_j} = \sqrt{MS_E \sum \left(\frac{c_i^2}{n_i}\right)}$$

where a = number of suppliers
b = number of lots within suppliers
n = number of replicates of lots within suppliers

Decision rule: If $|C_i| > S_{\alpha_j}$, reject H_0.

$$S_{c_j} = \sqrt{MS_E \sum \left(\frac{C^2}{n} \right)} = \sqrt{0.22 \left(\frac{1^2 + (-1)^2}{5} \right)} = 0.30$$

$$C_1 = |\bar{y}_{3(1)} - \bar{y}_{3(2)}| = |5.31 - 5.23| = 0.08$$

$$C_2 = |\bar{y}_{3(2)} - \bar{y}_{3(3)}| = |5.23 - 5.93| = 0.70$$

$$C_3 = |\bar{y}_{3(1)} - \bar{y}_{3(3)}| = |5.31 - 5.93| = 0.62$$

Because all three contrasts are the same, $S_{c_j} = 0.30$.
For $\alpha = 0.05$,

$$S_{\alpha_j} = S_{c_j}\sqrt{(b-1)F_{0.05(b-1;ab(n-1))}} = S_{c_j}\sqrt{(3-1)F_{0.05(2;3\cdot3(5-1))}}$$

$$= 0.30\sqrt{2F_{0.05(2;36)}}$$

$$S_{\alpha_j} = 0.30\sqrt{2(3.32)} = 0.30(2.58) = 0.77$$

If $|C_j| > 0.77$, reject H_0.

Because we know that none of the $|C_j|$ values is larger than 0.77, there is no reason to continue with the contrast procedure. But this example demonstrates just how one would do this if they were. In this case, if C_2 (lot 2 vs. lot 3) had been significant, we could look in the batch records as well as calibration/validation records to see what happened or simply report this to the supplier.

IV. LEAST SIGNIFICANT DIFFERENCE (LSD)

The least significant difference contrasts can also be used. The general procedure is the same as we have encountered over the previous chapters, and, like all other contrasts, it is not used unless F_C is significant.

A. Factor A

The LSD method is used to compare each possible combination of mean pairs. But note that use of the LSD contrast procedure is recommended against by a number of statisticians [34]. The test, for balanced designs where the sample size, n, values are equal, is:

$$\text{LSD} = t_{\alpha/2(\text{df denominator})} \sqrt{\frac{2(\text{MS}_{\text{denominator}})}{bn}}^{*}$$

The test is:

If $|\bar{y}_{i..} - \bar{y}_{j..}| > \text{LSD}$, reject H_0 at α

Let us compare all possible $[a(a-1)]/2 = (3 \cdot 2)/2 = 3$ combinations of factor A means.

$\bar{y}_{1..} = 5.18$

$\bar{y}_{2..} = 5.63$

$\bar{y}_{3..} = 5.49$

Set α at 0.05

$$\text{LSD} = t_{0.05/2;\ (a(b-1))} \sqrt{\frac{2(\text{MS}_{B(A)})}{bn}}$$

$$\text{LSD} = t_{0.025;6} \sqrt{\frac{2(0.44)}{3 \cdot 5}} = 2.447\sqrt{0.06} = 0.59$$

The three possible combinations of LSD are:

$|\bar{y}_{1..} - \bar{y}_{2..}| = |5.18 - 5.63| = 0.45 \not> 0.59$ Not significant

$|\bar{y}_{1..} - \bar{y}_{3..}| = |5.18 - 5.49| = 0.31 \not> 0.59$ Not significant

$|\bar{y}_{2..} - \bar{y}_{3..}| = |5.63 - 5.49| = 0.14 \not> 0.59$ Not significant

Hence, as before, none of the suppliers is different from any of the others at $\alpha = 0.05$. Again, this test was performed only as a demonstration and would be used only if F_C for factor A was significant.

B. Factor $B_{(A)}$

As with examples demonstrated earlier, when $B_{(A)}$ is random, which it often is, the individual mean tests are pretty much without value. The proper

---

*Again, the denominator used depends upon whether the factors are fixed or random (see Table 2). In this example, recall that factor A is fixed and factor $B_{(A)}$ is random. So F_C for factor A is $\text{MS}_A/\text{MS}_{B(A)}$. $\text{MS}_{B(A)}$ is the denominator in this case, which corresponds to $a(b-1)$ degrees of freedom.

interpretation of a significant F_C for $B_{(A)}$, when random, is that the groups $[B_{(A)}]$ do not have the same variance.

However, if $B_{(A)}$ is fixed, a test can be used to compare means. And, if $B_{(A)}$ is significant, the strategy is to perform F_C tests on the individual $B_{(A)}$ groups. The groups that are significantly different can then be compared with the LSD test.

Using our example, suppose that as in the Scheffe example, $B_{(A3)}$ was fixed and was significant in the F_C calculations, as presented in Table 7. Hence, the researcher knows that suppliers (factor A) do not differ, but do the mean microbial counts per lot from suppliers differ significantly? If so, perhaps a quality assurance problem exists in interlot (lot-to-lot) variability.

Now, if interlot variability makes sense only on the basis of the range, or variance, the range evaluation discussed in the Bonferroni section would be more useful. But suppose comparisons of growth characteristics in terms of the mean makes intuitive sense. And suppose $B_{(A3)}$ is significantly different, that is, $F_C > F_T$. The $\log_{10}$ sum totals and means for the three lots are:

$\text{Lot}_1 = 26.54$, with a mean of $26.54/5 = 5.31$
$\text{Lot}_2 = 26.15$, with a mean of $26.15/5 = 5.23$
$\text{Lot}_3 = 29.64$, with a mean of $29.64/5 = 5.93$

The researcher then compares all $[b(b-1)]/2 = 3$ combinations. The LSD value is:

$$t_{\alpha/2;(ab[n-1])}\sqrt{\frac{2\text{MS}_E}{n}}, \qquad \text{where MS}_E = 0.22 \text{ (Table 7)}.$$

If $|\bar{y}_{ij.} - \bar{y}_{ji.}| > \text{LSD}$, reject H_0 at α.

$$\text{LSD} = t_{(0.05/2; ab(n-1))}\sqrt{\frac{2\text{MS}_E}{n}}$$

$$= t_{(0.025;36)}\sqrt{\frac{2(0.22)}{5}} = 2.042(0.30) = 0.61$$

The three lot-to-lot combinations:

$c_1 = |\bar{y}_{31.} - \bar{y}_{32.}| = |5.31 - 5.23| = 0.08 \not> 0.61 \qquad$ Not significant

$c_2 = |\bar{y}_{31.} - \bar{y}_{33.}| = |5.31 - 5.93| = 0.62 > 0.61 \qquad$ Significant

$c_3 = |\bar{y}_{32.} - \bar{y}_{33.}| = |5.23 - 5.93| = 0.70 > 0.61 \qquad$ Significant

Notice that for this test, contrasts c_2 and c_3 are significantly different when the F_C value was not. This may reflect why there are recommendations against the LSD test. This does not usually occur, particularly because the LSD method tends to lack power as the number of contrasts increases. The researcher had already concluded that no significant difference exists at $\alpha = 0.05$ but if the F_C had been significant, the researcher would have noted that the mean variability among the lots provided by supplier C was excessive.

V. DUNCAN'S MULTIPLE RANGE TEST

Duncan's multiple range test is another that can be used to evaluate nested designs. As before, the test, however, is performed only if the F_C value is significant and if the factor evaluated is fixed effects.

A. Factor *A*

For demonstration purposes, we will evaluate factor A, despite the nonsignificant F_C. The goal is to determine whether any factor levels (suppliers) are significantly different from the others.

For a balanced design, the test formula is:

$$S_{\bar{y}_{i..}} = \sqrt{\frac{MS_{\text{denominator}}}{bn}}$$

where MS denominator for this example (factor A fixed, factor $B_{(A)}$ random) from Table 2 is $MS_{B(A)}$, which is 0.44 (Table 7 in this chapter).

Recall from LSD testing that $\bar{y}_{1..} = 5.18, \bar{y}_{2..} = 5.63,$ and $\bar{y}_{3..} = 5.49.$

$$S_{\bar{y}_{i..}} = \sqrt{\frac{0.44}{3 \cdot 5}} = 0.17$$

For Duncan's multiple range test, one obtains the critical values $[r_{\alpha(p,f)}]$ for $p = 2, \ldots, a$ (Appendix, Table E). Let $\alpha = 0.05$ and $f =$ degrees of freedom for MS denominator $= a(b-1) = 6$. The set of $a - 1$ least significant ranges, as before, is calculated for $p = 2, 3, \ldots, a$.

The least significant range calculation is:

$$R_p = r_{\alpha(p,f)} S_{\bar{y}_{i..}}$$

The observed differences between the means are then determined, beginning with contrasting the largest and the smallest, and comparing the result with R_p at a. Next, the largest is contrasted to the second smallest and the result compared with the R_p at $(a - 1)$. This process is continued until all of the $[a(a-1)]/2$ combinations have been compared. If an observed pair difference is greater than the R_p value, the pairs are considered significantly different from each other at α.

$$R_2 = r_{(0.05)(2,6)_{0.17}} \qquad R_3 = r_{(0.05)(3,6)_{0.17}}$$
$$= 3.46(0.17) \qquad\qquad = 3.58(0.17)$$
$$= 0.59 \qquad\qquad\quad = 0.61$$

The means are written in ascending order, $\bar{y}_{1..} = 5.18$, $\bar{y}_{3..} = 5.49$, and $\bar{y}_{2..} = 5.63$, .. and the smallest is subtracted from the largest, etc. The differences for the three contrasts are compared with the R_p values, as follows.

2 vs. 1	$5.63 - 5.18 = 0.45 < 0.61$	(R_3)
2 vs. 3	$5.63 - 5.49 = 0.14 < 0.59$	(R_2)
3 vs. 1	$5.49 - 5.18 = 0.31 < 0.59$	(R_2)

Notice that none of the factor A suppliers are significantly different at $\alpha = 0.05$, the result that was expected.

B. Factor $B_{(A)}$

The same process presented concerning factor A is relevant for testing $B_{(A)}$, using Duncan's multiple range test. Random effects for $B_{(A)}$ are not individually evaluated because the experimenter is concerned with variances, not means. However, as before, if F_C is significant, as presented in Table 7, the researcher can ascertain the individual levels of $B_{(A)}$ that are significantly different from one another if the $B_{(A)}$ factor is fixed. The range comparison could also be used, as in the Bonferroni procedure, to get an idea of what is going on in terms of variability [26,27].

Example cont. Assume, for demonstration purposes, that the appraisal of the population growth characteristic through the mean makes sense and that factor $B_{(A)}$, a fixed factor, was significant. Partitioning (Table 7) further showed that $B_{(A3)}$ was significantly different, that is, $F_C > F_T$. The researcher could then use the Duncan's multiple range test to evaluate the individual lots within a supplier.

$$S_{\bar{y}_{B_{(A)}}} = \sqrt{\frac{MS_E}{n}}, \qquad \text{where } MS_E = 0.22 \text{ (Table 7)}$$

Recall from the LSD testing that the means for supplier C were lot 1 = 5.31, lot 2 = 5.23, and lot 3 = 5.93

$$S_{\bar{y}_{B_{(A)}}} = \sqrt{\frac{0.22}{5}} = 0.21$$

From Duncan's multiple range test (Appendix, Table E), one can obtain the critical values of $r_{\alpha(p,f)}$ for $p = 2, 3, \ldots, b$. Let $\alpha = 0.05$ and $f =$ degrees of freedom for $MS_E = ab(n - 1) = 36$.

The least significant range calculation is:

$$r_{\alpha(p,f)}S_{\bar{y}_{j(i)}} \qquad \text{for } p = 2, 3, \ldots, b$$

The observed differences between the means are then evaluated, beginning with the largest versus the smallest, and the difference is compared with R_b. Next, the largest is compared with the second smallest and the result compared with $R_{(b-1)}$. This process is continued until all of the $[b(b-1)]/2$ combinations have been compared. If an observed pair difference is greater than the R_p value, the pair is considered significantly different at α.

As before, the two R_p values are computed:

$$R_2 = r_{(0.05)(2,36)}(0.21) \qquad R_3 = r_{(0.05)(3,36)}(0.21)$$

$$R_2 = 2.89(0.21) \qquad\qquad R_3 = 3.04(0.21)$$

$$R_2 = 0.61 \qquad\qquad\qquad R_3 = 0.64$$

The means are written in ascending order, $\bar{y}_{3(2)} = 5.23$, $\bar{y}_{3(1)} = 5.31$, $\bar{y}_{3(3)} = 5.93$, and the mean differences are then compared with the R_p values:

3 vs. 2	$5.93 - 5.23 = 0.70 > 0.64 \ (R_3)$
3 vs. 1	$5.93 - 5.31 = 0.62 > 0.61 \ (R_2)$
1 vs. 2	$5.31 - 5.23 = 0.08 < 0.61 \ (R_2)$

Notice that two of the individual contrasts are significantly different even though the F_C for $B_{(A)}$ was not. In this case, one would ignore the individual contrasts and consider the F_C not being significant for factor $B_{(A)}$ at $\alpha = 0.05$.

Often, Duncan's multiple range test is excessively conservative. But in this case, because MS_E was a relatively small value, had a large number of degrees of freedom [33,35], and only three contrasts were performed, it was "overly" sensitive. In other words, because factor $B_{(A)}$ was not significant at $\alpha = 0.05$, the individual contrasts were not "practically" significant.

VI. NEWMAN–KEULS TEST

The application of this contrast test is very much as described in previous chapters. The test can be conducted on both factors A and $B_{(A)}$ for all possible pairwise contrasts. The contrasts should not be made, however, if F_C (for factor A or factor $B_{(A)}$) is not significant.

A. Factor A

As before, the formula is $K_p = q_{\alpha(p,f)}S_{\bar{y}_{i..}}$ for $p = 2, 3, \ldots, a$, and $f =$ degrees of freedom for denominator

$$S_{\bar{y}_{i.}} = \sqrt{\frac{MS_{denominator}}{bn}}$$

In our example, factor A is fixed and $B_{(A)}$ is random. So, as before (Table 2), we note that the denominator is $MS_{B(A)}$ ($= 0.44$, from Table 7).

$$S_{\bar{y}_{i.}} = \sqrt{\frac{MS_{B(A)}}{3 \cdot 5}} = \sqrt{\frac{0.44}{15}} = 0.17$$

The three factor A means are $\bar{y}_{1..} = 5.18, \bar{y}_{2..} = 5.63,$ and $\bar{y}_{3..} = 5.49$.

For this example, $p = 2, 3,$ and $\alpha = 0.05$ with df $= f = a(b-1) = 6$.

From the Studentized range table, the q values are found (Table A.12).

$$q_{0.05(2,6)} = 3.46$$

$$q_{0.05(3,6)} = 4.34$$

The K values are computed, multiplying the q values and the $S_{\bar{y}}$ values.

$$K_p = q_{\alpha(p,f)} S_{\bar{y}_{..}}$$

$$K_2 = 3.46(0.17) = 0.59$$

$$K_3 = 4.34(0.17) = 0.74$$

The factor A means are ordered in ascending order $\bar{y}_{1..} = 5.18, \bar{y}_{3..} = 5.49,$ and $\bar{y}_{2..} = 5.63$.

The comparison procedure used in Duncan's multiple range test is also used here.

2 vs. 1	$5.63 - 5.18 = 0.45 < 0.74$	(K_3)
2 vs. 3	$5.63 - 5.49 = 0.14 < 0.59$	(K_2)
3 vs. 1	$5.49 - 5.18 = 0.31 < 0.59$	(K_2)

Hence, for the Newman–Keuls test, none of these contrasts are significant at $\alpha = 0.05$, which is as expected.

B. Factor $B_{(A)}$

Factor $B_{(A)}$ contrasts are performed in nearly the same fashion as those for factor A. However, random effects for $B_{(A)}$ are usually not pairwise compared because the experimenter is concerned not with mean variation but with variability. When $B_{(A)}$ is fixed, however, and if F_C is significant, the researcher can partition factor $B_{(A)}$ into individual $B_{j(i)}$ components to discover which ones are significant. And, too, range comparisons can be conducted, as in the Bonferroni example, to get an idea of what is going on.

As before, the Newman–Keuls test assumes that it makes sense to evaluate the mean differences in our example (assuming the factor is fixed) and that supplier C is significantly different, $F_C > F_T$. The researcher then uses the Newman-Keuls test to evaluate the lots within supplier C.

The formula is $K_p = q_{\alpha(p,f)}S_{\bar{y}_{j(i)}}$, for $p = 2, 3, \ldots, b$, where $MS_E = 0.22$ (Table 7), and $f =$ degrees of freedom for $MS_E = ab(n-1) = 36$.

$$S_{\bar{y}_{j(i)}} = \sqrt{\frac{MS_E}{n}} = \sqrt{\frac{0.22}{5}} = 0.21$$

The three lot means for supplier C are ordered in ascending order, $\text{Lot}_1 = \bar{y}_{C(2)} = 5.23$, $\text{Lot}_2 = \bar{y}_{C(1)} = 5.31$, and $\text{Lot}_3 = \bar{y}_{C(3)} = 5.93\ldots$ and the q values are determined using Table A.1, Studentized range table.

$$q_{0.05(2,36)} = 2.89$$

$$q_{0.05(3,36)} = 3.48$$

The K_p values are then calculated.

$$K_p = q_{\alpha(p,f)}S_{\bar{y}_{j(i)}}$$
$$K_2 = 2.89(0.21) = 0.61$$
$$K_3 = 3.48(0.21) = 0.73$$

The same comparison procedure as used in Duncan's multiple range test is used here.

3 vs. 2	$5.93 - 5.23 = 0.70 < 0.73$	(R_3)
3 vs. 1	$5.93 - 5.31 = 0.62 > 0.61$	(R_2)
1 vs. 2	$5.31 - 5.23 = 0.08 < 0.61$	(R_2)

Again, this test comparison generally would not be used when neither $B_{(A)}$ nor any of the individuals $B_{j(i)}$ components were found to be significant in the ANOVA. So, although 3 vs. 1 is significant here, it is not practically so.

VII. TUKEY METHOD

The Tukey test for the nested design is, again, a straightforward means for investigating factors A and $B_{(A)}$. Before using it, the researcher will want to ensure that the F_C values are significant at the selected α level. For instructive purposes, we will assume that they are.

A. Factor A

The formula for the Tukey test is:

$$T_\alpha = q_{\alpha(a,f)}S_{\bar{y}_{i..}}$$

where $S_{\bar{y}_{i..}} = \sqrt{MS_{\text{denominator}}/bn}$, f = degrees of freedom, and a = number of treatments in factor A. All $[a(a-1)]/2$ factor A treatments are contrasted.

In our example, factor A is fixed and factor $B_{(A)}$ is random. So, as can be seen from Table 2, $MS_{B(A)}$ is the denominator, with $a(b-1)$ degrees of freedom. $q_{\alpha(a,f)} = q_{(0.05)(3,6)}$, which from the Studentized range table (Table A.1) = 4.34.

$$S_{\bar{y}_{i..}} = \sqrt{\frac{MS_{B(A)}}{bn}} = \sqrt{\frac{0.44}{3 \cdot 5}} = 0.17$$

$$T_\alpha = q_{0.05, (3,6)}(S_{\bar{y}_{i..}}) = 4.34(0.17) = 0.74$$

If $|\bar{y}_{i..} - \bar{y}_{j..}| > t_\alpha$, reject H_0 at α.

The largest and the smallest means, followed by the largest and second smallest means and the second largest and smallest means, are contrasted.

$$\text{2 vs. 1} \qquad |5.63 - 5.18| = 0.45 < 0.74$$

$$\text{2 vs. 3} \qquad |5.63 - 5.49| = 0.14 < 0.74$$

$$\text{3 vs. 1} \qquad |5.49 - 5.18| = 0.31 < 0.74$$

As expected, none of the three suppliers are different at α.

B. Factor $B_{(A)}$

Factor $B_{(A)}$ contrast procedures are also similar to those already conducted. Random effects for $B_{(A)}$ are usually not contrasted. However, if F_C for $B_{(A)}$ was significant and if it was a fixed-effects model, the individual $B_{j(i)}$ could be evaluated with the Tukey test.

Let us, for demonstration purposes, assume that F_C was significant for the lots nested in supplier C.

$$T_\alpha = q_{\alpha(b, f)}S_{\bar{y}_{j(i)}}$$

where $S_{\bar{y}_{j(i)}} = \sqrt{MS_E/n}$, $b = 3$, and $f = ab(n-1) = 36$.

All $[b(b-1)]/2$ contrasts within a specific and significant factor A are compared.

$q_{\alpha(b, ab[n-1])}$, and using Table A.1, $q_{0.05(3,36)} = 3.48$

$$S_{\bar{y}_{j(i)}} = \sqrt{\frac{MS_E}{n}} = \sqrt{\frac{0.22}{5}} = 0.21$$

$$t_\alpha = q_{\alpha(p,f)}S_{\bar{y}_{j(i)}} = 3.48(0.21) = 0.73$$

If $|\bar{y}_{k(i)} - \bar{y}_{k(j)}| > t_\alpha$, reject H_0 at α.

3 vs. 2 $|5.93 - 5.23| = 0.70 < 0.73$

3 vs. 1 $|5.93 - 5.31| = 0.62 < 0.73$

3 vs. 1 $|5.31 - 5.23| = 0.08 < 0.73$

None of the three contrasts is statistically significant at α. This is expected because F_C was not significant for factor B.

VIII. DUNNETT'S METHOD

Dunnett's method is used when a researcher is comparing multiple test products with a single control or reference product. In our example, if the researcher had compared the new suppliers with the standard supplier, Dunnett's method could be used, but she should note that the test would be limited to factor A because factor $B_{(A)}$ is concerned with the intrasupplier variability of a specific supplier. One of the other contrasts, such as Tukey's, LSD, or Scheffe's, could be used to evaluate intraconfiguration variability.

A. Factor A

Let us perform an exercise in comparing the "control," say supplier A, with the two test suppliers, B and C, using Dunnett's method, although, as before, if F_C for factor A is not significant, neither Dunnett's method nor any other contrast method would be applied. We perform the exercise here for demonstration purposes only. For Dunnett's method, factor A must always be fixed effects.

Here $\bar{y}_{1..} = \bar{y}_{c..}$ = control, $\bar{y}_{2..}$ and $\bar{y}_{3..}$ = test configurations, and $a = 3$, $b = 3$, $n = 5$, and $\alpha = 0.05$. There are $a - 1 = 2$ contrasts, $\bar{y}_{2..}$ and $\bar{y}_{3..}$, and each is compared with, $\bar{y}_{c..}$, the control, as $\bar{y}_{2..} - \bar{y}_{c..}$ and $\bar{y}_{3..} - \bar{y}_{c..}$.

The test hypotheses are $H_0: \mu_{i..} = \mu_{control}$ and $H_A: \mu_{i..} \neq \mu_{control}$.

Decision Rule:

If

$$| \bar{y}_{i..} - \bar{y}_{c..} | > d_{\alpha(a-1, f)} \sqrt{\frac{2MS_{denominator}}{bn}}, \qquad \text{reject } H_0 \text{ at } \alpha$$

Because factor A is fixed and factor $B_{(A)}$ is random, from Table 2, we see that $MS_{B(A)}$ is the denominator, with $a(b-1) = 6$ degrees of freedom $= f$, and from Dunnett's table (Appendix, Table A.13), $d_{(a-1, f)} = d_{0.05\,(2, 6)} = 2.86$.

$$\sqrt{\frac{2MS_{B(A)}}{bn}} = \sqrt{\frac{2(0.44)}{3 \cdot 5}} = 0.24$$

so

$$d_{\alpha,(a-1,f)}\sqrt{\frac{2MS_{B(A)}}{bn}} = 2.86(0.24) = 0.69$$

$$|\bar{y}_{2..} - \bar{y}_{c..}| = |5.23 - 5.31| = 0.08 < 0.69 \qquad \text{Not significant}$$

$$|\bar{y}_{3..} - \bar{y}_{c..}| = |5.93 - 5.31| = 0.62 < 0.69 \qquad \text{Not significant}$$

The conclusion reached, then, is that the test configurations (suppliers B and C) are not significantly different from the control (supplier A) at $\alpha = 0.05$.

IX. NESTED DESIGNS BY MEANS OF A COMPUTER PROGRAM

The nested design can be generated with a software subroutine that allows nesting or a two-factor ANOVA with $A \times B$ interaction. When using a general linear model, for example, one would input the data as A (supplier) and B (lots within suppliers). Then one would merely add the B and $A \times B$ rows in the df column and B and $A \times B$ in the sum-of-squares column. Factor B plus the interaction of $A \times B$ is $B_{(A)}$ (Table 8).

Adding the degrees of freedom, $2 + 4 = 6$ for $B_{(A)}$, the sum of squares $B_{(A)}$ is $SS_B + SS_{A \times B} = 0.0670 + 2.5438 = 2.61$. The value for $MS_{B(A)}$ is $2.61/6 = 0.44$.

The residual values are determined by taking the fitted value, $\hat{y}_{ijk}$, and subtracting it from the actual value (y). For our purposes,

$$\hat{y}_{ijk} = \bar{y}_{ij.}$$

Recall that the $y_{ij.}$ values are the total values of each lot within suppliers (Table 4), and $\bar{y}_{ij.} = \sum(y_{ij.}/n)$. For example, $\bar{y}_{11.} = \hat{y}_{11.} = 26.94/5 \approx 5.39$ or 5.388 carried out three places to the right of the decimal point.

TABLE 8 Computerized ANOVA with $A \times B$ Interaction (Example 1 Data)

Source	DF	Seq SS	Adj SS	Adj MS	F	P
A	2	1.5916	1.5916	0.7958	3.58	.038
B	2	0.0670	0.0670	0.3335	0.15	.861
A × B	4	2.5438	2.5438	0.6360	2.86	.037
Error	36	7.9974	7.9974	0.2221		
Total	44	12.1998				

$B_{(A)}$ a spanning B, A × B rows; 6 and 2.61 spanning Seq SS for those rows.

[a]degrees of freedom for $B_{(A)} = 2 + 4 = 6$, $SS_{B(A)} = 0.0670 + 2.5438 = 2.61$, $MS_{B(A)} = 2.61 \div 6 = 0.44$.

Table 9 presents a code table of columns A and $B(A)$ as well as the actual values (y_{ijk}), the predicted values ($\hat{y}_{ijk}$), and the error (e_{ijk}).

Figure 5 provides a stem-and-leaf display of the residual values. They seem to approximate the requirements of a normal distribution.

Figure 6, a letter-value display of the residual values, appears to be normal. The midrange values are not consistently increasing or decreasing.

Figure 7 is a boxplot of the residuals. This, too, appears approximately normal.

Two other useful displays are plots of the residuals versus suppliers (Fig. 8) and residual versus predict values (Fig. 9). In both cases, these distributions appear normal.

X. VARIANCE COMPONENTS

Whenever the main factors (A or $B_{(A)}$ or both) fit a random-effects model, it is often useful to estimate the variance component. The variance component can be estimated for σ^2, $\sigma^2_{B(A)}$, and σ^2_A.

$$\sigma^2 = \text{the error term} = MS_E$$

$$\sigma^2_{B(A)} = \frac{MS_{B(A)} - MS_E}{n}$$

$$\sigma^2_A = \frac{MS_A - MS_{B(A)}}{bn}$$

In our example, $B_{(A)}$ is a random-effects component and A is fixed, a configuration commonly used in nested designs. We will estimate the variance for main factor $B_{(A)}$ using data from Table 7.

$$\sigma^2 = MS_E = 0.22$$

$$\sigma^2_{B(A)} = \frac{MS_{B(A)} - MS_E}{n} = \frac{0.44 - 0.22}{5} = 0.04$$

By the way, each level effect of factor A can be estimated using data from Table 4:

The formula is: $\bar{y}_{i..} - \bar{y}_{...}$ and $\bar{y}_{...} = \frac{244.51}{45} = 5.43$

$$\bar{y}_{1..} = \frac{y_{1..}}{15} = \frac{77.71}{15} = 5.18$$

$$\bar{y}_{2..} = \frac{y_{2..}}{15} = \frac{84.47}{15} = 5.63$$

$$\bar{y}_{3..} = \frac{y_{3..}}{15} = \frac{82.33}{15} = 5.49$$

TABLE 9 Code Table of Columns *A* and *B*

Row	A	$B_{(A)}$	y_{ijk}	$\hat{y}_{ijk}$	e_{ijk}
1	1	1	5.69	5.388	0.302000
2	1	1	4.79	5.388	−0.598000
3	1	1	5.23	5.388	−0.158000
4	1	1	5.51	5.388	0.122000
5	1	1	5.72	5.388	0.332000
6	1	2	4.38	5.356	−0.976000
7	1	2	6.21	5.356	0.854000
8	1	2	5.48	5.356	0.124000
9	1	2	5.92	5.356	0.564000
10	1	2	4.79	5.356	−0.566000
11	1	3	4.44	4.798	−0.358000
12	1	3	4.15	4.798	−0.648000
13	1	3	5.39	4.798	0.592000
14	1	3	5.29	4.798	0.492000
15	1	3	4.72	4.798	−0.078000
16	2	1	5.82	5.670	0.150000
17	2	1	5.97	5.670	0.300000
18	2	1	5.81	5.670	0.140000
19	2	1	5.32	5.670	−0.350000
20	2	1	5.43	5.670	−0.240000
21	2	2	5.32	5.552	−0.232000
22	2	2	6.21	5.552	0.658000
23	2	2	5.73	5.552	0.178000
24	2	2	4.91	5.552	−0.642000
25	2	2	5.59	5.552	0.038000
26	2	3	5.73	5.672	0.058000
27	2	3	5.81	5.672	0.138000
28	2	3	6.13	5.672	0.458000
29	2	3	5.13	5.672	−0.542000
30	2	3	5.56	5.672	−0.112000
31	3	1	5.36	5.308	0.052000
32	3	1	5.32	5.308	0.012000
33	3	1	4.79	5.308	−0.518000
34	3	1	5.15	5.308	−0.158000
35	3	1	5.92	5.308	0.612000
36	3	2	5.38	5.230	0.150000
37	3	2	4.29	5.230	−0.940000
38	3	2	5.71	5.230	0.480000
39	3	2	5.62	5.230	0.390000
40	3	2	5.15	5.230	−0.080000
41	3	3	6.01	5.928	0.082000

TABLE 9 Continued

Row	A	$B_{(A)}$	y_{ijk}	$\hat{y}_{ijk}$	e_{ijk}
42	3	3	6.23	5.928	0.302000
43	3	3	5.82	5.928	−0.108000
44	3	3	5.89	5.928	−0.038000
45	3	3	5.69	5.928	−0.238000

Hence

$$A_A = \bar{y}_{1..} - \bar{y}_{...} = 5.18 - 5.43 = -0.25$$
$$A_B = \bar{y}_{2..} - \bar{y}_{...} = 5.49 - 5.43 = 0.06$$
$$A_C = \bar{y}_{3..} - \bar{y}_{...} = 5.63 - 5.43 = 0.20$$

XI. POWER COMPUTATION FOR THE NESTED DESIGN

For nested designs, the power of the fixed portion of the test can be calculated before the analysis is performed. In our example, the fixed portion is the factor A effect.

Leaf Unit = 0.10

```
 2    -0 | 99
 4    -0 | 66
 8    -0 | 5555
12    -0 | 33222
20    -0 | 1111000
(12)   0 | 000001111111
13     0 | 33333
 8     0 | 44455
 2     0 | 66
 1     0 | 8
```

FIGURE 5 Stem-and-leaf display.

	DEPTH	LOWER	UPPER	MID	SPREAD
N=	45				
M	23.0		0.052	0.052	
H	12.0	-0.238	0.302	0.032	0.540
E	6.5	-0.554	0.486	-0.034	1.040
D	3.5	-0.645	0.602	-0.021	1.247
C	2.0	-0.940	0.658	-0.141	1.598
	1	-0.976	0.854	-0.061	1.830

FIGURE 6   Letter-value display.

A. Basic Formula for Power of the Test (Performed Before Conducting the Test)

The basic formula for calculation of the power of the test is:

$$\phi = \sqrt{\frac{n' \sum_{m=1}^{k'} (\mu_m - \mu)^2}{k' S^2}}$$

where   grand population mean $= \mu = \dfrac{\sum_{m=1}^{k'} \mu_m}{k'}$ and $\mu_m =$ factor mean m

$k' = a$, or ab for factor $B_{(A)}$ when fixed
$n' = bn$, if factor A, or n, if factor $B_{(A)}$
$s^2 = $ MS denominator for factor A or MS_E for $B_{(A)}$

These values would generally not be known, but would to be estimated on the basis of historical data.

1. Factor A

Using data from Table 6, the power calculation for factor A is as follows.

$k' = a = 3$
$n' = bn = 3 \times 5 = 15$
$v_1 = k'-1 = a-1 = 2 = $ df numerator
$v_2 = $ df denominator $= 6$

   [denominator is $MS_{B(A)}$ with $a(b - 1)$ degrees of freedom]

$$\mu = \frac{\sum_{m=1}^{a} \mu_m}{3} = \frac{1}{3}(5.18 + 5.63 + 5.49) = 5.43$$

```
                              -------------------
-----------------------------I  (    +  )  I -----------------------
                              -------------------
 -+------------+-------------+------------+------------+------------
 -1.05       -0.70       -0.35        0.00        0.35        0.70
```

FIGURE 7   Character box plot.

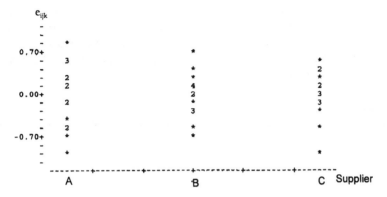

FIGURE 8 Residual values versus suppliers.

(In reality, the valuer would not be known but estimated from previous experience).

where $s^2 = \text{MS}_{\text{denominator}} = \text{MS}_{B(A)} = 0.44$

$$\phi = \sqrt{\frac{bn \sum (\mu_m - \mu)^2}{a \cdot s^2}}$$

$$= \sqrt{\frac{3.5[(5.18 - 5.43)^2 + (5.63 - 5.43)^2 + (5.49 - 5.43)^2]}{3(0.44)}} = 1.10$$

From the power table, Table A.4, read the $\alpha = 0.05$ table where $v_1 = 2$, $v_2 = 6$, and $\phi = 1.10$. We note that $1 - \beta \approx 0.25$.

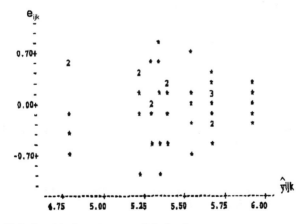

FIGURE 9 Plot of residuals versus predicted values.

Hence, from this experiment, the researcher has about a 75% chance of committing a type II error (stating that H_0 is true when it is actually false), that is, concluding that the suppliers are the same when they really are not. To differentiate them with greater confidence, the researcher will be wise to select a larger sample size.

2. Factor $B_{(A)}$

If factor $B_{(A)}$ was fixed, the power of the test could also be estimated, where

$$k' = ab = (3)(3) = 9$$
$$n' = n = 5$$
$$v_1 = b - 1 = 3 - 1 = 2$$
$$v_2 = df\, MS_E = 36$$
$$\alpha = 0.05$$

$$\mu = \frac{\sum_{m=1}^{ab} \mu_m}{ab} = \frac{5.39 + 5.36 + 4.80 + 5.67 + 5.55 + 5.67 + 5.31 + 5.23 + 5.93}{9}$$
$$= 5.43$$

(Again, in practice, these values would not be known, but estimated from previous experiments)

Where $s^2 = MS_{\text{denominator}} = MS_E = 0.22$,

$$\phi = \sqrt{\frac{n \sum_{m=1}^{ab} (\mu_m - \mu)^2}{ab(s^2)}}$$

$$\phi = \sqrt{\frac{\begin{array}{c} 5[(5.39 - 5.43)^2 + (5.36 - 5.43)^2 + (4.80 - 5.43)^2 + (5.67 - 5.43)^2 \\ + (5.55 - 5.43)^2 + (5.67 - 5.43)^2 + (5.31 - 5.43)^2 \\ + (5.23 - 5.43)^2 + (5.93 - 5.43)^2] \end{array}}{9(0.22)}}$$

$$\phi = 1.45$$

and from Table A.4, $1 - \beta \approx 0.76$.

Hence, the researcher will fail to reject H_0 when H_0 is false 24 times out of 100. Again, the solution to this is to increase lot samples.

B. Alternative Method for Determining Power of the Test Before Conducting the Test

Recall that ϕ can also be computed for fixed-effects components using the following formula:

$$\phi = \sqrt{\frac{n'\delta^2}{2k'S^2}}$$

where $n' = bn$ if A and n if B
$k' = a$ if A and b if B
$s^2 = $ MS denominator
$\delta = $ specific numerical difference one wishes to detect

1. Factor A (Using Data from Table 6)

$n' = 3 \times 5 = 15$
$k' = a = 3$
$s^2 = $ MS denominator, which is $MS_{B(A)} = 0.44$. This normally would not be known and would need to be estimated.
$\delta = $ set arbitrarily at 0.5 $\log_{10}$ scale

$$\phi = \sqrt{\frac{15(0.5)^2}{2(3)(0.44)}} = 1.19$$

Entering the power table, Table A.4, at $\alpha = 0.05$, $v_1 = a - 1 = 2$, $v_2 = $ degrees of freedom, $MS_{B(A)} = a(b-1) = 6$, we find that $1 - \beta = 0.20$. Hence, there is about a 4-in-5 chance of failing to reject a false null hypothesis. The investigator will want to increase the sample size.

2. Factor $B_{(A)}$

Factor $B_{(A)}$ would not be evaluated because it is a random-effects component. But supposing it was fixed effects, then:

$n' = n = 5$
$k' = b = 3$
$s^2 = MS_E = 0.22$ (This normally would not be known, but would be estimated.)
$\delta = $ set arbitrarily at 0.5 $\log_{10}$ scale

$$\phi = \sqrt{\frac{n'\delta^2}{2k's^2}} = \sqrt{\frac{5(0.5)^2}{2(3)(0.22)}} = 0.97$$

Entering the power table, Table A.4, at $\alpha = 0.05$, $v_1 = k - 1 = 3 - 1 = 2$, and $v_2 = $ df $MS_E = 36$, the value of $\beta \approx 0.75$ and $1 - \beta \approx 0.25$. There is approximately a three-out-of-four chance of failing to reject a false H_0 hypothesis. The sample size should be increased.

XII. POWER OF TEST DETERMINED AFTER EXPERIMENT HAS BEEN CONDUCTED

Once again, the power of the statistic is computed only for fixed effects. The general formula is:

$$\phi = \sqrt{\frac{(k')(\text{numerator MS}) - (\text{denominator MS})}{k'(\text{denominator MS})}}$$

1. Factor A (Using Data from Table 6)

Here $k' = a - 1 = 3 - 1 = 2$, MS numerator $= MS_A = 0.80$, and MS denominator $= MS_{B(A)}$ for this mixed model example $= 0.44$.

For $\alpha = 0.05$, $v_1 = k'$ degrees of freedom $= a - 1 = 3 - 1 = 2$ df, and $v_2 =$ denominator df; for this mixed model, the degrees of freedom $= a(b-1) = 3 \times 2 = 6$,

$$\phi = \sqrt{\frac{2(0.80 - 0.44)}{6(0.44)}} = 0.52$$

From the power table, Table A.4, at $\alpha = 0.05$, $v_1 = 2$ and $v_2 = 6$, the power of the statistic, $(1 - \beta) < 0.20$. Again, the investigator would want to increase the sample sizes, for there will be a four-in-five occurrence of failing to reject a false H_0 hypothesis. For this example, where the study is a validation study, it is critical that the power of the statistic be increased because with the model as is, the suppliers are likely to be considered equivalent when they are not.

2. Factor $B_{(A)}$

If factor $B_{(A)}$ was fixed effects, the calculation would be equally straight forward.

$$\phi = \sqrt{\frac{(k')(MS_{B(A)} - S^2)}{k'S^2}} = \sqrt{\frac{(b - 1)(MS_{B(A)} - MS_E)}{(b - 1)MS_E}}$$

The degrees of freedom for a specific α are:

$v_1 = b - 1$

$v_2 = ab(n - 1)$, the degrees of freedom for MS_E

XIII. SAMPLE SIZE REQUIREMENTS

Prior to conducting a study or experiment, such as the example we have been using, one should calculate whether the sample size is adequate to detect a statistical difference, given that one is present. In order to do this, the researcher must:

1. Select a desired statistical power $(1 - \beta)$.
2. Specify an α level (significance level).
3. Specify an estimated error term (σ^2) that is representative of the actual σ^2.
4. Specify a minimum detectable difference.

As we demonstrated in earlier chapters, this process is iterative, and generally the process is applied to the most important effect, which is factor A in Example 1. In addition, if the investigator suspects greater variability than she estimates, it would be wise to inflate the error term (denominator) so that one has a safety margin built into the statistic. This is particularly true when it is important for a study, such as our example, to show a difference between factors if one exists. In our example, an investigator is interested in "validating" alternative media suppliers. However, as we have shown, there was so little power in the statistic due to low sample size that it would have been very difficult to detect a true difference in the suppliers unless the difference was huge.

Calculation of sample size requirements is limited to fixed-effects components, using the formula:

$$\phi = \sqrt{\frac{n'\delta^2}{2k'S^2}}$$

where $n' = bn$, if factor A, and n, if factor $B_{(A)}$
$k' = a$, if factor A, and b, if factor B
$s^2 = $ estimate of σ^2
$v_1 = (a-1)$ degrees of freedom, factor A, and $(b-1)$ degrees of freedom, factor B
$v_2 = $ degrees of freedom denominator
δ = minimum desired detection limit between means in the factor being evaluated

1. Factor A (Using Data from Table 6)

Assume $\delta = 0.5 \log_{10}$ scale. Rewriting the formula:

$$\phi = \sqrt{\frac{bn\delta^2}{2as^2}}$$

let us estimate s^2 as 0.44 (which it really is), and set $\alpha = 0.05$ and $1-\beta = 0.80$. Let us begin with $n = 5$.

$$\phi = \sqrt{\frac{(3 \cdot 5)(0.5)^2}{2 \cdot 3(0.44)}} = 1.19$$

Looking at Table D (Appendix), for $v_1 = a-1 = 3-1 = 2$ and $v_2 = a(b-1) = 3 \times 2 = 6$, we see this is far too low, for $1 - \beta \sim 0.30$, so we increase the sample size to $n = 10$.

$$\phi = \sqrt{\frac{(3 \cdot 10)(0.5)^2}{2 \cdot 3(0.44)}} = 1.69$$

For $v_1 = 2$, and $v_2 = a(b-1) = 6, 1-\beta \sim 0.45$ is still too low, so we increase the sample size to, say, 15.

$$\phi = \sqrt{\frac{(3 \cdot 15)(0.5)^2}{2 \cdot 3(0.44)}} = 2.06$$

$1-\beta \approx 0.68$, which is too small. The researcher would continue testing larger sample sizes until $1-\beta \approx 0.80$.

2. Factor $B_{(A)}$

With respect to detecting intralot variation, there are times the researcher may want to evaluate $B_{(A)}$, given that it is a fixed-effects model. Suppose, in our model, it is. Then:

$$\phi = \sqrt{\frac{n\delta^2}{2(b)s^2}} = \sqrt{\frac{n(0.5)^2}{2(3)(0.22)}}$$

and $v_1 = b-1, v_2 = ab(n-1)$.

Suppose the researcher begins the sample estimate with $n = 15$. Suppose also that she estimates s^2 as 0.22 (which it was, from Table 6).

$$\phi = \sqrt{\frac{15(0.5)^2}{2(3)(0.22)}} = 1.69$$

For $v_1 = 2$ and $v_2 = ab(n-1) = 3 \times 3(14) = 126, 1-\beta = 0.74$, which is low. So, we increase, say, to $n = 20$

$$\phi = \sqrt{\frac{(20)(0.5)^2}{2(3)(0.22)}} = 1.95$$

For $v_1 = 2$, and $v_2 = ab(n-1) = 3 \times 3(19) = 171, 1-\beta = 0.88$. The researcher can now cut back the sample size to approximate $1-\beta = 0.80$.

XIV. MINIMUM DETECTABLE DIFFERENCE

Many times it is useful to determine the minimum detectable difference of a statistic before or after the test has been conducted. As discussed in earlier chapters, the minimum detectable difference informs the researcher about the numerical difference between means that can be detected using this nested design, at a specified α, β, sample size, and σ_2. Both factors A and $B_{(A)}$ can be evaluated, given that each is a fixed-effects model. The formula for this test is:

$$\delta = \sqrt{\frac{2ks^2\phi^2}{n'}}$$

where $k' = a$, if A, and b, if $B_{(A)}$
   $n' = bn$, if A, and n, if $B_{(A)}$
   $s^2 =$ for factor A: MS_E, if $MS_{B(A)}$ is fixed; $MS_{B(A)}$, if $MS_{B(A)}$ is random
        for factor B: MS_E, but only if factor $B_{(A)}$ is fixed
   $\phi =$ can be determined by reading it from Table A.4 (Power Table) at a specified α, v_1, v_2, and β, or by using the value previously computed when determining the power of the statistic.

1. Factor A

   $k' = a = 3$
   $s^2 =$ estimated variance or actual variance. When actual, use $MS_{B(A)}$ because factor A is fixed and factor $B_{(A)}$ is random. Factor $B_{(A)}$ is the denominator term used in calculating F_C for factor A (i.e., $F_C = MS_A/MS_{B(A)}$).
   $v_1 = a - 1 = 3 - 1 = 2$
   $v_2 = a(b - 1)$, which is the denominator term degrees of freedom $3(3 - 1) = 6$

   First, find v_2 in Table D corresponding to $\alpha = 0.05$, v_1, $1 - \beta$, and read ϕ. So $v_1 = 2$, $v_2 = 6$, $\alpha = 0.05$, and $\phi \approx 2.35$. Then calculate the δ formula:

$$\delta = \sqrt{\frac{2(3)(0.44)(2.35)^2}{3 \cdot 5}} = 0.99$$

   That is, with a replicate size of five for each of the three lots per supplier, the investigator can detect only 1 $\log_{10}$ difference. The researcher will need to increase the sample size, n, if she wants to get a $\delta = 0.5$.

2. Factor $B_{(A)}$

This procedure is done in the same way for $B_{(A)}$, given it is a fixed effect. Let us assume that it is for the moment.

$k' = b = 3$

s^2 = estimated MS_E or, if done after the experiment has been conducted, MS_E. We will use the actual $MS_E = 0.22$.

$v_1 = b - 1 = 3 - 1 = 2$

$v_2 = ab(n - 1) = 3 \times 3(4) = 36$

$\alpha = 0.05$

β = set at 0.20, so $1 - \beta = 0.80$

First, find v_1, v_2, α, and $1 - \beta$ in Table A.4 and read ϕ. So, for $v_1 = 2, v_2 = 36, \alpha = 0.05, 1 - \beta = 0.80, s^2 = 0.22$, the value of $\phi \approx 1.85$.

$$\delta = \sqrt{\frac{2k's^2\phi^2}{n'}} = \sqrt{\frac{2(3)(0.22)(1.85)^2}{5}} = 0.95$$

With the current statistic, the desired δ of $0.5 \log_{10}$ scale is grossly underestimated. The researcher, in reality, can get only a one log detection limit.

With the information from this chapter, the applied researcher is in an empowered position, for there are now many ways to design his or her research studies. Although we will not be evaluating more complex nested designs, the basic principles remain the same. The only major concepts remaining to be evaluated are regression analysis and nonparametrics equivalent to parametrics.

11

Linear Regression

Regression analyses are tools essential to the applied researcher in many instances. Regression is a statistical methodology that uses the relationship between two or more quantitative variables such that the value of one variable can be predicted based on the value(s) of the other(s) [25]. Determining the relationship between two variables, such as exposure time and lethality or wash time and $\log_{10}$ microbial reductions, is very common in applied research. From a mathematical perspective, two relationships are worth discussing: (1) a functional relationship and (2) a statistical relationship.

Recall from college algebra that a functional relationship has the form:

$$y = f(x)$$

where y is the resultant value, on the function of x, and $f(x)$ is any set mathematical procedure or formula such as $x + 1$, $2x + 10$, $4x^3 - 2x^2 + 5x - 10$, and so on.

Let us look at an example in which $y = 3x$.
Hence,

y	x
3	1
6	2
9	3

and graphing y on x, we have a linear graph (Fig. 1). Given a particular value of x, y is said to be determined by x.

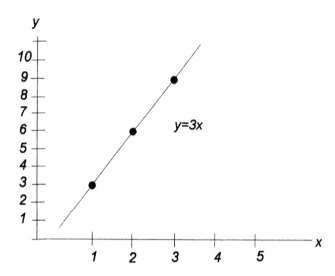

FIGURE 1   Linear graph.

A statistical relationship is not an exact or "perfect" one as a functional one is; y is not determined exactly by x. Even in the best of conditions, y is composed of the estimate of x as well as some amount of unexplained variance called statistical error. That is,

$$y = f(x) + \epsilon$$

So, using the previous example, $y = 3x$, now $y = 3x + \epsilon$ (Fig. 2). Here, the estimates of y on x actually do not fit the data estimate precisely.

1. GENERAL PRINCIPLES OF REGRESSION ANALYSIS

A. Regression and Causality

A statistical relationship demonstrated between two variables, y (the response, or dependent variable) and x (the independent variable), is not necessarily a causal one but can be. Ideally, it is, but unless one knows this for sure, y and x are said to be *associated* [25,28].

The fundamental regressional model is a simple regression model.

$$y_i = \beta_0 + \beta_1 x_i + \epsilon_i \tag{1}$$

where y = the response, or dependent variable for the ith observation

β_0 = population y intercept, when $x = 0$
β_1 = population regression parameter (SLOPE, or $\frac{\text{rise}}{\text{run}}$)
x_i = independent variable
ϵ_i = random error for the ith observation
$\epsilon = N(0, \sigma^2)$; that is, the errors are normally and independently distributed with a mean of zero and a variance of
σ^2; ϵ_i and ϵ_j are assumed not to be correlated (which simply
means that the errors are not influenced by the magnitude
of the previous or other error terms), so the covariance =
0, for all $i, j, i \neq j$.

This model is linear in the parameters (β_0, β_1) as well as in the x_i values,
and there is only one predictor value, x_i, in only a power of 1. In actually applying the regression function to sample data, we will use the form
$\hat{y}_i = b_0 + b_1 + \epsilon_i$. Often, this function also is written as $\hat{y}_i = a + bx + \epsilon_i$. This
form is also known as a first-order model. As previously stated, the actual y
value is composed of two components: (1) $b_0 + b_1 x$, the constant term, and
(2) ϵ, the random variable term. The expected value of y is $E(Y) = \beta_0 + \beta_1 x$.
The variability of σ is assumed to be constant and equidistant over the regression function's entirety (Fig. 3). Examples of nonconstant, nonequidis-
tant variability are presented in Fig. 4.

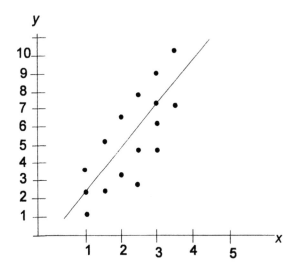

FIGURE 2   Linear graph.

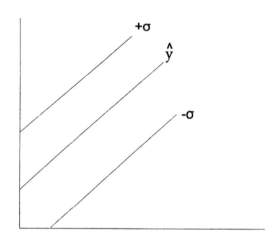

FIGURE 3   Constant variability.

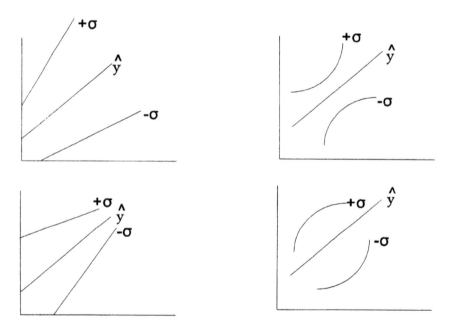

FIGURE 4   Nonconstant variability.

B. Meaning of Regression Parameters

A researcher is performing a steam-heat thermal-death curve calculation on a 10^6 microbial population of *Bacillus stearothermophilus*, where the steam sterilization temperature is 121 °C. Generally, a $\log_{10}$ reexpression is used to linearize the microbial population. In $\log_{10}$ scale, 10^6 is 6. In this example, assume the microbial population is reduced 1 $\log_{10}$ for every 30 seconds of exposure to steam. This example is presented graphically in Fig. 5.

$$\hat{y} = b_0 + b_1 x$$

b_1 represents the slope of the regression line, which is the rise/run or tangent. This rise is negative because the value is decreasing over exposure time, so

$$b_1 = \frac{\text{rise}}{\text{run}} = \frac{-1}{30} = -0.0333$$

b_0 represents the value of $\hat{y}$ when $x = 0$, which is $\hat{y} = 6 - 0.0333(0) = 6$ in this example.

$$\hat{y} = 6 - 0.0333(x)$$

For $x = 60$ seconds, $\hat{y} = 6 - 0.0333(60) = 4$.

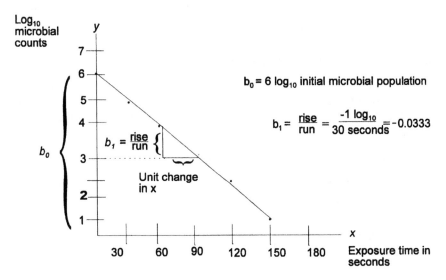

FIGURE 5 Regression parameters.

For every second of exposure time, the $\log_{10}$ reduction in microorganisms is $0.0333 \log_{10}$.

C. Data for Regression Analysis

The researcher ordinarily will not know the population values of β_0 or β_1. They will have to be estimated by a b_0 and b_1 computation, termed the method of least squares. In this calculation, data relevant to the response, or dependent variable (y_i), and the independent variable (x_i) are used. These data can be obtained by observation, by experiment, or by complete randomization.

Observational data are obtained by "nonexperimental" study. There are times a researcher may collect data (x and y) within the environment to perform a regression evaluation. For example, a quality assurance person may suspect a relationship exists between warm weather (winter to spring to summer) and microbial contamination levels of the laboratory. The microbial counts (y) are then compared with the months, x (1–6), to determine whether this theory holds up (Fig. 6).

In experimental designs, usually the values of x are *selected* or set at specific levels and the y values corresponding to these are dependent on the x levels set. This provides y or x values, and a controlled regimen or process is enacted. Generally, multiple observations of y at a specific x value are conducted to increase the precision of the error term estimate.

In the completely randomized regression designs, the actual values of x are selected randomly, not specifically set. Hence, both x and y are random variables. This design, although useful, is not as common as the other two.

D. Regression Parameter Calculation

To find the estimates of both b_0 and b_1, we use the least squares method. This method provides the best estimate (the one with the least error) by minimizing the difference between the actual and predicted values from the set of collected values.

$$(y - \hat{y})^2 \qquad \text{or} \qquad (y - (b_0 + b_1 x))^2$$

The computation utilizes all the observations in a set of data. The sum of the squares is denoted by Q. That is,

$$Q = \sum_{i=1}^{n} (y_i - b_0 - b_1 x_i)^2$$

where Q is the smallest possible number, as determined by the least squares

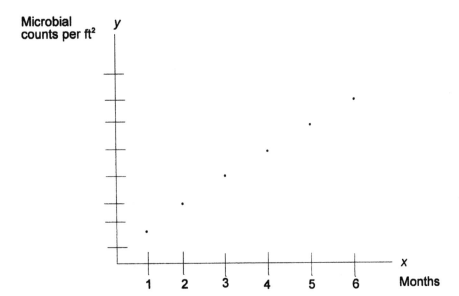

FIGURE 6   Microbial counts vs. months.

method [34]. The actual computational formulas are:

$$b_1 = \text{slope} = \frac{\sum\limits_{i=1}^{n}(x_i - \bar{x})(y_i - \bar{y})}{\sum\limits_{i=1}^{n}(x_i - \bar{x})^2} \tag{2}$$

$$b_0 = y \text{ intercept} = \frac{\sum\limits_{i=1}^{n} y_i - b_1 \sum\limits_{i=1}^{n} x_i}{n} \tag{3}$$

or

$$b_0 = \bar{y} - b_1\bar{x}$$

E. Properties of the Least Squares Estimation

The expected value of $b_0 = E[b_0] = \beta_0$. The expected value of $b_1 = E[b_1] = \beta_1$. The least squares estimators of b_0 and b_1 are unbiased estimators and have the minimum variance of all other possible linear combinations [36].

Example 1:   An experimenter exposes 1×10^6 *Staphylococcus aureus* microorganisms to a benzalkonium chloride disinfectant for a series of timed exposures. As noted before, exponential microbial colony counts are customarily linearized via a $\log_{10}$ scale transformation, which has been

TABLE1   Data from Regression Analysis

n	x	y
1	0	6.09
2	0	6.10
3	0	6.08
4	15	5.48
5	15	5.39
6	15	5.51
7	30	5.01
8	30	4.88
9	30	4.93
10	45	4.53
11	45	4.62
12	45	4.49
13	60	3.57
14	60	3.42
15	60	3.44

performed in this example. The resultant data are presented in Table 1. The researcher would like to perform regression analysis on the data in order to construct a chemical microbial inactivation curve.

x = exposure time in seconds
y = $\log_{10}$ colony-forming units recovered

Notice that the data are replicated in triplicate for each exposure time, x. First, we will compute the slope of the data.

$$b_1 = \frac{\sum_{i=1}^{n}(x_i - \bar{x})(y_i - \bar{y})}{\sum_{i=1}^{n}(x_i - \bar{x})^2}$$

where

$$\bar{x} = 30$$

$$\bar{y} = 4.90$$

$$\sum_{i=1}^{15}(x_i - \bar{x})(y_i - \bar{y}) = (0-30)(6.09-4.90) + (0-30)(6.10-4.90)$$

$$+ \cdots + (60-30)(3.42-4.90) + (60-30)(3.44-4.90)$$

$$= -276.60$$

$$\sum_{i=1}^{15}(x_i - \bar{x})^2 = (0 - 30)^2 + (0 - 30)^2$$
$$+ \cdots + (60 - 30)^2 + (60 - 30)^2 + (60 - 30)^2$$
$$= 6750$$

$$b_1 = \frac{-276.60}{6750} = -0.041^*$$

The negative sign means that the regression line estimated by $\hat{y}$ is descending, from the y intercept.

$$b_0 = \bar{y} - b_1\bar{x} = 4.90 - (-0.041)30$$

$b_0 = 6.13$ is the y intercept point when $x = 0$

The complete regression equation is:

$$\hat{y}_i = b_0 + b_1 x_i$$
$$\hat{y}_i = 6.13 - 0.041x_i \tag{4}$$

This regression equation can then be used to predict each $\hat{y}$, a procedure known as point estimation.

$$\text{For example, for } x = 0, \quad \hat{y} = 6.13 - 0.041(0) \ = 6.130$$
$$15, \quad \hat{y} = 6.13 - 0.041(15) = 5.515$$
$$30, \quad \hat{y} = 6.13 - 0.041(30) = 4.900$$
$$60, \quad \hat{y} = 6.13 - 0.041(60) = 3.670$$

From these data, we can now make a regression diagrammatic table to see how well the model fits the data. Regression functions are standard on most scientific calculators and computer software packages. One of the statistical software packages that is easiest to use and has a considerable number of options is MiniTab®. We will first learn to perform the computations by hand and then switch to this software package because of its simplicity and efficiency. Table 2 presents the data.

It is also very useful in regression to plot the predicted regression values, $\hat{y}$, with the actual observations, y, superimposed. And, too, exploratory

---

*There is a faster "machine" computational formula for b_1, useful with a hand-held calculator, although many scientific calculators provide b_1 as a standard routine. It is:

$$b_1 = \frac{\sum_{i=1}^{n} x_i y_i - \left(\sum_{i=1}^{n}\right)\left(\sum_{i=1}^{n} y_i\right)/n}{\sum_{i=1}^{n} x_i^2 - \left(\sum_{i=1}^{n} x_i\right)^2/n}$$

TABLE 2   Data

n	x = time	y = actual $\log_{10}$ values	$\hat{y}$ = predicted $\log_{10}$ values	$e = y - \hat{y}$ (e = actual − predicted)
1	0.00	6.0900	6.1307	−0.0407
2	0.00	6.1000	6.1307	−0.0307
3	0.00	6.0800	6.1307	−0.0507
4	15.00	5.4800	5.5167	−0.0367
5	15.00	5.3900	5.5167	−0.1267
6	15.00	5.5100	5.5167	−0.0067
7	30.00	5.0100	4.9027	0.1073
8	30.00	4.8800	4.9027	−0.0227
9	30.00	4.9300	4.9027	0.0273
10	45.00	4.5300	4.2887	0.2416
11	45.00	4.6200	4.2887	0.3313
12	45.00	4.4900	4.2887	0.2013
13	60.00	3.5700	3.6747	−0.1047
14	60.00	3.4200	3.6747	−0.2547
15	60.00	3.4400	3.6747	−0.2347

data analysis (EDA) is useful, particularly when using regression methods with the residual values ($e = y - \hat{y}$) to ensure that no pattern or trending is seen that would suggest inaccuracy. Although regression analysis can be extremely valuable, it is particularly prone to certain problems, as follow.

1. The regression line, $\hat{y}$, computed will be straight line or linear. Often experimental data are not linear and must be transformed to a linear scale, if possible, so that the regression analysis provides an accurate and reliable model of the data. The EDA methods described in Chap. 3 are particularly useful in this procedure. However, some data transformations may confuse the intended audience. For example, if the y values are transformed to a cube root ($\sqrt[3]{}$) scale, the audience receiving the data analysis may have trouble understanding the regression's meaning in "real life" because they cannot translate the original scale to a cube root scale "in their heads." That is, they cannot make sense of the data. In this case, the researcher is in a dilemma. Although it would be useful to perform the cube root transformation to linearize the data, the researcher may then need to take the audience verbally and graphically through the transformation process in an attempt to enlighten them. As an alternative, however, a nonparametric

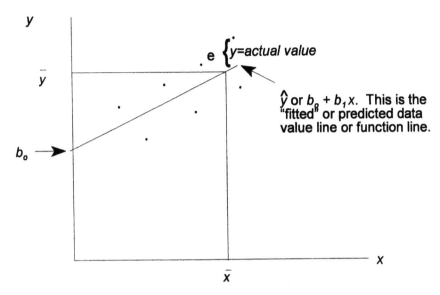

FIGURE 7   Regression model. Note: $e = y - \hat{y}$, or the error term, which is merely the actual y value less the predicted $\hat{y}$ value.

method could be applied to analyze the nonlinear data. Unfortunately, this, too, is likely to require a detailed explanation.

2. Sometimes, a model must be expanded in the b_i parameters in order to better estimate the actual data. For example, the regression equation may expand to:

$$\hat{y} = b_0 + b_1 x_1 + b_2 x_2 \tag{5}$$

or

$$\hat{y} = b_0 + b_1 x_1 + \cdots b_k x_k \tag{6}$$

where the b values will always be linear values.

We will, however, concentrate on simple linear regression procedures, that is, $\hat{y} = b_0 + b_1 x_i$.

Before continuing, let us look at a regression model to understand better what $\hat{y}, y$, and ϵ represent. Figure 7 portrays them.

F. Diagnostics

One of the most important steps in regression analysis is to plot the actual data values (y_i) and the fitted data ($\hat{y}_i$) on the same graph to visualize clearly how closely the regression line ($\hat{y}_i$) fits, or predicts the actual data (y_i).

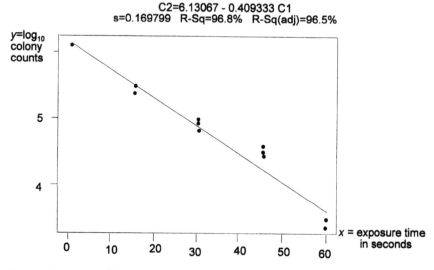

FIGURE 8   MiniTab® regression plot.

Figure 8 presents a MiniTab® graphic plot of this as an example. In the figure, R^2 ("R-Sq") is the coefficient of determination, a value used to evaluate the adequacy of the model, which in this example indicates that the regression equation is about a 96.8% better predictor of y than using $\bar{x}$. An R^2 of 1.00, or 100%, is a perfect fit (the $\hat{y} = y$). We will discuss both R and R^2 later in this chapter.

Notice that, on examining the regression plot (Fig. 8), it appears that the data seem to be adequately "modeled" by the linear regression equation used. The researcher next should perform a stem–leaf display, a letter-value display, and a boxplot display of the residuals, or $y - \hat{y} = e$ values. Also, it is often useful to plot the y values and the residual values, e and the $\hat{y}$ values and the residual values, e.

Figure 9 presents a stem–leaf display of the residual data $(y_i - \hat{y}_i)$. The stem-leaf display of the residual data $(y_i - \hat{y}_i)$ portrays nothing of great concern, that is, no abnormal patterns. Recall that residual value plots should be patternless if the model is adequate. The residual mean is not precisely 0 but very close to it.

Figure 10 presents the letter-value display of the residual data. Notice that the letter-value display "Mid" column is tending toward increased value (a phenomenon we discussed in Chap. 3), meaning that the residual values are skewed slightly to the right or to the values greater than the mean value. In regression analysis, this is a clue that the predicted regression line

STEM-AND-LEAF DISPLAY OF RESID   N=15

LEAF UNIT = 0.010

2	-2	53
4	-1	20
(6)	-0	543320
5	0	2
4	1	0
3	2	04
1	3	3

FIGURE 9   Stem-and-leaf display.

function may not adequately model the data. The researcher will next want to examine a residual value (ϵ) versus actual y value graph (Fig. 11) and a residual versus predicted ($\hat{y}$) value graph (Fig. 12) and to review the actual regression graph (Fig. 8). Looking closely at these graphs and the letter-value display, we see clearly that the regression model does not completely describe the data. The actual data appear not quite $\log_{10}$ linear. For example, note that beyond time $x_i = 0$, the regression model overestimates the actual $\log_{10}$ microbial kill by about 0.25 $\log_{10}$, underestimates the actual $\log_{10}$ kill at

	Depth	Lower		Upper	Mid	Spread
N=	15					
M	8.0		-0.031		-0.031	
H	4.5	-0.078		0.067	-0.005	0.145
E	2.5	-0.181		0.221	0.020	0.402
D	1.5	-0.245		0.286	0.021	0.531
	1	-0.255		0.331	0.038	0.586

FIGURE 10   Letter-value display.

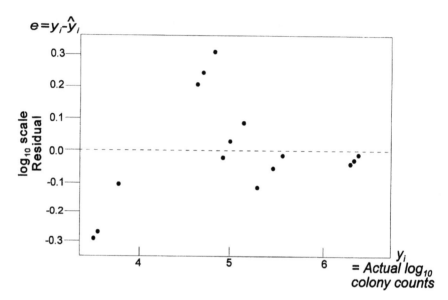

FIGURE 11   Residual vs. actual y value graph.

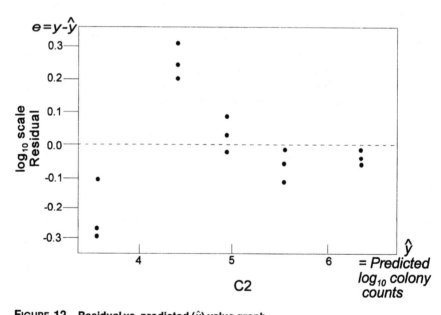

FIGURE 12   Residual vs. predicted ($\hat{y}$) value graph.

$x_i = 45$ seconds by about $0.25 \log_{10}$, and again overestimates at $x_i = 60$ seconds. Is this significant or not?

The researcher can draw on his or her primary field knowledge to determine this, whereas a card-carrying statistician usually cannot. The statistician may decide to use a polynomial regression model and is sure that, with some manipulation, it can model the data better, particularly in that the error at each observation is considerably reduced (as supported by several indicators we have yet to discuss, the regression f-test and the coefficient of determination, r^2). However, the applied microbiology researcher has an advantage over the statistician, knowing that, often, the initial value at time 0 ($x = 0$) is not reliable in microbial death rate kinetics and, in practice, is often dropped from the analysis. In addition, the applied microbiology researcher, from experience, knows that, once the data drop below four $\log_{10}$, a different inactivation rate (i.e., slope of b_i) occurs with this microbial species until the population reaches about two logs, where the microbial inactivation rate slows due to survivors genetically resistant to the drug. Hence, the microbial researcher may decide to perform a "piecewise" regression (to be explained later) to better model the data and explain the inactivation properties at a level more basic than provided by a polynomial regression [27,30]. The final regression, when carried out over sufficient time, could be modeled using a form such as that in Fig. 13.

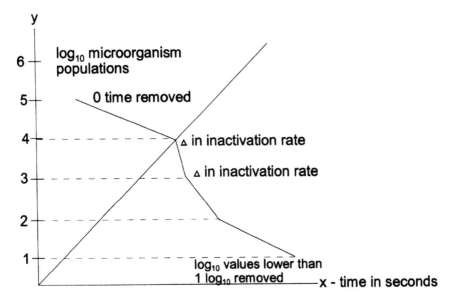

FIGURE 13   Final regression model.

In conclusion, the field microbiology researcher generally has a definite advantage over a statistician in understanding and modeling the data, because the researcher grounds the interpretation in basic knowledge of the field.

G. Estimation of the Error Term

As before, the variance (σ^2) of the error term (written as either e or ϵ) needs to be estimated. Recall from earlier chapters that the sample variance (s^2) was obtained by measuring the squared deviation between each of the actual values, x_i, and the average value, $\bar{x}$.

$$\sum_{i=1}^{n}(x_i - \bar{x})^2 = \text{sum of squares}$$

From this equation, we computed the sample variance by dividing the sum of squares by the degrees of freedom ($n - 1$).

$$s^2 = \frac{\sum_{i=1}^{n}(x_i - \bar{x})^2}{n-1} \tag{7}$$

This concept is applicable to the regression model, particularly as discussed in the previous chapters using analysis of variance (ANOVA) procedures. Hence, the sum of squares for the error term in the regression method is:

$$SS_E = \sum_{i=1}^{n}(y_i - \hat{y})^2 = \sum_{i=1}^{n}\epsilon^2 = \text{sum of squares error term} \tag{8}$$

Recall that the mean square error (MS_E) was used to predict σ^2. Hence,

$$E(MS_E) = \sigma^2 \tag{9}$$

where

$$MS_E = \frac{SS_E}{n-2} \tag{10}$$

Two degrees of freedom are lost because both b_0 and b_1 are estimated in the model, ($b_0 + b_1 x_i$), to predict $\hat{y}$. The standard deviation of the y values can be computed directly from

$$S = \sqrt{MS_E} \tag{11}$$

The value, S, is considered to be constant for any y value range on its corresponding x values.

H. Regression Inferences

Recall that the simple regression model equation is

$$y_i = \beta_0 + \beta_1 x_i + \epsilon_i$$

where β_0 and β_1 are regression parameters

   x_i = known (set) independent values

   $\epsilon = (y - \hat{y})$, normally and independently distributed, $N(0, \sigma^2)$

Frequently, the investigator will want to know whether the slope, β_1, is significant, i.e., whether $\beta_1 \neq 0$. If $\beta_1 = 0$, then regression analysis should not be used. The inference test for β_1 is:

H_0: $\beta_1 = 0$ (slope is not significantly different from 0)

H_A: $\beta_1 \neq 0$ (slope is significantly different from 0)

The conclusions that are drawn when $\beta_1 = 0$ are these:

1.   There is no linear association between y and x.
2.   There is no relationship of any type between y and x.

Recall that β_1 is estimated by b_1, which is:

$$b_1 = \frac{\displaystyle\sum_{i=1}^{n}(x_i - \bar{x})(y_i - \bar{y})}{\displaystyle\sum_{i=1}^{n}(x_i - \bar{x})^2}$$

and b_1, the mean slope value, is an unbiased estimator of β_1.
   The variance of β_1 is:

$$\sigma_{\beta_1}^2 = \frac{\sigma^2}{\displaystyle\sum_{i=1}^{n}(x_i - \bar{x})^2} \tag{12}$$

In practice, $\sigma_{\beta_1}^2$ will be estimated by:

$$S_{b_1}^2 = \frac{MS_E}{\displaystyle\sum_{i=1}^{n}(x_i - \bar{x})^2} \tag{13}$$

$$\sqrt{S_{b_1}^2} = S_{b_1} \text{ or the standard deviation value for } \beta_1. \tag{14}$$

Returning to the β_1 test, to evaluate whether β_1 is significant ($\beta_1 \neq 0$), the researcher will set up a two-tail hypothesis, using the six-step procedure.

Step 1.   Determine the hypothesis.

$H_0 : \beta_1 = 0$
$H_A : \beta_1 \neq 0$

Step 2.   Set the α level.
Step 3.   Select the test statistic.

$$t_{\text{calculated}} = t_c = \frac{b_1}{S_{b_1}} \qquad (15)$$

where:

$$b_1 = \frac{\sum_{i=1}^{n}(x_i - \bar{x})(y_i - \bar{y})}{\sum_{i=1}^{n}(x_i - \bar{x})^2}$$

and

$$S_{b_1} = \sqrt{\frac{MS_E}{\sum_{i=1}^{n}(x_i - \bar{x})^2}}$$

Step 4.   Write the decision rule.

If $| t_c | > t_{(\alpha/2,n-2)}$, reject H_0; the slope β_1 differs significantly from 0.
If $| t_c | \leq t_{(\alpha/2,n-2)}$, the researcher cannot reject the null H_0 hypothesis at α.

Step 5.   Compute the calculated test statistic (t_c).
Step 6.   State the conclusion.

Let us now calculate whether or not the slope is 0 for data presented in Example 1.

Step 1.   Establish the hypothesis.

$H_0 : B_1 = 0$
$H_A : B_1 \neq 0$

Step 2.   Set α. Let us set α at 0.05.
Step 3.   Select the test statistic.

$$t_c = \frac{b_1}{S_{b_1}}$$

where:

$$S_{b_1} = \frac{MS_E}{\displaystyle\sum_{i=1}^{n}(x_i - \bar{x})^2}$$

Step 4.   Decision rule.

If $|\ t_c\ | > t_{(\alpha/2,n-2)}$ one rejects the null hypothesis (H_0) at $\alpha = 0.05$. Using Student's t table (Table A.2) $t_{(0.05/2,15-2)} = t_{0.025,13} = 2.160$. So if $|\ t_{\text{calculated}}\ | > 2.160$, reject H_0 at $\alpha = 0.05$.

Step 5. Calculate the test statistic, $t_c = b_1/S_{b_1}$.

Recall from Example 1 that $b_1 = -0.041$. Also recall from the initial computation of b_1 that $\sum_{i=1}^{n}(x_i - \bar{x})^2 = 6,750$.

$$MS_E = \frac{\displaystyle\sum_{i=1}^{n}(y_i - \hat{y})^2}{n-2} = \frac{\displaystyle\sum_{i=1}^{n}e_i^2}{n-2}$$

$$= \frac{(-0.0407)^2 + (-0.0307)^2 + \cdots + (-0.2547)^2 + (-0.2347)^2}{13}$$

$$= \frac{0.3750}{13} = 0.0288$$

$$S_{b_1} = \sqrt{\frac{MS_E}{\displaystyle\sum_{i=1}^{n}(x_i - \bar{x})^2}} = \sqrt{\frac{0.0288}{6750}} = 0.0021$$

$$t_c = \frac{b_1}{S_{b_1}} = \frac{-0.041}{0.0021} = -19.5238$$

Step 6.   Draw conclusion.

Because $|\ t_c\ | = -19.5238 > 2.160$, the researcher will reject H_0, that the slope (rate of bacterial destruction per second) is 0 at $\alpha = 0.05$.

Note that one-sided tests (upper or lower tail) for b_1 are also possible. If the researcher wanted to conduct an upper tail test (hypothesize that B_1 is significantly positive, that is, an ascending regression line), the hypothesis would be

$$H_0: \ B_1 \leq 0$$
$$H_A: \ B_1 > 0$$

with the same test statistic as used in the two-tail test,

$$t_c = \frac{b_1}{S_{b_1}}$$

The test is:

If $t_c > t_{(\alpha, n-2)}$, reject H_0 at α.

Note: The upper tail value from Table A.2, which is a positive value, will be used.

For the lower tail test, the test hypothesis for B_1 will be a negative value (descending regression line):

$$H_0: \ B_1 \geq 0$$
$$H_A: \ B_1 < 0$$

with the test calculated value

$$t_c = \frac{b_1}{S_{b_1}}$$

If $t_c < t_{(\alpha, n-2)}$, reject H_0 at α.

Note: The lower tail value from Table B, which is negative, is used, to find the $t_{(\alpha, n-2)}$ value.

Finally, if the researcher wants to compare B_1 with a specific value, k, that, too, can be accomplished using a two-tail or one-tail test. For the two-tail test, the hypothesis is

$$H_0: \ B_1 = k$$
$$H_A: \ B_1 \neq k$$

where k is a set value.

$$t_c = \frac{b_1 - k}{S_{b_1}}$$

If $| \ t_c \ | > t_{(\alpha/2, n-2)}$, reject H_0.

Both upper and lower tail tests can be evaluated for a k value using the lower and upper tail procedures just described. The only modification is that $t_c = (b_1 - k)/S_{b_1}$.

I. Computer Output

Generally, it will be most efficient to use a computer for regression analyses. A regression analysis using MiniTab®, a common software program, is presented in Table 3, using the data from Example 1.

J. Confidence Interval for B_1

A $1 - \alpha$ confidence interval for β_1 is a straightforward computation.

$$\beta_1 = b_1 \pm t_{(\alpha/2, n-2)} S_{b_1}$$

Example 1 (continued)   To determine the 95% confidence interval for B_1, using the data from Example 1 and our regression analysis data, we find:

$t_{(0.05/2, 15-2)}$ (from Table A.2, Student's t table) $= \pm 2.16$

$b_1 = -0.0409$

$$S_{b_1} = \sqrt{\frac{MS_E}{\sum (x - \bar{x})^2}} = \sqrt{\frac{0.0288}{6750}} = 0.0021$$

TABLE 3   Computer Printout of Regression Analysis

The regression equation is
① C2 = 6.13 − 0.0409 C1

Predictor	Coef	SE Coef	T	P
② Constant	6.13067	0.07594	80.73	0.000
③ C1	−0.040933	0.002057	−19.81	0.000
⑤ S = 0.1698	④ R-Sq = 96.8%			

where:
 c2 = y
 c3 = x

NOTE: ① = regression equation.
② = b_o value row = constant = y intercept when $x = 0$. The value below the Coef is b_o (6.13067); the values below SE Coef (0.07594) is the standard error of b_o. The value below T (80.73) is the T test calculated value for b_o hypothesizing it as 0, from H_o. The value (0.00) below P (0.00) is the probability, when H_o is true, of seeing a value of T greater than or the same as 80.73, and this is essentially 0.
③ = b_1 value row = slope. The value below Coef (−0.040933) is b_1; the value below SE Coef (0.002057) is the standard error of b_1; the value below T (−19.81) is the T test calculated value for the null hypothesis that $b_1 = 0$. The value below P (0.00) is the probability of computing a value of −19.81 or more extreme, given the b_1 value is actually 0.
④ = r^2, or coefficient of determination.
⑤ = $s = \sqrt{MS_E}$.

$$b_1 + t_{\alpha/2}S_{b_1} = -0.0409 + (2.16)(0.0021) = -0.0364$$

$$b_1 - t_{\alpha/2}S_{b_1} = -0.0409 - (2.16)(0.0021) = -0.454$$

$$-0.0454 \le \beta_1 \le -0.0364$$

The researcher is confident at the 95% level that the true slope (β_1) lies within this confidence interval. In addition, the researcher can determine whether $\beta_1 = 0$ from the confidence interval. If the confidence interval includes 0 (which it does not), the H_0 hypothesis, $B_1 = 0$, cannot be rejected at α.

K. Inferences with B_0

The point estimator of B_0, the y intercept, is

$$b_0 = \bar{y} - b_1\bar{x} \tag{16}$$

The expected value of b_0 is

$$E(b_0) = B_0 \tag{17}$$

The expected variance of B_0 is:

$$\sigma_{b_0}^2 = \sigma^2 \left[\frac{1}{n} + \frac{\bar{x}^2}{\sum\limits_{i=1}^{n}(x_i - \bar{x})^2} \right] \tag{18}$$

which is estimated by $S_{b_0}^2$:

$$S_{b_0}^2 = MS_E \left[\frac{1}{n} + \frac{\bar{x}^2}{\sum\limits_{i=1}^{n}(x_i - \bar{x})^2} \right] \tag{19}$$

where

$$MS_E = \frac{\sum\limits_{i=1}^{n}(y_i - \hat{y})^2}{n-2} = \frac{\sum \epsilon^2}{n-2}$$

Probably the most useful procedure for evaluating B_0 is to determine a $1 - \alpha$ confidence interval for its true value. The procedure is straightforward. Using our previous Example 1:

$$B_0 = b_0 \pm t_{(\alpha/2, n-2)}S_{b_0}$$

$$b_0 = 6.1307$$

$$t_{(0.05/2, 15-2)} = \pm 2.16 \text{ from Table A.2 (Student's } t \text{ table).}$$

$$S_{b_0} = \sqrt{MS_E \left[\frac{1}{n} + \frac{\bar{x}^2}{\sum\limits_{i=1}^{n}(x_i - \bar{x})^2} \right]}$$

$$S_{b_0} = \sqrt{0.0288 \left[\frac{1}{15} + \frac{30^2}{6750} \right]} = 0.0759$$

$$b_0 + t_{(\alpha/2, n-2)} S_{b_0} = 6.1307 + 2.16(0.0759) = 6.2946$$

$$b_0 - t_{(\alpha/2, n-2)} S_{b_0} = 6.1307 - 2.16(0.0759) = 5.9668$$

$$5.9668 \leq \beta_0 \leq 6.2946 \quad \text{at } \alpha = 0.05.$$

The researcher is $1 - \alpha$ (95%) confident that the true B_0 value lies within the confidence interval, 5.9668 to 6.2946.

Notes:

1. In making inferences about B_0 and/or B_1, the distribution of the y_i values, as with our previous work with the x_i values using Student's t-test or ANOVA, does not have to be perfectly normal. It can approximate normality. Even if the distribution is rather far from normal, the estimators b_0 and b_1 are said to be asymptotically normal. That is, as the sample size increases, the y distribution used to estimate both b_0 and b_1 approaches normality. In cases in which the y_i data are clearly not normal, however, the researcher can use nonparametric regression approaches (see Chap. 12).

2. The regression procedure we have been using assumes that the x_i values are fixed and have not been collected at random. The confidence intervals and tests concerning B_0 and B_1 are interpreted with respect to the range the x values cover. They do not purport to estimate B_0 and B_1 outside that range.

3. As with the t-test, the $1 - \alpha$ confidence level should not be interpreted that one is "95% confident the true B_0 or B_1 lies within the $1 - \alpha$ confidence interval." Instead, over 100 runs, one will observe the b_0 or b_1 contained within that interval $(1 - \alpha)$ times. At $\alpha = 0.05$, for example, if one performed the experiment 100 times, 95 times out of 100 the calculated b_0 or b_1 would be contained within that calculated interval.

4. It is important for the researcher to know that the greater the range covered by the x_i values selected, the more generally useful will be

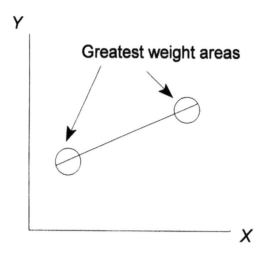

FIGURE 14   Greatest weight in regression computation.

the regression equation. In addition, the greatest weight in the regression computation lies with the outer values (Fig. 14). The researcher generally will benefit from taking great pains to ensure that the outer data regions are representative of the true condition. Recall that in our discussion of the example data set, when we noted the importance in the $\log_{10}$ linear equation of death curve kinetics, the first value (time zero) and the last value are known to have undue influence on the data, so we dropped them. This sort of insight, afforded only by experience, must be drawn on constantly by the researcher. In research, it is often, but not always, wise to take the worst-case approach to making decisions. Hence, the researcher should constantly interplay statistical theory with field knowledge and experience.

5. The greater the spread of the x values, the greater the value $\sum_{i=1}^{n}(x_i - \bar{x})^2$ which is the denominator of S_{b_1} and a major portion of the denominator for β_0, and the smaller the variance of values for b_1 and b_0 will be. This is particularly important for statistical inferences concerning β_1.

L. Power of the Tests for β_0 and β_1

To compute the power of the tests concerning β_0 and β_1, the approach is relatively simple.

$$H_0 : \beta = \beta_x$$
$$H_A : \beta \neq \beta_x$$

where $\beta = \beta_1$ or β_0, and

β_x = any constant value. If the test is to evaluate the power relative to 0 (e.g., $\beta_1 \neq 0$), the β_x value should be set at zero. As always, the actual sample testing uses lowercase b_i values.

$$t_c = \frac{b_i - B_x}{S_{b_i}} \qquad (20)$$

is the test statistic to be employed, where

b_i = the ith regression parameter;
$i = 0$ if b_0 and 1 if b_1
B_x = constant value, or 0
S_{b_i} = standard error of β_i; $i = 0$ if b_0 and 1 if b_1

The power computation of the statistic is

$$\delta = \frac{|B_i - B_x|}{\sigma_{b_i}} \qquad (21)$$

where σ_{b_i} = standard error of b_i

If $\beta_i = \beta_0$, $\qquad \sigma_{(\beta_0)} = \sqrt{\sigma^2 \left[\dfrac{1}{n} + \dfrac{\bar{x}^2}{\sum\limits_{i=1}^{n}(x_i - \bar{x})^2} \right]}$

which, in practice, is

$$S_{b_0} = \sqrt{MS_E \left[\frac{1}{n} + \frac{\bar{x}^2}{\sum\limits_{i=1}^{n}(x_i - \bar{x})^2} \right]}$$

Note: Generally, the power of the test is calculated prior to the evaluation to ensure that the sample size is adequate. Typically, σ^2 is estimated from previous experiments because MS_E cannot be known if the power is computed prior to performing the experiment. The value of σ^2 is estimated using MS_E when the power is computed after the sample data have been collected.

If $\beta_i = \beta_1$, $\qquad \sigma_{(\beta_1)} = \sqrt{\dfrac{\sigma^2}{\sum\limits_{i=1}^{n}(x_i - \bar{x})^2}}$

which is estimated by

$$S_{\beta_1} = \sqrt{\frac{MS_E}{\sum_{i=1}^{n}(x_i - \bar{x})^2}}$$

Let us work an example. The researcher wants to compute the power of the statistic for β_1.

$H_0: \beta_1 = \beta_x$

$H_A: \beta_1 \neq \beta_x$

Let $\beta_x = 0$, in this example.

Recall $b_1 = -0.0409$. Let us estimate σ^2 with MS_E and assume we want to evaluate the power (δ) after the study has been conducted instead of before.

$$S_{b_1}^2 = \frac{MS_E}{\sum_{i=1}^{n}(x_i - \bar{x})^2}$$

$$S_{b_1}^2 = \frac{0.0288}{6750}$$

$$S_{b_1} = \sqrt{\frac{0.0288}{6750}} = 0.0021$$

$$\delta = \frac{0.0409 - 0}{0.0021} = \frac{0.0409}{0.0021} = 19.4762$$

Using Table A.17 (power table for two-tail t-test), df $= n-2 = 15-2 = 13$, $\alpha = 0.05$, $\delta = 19.4762$, the power $= 1 - \beta \approx 1.00$ or $\approx 100\%$ at $\delta = 9$, which is the largest value of δ available in the table. Hence, the researcher is assured that the power (δ) of the test is adequate to determine that the slope (B_1) is not 0, given it is not 0, at a σ of 0.0021 and $n = 15$.

M. Estimating $\hat{y}$ from Confidence Intervals

A common aspect of interval estimation involves estimating the regression line value $\hat{y}$ with simultaneous confidence intervals for a specific value of x. That value $\hat{y}$ can be further subcategorized as an average predicted $\hat{y}$ value or a specific $\hat{y}$. Figure 15 shows which regions on the regression plot can and cannot be estimated reliably through point and interval measurements.

The region—interpolation range—based on actual x, y values can be predicted confidently by regression methods. If gaps between the y values

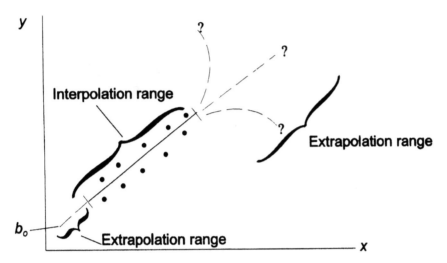

FIGURE 15 Regions on the regression plot.

are small, the prediction is usually more reliable than if they are extended [25,29]. In my view, the determining factor is background—field—experience. If one, for example, has worked with lethality curves and has an understanding of a particular microorganism's death rate, the reliability of the model is greatly enhanced if the statistical data are grounded in this knowledge [17]. Any region not represented by both smaller and larger actual values of x, y is a region of extrapolation. It is usually *very dangerous* to assume accuracy and reliability of an estimate in an extrapolation region because this assumes the data respond identically to the regression function computed from the observed x, y data [34,35]. Because that usually cannot be safely assumed, it is better not to attempt extrapolation at all. That is better dealt with by forecasting and time series procedures [31]. The researcher should focus exclusively on the region of the regression, the interpolation region, where actual x, y data have been collected, and so we shall in this text.

Up to this point, we have considered the sampling regions of both b_0 and b_1 but not $\hat{y}$ itself. Recall that the expected value of a predicted $\hat{y}$ at a givn x is

$$E(\hat{y}) = b_0 + b_1 x \qquad (22)$$

The variance of $E(\hat{y})$ is

$$\sigma_{\hat{y}}^2 = \sigma^2 \left[\frac{1}{n} + \frac{(x_i - \bar{x})^2}{\sum_{i=1}^{n}(x_i - \bar{x})^2} \right]$$

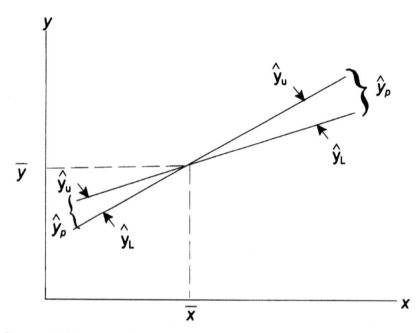

FIGURE 16   Regression line pivots.

As stated earlier, the greater the numerical spread of the x_i values, the smaller the corresponding $\sigma_{\hat{y}}^2$ value is. However, notice that the $\sigma_{\hat{y}}^2$ value is for one x_i point, and the farther the individual x_i is from the mean, $\bar{x}$, the larger $\sigma_{\hat{y}}^2$ will be. This phenomenon is important from a practical as well as a theoretical point of view. In the regression equation, $b_0+b_1x_i$, there will always be some error in b_0 and b_1 estimates. In addition, the regression line will always go through $(\bar{x},\bar{y})$, the pivot points. The more variability in $\sigma_{\hat{y}}^2$, the greater the swing on the pivot points $(\bar{x},\bar{y})$. Figure 16 illustrates this. The true regression equation, y_p, is somewhere between $\hat{y}_L$ and $\hat{y}_U$ (estimate of y upper and lower). The regression line can pivot on the $\bar{x}$ axis to a certain degree, with both b_0 and b_1 varying.

Because the researcher does not know exactly what the true regression linear function is, it must be estimated. Any of the $\hat{y}$ (y predicted values) on some particular x value will be wider, the farther away from the mean ($\bar{x}$) one estimates in either direction. This, of course, means that the $\hat{y}$ confidence interval is not parallel to the regression line but curvilinear (see Fig. 17).

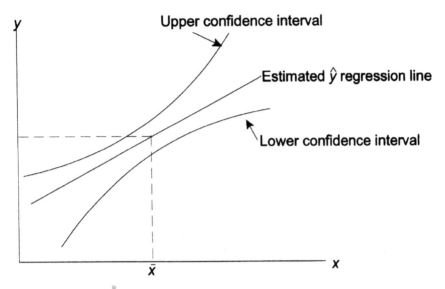

FIGURE 17 Confidence intervals.

N. Confidence Interval of $\hat{y}$

A $1-\alpha$ confidence interval for the expected value—average value—of $\bar{y}$ for a specific x is calculated using the following equation.

$$\hat{y} + t_{(\alpha/2;n-2)}S_{\bar{y}} \tag{23}$$

where:

$$\hat{y} = b_0 + b_1x$$

and

$$S_{\bar{y}} = \sqrt{MS_E\left[\frac{1}{n} + \frac{(x_i - \bar{x})^2}{\sum\limits_{i=1}^{n}(x_i - \bar{x})^2}\right]} \tag{24}$$

and where x_i is the set x value on which to predict $\hat{y}_i$.

$$MS_E = \frac{\sum\limits_{i=1}^{n}(y_i - \hat{y}_i)^2}{n-2} = \frac{\sum\limits_{i=1}^{n}\varepsilon_i^2}{n-2}$$

Example 1 (continued)   Using the data in Table 1 and from Eq. (1), we see that the regression equation is $\hat{y} = 6.13 - 0.041x$. Suppose the researcher would like to know the expected (average) value of y, as predicted by x_i, when

$x_i = 15$ seconds. What is the 95% confidence interval (CI) for the expected $\hat{y}$ (mean) value?

$$\hat{y}_{15} = 6.13 - 0.041(15) = 5.515$$

$$n = 15$$

$$\bar{x} = 30$$

$$\sum_{i=1}^{n}(x_i - \bar{x})^2 = 6750$$

$$MS_E = \frac{\sum_{i=1}^{n}(y_i - \hat{y}_i)^2}{n-2} = 0.0288$$

$$S_y^2 = MS_E\left[\frac{1}{n} + \frac{(x_i - \bar{x})^2}{\sum_{i=1}^{n}(x_i - \bar{x})^2}\right] = 0.0288\left[\frac{1}{15} + \frac{(15 - 30)^2}{6750}\right]$$

$$S_{\hat{y}_{15}}^2 = 0.0029$$

$$S_{\hat{y}_{15}} = 0.0537$$

$$t_{(\alpha/2;n-2)} = t_{(0.025;15-2)} = 2.16$$

from Table A.2, Student's t-table. The 95%CI $= \hat{y} \pm t_{(\alpha/2;n-2)}\ S_{\hat{y}} = 5.515 \pm 2.16(0.0537) = 5.515 \pm 0.1160$, or $5.40 \leq \hat{y}_{15} \leq 5.63$, at $\alpha = 0.05$.

Hence, the expected or average $\log_{10}$ population of microorganisms remaining after exposure to a 15-second treatment with an antimicrobial is between 5.40 and 5.63 $\log_{10}$ at the 95% confidence level. This confidence interval is a prediction for one value, not multiple ones. Multiple estimation will be discussed later.

O. Prediction of a Specific Observation

Many times a researcher is not interested in an "expected" (mean) value or mean value confidence interval. The researcher instead wants an interval for a specific y_i value corresponding to a specific x_i.

The process for this is very similar to that for the expected (mean) value procedure, but the confidence interval for a single, new y_i value results in a wider confidence interval than does predicting for an average y_i value. The formula for a specific y_i value is:

$$\hat{y} \pm t_{(\alpha/2;n-2)}\ S_{\hat{y}} \tag{25}$$

where:

$$\hat{y} = b_0 + b_1 x$$

$$S_{\hat{y}}^2 = MSE \left[1 + \frac{1}{n} + \frac{(x_i - \bar{x})^2}{\sum\limits_{i=1}^{n}(x_i - \bar{x})^2} \right] \tag{26}$$

and

$$MSE = \frac{\sum\limits_{i=1}^{n}(y_i - \hat{y}_i)^2}{n - 2} = \frac{\sum\limits_{i=1}^{n}\epsilon^2}{n - 2}$$

Example 1(continued)   Again, using data from Table 1 and Eq. (1), suppose the researcher wants to construct a 95% confidence interval for an individual value, y_i, at a specific x_i, say 15 seconds.

$\hat{y} = b_0 + b_1 x$ and $\hat{y}_{15} = 6.13 - 0.041(15) = 5.515$ as before

$n = 15$

$\bar{x} = 30$

$$\sum_{i=1}^{n}(x_i - \bar{x})^2 = 6750$$

$$MSE = \frac{\sum\limits_{i=1}^{n}(y - \hat{y})^2}{n - 2} = 0.0288$$

$S_{\hat{y}}^2 =$ standard error of a specific y on x

$$S_{\hat{y}}^2 = MSE \left[1 + \frac{1}{n} + \frac{(x_i + \bar{x})^2}{\sum(x_i - \bar{x})^2} \right] = 0.0288 \left[1 + \frac{1}{15} + \frac{(15 - 30)^2}{6750} \right]$$

$S_{\hat{y}}^2 = 0.0317$

$S_{\hat{y}} = 0.1780$

$t_{(\alpha/2; n-2)} = t_{(0.025; 15-2)} = 2.16$, from Table A.2, Student's t table.
        The   95%   CI$= \hat{y} \pm t_{(\alpha/2; n-2)}S_{\hat{y}} = 5.515 \pm 2.16(0.1780) = 5.515\pm$
0.3845, or $5.13 \le \hat{y}_{15} \le 5.90$, at $\alpha = 0.05$.
        Hence, the researcher can expect the value $\hat{y}_i$ ($\log_{10}$ microorganisms) to be contained within the interval 5.13 to 5.90 $\log_{10}$ for a 15-second exposure at a 95% confidence level. This does not mean that there is a 95% chance of the value being within the confidence interval. It means that if the experimental procedure was conducted 100 times, approximately 95 times out of 100 the value would lie within this interval. Again, this interval is a prediction interval of one y_i value on one x_i value.

P. Confidence Interval for Entire Regression Model

There are many cases in which a researcher would like to map out the entire regression model with a $1 - \alpha$ confidence interval [32]. If the data have excess variability, the confidence interval will be wide. In fact, it may be too wide to be useful. If this occurs, the experimenter may want to rethink the entire experiment or conduct it in a more controlled manner. Perhaps more observations—particularly replicate observations—will be needed. In addition, if the error, $(y - \hat{y}) = \epsilon$, values are not patternless, the experimenter might transform the data to better fit the regression model to the data or add additional variables (e.g., $b_2 + \cdots + b_k$) to the model.

Given that these problems are insignificant, one straightforward way to compute the entire regression model is the Working–Hotelling method [25], which enables the researcher not only to plot the entire regression function, but also to find the upper and lower confidence interval limits for $\hat{y}$ on any or all x_i values using the formula

$$\hat{y} \pm W S_{\bar{y}} \tag{27}$$

The F distribution (Table A.3) is used in this procedure, instead of the t table, where:

$$W^2 = 2F_{\alpha;(2,n-2)}$$

and as before,

$$\hat{y}_i = b_0 + b_1 x_i \text{ and}$$

$$S_{\bar{y}} = \sqrt{MS_E \left[\frac{1}{n} + \frac{(x_i - \bar{x})^2}{\sum_{i=1}^{n}(x_i - \bar{x})^2} \right]} \tag{28}$$

Note that the latter is the same formula used previously to obtain a $1 - \alpha$ confidence interval for the expected (mean) value of a specific y_i on a specific x_i. However, the confidence interval in this procedure is wider than the expected value because it accounts for all x_i values simultaneously.

Example 1 (continued)   Suppose the experimenter wants to determine the 95% confidence interval for Example 1 and know the $\hat{y}_i$ on $x_i = 0$, 15, 30, 45, and 60 seconds. The $\hat{y}_i$ values predicted are expected (mean) values, not actual values.

$$\hat{y} = 6.13 - 0.041(x_i)$$

where

$$x = 0; \quad \hat{y} = 6.13 - 0.041(0) = 6.13$$
$$x = 15; \quad \hat{y} = 6.13 - 0.041(15) = 5.52$$
$$x = 30; \quad \hat{y} = 6.13 - 0.041(30) = 4.90$$
$$x = 45; \quad \hat{y} = 6.13 - 0.041(45) = 4.29$$
$$x = 60; \quad \hat{y} = 6.13 - 0.041(60) = 3.67$$

$W^2 = 2F_{(0.05;2,15-2)}$ (where the F tabled distribution value may be found in Table A.3)

The F-tabled value (Table A.3) $= 3.81$

$$W^2 = 2(3.81) = 7.62$$

$$W = \sqrt{2F} = \sqrt{7.62} = 2.76$$

$$S_{(\bar{y})} = \sqrt{MS_E \left[\frac{1}{n} + \frac{(x_i - \bar{x})^2}{\sum\limits_{i=1}^{n} (x_i - \bar{x})^2} \right]} \quad \text{for } x_i = 0, 15, 30, 45, 60$$

$$S_{(\bar{y}_0)} = \sqrt{0.0288 \left[\frac{1}{15} + \frac{(0 - 30)^2}{6750} \right]} = 0.0759$$

$$S_{(\bar{y}_{15})} = \sqrt{0.0288 \left[\frac{1}{15} + \frac{(15 - 30)^2}{6750} \right]} = 0.0537$$

$$S_{(\bar{y}_{30})} = \sqrt{0.0288 \left[\frac{1}{15} + \frac{(30 - 30)^2}{6750} \right]} = 0.0438$$

$$S_{(\bar{y}_{45})} = \sqrt{0.0288 \left[\frac{1}{15} + \frac{(45 - 30)^2}{6750} \right]} = 0.0537$$

$$S_{(\bar{y}_{60})} = \sqrt{0.0288 \left[\frac{1}{15} + \frac{(60 - 30)^2}{6750} \right]} = 0.0759$$

Putting these together, one can construct a simultaneous $1 - \alpha$ confidence interval for each x_i.

$$\hat{y} \pm WS_{\hat{y}} \quad \text{for each } x_i$$

For $x_i = 0$

$$6.13 \pm 2.76(0.0759)$$

$$6.13 \pm 0.2095$$

$$5.92 \leq \hat{y}_0 \leq 6.34$$

when $x = 0$ at $\alpha = 0.05$ for the expected (mean) value of y.
    For $x_i = 15$

$$5.52 \pm 2.76(0.0537)$$

$$5.52 \pm 0.1482$$

$$5.37 \leq \hat{y}_{15} \leq 5.67$$

when $x = 15$ at $\alpha = 0.05$ for the expected (mean) value of y.
    For $x_i = 30$

$$4.90 \pm 2.76(0.0438)$$

$$4.90 \pm 0.1209$$

$$4.78 \leq \hat{y}_{30} \leq 5.02$$

when $x = 30$ at $\alpha = 0.05$ for the expected (mean) value of y.
    For $x_i = 45$

$$4.29 \pm 2.76(0.0537)$$

$$4.29 \pm 0.1482$$

$$4.14 \leq \hat{y}_{45} \leq 4.44$$

when $x = 45$ at $\alpha = 0.05$ for the expected (mean) value of y.
    For $x_i = 60$

$$3.67 \pm 2.76(0.0759)$$

$$3.67 \pm 0.2095$$

$$3.46 \leq \hat{y}_{60} \leq 3.88$$

when $x = 60$ at $\alpha = 0.05$ for the expected (mean) value of y.
    Another way to do this is with a software computer program.
    Figure 18 provides a MiniTab® computer graph of the 95% confidence interval (outer two lines) as well as the predicted $\hat{y}_i$ values (inner line).

Log₁₀ Microbial Counts

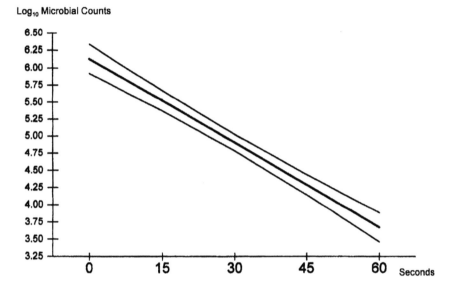

FIGURE 18   MiniTab® computer graph of the confidence interval and predicted values.

Notice that, although not dramatic, the confidence intervals widen for the $\hat{y}_i$ regression line as the data points move away from the mean ($\bar{x}$) value of 30. That is, the confidence interval is the most narrow where $x_i = \bar{x}$ and increases in size as the values of x_i become farther from $\bar{x}$ in either direction [35]. In addition, one is not restricted to the values of x for which one has corresponding y data. One can interpolate for any value between and including 0 to 60 seconds. The assumption, however, is that the actual y_i values for $x = (0, 60)$ follow the $\hat{y} = b_0 + b_1 x$ equation. Given that one has field experience, is familiar with the phenomena under investigation (here, antimicrobial death kinetics), and is sure the death curve remains log linear, there is no problem. If not, the researcher could make a huge mistake in thinking the interpolated data follow the computed regression line when they actually oscillate around the predicted regression line. Figure 19 illustrates this point graphically.

II. ANOVA AND REGRESSION

Analysis of variance (ANOVA) is a statistical methodology commonly used for checking the significance and adequacy of the calculated linear regression model. In simple linear—straight line—regression models, such as we are discussing now, ANOVA can be used for evaluating whether or not β_1 (slope) is 0. But it is particularly useful for evaluating models involving two

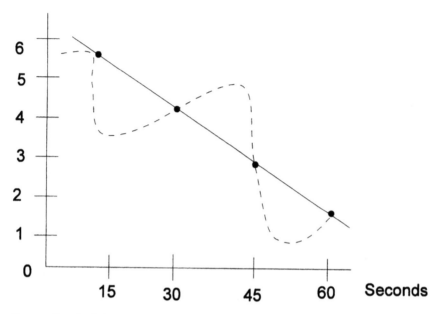

FIGURE 19 Antimicrobial death kinetics curve. (•) Actual collected data points; (—) predicted data points (regression analysis) that should be confirmed by the researcher's field experience; (- - -) actual data points unknown to the researcher. This example is exaggerated but emphasizes that statistics must be grounded in field science.

or more β_i, for example, determining whether extra β_i (e.g., β_2, β_3, β_k) are of statistical value [33–38]. However, in this text we will not explore its application to multiple β_i values.

The application of the ANOVA model to analysis of simple linear regression is similar to our previous work with ANOVA. In regression, three primary sum-of-squares values are needed: the total sum of squares, SS_T; the sum of squares explained by the regression, SS_R; and the sum of squares due to the random error, SS_E. The total sum of squares is merely the sum of squares of the differences between actual y_i observations and the $\bar{y}$ mean.

$$SS_{TOTAL} = \sum_{i=1}^{n}(y_i - \bar{y})^2 \qquad (29)$$

Graphically, the total sum of squares $(y_i - \bar{y})$ includes both the regression and error effects in that it does not distinguish between them (Fig. 20).

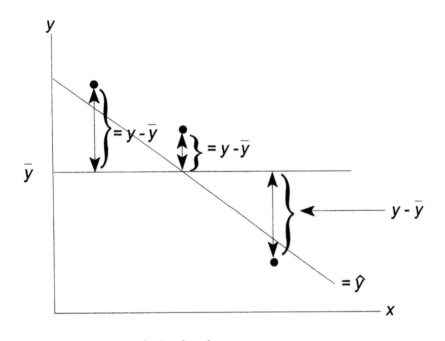

•●• **Actual values**

FIGURE 20   Total sum of squares.

The total sum of squares, to be useful, is partitioned into the sum of squares due to regression (SS_R) and the sum of squares due to error (SS_E), or random variability.

The sum of squares due to regression (SS_R) is the sum of squares value of the predicted values ($\hat{y}_i$) minus the $\bar{y}$ mean value.

$$SS_R = \sum_{i=1}^{n}(\hat{y}_i - \bar{y})^2 \qquad (30)$$

Figure 21 portrays this graphically. If the slope is 0, the SS_R value is 0 because the regression parameters $\hat{y}$ and $\bar{y}$ are the same values.

Finally, the sum of the squares error term, SS_E, is the sum of the squares of the actual Y_i values minus the predicted $\hat{y}_i$ value.

$$SS_E = \sum_{i=1}^{n}(y_i - \hat{y}_i)^2 \qquad (31)$$

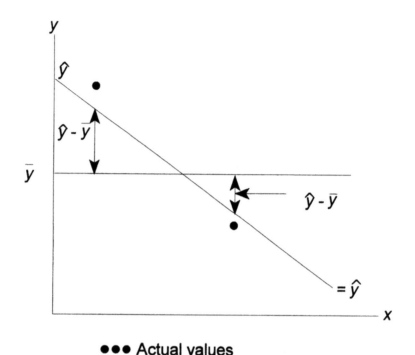

●●● Actual values

FIGURE 21   Sum of squares regression.

Figure 22 portrays this graphically. As before, the sums of SS_E and SS_R equal SS_{TOTAL}.

$$SS_R + SS_E = SS_{TOTAL} \tag{32}$$

The degrees of freedom for these three parameters and as the mean square error are presented in Table 4.

The entire ANOVA table is presented in Table 5.

The six-step procedure can easily be applied to the regression ANOVA for determining whether $\beta_1 = 0$. Let us now use the data in Example 1 to construct an ANOVA table.

Step 1.   Establish the hypothesis.

$H_0: \beta_1 = 0$

$H_A: \beta_1 \neq 0$

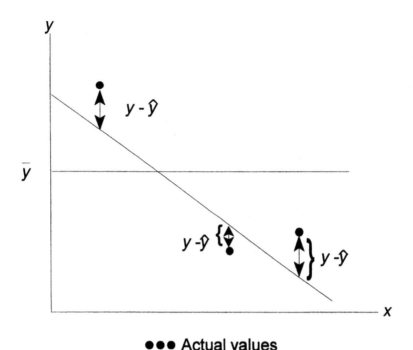

●●● Actual values

FIGURE 22   Sum-of-squares error term.

Step 2.   Select the α significance level. Let us set α at 0.10.
Step 3.   Specify the test statistic. The test statistic used to determine whether $B_1 = 0$ is found in Table 5.

$$F_C = \frac{MS_R}{MS_E}$$

TABLE 4   Degrees of Freedom and Mean Square Error

Sum of squares (SS)	Degrees of freedom (df)	Mean square
SS_R	1	$SS_R/1$
SS_E	$n-2$	$SS_E/n-2$
SS_{TOTAL}	$n-1$	Not calculated

TABLE 5 ANOVA Table

Source	SS	df	MS	F_C	F_T	Significant/ not Significant
Regression	$SS_R = \sum_{i=1}^{n}(\hat{y}_i - \bar{y})^2$	1	$\frac{SS_R}{1} = MS_R$ [a]	$\frac{MS_R}{MS_E}$	$F_{(\alpha;1,n-2)}$	If $F_c > F_T$, reject H_0
Error	$SS_E = \sum_{i=1}^{n}(y_i - \hat{y}_i)^2$	$n-2$	$\frac{SS_E}{n-2} = MS_E$			
Total	$SS_{TOTAL} = \sum_{i=1}^{n}(y_i - \bar{y})^2$	$n-1$				

[a] An alternative that is often useful for calculating MS_R is $b_1^2 \sum_{i=1}^{n}(y_i - \bar{x})^2$.

Step 4. Decision rule: if $F_C > F_T$, reject H_0 at α.
$F_T = F_{(\alpha;1,n-2)} = F_{0.10(1,13)} = 3.14$, from Table A.3, the F distribution.
If $F_C > 3.14$, reject H_0 at $\alpha = 0.10$.

Step 5. Compute ANOVA model. Recall from our calculations earlier, $\bar{y} = 4.90$.

$$SS_{TOTAL} = \sum_{i=1}^{n}(y_i - \bar{y})^2$$

$$= (6.09 - 4.90)^2 + (6.10 - 4.90)^2 + \cdots + (3.42 - 4.90)^2$$
$$+ (3.44 - 4.90)^2$$

$$= 11.685$$

SS_R (using the alternate formula): Recall that $\sum_{i=1}^{n}(x_i - \bar{x})^2 = 6750$ and $b_1 = -0.040933$.

$$SS_R = b_1^2 \sum_{i=1}^{n}(x_i - \bar{x})^2 = -0.040933^2(6750) = 11.3097$$

$$SS_E = SS_{TOTAL} - SS_R = 11.685 - 11.310 = 0.375$$

TABLE 6 ANOVA Table

Source	SS	df	MS	F_C	F_T	Significant/ not significant
Regression	$SS_R = 11.310$	1	11.310	392.71	3.14	Significant
Error	$SS_E = 0.375$	13	0.0288			
Total	11.685	14				

TABLE 7   MiniTab® Printout ANOVA Table

Analysis of Variance Source	DF	SS	MS	F	P
Regression	1	11.310	11.310	390.0	0.000
Residual error	13	0.375	0.029		
Total	14	11.685			

Step 6.   The researcher sees clearly that the regression slope b_1 is not equal to 0. That is, $F_C = 392.70 > F_T = 3.14$. Hence, the null hypothesis is rejected.

Table 6 provides the completed ANOVA model of this evaluation. Table 7 provides a MiniTab® version of this table.

A.   Linear Model Evaluation of Fit of the Model

The ANOVA F-test to determine the significance of the slope ($\beta_1 \neq 0$) is useful, but can it be expanded to evaluate the fit of the statistical model? That is, how well does the model predict the actual data? This procedure is often very important in multiple linear regression in determining whether increasing the number of variables (β_i) is statistically efficient and effective [25,29].

A lack-of-fit procedure, which is straightforward, can be used in this situation. However, it requires repeated measurements (i.e., replication) for at least some of the x_i values. The F-test for lack of fit is used to determine whether the regression model used (in our case, $\hat{y} = b_0 + b_1 x_i$) adequately predicts and models the data. If it does not, the researcher can (1) increase the beta variables, $\beta_2 \ldots \beta_n$, by collecting additional experimental information or (2) transform the scale of the data to linearize them.

For example, in Fig. 23, if the linear model is represented by a line and the data by dots, one can easily see that the model does not fit the data. In this case, a simple $\log_{10}$ transformation, without increasing the number of β_i values, may be the answer. Hence, a $\log_{10}$ transformation of the y values makes the simple regression model appropriate (Fig. 24).

In computing the lack-of-fit F-test, several assumptions about the data must be made [35]:

1. The y_i values corresponding to each x_i are independent of each other.
2. The y_i values are normally distributed and share the same variance.

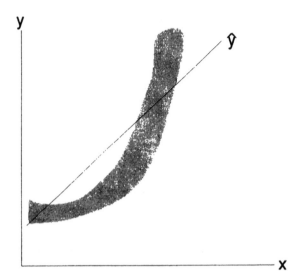

FIGURE 23   Inappropriate linear model.

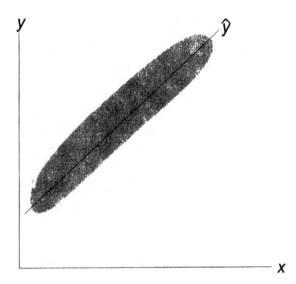

FIGURE 24   Simple regression model after $\log_{10}$ transformation.

In practice, assumption 1 is often difficult to ensure. For example, in a time–kill study, the exposure values y at 1 minute are related to the exposure values y at 30 seconds. This author has found that, even if the y values are correlated, the regression is still very useful and appropriate. However, it may be more useful to use a different statistical model (Box–Jenkins, weighted average, etc.) [31,33]. This is particularly so if values beyond the data range collected are predicted.

It is important to realize that the F-test for regression fit relies on replication of various x_i levels. These require actual replication of these levels, not just repeated measurements [27,30]. For example, if a researcher is evaluating the antimicrobial efficacy of an antimicrobial surgical scrub product by exposing a known number of microorganisms for 30 seconds to the antimicrobial compound, then neutralizing the antimicrobial and plating each dilution level three times would not constitute a triplicate replication. The entire procedure must be replicated, or repeated three times, to include initial population, exposure to the antimicrobial, neutralization, dilutions, and plating.

The model the F-test for lack of fit evaluates is $E[y] = b_0 + b_1 x_i$

$$H_0 : E[y] = b_0 + b_1 x_i$$

$$H_A : E[y] \neq b_0 + b_1 x_i \tag{33}$$

The statistical process utilizes a *full error* model and a *reduced error* model. The full model is evaluated first and often is represented by

$$y_{ij} = \mu_j + \epsilon_{ij} \tag{34}$$

where the μ_j are the parameters $j = 1, \ldots, k$.

The full model states that the y_{ij} values are made up of two components:

1. The expected "mean" response for the μ_j at a specific x_j value ($\mu_j = \bar{y}_j$)
2. The random error (ϵ_{ij})

The sum-of-squares error for the full model is considered "pure error," which will be used to determine the fit of the model. The pure error is any variation from $\bar{y}_j$ at a specific x_j level.

$$\text{SSE}_{\text{FULL}} = \text{SS}_{\text{PURE ERROR}} = \sum_{j=1}^{k} \sum_{i=1}^{n} (y_{ij} - \bar{y}_j)^2$$

The $\text{SS}_{\text{PURE ERROR}}$ is the variation of the replicate y_j values from the $\bar{y}_j$ value at each replicated x_j.

B. Reduced "Error" Model

The reduced model determines whether the actual regression model under the null hypothesis $(b_0 + b_1 x)$ is adequate to explain the data [36]. The reduced model is:

$$y_{ij} = b_0 + b_1 x_j + \epsilon_{ij} \tag{35}$$

That is, the amount that error is *reduced* due to the regression equation $(b_0 + b_1 x_i)$ in terms of

$$\epsilon = y - \hat{y} \tag{36}$$

or the actual value minus the predicted value is determined.

More formally:

Sum of squares reduced model

$$= SS_{(red)} = \sum_{i=1}^{k}\sum_{j=1}^{n}(y_{ij} - \hat{y}_{ij})^2 = \sum_{i=1}^{k}\sum_{j=1}^{n}[y_{ij} - (b_0 + b_1 x_j)]^2 \tag{37}$$

Note that

$$SS_{(red)} = SS_E. \tag{38}$$

It can be shown that the difference between SS_E and $SS_{\text{PURE ERROR}} = SS_{\text{lack of fit}}$.

$$SS_E = SS_{\text{PURE ERROR}} + SS_{\text{LACK OF FIT}} \tag{39}$$

$$(y_{ij} - \hat{y}_{ij})^2 = (y_{ij} - \bar{y}_j)^2 + (\bar{y}_j - \hat{y}_{ij})^2 \tag{40}$$
Total error   Pure error   Lack of fit

Let us look at this diagrammatically (Fig. 25). Pure error = difference of actual y values from $\bar{y}$ at a specific x (in this case, x_j, where $j = 4$).

$$y_i - \bar{y} = 23 - 21.33 = 1.67$$
$$21 - 21.33 = -0.33$$
$$20 - 21.33 = -1.33$$

Lack of fit = difference between the $\bar{y}$ value at a specific x and the predicted $\hat{y}$ at that specific x value, or $\bar{y}_4 - \hat{y}_4 = 21.33 - 16 = 5.33$.

The entire ANOVA procedure can be completed in conjunction with the previous F-test ANOVA by expanding the SS_E term to include both $SS_{\text{PURE ERROR}}$ and $SS_{\text{LACK OF FIT}}$. This procedure can be done only with replication of the x values (Table 8).

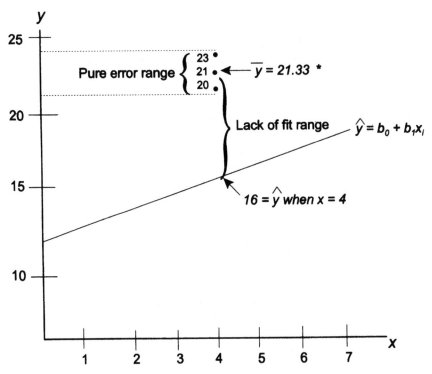

FIGURE 25 Lack-of-fit diagram. *21.33 is the average of $y_{1,4} = 23$, $y_{2,4} = 21$, and $y_{3,4} = 20$.

TABLE 8 ANOVA Table

Source	Sum of squares	Degrees of freedom	MS	F_c	F_T
Regression	$SS_R = \sum\limits_{i=n=1}^{n} \sum\limits_{j=k=1}^{k} (\hat{y}_{ij} - \bar{y})^2$	1	$\frac{SS_R}{1} = MS_R$	$\frac{MS_R}{MS_E}$	$F_{\alpha(1,n-2)}$
Error	$SS_E = \sum\limits_{i=1}^{n} \sum\limits_{j=1}^{k}(y_{ij} - \hat{y}_{ij})^2$	$n - 2$	$\frac{SS_E}{n-2} = MS_E$		
Lack-of-fit error	$SS_{LACK\ OF\ FIT}$ $= \sum\limits_{i=1}^{n} \sum\limits_{j=1}^{k}(\bar{y}_j - \hat{y}_{ij})^2$	$c - 2$	$\frac{SS_{LACK\ OF\ FIT}}{c-2}$ $= MS_{LF}$	$\frac{MS_{LF}}{MS_{PE}}$	$F_{\alpha(c-2,n-c)}$
Pure error	$SS_{PURE\ ERROR}$ $= \sum\limits_{i=1}^{n} \sum\limits_{j=1}^{k}(y_{ij} - \bar{y}_j)^2$	$n - c$	$\frac{SS_{PURE\ ERROR}}{n-c}$ $= MS_{PE}$		
Total	SS_{TOTAL} $= \sum\limits_{i=1}^{k} \sum\limits_{j=1}^{c}(y_{ij} - \bar{y})^2$	$n - 1$			

The test hypothesis for the lack of fit component is:

$H_0: E[y] = b_0 + b_1 x$ (linear regression adequately describes data)
$H_A: E[y] \neq b_0 + b_1 x$ (linear regression does not adequately describe data)
If $F_c = (MS_{LF}/MS_{PE}) > F_T[(F_{\alpha(c-2;n-c)})]$, reject H_0 at α.

where c = number of groups of data (replicated and nonreplicated), which is the number of different x_j levels
n = number of observations
Let us now work the data in Example 1.

The F-test for the lack of fit for the simple linear regression model is easily expressed in the six-step procedure.

Step 1. Determine the hypothesis.
$H_0: E[y] = b_0 + b_1 x$
$H_A: E[y] \neq b_0 + b_1 x$
Note: The null hypothesis for the lack of fit is that the simple linear regression model cannot be rejected at the specific α level.
Step 2. State the significance level (α). In this example, let us set α at 0.10.
Step 3. Write the test statistic to be used.

$$F_C = \frac{MS_{LACK\,OF\,FIT}}{MS_{PURE\,ERROR}}$$

Step 4. Specify the decision rule. If $F_C > F_T$, reject H_0 at α. In this example, the value for F_T is

$$F_{\alpha(c-2;n-c)} = F_{0.10;(5-2;15-5)} = F_{0.10(3,10)} = 2.73$$

So, if $F_c > 2.73$, reject H_0 at $\alpha = 0.10$.

Step 5. Perform the ANOVA. $n = 15$; $c = 5$

Level = j =	1	2	3	4	5
x_j	0	15	30	45	60
Replicate					
1	6.09	5.48	5.01	4.53	3.57
2	6.10	5.39	4.88	4.62	3.42
3	6.08	5.51	4.93	4.49	3.44
$\bar{y}_{.j}$ =	6.09	5.46	4.94	4.55	3.48

$$\text{SS}_{\text{PURE ERROR}} = \sum_{j=1}^{n}(y_{ij} - \bar{y}_j)^2 \text{ over the five levels of } x_j, c = 5.$$

$$\text{SS}_{\text{PE}} = (6.09 - 6.09)^2 + (6.10 - 6.09)^2 + (6.08 - 6.09)^2 + (5.48 - 5.46)^2$$
$$+ \cdots (3.57 - 3.48)^2 + (3.42 - 3.48)^2 + (3.44 - 3.48)^2$$
$$= 0.0388$$

$$\text{SS}_{\text{LACK OF FIT}} = \text{SS}_E - \text{SS}_{\text{PE}}$$
$$\text{SS}_E \text{ (from Table 6)} = 0.375$$
$$\text{SS}_{\text{LACK OF FIT}} = 0.375 - 0.0388 = 0.3362$$

In anticipation of this kind of analysis, it is often useful to include the lack of fit and pure error within the basic ANOVA table (Table 9). Note that the computations of lack of fit and pure error are a decomposition of SS_E.

Step 6. Decision. Because F_c (28.74) $> F_T$ (2.73), we reject H_0 at the α = 0.10 level. The rejection, i.e., the model is portrayed to lack fit, is primarily because there is too little variability within each of the j replicates used to obtain pure error. So, even though the actual data are reasonably well represented by the regression model, the model could be better.

The researcher must now weigh the pros and cons of the linear regression model. From a practical perspective, the model may very well be useful enough, even though the lack-of-fit error is significant [36,37]. In many situations experienced by this author, this model would be good enough. However, to a purist, perhaps a third variable (β_2) could be useful. But will a

TABLE 9 New ANOVA Table

Source	SS	df	MS	F_C	F_T	Significant/ not significant
Regression	11.3100	1	11.3100	392.71	3.14	Significant
Error	0.375	13	0.0288			
Lack-of-fit error	0.3362	3	0.1121	28.74	2.73	Significant
Pure error	0.0388	10	0.0039			
Total	11.6850	14				

third variable hold up in different studies? It may be better to collect more data and see if the simple linear regression model holds up in other cases. It is quite frustrating for the end user to have to compare different reports using different models to make decisions, let alone understand the underlying data. For example, if a decision maker reviews several death-rate kinetic studies of a specific product and specific microorganisms and the statistical model is different for each study, the decision-maker will probably not use the statistical analyst's services much longer. So, when possible, use general but robust models.

This author would elect to use the simple linear regression model to approximate the antimicrobial activity but would collect more data sets to see not only whether the H_0 hypothesis continues to be rejected but also whether the extra variable (β_2) model is adequate for the new data. In statistics, data pattern chasing can be an endless pursuit with no final conclusion ever reached.

If the simple linear regression model, in the researcher's opinion, does not model the data properly, there are several options:

1. Transform the data using EDA methods (to be discussed next).
2. Abandon the simple linear regression approach for a more complex one.
3. Use a nonparametric statistic analog.

When possible, transform the data because the simple (linear) regression model can still be used. However, there is certainly value in multiple regression procedures, in which the computations are done by matrix algebra [35,37]. The only practical approach to performing multiple regression is with a computer. Note that the replicate x_j values do not need to be consistent in number, as in our previous work in ANOVA. For example, if the data

TABLE 10   Lack-of-Fit Computation (ns Are Not Equal)

Level	j	1	2	3	4	5
	x value	0	15	30	45	60
	Corresponding y_{ij} values	6.09	5.48	5.01	4.53	3.57
			5.39	4.88	4.62	3.42
			5.51			3.44
	Mean $\bar{y}_j =$	6.09	5.46	4.95	4.58	3.48
	$n =$	1	3	2	2	3
where $n = 11, c = 5$						

collected were as in Table 10, the computation would be performed in the same way.

$$SS_{PURE ERROR} = (6.09 - 6.09)^2 + (5.48 - 5.46)^2 + (5.39 - 5.46)^2$$

$$+ (5.51 - 5.46)^2 + \cdots + (3.42 - 3.48)^2$$

$$+ (3.44 - 3.48)^2 = 0.0337$$

Degrees of freedom $= n - c = 11 - 5 = 6$
Given SS_E is 0.375, $SS_{LACK OF FIT}$ would equal:

$$SS_{LF} = SS_E - SS_{PURE ERROR} = 0.375 - 0.0337 = 0.3413$$

Source	SS	df	MS	F_c
SS_E	0.375	—	—	—
Error lack of fit	0.3413	3	0.1138	20.32
Pure error	0.0337	6	0.0056	

Let us now perform the lack-of-fit test with MiniTab® on the original data. Table 11 portrays this.

As one can see, the ANOVA consists of the regression and residual error (SS_E) term. The regression is highly significant, with an F_c of 392.27. The residual error (SS_E) is broken into lack of fit and pure error. As before, the researcher sees that the lack-of-fit component is significant. That is, the linear model is not a precise fit even though, from a practical perspective, the linear regression model may be adequate.

For many decision-makers, as well as applied researchers, it is one thing to generate a complex regression model but another entirely to explain its meaning in terms of variables grounded in one's field of expertise. For those interested in much more depth in regression, see *Applied Regression Analysis* by Kleinbaum et al. [35], *Applied Regression Analysis* by Draper and Smith [32], or *Applied Linear Statistical Models* by Neter et al. [33].

The vast majority of data can be linearized by merely performing a transformation. For the data that have nonconstant error variances, sigmoidal shapes, and other anomalies, the use of nonparametric regression is an option.

Let us now refocus on exploratory data analysis (EDA) as it applies to regression.

TABLE 11   MiniTab® Lack-of-Fit Test

Analysis of Variance Source P	D-	F	SS	MS	F
Regression	1	11.310	11.310	390.0	0.000
Residual error	13	0.375	0.029		
Lack of fit	3	0.336	0.112	28.0	0.000
Pure error	10	0.039	0.004		
Total	14	11.685			

C. Exploratory Data Analysis and Regression

Recall that, in Chap. 3, Table 5 provided a table of reexpressions as well as suggestions for what to do for nonnormal (skewed) data. A similar strategy works well for regression data. In simple (linear) regression, of the form $\hat{y} = b_0 + b_1 x$, the data must approximate a straight line. In practice, this often does not occur, so in order to use the regression equation, the data need to be "straightened." Four common nonlinear data patterns can be straightened very simply. Figure 26 portrays these patterns.

1. Pattern A

For pattern A, the researcher will "go down" in the reexpression power of either x or y or both. Often, audiences grasp the data more easily if the transformation is done on the y scale ($\sqrt{y}$, $\log_{10} y$, etc.) rather than on the x scale. The x scale is left at power 1; that is, it is not reexpressed. The regression is then "refit," using the transformed data scale and checked to assure the data have been straightened [14,15]. If the plotted data do not appear straight-line, the data are reexpressed again, say from $\sqrt{y}$ to $\log y$ or even $-1\sqrt{y}$ (see Chap. 3). This process is done iteratively. In cases in which one transformation almost straightens the data but the next power transformation over-straightens the data slightly, the researcher may opt to choose the reexpression that has the smallest F_c value for lack of fit.

2. Pattern B

Data appearing like pattern B may be linearized by increasing the power of the y values (e.g., y^2, y^3), increasing the power of the x values (e.g., x^2, x^3), or increasing the power of both (y^2, x^2). Again, it is often easier for the intended audience—decision-makers, business directors, or clients—to understand the data when y is reexpressed and x is left in the original scale. As before, the reexpression procedure is done sequentially (y^2 to y^3, etc.),

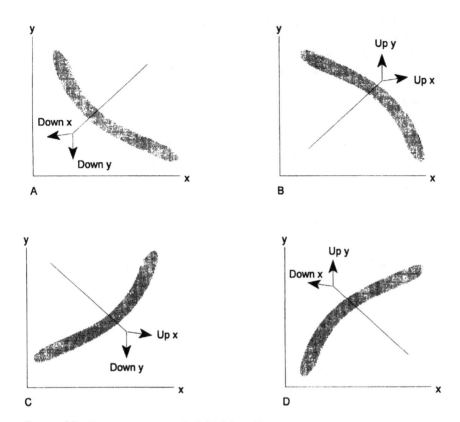

FIGURE 26   Four common nonstraight data patterns.

computing the F_c value for lack of fit each time. The smaller the F_c value, the better. I find it most helpful to plot the data after each reexpression procedure in order to select the best fit visually. The more linear the data are, the better.

3.   Pattern C

For data that resemble pattern C, the researcher needs to "up" the power scale of x (x^2, x^3, etc.) or "down" the power scale of y ($\sqrt{y}$, log y, etc.) to linearize the data. For reasons previously discussed, I tend to recommend transforming the y values only, leaving the x values in the original form. When the data have been reexpressed, plot them to help determine visually whether the reexpression adequately linearized them. If not, the next lower power transformation should be used, on the y value in this case. Once the data are reasonably linear, as determined visually, the F_c test for lack of fit can be used. The smaller the F_c value, the better. If, say, the data are not quite linearized by $\sqrt{y}$ but are slightly curved in the opposite direction with the log y transformation, pick the reexpression having the smaller F_c value in the lack-of-fit test.

4. Pattern D

For data that resemble pattern D, the researcher can go up the power scale in reexpressing y or down the power scale in reexpressing x, or do both. Again, I recommend reexpressing the y values (y^2, y^3, etc.) only. The same strategy previously discussed should be used in determining the most appropriate reexpression, based on the F_c value.

5. Data That Cannot Be Linearized by Reexpression

Data that are sigmoidal, or open up and down or down and up, cannot be easily transformed. A change to one area (making it linear) makes the other

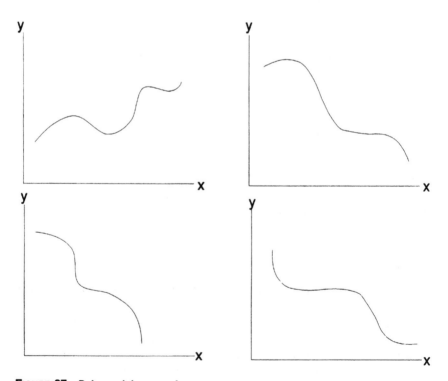

FIGURE 27   Polynomial regressions.

areas even worse. Polynomial regression, a form of multiple regression, can be used for modeling these types of data (see Fig. 27) [25, 33, 35, 37].

D. Exploratory Data Analysis to Determine the Linearity of a Regression Line Without Using the F_C Test for Lack of Fit

A relatively simple and effective way of determining whether a selected reexpression procedure linearizes the data can be completed with EDA pencil-and-paper techniques (Fig. 28). It is known as the method of half-slopes in EDA parlance [15,39].

> *Step* 1. Divide the data into thirds, finding the median (x,y) value of each group. Note that there is no need to be "ultra-accurate" when partitioning the data into the three groups. To find the left x, y medians (denoted x_L, y_L), use the left one third of the data. To find the middle x, y medians, use the middle one third of the data, and label these x_M, y_M. To find the right x, y medians, denoted x_R, y_R, use the right one third of the data.
>
> *Step* 2. Estimate the slope (b_1) for both the left and right thirds of the data set.

$$b_L = \frac{y_M - y_L}{x_M - x_L} \tag{41}$$

$$b_R = \frac{y_R - y_M}{x_R - x_M} \tag{42}$$

> where y_M = median of the y values in the middle third of the data set
> y_L = median of the y values in the left third of the data set
> y_R = median of the y values in the right third of the data set
> x_M = median of the x values in the middle third of the data set
> x_L = median of the x values in the left third of the data set
> x_R = median of the x values in the right third of the data set

> *Step* 3. Determine the slope coefficient b_R / b_L. (43)
>
> *Step* 4. If the b_R / b_L ratio is close to 1, the data are considered linear and "good enough." If not, reexpress the data and repeat steps 1 through 3. In practice, I suggest, when reexpressing a data set to approximate a straight line, that this EDA procedure be used rather than the F_c test for lack of fit.

Also note that, for any data set, approximations of β_1 (slope) and β_0 (y intercept) can be computed using the median values.

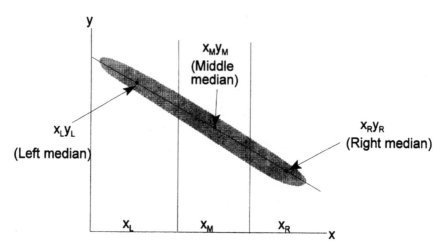

FIGURE 28   Halfslopes in EDA.

$$b_1 = \frac{y_R - y_L}{x_R - x_L} \tag{44}$$

$$b_0 = y_M - b_1(x_M) \tag{45}$$

Let us use the data in Example 1 to perform the EDA procedures just discussed. Because these data cannot be partitioned into equal thirds, the data will be approximately separated into thirds. Because the left and right thirds have more influence on this EDA procedure than the middle group, we will use $x = 0$ and 15 in the left group, only $x = 30$ in the middle group, and $x = 45$ and 60 in the right group.

Step 1.   Separate the data into thirds at the x levels.

Left group	Middle group	Right group
$x = 0$ and 15	$x = 30$	$x = 45$ and 60
$x_L = 7.5$	$x_M = 30$	$x_R = 52.50$
$y_L = 5.78$	$y_M = 4.93$	$y_R = 4.03$

Step 2.   Compute the slopes (β_1) for the left and right groups.

$$b_L = \frac{y_M - y_L}{x_M - x_L} = \frac{4.93 - 5.78}{30 - 7.5} = -0.0378$$

$$b_R = \frac{y_R - y_M}{x_R - x_M} = \frac{4.03 - 4.93}{52.5 - 30} = -0.0400$$

Step 3. Compute the slope coefficient, checking it to see if it equals 1.

$$\text{Slope coefficient} = \frac{b_R}{b_L} = \frac{-0.0400}{-0.0378} = 1.0582$$

Note, in this procedure, that it is just as easy to see if $b_R = b_L$. If they are not exactly equal, it is the same as the slope coefficient not equaling 1. Because the slope coefficient ratio in our example is very close to 1 (and the values b_R and b_L are nearly equal), we can say that the data set is approximately linear.

If the researcher wants a rough idea of what the slope (b_1) and y intercept (b_0) are, they can be computed using Eqs. (44) and (45).

$$b_1 = \frac{y_R - y_L}{x_R - x_L} = \frac{4.03 - 5.78}{52.5 - 7.5} = -0.0389$$

$$b_0 = y_M - b_1(x_M) = 4.93 - (-0.0389)30 = 6.097$$

Hence, before we have even opened discussion of nonparametric statistics, we have determined a "nonparametric" regression estimate of the regression equation, $\hat{y} = b_0 + b_1 x_1$, or $\hat{y} = 6.097 - 0.0389x$, which is very close to the parametric result, $\hat{y} = 6.13 - 0.041x$, computed using the formal regression procedure.

E. Correlation Coefficient

The correlation coefficient, r, is a statistic frequently used to measure the strength of association between x and y. A correlation coefficient of 1.00, or 100%, is a perfect fit (all of the predicted $\hat{y}$ values equal the actual y values), and a 0 value represents a completely random array of data (Fig. 29).

Theoretically, the range is -1 to 1, where -1 describes a perfect fit, descending slope (Fig. 30).

The correlation coefficient (r) is a dimensionless value independent of x and y. Note that, in practice, the value for r^2 (coefficient of determination) is generally more directly applicable. That is, knowing that $r = 0.80$ is not directly useful, but $r^2 = 0.80$ is, because the r^2 means that the regression equation is 80% better in predicting y than is the use of $\bar{y}$.

The more positive the r (closer to 1), the stronger the statistical association. That is, the accuracy and precision of predicting a y value from x increase. It also means that, as the values of x increase, so do the y values. Likewise, the more negative the r value (closer to -1), the stronger the statistical association. In this case, as the x values increase, the y values decrease. The closer the r value is to 0, the less linear association there is between x and y, meaning the

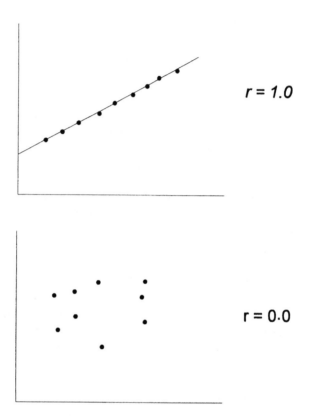

FIGURE 29   Correlation coefficients.

accuracy in predictions of a y value from an x value decreases. By association, I mean dependence of y and x. That is, one can predict y by knowing x.

The correlation coefficient value, r, is computed as:

$$r = \frac{\sum_{i=1}^{n}(x_i - \bar{x})^2(y_i - \bar{y})^2}{\sqrt{\sum_{i=1}^{n}(x_i - \bar{x})^2 \sum_{i=1}^{n}(y_i - \bar{y})^2}} \tag{46}$$

A simpler formula is often used for hand calculator computation:

$$r = \frac{\sum_{i=1}^{n} x_i y_i - \left(\sum_{i=1}^{n} x_i\right)\left(\sum_{i=1}^{n} y_i\right)/n}{\sqrt{\left[\sum_{i=1}^{n} x_i^2 - \left(\sum_{i=1}^{n} x_i\right)^2/n\right]\left[\sum_{i=1}^{n} y_i^2 - \left(\sum_{i=1}^{n} y_i\right)^2/n\right]}} \tag{47}$$

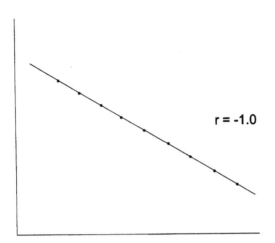

r = -1.0

FIGURE 30   Perfect descending slope.

Fortunately, even the less expensive scientific calculators usually have an internal program for calculating r.

Let us compute r from the data in Example 1.

$$\sum_{i=1}^{n} x_i y_i = \sum_{i=1}^{15}(0 \cdot 6.09)+(0 \cdot 6.10)+\cdots+(60 \cdot 3.57)+(60 \cdot 3.42)+(60 \cdot 3.44)$$
$$= 1929.90$$

$$\sum_{i=1}^{15} x_i = 450$$

$$\sum_{i=1}^{15} y_i = 73.54$$

$$\sum_{i=1}^{15} x_i^2 = 20250.00$$

$$\sum_{i=1}^{15} y_i^2 = 372.23$$

$$n = 15$$

$$r = \frac{1929.90 - (450)(73.54)/15}{\sqrt{[20250.00 - (450)^2/15][372.23 - (73.54)^2/15]}} = -0.9837$$

The correlation coefficient is -0.9837 or, as a percentage, 98.37%. This value represents a strong negative correlation. But the more useful value to use, in this author's view, is the coefficient of determination, r^2. In this example, $r^2 = (-0.9837)^2 = 0.9677$. This r^2 value translates directly to the strength of association. That is, 96.77% of the variability of the (x, y) data can be explained through the linear regression function. Notice in Table 3 that the r^2 is given as 96.8% (or 0.968) from the MiniTab® computer software regression routine. Also:

$$r^2 = \frac{SS_T - SS_E}{SS_T} = \frac{SS_R}{SS_T}$$

where

$$SS_T = \sum_{i=1}^{n}(y_i - \bar{y})^2$$

r^2 ranges between 0 and 1, or $0 \le r^2 \le 1$.

SS_R, as the reader will recall, is the amount of total variability directly due to the regression model. SS_E is the error not accounted for by the regression equation, which is generally called random error. Recall that $SS_T = SS_R + SS_E$. The larger SS_R is relative to error, SS_E, the greater the r^2 value. Likewise, the larger SS_E is relative to SS_R, the smaller (closer to 0) r^2 will be.

Again, r^2 is, in this author's opinion, the better of the two (r^2 vs. r) to use because r^2 can be applied directly to the outcome of the regression. If $r^2 = 0.50$, the researcher can conclude that 50% of the total variability is explained by the regression equation. This is no better than using the average $\bar{y}$ as predictor and dropping the need for the $\bar{x}$ dimension entirely. Note that when $r^2 = 0.50$, $r = 0.71$. The correlation coefficient can be deceptive in cases like this, for it can lead a researcher to conclude that a higher degree of statistical association exists than actually does.

Neither r^2 nor r is a measure of the magnitude of b_1, the slope. Hence, it cannot be said that the greater the slope value b_1, the larger r^2 or r will be (Fig. 31). If all the predicted values and actual values are the same, $r^2 = 1$, no matter what the slope and as long as there is a slope. If there is no slope, b_1 drops out and b_0 becomes the best estimate of y, which turns out to be $\bar{y}$. Instead, r^2 is a measure of how close the actual y values are to the $\hat{y}$ values (Fig. 32).

Finally, r^2 is not a measure of the appropriateness of the linear model (see Fig. 33). The $r^2 = 0.82$ for this model is high, but it is obvious that a linear model is not appropriate.

For Fig. 34, the $r^2 = 0.12$. Clearly, these data are not linear and not evaluated well by linear regression.

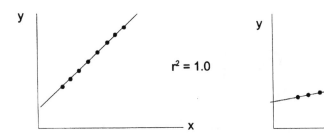

FIGURE 31   Correlation of slope rates.

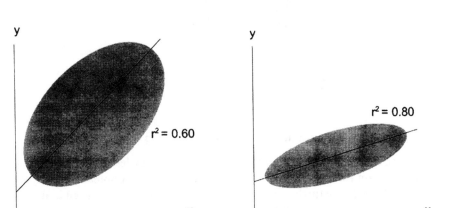

FIGURE 32   Degree of closeness of y to $\hat{y}$.

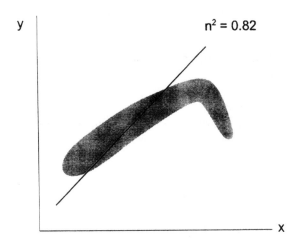

FIGURE 33   Inappropriate linear model.

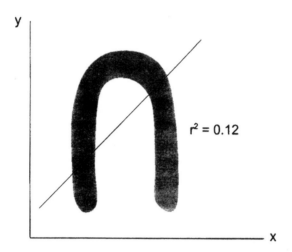

FIGURE 34   Nonlinear model.

F. Correlation Coefficient Hypothesis Testing

Because the researcher will undoubtedly be faced with describing the regression function via the correlation coefficient r, which is a popular statistic, we will develop its use further. The correlation coefficient can be used to determine whether $r = 0$ and, if $r = 0$, b_1 also equals 0. This computation can be performed with the six-step procedure.

Step 1.   Determine hypothesis.
   H_0: $R = 0$ (x and y are not associated)
   H_A: $R \neq 0$ (x and y are associated)
Step 2.   Set α level.
Step 3.   Write out the test statistic, which is a t-test presented in Eq. (48).

$$t_c = \frac{r\sqrt{n - 2}}{\sqrt{1 - r^2}} \quad \text{with } n - 2 \text{ degrees of freedom} \tag{48}$$

Step 4.   Decision rule.

   If $|t_c| > t_{(\alpha/2, n-2)}$, reject H_0 at α.

Step 5.   Perform computation.
Step 6.   Make the decision.

Example 1 (continued)   Using our chapter example (Example 1), let us
do the problem.

Step 1. H_0: $R=0$
          H_A: $R \neq 0$
Step 2.   Let us set $\alpha = 0.05$. Because this is a two-tail test, the t tabled
          (t_t) value will utilize $\alpha/2$ from Table A.2.
Step 3.   The test statistic is:

$$t_c = \frac{r\sqrt{n-2}}{\sqrt{1-r^2}}$$

Step 4.   If $|t_c| > t_{(0.05/2, 15-2)} = 2.16$, reject H_0 at $\alpha = 0.05$.
Step 5.   Perform computation.

$$t_c = \frac{-0.9837\sqrt{15-2}}{\sqrt{1-0.9677}} = \frac{-3.5468}{0.1797} = -19.7348$$

Step 6.   Decision. Because $|t_c| = 19.7348 > t_{(\alpha/2, 13)} = 2.16$, the H_0
hypothesis is rejected at $\alpha = 0.05$. The correlation coefficient is not
0, nor does the slope $b_1 = 0$.

G. Confidence Interval for R

A $1 - \alpha$ confidence interval can be derived using a modification of Fisher's Z
transformation [34]. The transformation has the form

$$\frac{1}{2} \ln \frac{1+r}{1-r}$$

The researcher also uses the normal Z table (Table A.1) instead of Student's t
table. The test is reasonably powerful as long as $n \geq 20$.
     The complete confidence interval is:

$$\frac{1}{2} \ln \frac{1+r}{1-r} \pm \frac{Z_{\alpha/2}}{\sqrt{n-3}} \tag{49}$$

The quantity $\frac{1}{2} \ln[(1+r)/(1-r)]$ approximates the mean and $Z_{\alpha/2}/\sqrt{n-3}$
the variance.

     Lower limit $= \dfrac{1}{2} \ln \dfrac{1+L_r}{1-L_r}$ $\tag{50}$

The lower limit value is then found in Table A.16 (Fisher Z transformation
table) for the corresponding r value.

     Upper limit $= \dfrac{1}{2} \ln \dfrac{1+U_r}{1-U_r}$ $\tag{51}$

The upper limit is also found in Table A.16 for the corresponding r value.

The $(1 - \alpha)$ 100% confidence interval is of the form $L_r < R < U_r$. Let us use Example 1. Four steps are required for the calculator.

Step 1. Compute basic interval, letting $\alpha = 0.05$, $Z_{0.05/2} = 1.96$ (Table A).

$$\frac{1}{2} \ln \frac{1 + 0.9837}{1 - 0.9837} \pm \frac{1.96}{\sqrt{15 - 3}}$$

2.4008 ± 0.5658

Step 2. Compute lower/upper limits.
$L_r = 2.4008 - 0.5658 = 1.8350$
$U_r = 2.4008 + 0.5658 = 2.9660$

Step 3. Find L_r (1.8350) in Table A.16 (Fisher's Z transformation table), and then find the corresponding value of r.
$r = 0.95$
Find U_r (2.9660) in Table A.16 (Fisher's Z transformation table), and again find the corresponding value of r.
$r = 0.994$

Step 4. Display $1 - \alpha$ confidence interval.

$0.950 < R < 0.994$

at $\alpha = 0.05$.

Note: This researcher has adapted the Fisher test to a t-table test, which is useful for smaller sample sizes. It is a more conservative test than the Z-test, so the confidence intervals will be wider until the sample size of the t table is large enough to equal the Z table value.

Basic modified interval:

$$\frac{1}{2} \ln \frac{1 + r}{1 - r} \pm \frac{t_{\alpha/2;(n-2)}}{\sqrt{n - 3}} \tag{52}$$

Everything else is the same as for the Z-based confidence interval example.

Example 1 (continued). Let $\alpha = 0.05$; $t_{(\alpha/2; n-2)} = t_{(0.05/2, 13)} = 2.16$, as found in Student's t table (Table A.2).

Step 1. Compute the basic interval.

$$\frac{1}{2} \ln \frac{1 + 0.9837}{1 - 0.9837} \pm \frac{2.16}{\sqrt{15 - 3}} = 2.4008 \pm 0.6235 \tag{53}$$

Step 2. Compute the lower/upper limits, as before.

$$L_r = 2.4008 - 0.6235 = 1.7773$$

$$L_u = 2.4008 + 0.6235 = 3.0243$$

Step 3. Find L_r (1.773) in Table A.16 (Fisher's Z table), and find the corresponding value of r.

$r = 0.944$

Find U_r (3.0243) in Table A.16 (Fisher's Z table), and find the corresponding value of r.

$r = 0.995$

Step 4. Display the $1 - \alpha$ confidence interval.

$0.944 < R < 0.995$

at $\alpha = 0.05$.

H. Prediction of a Specific *x* Value from a *y* Value

There are times when a researcher wants to predict a specific x value from a y value as well as generate confidence intervals for that estimated x value. For example, in microbial death kinetic studies (D values), a researcher often wants to know how much exposure time (x) is required to reduce a microbial population, say, three logs from the baseline value. In this situation, the researcher will predict x from y. Or a researcher may want to know how long an exposure time (x) is required for an antimicrobial sterilant to reduce the population to zero. Many microbial death kinetic studies, including those using dry heat, steam, ethylene oxide, and gamma radiation, can be computed in this way [1]. The most common procedure uses the D value, which is the time (generally in minutes) in which the initial microbial population is reduced by one $\log_{10}$ value.

The procedure is quite straightforward, requiring just basic algebraic manipulation of the linear regression equation, $\hat{y} = b_0 + b_1 x$. As rearranged, then, the regression equation used to predict the x value is

$$\hat{x} = \frac{y - b_0}{b_1} \tag{54}$$

The process requires that a standard regression, $\hat{y} = b_0 + b_1 x$, be computed to estimate β_0 and β_1. It is then necessary to ensure that the regression fit is adequate for the data described. At that point, the b_0 and b_1 values can be inserted into Eq. 54.

Equation (55) works from results of Eq. (54) to provide a confidence interval for $\hat{x}$. The $1 - \alpha$ confidence interval equation for $\hat{x}$ is:

$$\hat{x} \pm t_{\alpha/2;n-2} S_x \tag{55}$$

where:

$$S_x^2 = \frac{MSE}{b_1^2}\left[1 + \frac{1}{n} + \frac{(\hat{x} - \bar{x})^2}{\sum\limits_{i=1}^{n}(x_i - \bar{x})^2}\right] \tag{56}$$

Let us perform the computation using the data in Example 1 to demonstrate this procedure. The researcher's question is "how long an exposure to the test antimicrobial product is required to achieve a two $\log_{10}$ reduction from the baseline?"

Recall that the regression for this example has already been completed. It is $\hat{y} = 6.13067 - 0.040933x$, where $b_0 = 6.13067$ and $b_1 = -0.040933$. First, the researcher calculates the theoretical baseline, or beginning value of y when $x = 0$ time: $\hat{y} = b_0 + b_1 x = 6.13067 - 0.040933(0) = 6.13$. The two $\log_{10}$ reduction time is found by using Eq. (54), $\hat{x} = (y - b_0)/b_1$, where y is a two $\log_{10}$ reduction from $\hat{y}$ at time 0. We calculate this value as $6.13 - 2.0 = 4.13$. Then, using Eq. (54), we can determine $\hat{x}$, or the time in seconds for the example.

$$\hat{x} = \frac{4.13 - 6.13}{-0.041} = 48.78 \text{ seconds}$$

The confidence interval for this $\hat{x}$ estimate is computed as follows, where $\bar{x} = 30$, $n = 15$, $\sum_{i=1}^{n}(x_i - \bar{x})^2 = 6750$, and $MSE = 0.0288$. Using Eq. (55), $\hat{x} \pm t_{\alpha/2; n-2} S_x$, and $t_{(0.05/2, 15-2)} = 2.16$ (from Table A.2)

$$S_x^2 = \frac{MSE}{b_1^2}\left[1 + \frac{1}{n} + \frac{(\hat{x} - \bar{x})^2}{\sum\limits_{i=1}^{n}(x_i - \bar{x})^2}\right]$$

$$S_x^2 = \frac{0.0288}{(-0.041)^2}\left[1 + \frac{1}{15} + \frac{(48.78 - 30)^2}{6750}\right]$$

$$S_x^2 = 19.170 \quad \text{and} \quad S_x = 4.378$$

$$\hat{x} \pm t_{0.05/2,13} S_x$$

$$48.78 \pm 2.16(4.378)$$

$$48.78 \pm 9.46$$

$$39.32 \le \hat{x} \le 58.24$$

So, the actual new value, $\hat{x}$, on $y = 4.13$ is contained in the interval $39.32 \le \hat{x} \le 58.24$ when $\alpha = 0.05$. This is a 18.92-second spread, which may not be very useful to the researcher. The main reasons for the wide confidence interval are variability in the data and that one is predicting a specific, not an average, value. The researcher may want to increase the sample size to reduce the variability or may settle for the average expected value of x because the confidence interval will be narrower.

I. Predicting an Average $\hat{x}$

Often, a researcher is more interested in the average value of $\hat{x}$. In this case, the formula for determining x is the same as Eq. (54).

$$\hat{x} = \frac{y - b_0}{b_1} \tag{54}$$

The equation for calculating the $1 - \alpha$ confidence interval is nearly the same [Eq. (57)]. The difference is that the 1 is removed from Eq. (56) in order to calculate the value of $S_{\bar{x}}$, as can be seen in Eq. (58).

$$\hat{x} \pm t_{\alpha/2;n-2} S_{\bar{x}} \tag{57}$$

$$S_{\bar{x}} = \frac{MS_E}{b_1^2} \left[\frac{1}{n} + \frac{(\hat{x} - \bar{x})^2}{\sum\limits_{i=1}^{n}(x_i - \bar{x})^2} \right] \tag{58}$$

Let us use Example 1 again. Here, the researcher wants to know, on the average, what the 95% confidence interval is for $\hat{x}$ when y is 4.13 (or a two $\log_{10}$ reduction).

$\hat{x} = 48.78$ seconds, as before

$$S_x^2 = \frac{0.0288}{(-0.041)^2} \left[\frac{1}{15} + \frac{(48.78 - 30)^2}{6750} \right] = 2.037$$

$S_x = 1.427$

$\hat{x} \pm t_{(\alpha/2,n-2)} S_{\bar{x}} = \hat{x} \pm t_{0.025, \ 13} S_{\bar{x}}$

$48.78 \pm 2.16(1.427)$

48.78 ± 3.08

$45.70 \leq \hat{x} \leq 51.86$

So, on the average, the time required to reduce the initial population is between 45.70 and 51.86 seconds. For practical purposes, the researcher may round up to a 1-minute exposure.

J. D Value Computation

The D value is the time, usually in minutes, of exposure to steam, dry heat, or ethylene oxide that it takes to reduce the initial microbial population one $\log_{10}$.

$$\hat{y} = b_0 + b_1 x$$

$$\hat{x}_D = \frac{y - b_0}{b_1} \tag{59}$$

Note that, when we look at a one $\log_{10}$ reduction, $y - b_0$ will always be 1. Hence, the D value, $\hat{x}_D$, will always equal $|1/b_1|$.

The D value can also be computed for a new specific value. The complete formula is:

$$\hat{x}_D \pm t_{(\alpha/2, n-2)} S_x$$

where

$$S_x^2 = \frac{MS_E}{b_1^2}\left[1 + \frac{1}{n} + \frac{(\hat{x}_D - \bar{x})^2}{\sum\limits_{i=1}^{n}(x_i - \bar{x})^2}\right] \tag{60}$$

Or the D value can be computed for the average or expected value $E(x)$.

$$\hat{x}_D \pm t_{(\alpha/2; n-2)} S_{\bar{x}}$$

where

$$S_{\bar{x}}^2 = \frac{MS_E}{b_1^2}\left[\frac{1}{n} + \frac{(\hat{x}_D - \bar{x})^2}{\sum\limits_{i=1}^{n}(x_i - \bar{x})}\right] \tag{61}$$

Example 8.   Suppose the researcher wants to compute the average D value, or the time it takes to reduce the initial population one $\log_{10}$.

$$\hat{x}_D = \left|\frac{1}{b_1}\right| = \left|\frac{1}{-0.041}\right| = 24.39$$

$$S_{\bar{x}}^2 = \frac{MS_E}{b_1^2}\left[\frac{1}{n} + \frac{(\hat{x} - \bar{x})^2}{\sum\limits_{i=1}^{n}(x - \bar{x})^2}\right] = \frac{0.0288}{-0.041^2}\left[\frac{1}{15} + \frac{(24.39 - 30)^2}{6750}\right] = 1.222$$

$$S_{\bar{x}} = 1.11$$
$$\hat{x}_D \pm t_{\alpha/2, n-2} S_{\bar{x}}$$
$$24.39 \pm 2.16(1.11)$$
$$24.39 \pm 2.40$$
$$21.59 \le \hat{x}_D \le 26.79$$

Hence, the D value, on the average, is contained within the interval $21.59 \le \hat{x}_D \le 26.79$ at the 95% level of confidence.

K. Simultaneous MEAN Inference of B_0 and B_1

In certain situations, such as antimicrobial time-kill studies, an investigator may be interested in the average confidence intervals for both b_0 (initial population) and b_1 (rate of inactivation). In previous examples, confidence intervals were calculated for b_0 and b_1 separately. Now we will discuss how confidence intervals for both b_0 and b_1 can be achieved simultaneously. In some text books, this is known as joint confidence intervals [26,33,37,38]. We will use the Bonferroni method for this procedure.

Recall:

$$\beta_0 = b_0 \pm t_{(\alpha/2,n-2)}S_{b_0}$$
$$\beta_1 = b_1 \pm t_{(\alpha/2,n-2)}S_{b_1}$$

Because we are estimating two parameters, b_0 and b_1, we will use $\alpha/2 + \alpha/2 = \alpha/4$. So the revised formulas for b_0 and b_1 are:

$$\beta_0 = b_0 \pm t_{(\alpha/4,n-2)}S_{b_0} \tag{62}$$

$$\beta_1 = b_1 \pm t_{(\alpha/4,n-2)}S_{b_1} \tag{63}$$

where:

$b_0 = y$ intercept

$b_1 = $ slope

$$S_{b_0}^2 = MS_E\left[\frac{1}{n} + \frac{\bar{x}^2}{\sum\limits_{i=1}^{n}(x_i - \bar{x})^2}\right]$$

$$S_{b_1}^2 = \frac{MS_E}{\sum\limits_{i=1}^{n}(x_i - \bar{x})^2}$$

Let us now perform the computation using the data in Example 1. Recall that $b_0 = 6.13$, $b_1 = -0.041$, $MS_E = 0.0288$, $\sum_{i=1}^{n}(x_i - \bar{x})^2 = 6750$, $\bar{x} = 30$, $n = 15$, $\alpha = 0.05$. From Table A.2, Student's t table, $t_{\alpha/4,n-2} = t_{0.05/4,15-2} = t_{0.0125,13} \approx 2.5$.

$S_{b_1} = 0.0021$

$S_{b_0} = 0.0759$

$\beta_0 = b_0 \pm t_{(\alpha/4,n-2)}\left(S_{b_0}\right)$

$\quad = 6.13 + 0.1898 = 6.32$

$\quad = 6.13 - 0.1898 = 5.94$

$5.94 \leq \beta_0 \leq 6.32$

$$\beta_1 = b_1 \pm t_{(\alpha/4, n-2)}(S_{b_1})$$

$$= -0.041 + 0.0053 = -0.036$$

$$= -0.041 - 0.0053 = -0.046$$

$$-0.046 \leq \beta_1 \leq -0.036$$

Hence, the joint 95% confidence intervals for β_0 and β_1 are:

$$5.94 \leq \beta_0 \leq 6.32$$

$$-0.046 \leq \beta_1 \leq -0.036$$

The researcher can conclude, at the 95% confidence level, that the initial microbial population (β_0) is between 5.94 and 6.32 logs and the rate of inactivation (β_1) is between 0.046 and 0.036 $\log_{10}$ per second of exposure.

L. Simultaneous Multiple Mean Estimates of Y

There are times when a researcher wants to estimate the mean y values for multiple x values simultaneously. For example, suppose a researcher wants to predict the $\log_{10}$ microbial counts (y) at times 1, 10, 30, and 40 seconds after the exposures and wants to be sure of their overall confidence at $\alpha = 0.10$.

The Bonferroni procedure can again be used for $x_1, x_2, \ldots x_r$ simultaneous estimates.

$$\hat{y} \pm t_{(\alpha/2r, n-2)} S_{\bar{y}} \quad \text{(mean response)} \tag{64}$$

where

r = number of x_i values estimated.

$\hat{y} = b_0 + b_1 x_i \quad$ for $i = 1, 2, \ldots, r$ simultaneous estimates

$$S_{\bar{y}}^2 = MS_E \left[\frac{1}{n} + \frac{(x_i - \bar{x})^2}{\sum\limits_{i=1}^{n}(x_i - \bar{x})^2} \right]$$

Example 9. Using the data from Example 1, a researcher wants a 0.90 confidence interval for a series of estimates ($i = 0, 10, 30, 40$ and $r = 4$). What are they? Recall that $\hat{y} = 6.13 - 0.41 x_i$, $n = 15$, $MS_E = 0.0288$, and $\sum_{i=1}^{n}(x - \bar{x})^2 = 6750$.

$$S_{\bar{y}}^2 = MS_E \left[\frac{1}{n} + \frac{(x_i - \bar{x})^2}{\sum\limits_{i=1}^{n}(x_i - \bar{x})^2} \right] = 0.0288 \left[\frac{1}{15} + \frac{(x_i - 30)^2}{6750} \right]$$

$t_{(0.10/2(4),\,13)} = \approx 2.5$ from Table A.2 Student's t table

For $x = 0$:

$\hat{y}_0 = 6.13 - 0.041(0) = 6.13$

$S_{\hat{y}}^2 = 0.0288 \left[\dfrac{1}{15} + \dfrac{(0 - 30)^2}{6750} \right] = 0.0058$

$S_{\hat{y}} = 0.076$

$\hat{y}_0 \pm t_{0.10/2(4),\,13}(S_{\hat{y}})$

$6.13 \pm 2.5(0.076)$

6.13 ± 0.190

$5.94 \le \hat{y}_0 \le 6.32$ for $x = 0$, or no exposure, at $\alpha = 0.10$

For $x = 10$:

$\hat{y}_{10} = 6.13 - 0.041(10) = 5.72$

$S_{\hat{y}}^2 = 0.0288 \left[\dfrac{1}{15} + \dfrac{(10 - 30)^2}{6750} \right] = 0.0036$

$S_{\hat{y}} = 0.060$

$\hat{y}_{10} \pm t_{0.10/2(4),\,13}(S_{\hat{y}})$

$5.72 \pm 2.5(0.060)$

5.72 ± 0.150

$5.57 \le \hat{y}_{10} \le 5.87$ for $x = 10$ seconds, at $\alpha = 0.10$

For $x = 30$:

$\hat{y}_{30} = 6.13 - 0.041(30) = 4.90$

$S_{\hat{y}}^2 = 0.0288 \left[\dfrac{1}{15} + \dfrac{(30 - 30)^2}{6750} \right] = 0.0019$

$S_{\hat{y}} = 0.044$

$\hat{y}_{30} \pm t_{0.10/2(4),\,13}(S_{\hat{y}})$

$4.90 \pm 2.5(0.044)$

4.90 ± 0.11

$4.79 \le \hat{y}_{30} \le 5.01$ for $x = 30$ seconds exposure, at $\alpha = 0.10$

For $x = 40$:

$\hat{y}_{40} = 6.13 - 0.041(40) = 4.49$

$S_{\bar{y}}^2 = 0.0288 \left[\dfrac{1}{15} + \dfrac{(40 - 30)^2}{6750} \right] = 0.0023$

$S_{\bar{y}} = 0.048$

$\hat{y}_{40} \pm t_{0.10/2(4), \, 13}(S_{\bar{y}})$

$4.49 \pm 2.5(0.048)$

4.49 ± 0.12

$4.37 \leq \hat{y}_{40} \leq 4.61 \quad$ for $x = 40$ seconds exposure, at $\alpha = 0.10$

Note: Individual simultaneous confidence intervals can be made on not only the mean values but also the individual values. The procedure is identical to that already shown except that $S_{\bar{y}}$ is replaced by $S_{\hat{y}}$, where:

$$S_{\hat{y}} = MS_E \left[1 + \frac{1}{n} + \frac{(x_i - \bar{x})^2}{\sum\limits_{i=1}^{n}(x_i - \bar{x})^2} \right] \tag{65}$$

III. SPECIAL PROBLEMS

A. Piecewise Regression

There are times when it makes no sense to perform a transformation. This is true, for example, when the audience will not make sense of the transformation or when the data are too complex. The data displayed in Fig. 35 exemplify the latter circumstance.

Figure 35 is a complicated data display that easily can be handled using multiple regression procedures with dummy variables. Yet the data can also be approximated by simple linear regression techniques using three separate regression functions (see Fig. 36). Here:

$\hat{y}_a$ covers the range x_a, $b_0 = $ initial a value when $x = 0$,
$\quad b_1 = $ slope of y_a over the x_a range
$\hat{y}_b$ covers the range x_b, $b_0 = $ initial b value, when $x = 0$,
$\quad b_1 = $ slope of y_b over the x_b range
$\hat{y}_c$ covers the range x_c, $b_0 = $ initial c value, when $x = 0$,
$\quad b_1 = $ slope of y_c over the x_c range

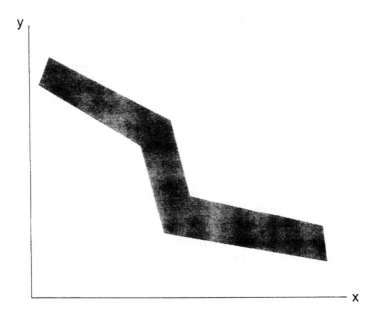

FIGURE 35   Complex data.

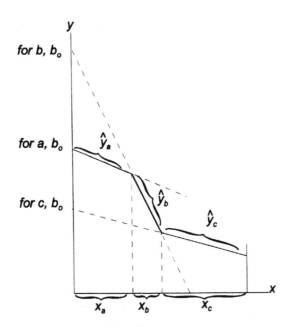

FIGURE 36   Piecewise regression functions.

A regression of this kind is rather simple to perform, yet is time consuming. The process is greatly facilitated by use of a computer while consulting certain technical texts [26,33,35,36].

The researcher can always take each x point and obtain a t-test confidence interval, and this is often the course chosen. Although from a probability perspective, this is not correct, from a practical perspective it is easy, useful, and more readily understood by audiences.

B. Comparison of Multiple Simple Linear Regression Functions

There are many times when a researcher would like to compare multiple regression function lines. A researcher can construct a series of 95% confidence intervals for each of the $\hat{y}$ values at specific x_i values. If the confidence intervals overlap, from regression line A to regression line B, the researcher simply states that no difference exists; if the confidence intervals do not overlap, the researcher states that the y points are significantly different from each other at α (see Fig. 37).

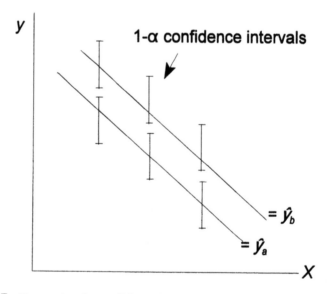

FIGURE 37   Nonoverlapping confidence intervals. Note: If the confidence intervals of $\hat{y}_a$ and $\hat{y}_b$ overlap, the $\hat{y}$ values on a specific x value are considered equivalent at α. Notice that the confidence intervals in this figure do not overlap, so the two regression functions are considered to differ at α.

When a researcher must be more accurate and precise in deriving conclusions, a more sophisticated procedure is necessary. Using the $1 - \alpha$ confidence interval approach, the $1 - \alpha$ confidence interval (CI) is not $1 - \alpha$ in probability. Moreover, the CI approach does not compare rates (b_1) or intercepts (b_0) but merely indicates whether the y values are the same or different. Hence, although the confidence interval procedure certainly has a place in describing regression functions, it is finite. There are other possibilities (see Fig. 38).

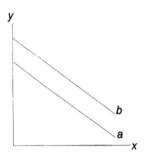

1
Slopes are equivalent ($b_{1a} = b_{1b}$), but intercepts are not ($b_{oa} \neq b_{ob}$).

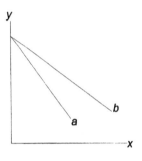

2
Slopes are not equivalent ($b_{1a} \neq b_{1b}$), but intercepts are ($b_{oa} = b_{ob}$).

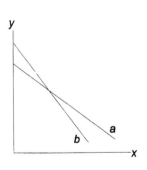

3
Slopes are not equivalent ($b_{1a} \neq b_{1b}$), and intercepts are not equivalent ($b_{oa} \neq b_{ob}$).

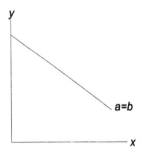

4
Slopes and intercepts are equivalent ($b_{1a} = b_{1b}$ and $b_{oa} = b_{ob}$).

FIGURE 38 Other possible comparisons between regression lines.

C. Evaluating Two Slopes (b_{1a} and b_{1b}) for Equivalence in Values

At the beginning of this chapter, we learned to evaluate b_1 to ensure that the slope was not 0. Now we will expand this process slightly to compare two slopes, b_{1a} and b_{1b}.

The test hypothesis for a two-tail test will be:

H_0: $\beta_{1a} = \beta_{1b}$

H_A: $\beta_{1a} \neq \beta_{1b}$

However, the test can be adapted to perform one-tail tests too.

Lower tail	Upper tail
H_0: $\beta_{1a} \geq \beta_{1b}$	H_0: $\beta_{1a} \leq \beta_{1b}$
H_A: $\beta_{1a} < \beta_{1b}$	H_A: $\beta_{1a} > \beta_{1b}$

The statistical procedure is an adaptation of Student's t-test.

$$t_c = \frac{b_{1a} - b_{1b}}{S_{b_{a-b}}} \qquad (66)$$

where:

b_{1a} = slope of regression function a $(\hat{y}_a)$

b_{1b} = slope of regression function b $(\hat{y}_b)$

$$S_{b_{a-b}}^2 = S_{\text{pooled}}^2 \left[\frac{1}{(n_a - 1)S_{x_a}^2} + \frac{1}{(n_b - 1)S_{x_b}^2} \right]$$

where:

$$S_{x_i}^2 = \frac{\sum\limits_{i=1}^{n} x_i^2 - \left(\sum\limits_{i=1}^{n} x_i \right)^2 / n}{n - 1}$$

$$S_{\text{pooled}}^2 = \frac{(n_a - 2)\text{MSE}_a + (n_b - 2)\text{MSE}_b}{n_a + n_b - 4}$$

$$\text{MSE}_a = \frac{\sum\limits_{i=1}^{n}(y_{ia} - \hat{y}_a)^2}{n - 2} = \frac{\text{SSE}_a}{n - 2}$$

$$MSE_b = \frac{\sum_{i=1}^{n}(y_{ib} - \hat{y}_b)^2}{n-2} = \frac{SSE_b}{n-2}$$

This procedure can easily be used in the standard six-step procedure.

Step 1.   Formulate hypothesis (one of three):

Two tail	Lower tail	Upper tail
H_0: $\beta_{1a} = \beta_{1b}$	H_0: $\beta_{1a} \geq \beta_{1b}$	H_0: $\beta_{1a} \leq \beta_{1b}$
H_A: $\beta_{1a} \neq \beta_{1b}$	H_A: $\beta_{1a} < \beta_{1b}$	H_A: $\beta_{1a} > \beta_{1b}$

Step 2.   State the α level.
Step 3.   Write out the test statistic, which is:

$$t_c = \frac{b_{1a} - b_{1b}}{S_{b_{a-b}}}$$

where:

$b_{1a} =$ slope estimate of the ath regression line
$b_{1b} =$ slope estimate of the bth regression line

Step 4.   Determine hypothesis rejection criteria used on one of the three options:

Two tail	Lower tail	Upper tail
H_0: $\beta_{1a} = \beta_{1b}$	H_0: $\beta_{1a} \geq \beta_{1b}$	H_0: $\beta_{1a} \leq \beta_{1b}$
H_A: $\beta_{1a} \neq \beta_{1b}$	H_A: $\beta_{1a} < \beta_{1b}$	H_A: $\beta_{1a} > \beta_{1b}$

For a two-tail test (Fig. 39):
Decision rule: If $|t_c| \neq t_t = t_{\alpha/2,[(n_a-2)+(n_b-2)]}$, reject H_0 at α.
For a lower tail test (Fig. 40)
Decision rule: If: $t_c < t_t = t_{-\alpha,[(n_a-2)+(n_b-2)]}$, reject H_0 at α.
For an upper tail test (Fig. 41)
Decision rule: If: $t_c > t_t = t_{\alpha,[(n_a-2)+(n_b-2)]}$, reject H_0 at α.
Step 5.   Perform statistical evaluation to determine t_c.
Step 6.   Make decision based on comparing t_c and t_t.

Let us look at an example.

Example 2.   Suppose the researcher exposed agar plates inoculated with *Escherichia coli* to forearms of human subjects that were treated with an antimicrobial formulation, as in an agar patch test [1]. In the study, four

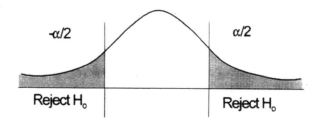

FIGURE 39   Step 4, decision rule for two-tail test.

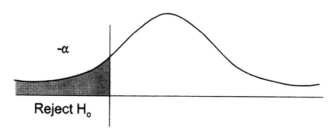

FIGURE 40   Step 4, decision rule for lower tail test.

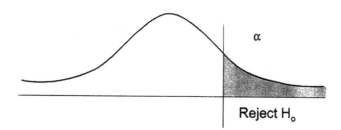

FIGURE 41   Step 4, decision rule for upper tail test.

plates were attached to each of the treated forearms of each subject. In addition, one inoculated plate was attached to untreated skin on each forearm to provide baseline determinations of the initial microbial population exposed. A random selection schema was used to determine the order in which the plates would be removed from the treated forearms. Two plates were removed and incubated after exposure for 15 minutes to the antimicrobially treated forearms, two were removed and incubated after 30 minutes, two were removed and incubated after 45 minutes, and the remaining two were removed and incubated after 60 minutes. Two test groups of five subjects each were used, one for antimicrobial product A and one for antimicrobial product B, for a total of 10 subjects. The agar plates were removed from 24 hours of incubation at $35°C \pm 2°C$ and the colonies counted. The duplicate plates at each time point for each subject were averaged to provide one value for each subject at each time.

The final average raw data provided the results shown in Table 12. The experimenter, we assume, has completed the model selection procedures, as previously discussed, and the linear regression models used are adequate. Figure 42 portrays the $\hat{y}$ (regression line) as well as the actual data at a 95% confidence interval for product A. Figure 43 portrays the same data for product B.

Hence, using the methods previously discussed throughout this chapter, the following data have been collected.

	Product A	**Product B**
Regression equation:	$\hat{y}_a = 5.28 - 0.060x$	$\hat{y}_b = 5.56 - 0.051x$
	$r^2 = 0.974$	$r^2 = 0.984$
	$MS_E = \frac{SS_E}{n-2} = 0.216$	$MS_E = \frac{SS_E}{n-2} = 0.145$
	$n_a = 25$	$n_b = 25$
	$SS_E = \sum_{i=1}^{n}(y_i - \hat{y})^2 = 1.069$	$SS_E = \sum_{i=1}^{n}(y_i - \hat{y})^2 = 0.483$

The experimenter wants to compare the regression models of products A and B. She or he would like to know not only the $\log_{10}$ reduction values at specific times, as provided by each regression equation, but also whether the death kinetic rates (b_{1a} and b_{1b}) — the slopes— are equivalent. The six-step procedure is used in this determination.

TABLE 12 Final Average Raw Data

Exposure time in minutes (x)	$\log_{10}$ average microbial counts (y), product A					$\log_{10}$ average microbial counts (y), product B				
Subject	5	1	3	4	2	1	3	2	5	4
0 (baseline counts)	5.32	5.15	5.92	4.99	5.23	5.74	5.63	5.52	5.61	5.43
15	4.23	4.44	4.18	4.33	4.27	4.75	4.63	4.82	4.98	4.62
30	3.72	3.25	3.65	3.41	3.37	3.91	4.11	4.05	4.00	3.98
45	3.01	2.75	2.68	2.39	2.49	3.24	3.16	3.33	3.72	3.27
60	1.55	1.63	1.52	1.75	1.67	2.47	2.40	2.31	2.69	2.53

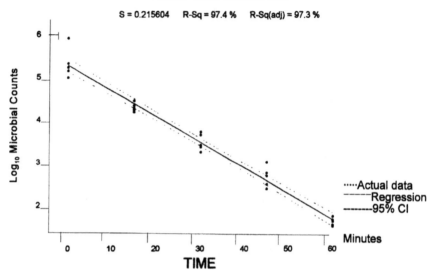

FIGURE 42   Linear regression model (product A).

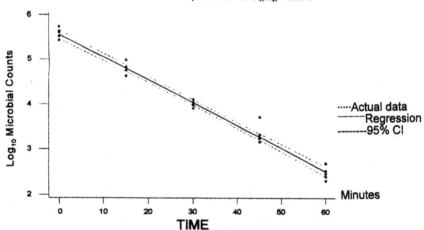

FIGURE 43   Linear regression model (product B).

Step 1.   Formulate the hypothesis. Because the researcher wants to know whether the rates of inactivation are different, a two-tail test is performed.

H_0: $\beta_{1A} = \beta_{1B}$ (inactivation rates of products A and B are the same)
H_A: $\beta_{1A} \neq \beta_{1B}$ (inactivation rates of products A and B are different)

Step 2.   Select α level. The researcher selects an α level of 0.05.

Step 3. Write out the test statistic.

$$t_{calculated} = \frac{\beta_{1a} - \beta_{1b}}{S_{\beta_{a-b}}}$$

$$S_{b_{a-b}}^2 = S_{pooled}^2 \left[\frac{1}{(n_a - 1)S_{x_a}^2} + \frac{1}{(n_b - 1)S_{x_b}^2} \right]$$

$$S_x = \sqrt{\frac{\sum_{i=1}^{n} x_i^2 - \left(\sum_{i=1}^{n} x_i\right)^2 / n}{n-1}}$$

$$S_{pooled}^2 = \frac{(n_a - 2)MSE_a + (n_b - 2)MSE_b}{n_a - n_b - 4}$$

$$MSE = S_y^2 = \frac{SS_E}{n-2} = \frac{\sum_{i=1}^{n}(y_i - \hat{y})^2}{n-2} = \frac{\sum_{i=1}^{n} \epsilon^2}{n-2}$$

Step 4.   Decision rule (Fig. 44).

$t_{tabled} = t_{(\alpha/2; n_a + n_b - 4)}$, using Table A.2, Student's t table.

$$= t_{(0.05/2; 25+25-4)} = t_{(0.025; 46)} = 2.021$$

If $|t_{calculated}| > 2.021$, reject H_0.

Step 5.   Perform calculation of t_c.

$$S_{\beta_{a-b}}^2 = S_{pooled}^2 \left[\frac{1}{(n_a - 1)S_{x_a}^2} + \frac{1}{(n_b - 1)S_{x_b}^2} \right]$$

$$S_{pooled}^2 = \frac{(n_a - 2)MSE_a + (n_b - 2)MSE_b}{n_a + n_b - 4}$$

$$= \frac{(25 - 2)0.216 + (25 - 2)0.145}{25 + 25 - 4} = 0.1805$$

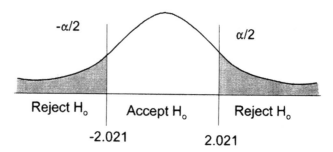

FIGURE 44 Step 4, decision rule.

$$S_{x_a}^2 = \frac{\sum\limits_{i=1}^{n} x_i^2 - \left(\sum x_i\right)^2 / n}{n-1}, \quad \text{where } \sum\limits_{i=1}^{n} x_i^2 = 33750$$

$$\text{and } \left(\sum\limits_{i=1}^{n} x_i\right)^2 = (750)^2 = 562,500$$

$$S_{x_a}^2 = \frac{33750 - (562,500/25)}{25-1} = 468.75$$

$$S_{x_a} = 21.65$$

$$S_{x_b}^2 = \frac{\sum\limits_{i=1}^{n} x_i^2 - \left(\sum\limits_{i=1,x_i}^{n}\right)^2 / n}{n-1} \quad \text{where, } \sum\limits_{i=1}^{n} x_i^2 = 33750 \text{ and}$$

$$\left(\sum\limits_{i=1}^{n} x_i\right)^2 = (750)^2 = 562,500$$

$$S_{x_b}^2 = 468.75 \quad \text{and } S_{x_b} = 21.65$$

$$S_{b_{a-b}}^2 = S_{pooled}^2\left[\frac{1}{(n_a-1)S_{x_a}^2} + \frac{1}{(n_b-1)S_{x_b}^2}\right]$$

$$= 0.1805\left[\frac{1}{(25-1)(468.75)} + \frac{1}{(25-1)(468.75)}\right]$$

$$S_{b_{a-b}}^2 = 3.21 \times 10^{-5}$$

$S_{b_{a-b}} = 0.0057$

For $b_{1a} = -0.060$ and $b_{1b} = -0.051$

$$t_c = \frac{b_{1a} - b_{1b}}{S_{b_{a-b}}} = \frac{-0.060 - (-0.051)}{0.0057} = -1.58$$

Step 6. Because $|t_c| \; (|-1.58|) < F_{\text{tabled}}$ (2.021), one cannot reject the null (H_0) hypothesis at $\alpha = 0.05$. We cannot conclude that the slopes (b_1) are significantly different from each other at $\alpha = 0.05$.

D. Evaluating the Two *Y* Intercepts (β_0) for Equivalence

There are times in regression evaluations when a researcher wants to be assured that the y intercepts of the two regression models are equivalent. For example, in microbial inactivation studies, if a researcher is comparing $\log_{10}$ reductions attributable to antimicrobials directly, the researcher wants to be assured that they begin at the same y intercept—have the same baseline.

Using a *t*-test procedure, this can be done, with a slight modification to what we have already done in determining a $1 - \alpha$ confidence interval for β_0.

The two separate β_0 values can be evaluated as a two-tail test, a lower tail test, or an upper tail test.

The test statistic used is:

$$t_{\text{calculated}} = t_c = \frac{\beta_{0a} - \beta_{0b}}{S_{0_{a-b}}}$$

$$S_{0_{a-b}}^2 = S_{\text{pooled}}^2 \left[\frac{1}{n_a} + \frac{1}{n_b} + \frac{\bar{x}_a^2}{(n_a - 1)S_{x_a}^2} + \frac{\bar{x}_b^2}{(n_b - 1)S_{x_b}^2} \right]$$

where:

$$S_x^2 = \frac{\sum\limits_{i=1}^{n} x_i^2 - \left(\sum\limits_{i=1}^{n} x_i \right)^2 / n}{n - 1}$$

$$S_{\text{pooled}}^2 = \frac{(n_a - 2)MSE_a + (n_b - 2)MSE_b}{n_a + n_b - 4}$$

This test can also be framed in the six-step procedure.

Step 1.   Formulate test hypothesis (one of three)

Two tail	Lower tail	Upper tail
$H_0: \beta_{0a} = \beta_{0b}$	$H_0: \beta_{0a} \geq \beta_{0b}$	$H_0: \beta_{0a} \leq \beta_{0b}$
$H_A: \beta_{0a} \neq \beta_{0b}$	$H_A: \beta_{0a} < \beta_{0b}$	$H_A: \beta_{0a} > \beta_{0b}$

Note: The order of *a* or *b* makes no difference; the three hypotheses could be written in reverse order.

Two tail	Lower tail	Upper tail
$H_0: \beta_{0b} = \beta_{0a}$	$H_0: \beta_{0b} \geq \beta_{0a}$	$H_0: \beta_{0b} \leq \beta_{0a}$

Step 2.   State the α.
Step 3.   Write the test statistic.
$$t_c = \frac{b_{0a} - b_{0b}}{S_{0_{a-b}}}$$

Step 4.   Determine the decision rule (Fig. 45). For a two-tail test:
$H_0: \beta_{0a} = \beta_{0b}$

$H_A: \beta_{0a} \neq \beta_{0b}$

If $|t_c| > t_t = t_{\alpha/2,(n_a+n_b-4)}$, reject H_0 at α.

For a lower-tail test (Fig. 46):
$H_0: \beta_{0a} \geq \beta_{0b}$

$H_A: \beta_{0a} < \beta_{0b}$

If $t_c < t_t = t_{-\alpha,(n_a+n_b-4)}$, reject H_0 at α.

For upper-tail test (Fig. 47):
$H_0: \beta_{0a} \leq \beta_{0b}$

$H_A: \beta_{0a} > \beta_{0b}$

If $t_c > t_t = t_{\alpha,(n_a+n_b-4)}$, reject H_0 at α

Step 5.   Perform statistical evaluation to determine t_c.

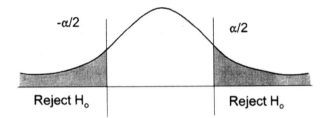

FIGURE 45   Step 4, decision rule for two-tail test.

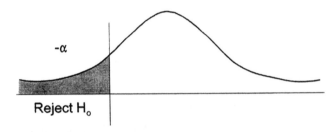

FIGURE 46   Step 4, decision rule for lower tail test.

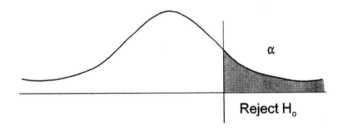

FIGURE 47   Step 4, decision rule for upper tail test.

Step 6.   Draw conclusions based on comparing t_c and t_t.

Let us now work Example 2 where the experimenter wants to compare the initial populations (times = 0) for equivalence.

Step 1.   This would, again, be a two-tail test:
H_0: $\beta_{0a} = \beta_{0b}$

H_A: $\beta_{0a} \neq \beta_{0b}$ (the initial populations—y intercepts—are not equivalent)

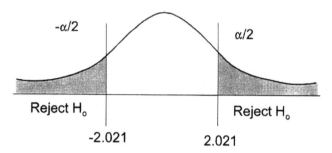

FIGURE 48   **Step 4, decision rule.**

Step 2.   Let us set α at 0.05, as usual.
Step 3.   The test statistic is:

$$t_c = \frac{b_{0a} - b_{0b}}{S_{0_{a-b}}}$$

Step 4.   Decision rule (Fig. 48)

$t_{(\alpha/2, n_a + n_b - 4)} - t_{(0.05/2, [25+25-4])} \approx 2.021$, from Table A.2, Student's t table

If $|t_c| > 2.021$, reject H_0

Step 5.   Perform statistical evaluation to derive t_c.

$$t_c = \frac{b_{0a} - b_{0b}}{S_{b_{a-b}}}$$

$$b_{0a} = 5.28$$

$$b_{0b} = 5.56$$

$$S_{0_{a-b}}^2 = S_{pooled}^2 \left[\frac{1}{n_a} + \frac{1}{n_b} + \frac{\bar{x}_a^2}{(n_a - 1)S_{x_a}^2} + \frac{\bar{x}_b^2}{(n_b - 1)S_{x_b}^2} \right]$$

$$S_{x.}^2 = \frac{\sum\limits_{i=1}^{n} x_i^2 - \left(\sum\limits_{i=1}^{n} x_i \right)^2 / n}{n - 1} = \frac{33750 - (750)^2/25}{25 - 1} = 468.75$$

$$S_{0_{a-b}}^2 = S_{pooled}^2 \left[\frac{1}{25} + \frac{1}{25} + \frac{30^2}{24(468.75)} + \frac{30^2}{24(468.75)} \right]$$

where:

$$S_{\text{pooled}}^2 = \frac{(n_a - 2)MS_{E_a} + (n_b - 2)MS_{E_b}}{n_a + n_b - 4} = \frac{(25 - 2)0.216 + (25 - 2)0.145}{25 + 25 - 4}$$

$$S_{\text{pooled}}^2 = 0.1805$$

$$S_{0_{a-b}}^2 = 0.1805\left[\frac{1}{25} + \frac{1}{25} + \frac{30^2}{24(468.75)} + \frac{30^2}{24(468.75)}\right] = 0.0433$$

$$S_{0_{a-b}} = 0.2081$$

$$t_c = \frac{5.28 - 5.56}{0.2081} = -1.35$$

Step 6. Because $|t_c| = |-1.35| < t_t = 2.021$, one cannot reject H_0 at $\alpha = 0.05$. The baseline values are equivalent.

E. Multiple Regression

Multiple regression procedures are easily accomplished using software packages such as MiniTab®. However, in much of applied research, they can become less useful for several reasons: they are more difficult to understand, the cost–benefit ratio is often low, and the underlying experiment is often poorly thought out.

1. More Difficult to Understand

As the variable numbers increase, so does the complexity of the statistical model and its comprehension. If comprehension becomes more difficult, interpretation becomes nebulous.

For example, if a researcher has a four- or five-variable model, trying to visualize what a fourth or fifth dimension represents—would look like—is impossible. If a researcher works in industry, no doubt his or her job will soon be in jeopardy for nonproductivity. The key is not that the models fit the data better with an r^2 or F test fit, it is whether the investigator can truly comprehend and describe the model's meaning in nonequivocal terms. In this author's view, it is far better to utilize a weaker model (lower r^2 or F value) and understand the relationship between fewer variables than hide behind a complex model that is applicable only to a specific data set and is not robust enough to hold up for other data collected under similar circumstances.

2. Cost–Benefit Ratio Low

Generally speaking, the more variables, the greater the experimental costs, and the relative value of the extra variables often diminishes. The developed model simply cannot produce valuable and tangible results in developing new drugs, new methods, or new processes with any degree of repeatability. Generally, this is due to lack of robustness. A complex model simply does not hold true if even minute changes occur.

It is far better to control variables—temperature, weight, mixing, flow, drying, etc.—than to produce a model in an attempt to account for them. In practice, no quality control or assurance group is prepared to track a "four-dimensional" control chart, and government regulatory agencies would not support them.

3. Poorly Thought-Out Study

It has been my experience that most multiple regression models applied in research are merely the result of a poorly controlled experiment or process. When I first began my industrial career in 1981, I headed a solid dosage validation group. My group's goal was to predict the quality of a drug batch before it was made by measuring mixing times, drying times, hardness, temperatures, tableting press variability, friability, dissolution rates, compaction, and hardness of similar lots, as well as other variables. Computationally, it was not difficult; time series and regression model development were not difficult either. The final tablet prediction confidence interval was useless. A 500 ± 50 mg tablet became 500 ± 800 mg at a 95% confidence interval. Remember then, the more variables, the more error.

F. Conclusion

With this said, multiple regression is valuable under certain conditions, experience being paramount. We will discuss them in the sister volume to this book, *Complex Applied Statistical Designs for the Researcher*, which begins where this book stops.

The applied researcher now has quite an arsenal of parametric methods at his or her disposal.

12

Nonparametric Statistics

Up to this point, Chaps. 1 through 11, we have discussed parametric statistics and have become quite knowledgeable in their applications. Now, we will focus on nonparametric statistical methods. Parametric statistics, although generally more powerful, require that more assumptions be met than do non-parametric methods. For example, in situations in which the experimenter has no previous understanding of the data (e.g., has not worked in this area before), it is not known whether the data are normally distributed or fall under another distribution. Although increasing the sample size tends to normalize any distribution, an experimenter is often restrained by a budget to a small sample size. Nonparametric statistics can be useful here, for they do not require a normal distribution. Nonparametric statistics are so termed because they do not utilize parameters, e.g., the mean, the variance, or the standard deviation.* Instead, the median—midpoint of the data—is generally utilized. The biggest advantage of using nonparametric statistics is that they remain valid under very general and limited assumptions [40,41].

There are also many times when an experimenter cannot use ratio scale data (e.g., 1.237, 156.21) but instead must use ordinal and even nominal data. Ordinal data, recall, are data that can be *ranked* and often are of a subjective nature (e.g., good, average, or bad or high, medium, or low). Nominal data are essentially nonrankable classification data, consisting of numbers or letters assigned to particular qualities (e.g., male/female, brown/green, growth/no

---

*This is not always the case. When we compute the Moses test for dispersion, we will calculate both the mean and a portion of the variance.

growth for *Staphylococcus aureus*, or 1/0). Nonparametric statistics are applicable to these two types of data, whereas parametric statistics are not.

A number of authors subdivide nonparametric statistics into two categories: true nonparametric methods and distribution-free procedures [42, 45]. This work will refer to both as nonparametric statistics without any distinction between them.

Advantages of nonparametric statistics:

1. Statistical assumptions are minimal, so the probability of using them improperly is relatively small.
2. The statistical concepts are relatively easy to understand.
3. They can be applied to all data types, including *nominal* and *ordinal* scale data.

Disadvantages: Because nonparametric statistics do not require set parameters, they generally lack the power of parametric statistics [42–49]. If the null hypothesis is rejected by a parametric procedure, it may not be by a nonparametric procedure because the latter lacks power. In general, to attain the same power as parametric statistics, nonparametrics require a larger sample size. This is a definite disadvantage, particularly in pilot studies, because the researcher will require greater location differences in the sample medians to detect statistically significant differences. This requirement, however, can be partially mitigated by increasing the significance level (e.g., to 0.10 instead of 0.05), a strategy this author uses when looking for potential new antimicrobial products through small screening studies.

Nonparametric studies also offer certain advantages. For example, in screening studies in which a new product must be distinctly better (e.g., more effective than a standard), using a nonparametric statistic at $\alpha = 0.05$ (standard α level) provides insurance against accepting a marginally more effective product as truly better. If superiority can be demonstrated nonparametrically, the product is truly better.

The format of this chapter will be to provide a nonparametric statistic—insofar as possible—analogous to each parametric test already discussed in earlier chapters. We will construct test statistics relative to the three types of data: nominal, ordinal, and interval. Let us begin with the nonparametric statistical methods corresponding to the independent two-sample Student's *t*-test.

I. NOMINAL SCALE (COUNT AND CATEGORY DATA): TWO INDEPENDENT SAMPLES

In experimental situations where two independent samples are to be compared and nominal data are to be collected, a particularly useful

	Treatment A	Treatment B	Total
Sample Group 1	a	b	a + b
Sample Group 2	c	d	c + d
Total	a + c	b + d	N

FIGURE 1 2 × 2 chi square table.

nonparametric method is the 2×2 chi square (χ^2) contingency table test. This method is also called Fisher's exact test for 2×2 tables [40, 41].

The study design requires two independent test conditions—the treatments and the sample groups. Figure 1 portrays this design. The assumptions for this test are that:

1. Each sample is selected randomly.
2. The two test groups are independent.
3. Each observation can be categorized as A or B.

The six-step procedure is as follows:

Step 1.   Formulate hypothesis:

Two-tail	Upper tail	Lower tail
H_0: $A = B$	H_0: $A \leq B$	H_0: $A \geq B$
H_A: $A \neq B$	H_A: $A > B$	H_A: $A < B$

Step 2.   Select α level. Note that the two-tail test is a chi square test and one-tail tests are t-tests.

Step 3.   Write the test statistic formula.

Two tail:

$$\chi_c^2 = \frac{N(ad - bc)}{(a + b)(c + d)(a + c)(b + d)} \tag{1}$$

Single tail:

$$t_c = \frac{\sqrt{N}(ad - bc)}{\sqrt{(a + b)(c + d)(a + c)(b + d)}} \tag{2}$$

Step 4.   Decision rule.

Two tail	Upper tail	Lower tail
Reject H_0, if $\chi_c^2 = \chi_{t(\alpha,1\,df)}^2$	Reject H_0, if $t_c > t_{t(\alpha,N-1)}$	Reject H_0, if $t_c < t_{t(-\alpha,N-1)}$

Step 5.   Compute the test statistic.

$$\chi_c^2 \quad \text{or} \quad t_c$$

Step 6.   Make decision to accept or reject H_0 at α.

Example 1: Defective equipment is a problem typically encountered in nearly all industries. A quality control manager is interested in determining whether supplier A provides equipment with more defective parts than does supplier B. Her company bought the lot samples from the two suppliers shown in Table 1.

The quality control manager has two categories for items in each lot: usable or defective. A test using the Poisson distribution for rare events could be used to explore differences between the suppliers, but this 2×2 test, I find, also performs well. This process can be structured easily into the six-step procedure.

Step 1.   Formulate hypothesis. In Example 1, the research question is "are there more defects coming from supplier A than B?" This can be written in two ways as a one-tail test.

TABLE 1   Lot Numbers

	Supplier A			Supplier B	
Sample	Lot size	Defective	Sample	Lot size	Defective
1	100	3	1	300	13
2	700	21	2	513	17
3	221	7	3	250	3
4	53	5	4	910	22
	1074	36		1973	55

Upper tail:

H_0: Number of defects from supplier A is less than or equal to ($\leq$) that from supplier B.

H_A: Number of defects from supplier A is more than ($>$) that from supplier B.

or:

$H_0: A \leq B$
$H_A: A > B$

Lower tail:

H_0: Number of defects from supplier B is greater than or equal to ($\geq$) that from supplier A.

H_A: Number of defects from supplier B is less than ($<$) that from supplier A.

or:

$H_0 : B \geq A$
$H_A : B < A$

For this example, we will use the upper tail hypothesis.

Step 2. We will use $\alpha = 0.05$.

Step 3. The decision rule is:

If $t_c > t_{t(0.05, N-1)}$, reject H_0 at α.

$N = 1074 + 1973 = 3047$

$t_{t(0.05, 3046)} = 1.645$

So, if $t_c > 1.645$, reject H_0 at α (Fig. 2).

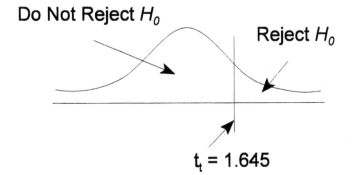

FIGURE 2   Example 1, step 3.

Step 4.   Write the test statistic.

$$t_c = \frac{\sqrt{N}(ad - bc)}{\sqrt{(a + b)(c + d)(a + c)(b + d)}}$$

	Nondefective	Defective	
Supplier A	*a*	*b*	*a* + *b*
Supplier B	*c*	*d*	*c* + *d*
	a + *c*	*b* + *d*	*N*

a = number not defective from supplier A
b = number defective from supplier A
$a + b$ = total lot size (nondefective + defective), supplier A
c = number not defective from supplier B
d = number defective from supplier B
$c + d$ = total lot size (nondefective + defective), supplier B
$a + c$ = number not defective from suppliers A and B
$b + d$ = number defective from suppliers A and B

	Nondefective	Defective	
Supplier A	*a* = 1038	*b* = 36	*a* + *b* = 1074
Supplier B	*c* = 1918	*d* = 55	*c* + *d* = 1973
	a + *c* = 2956	*b* + *d* = 91	*N* = 3047

Step 5.   Compute test statistic.

$$t_c = \frac{\sqrt{3047}[(1038 \cdot 55) - (1918 \cdot 36)]}{\sqrt{1074 \cdot 1973 \cdot 2956 \cdot 91}} = -0.8743$$

Step 6.   Make decision rule. Because t_c $(-0.8743) \ngtr t_t$ (1.645), one cannot reject H_0 at $\alpha = 0.05$.

Supplier A does not provide equipment with proportionately more defective parts than supplier B.

A. Computer Output

A 2×2 contingency table can also be computed with statistical software such as MiniTab®. It is recommended, however, that the researcher perform all six steps by hand, except step 5, which can be done by computer with

TABLE 2   2 × 2 MiniTab® Contingency Table: Expected Counts are Printed Beneath Observed Counts

	Nondefective	Defective	Total
Supplier A	1038	36	1074
	1041.92	32.08	
Supplier B	1918	55	1973
	1914.08	58.92	
Total	2956	91	3047
Chi square =	0.015 + 0.480 + 0.008		
	+ 0.261 = 0.764		
DF = 1, P value = 0.382			

results provided on a printout (Table 2). Because P value $= 0.382 > 0.05$, one cannot reject H_0.

Note: This program uses a chi square test for one-tail tests instead of a t-tabled test. Results are given as a P value and a χ^2 value.

II. ORDINAL SCALE (DATA THAT CAN BE RANKED): TWO INDEPENDENT SAMPLES

For ordinal data (or interval data, for that matter), the Mann–Whitney U-test can be used. The Mann–Whitney U-test, sometimes referred to as the Mann–Whitney–Wilcoxon test, is the nonparametric equivalent of the two-sample independent Student's t-test, and the statistic is used to compare two independent samples [40,43].

There are several requirements in using this statistic.

1. The data must be at least ordinal, that is, rankable. If interval data are used, they are reduced to ranked ordinal data.
2. Sampling is conducted randomly.
3. There is independence between the data of the two tested groups. If the data are paired, there is a better nonparametric statistic to use.

As with the two-sample independent t-test, upper, lower, and two-tail tests can be conducted. The Mann–Whitney U-test is based upon ranking. The sample sizes do not have to be equal, but if there are many ties among values, adjustment factors should be used.

In short, the Mann–Whitney U-test is statistically powerful and a very useful alternative to the two-sample independent t-test.

Let us use the six-step procedure to perform this test.

Step 1.   Formulate the hypothesis.

Two tail	Upper tail	Lower tail
$H_0 : x_A = x_B$	$H_0 : x_A \leq x_B$	$H_0 : x_A \geq x_B$
$H_A : x_A \neq x_B$	$H_A : x_A > x_B$	$H_A : x_A < x_B$

Step 2.   Select α level.

Two tail	Upper tail	Lower tail
$\alpha/2$	α	$-\alpha$

Step 3.   Write out the test statistic to be used.

$$t_c = \sum_{i=1}^{n} R_i - \frac{n_A(n_A + 1)}{2} \tag{3}$$

where: $\sum_{i=1}^{n} R_i$ = sum of the ranks of sample group A or x_A

n_A = sample size of sample group A

t_c = test statistic calculated

Step 4.   Make the decision rule.

Two tail	Upper tail	Lower tail
Reject H_0, if $t_c < M_{(\alpha/2)}$ or $t_c > M_{(1-\alpha/2)}$ where $M_{(\alpha/2)}$ is the tabled Mann–Whitney value at $M_{(\alpha/2;n_A,n_B)}$ and $M_{(1-\alpha/2)} = n_A n_B - M_{(\alpha/2;n_A,n_B)}$	Reject H_0, if $t_c > M_{(1-\alpha)}$ where $M_{(1-\alpha)} = n_A n_B - M_{(\alpha)}$	Reject H_0, if $t_c < M_{(\alpha)}$ where $M_{(\alpha)} = M_{(\alpha;n_A,n_B)}$

Note: Table A.6 (Mann–Whitney table) is used for all determinations of M.

Step 5.   Compute statistic.

Step 6. Decision.

Example 2: Suppose a researcher wants to compare the nosocomial infection rates in hospitals from two separate regions, A and B. The researcher wants to determine whether they differ. Table 3 presents the data obtained over a specified 1-month period.

Step 1. Formulate the hypothesis. This is a two-tail test.

$H_0 : x_A = x_B$

$H_A : x_A \neq x_B$

where $x_A =$ hospital region A nosocomial infection rate
$\quad\quad x_B =$ hospital region B nosocomial infection rate

Step 2. Select α level.

$\alpha = 0.05$, so $\alpha/2 = 0.025$

Step 3. Write out the test statistic (t_c).

$$t_c = \sum_{i=1}^{n} R_i - \frac{n_A(n_A + 1)}{2}$$

Note that both groups A and B will be ranked, but only A will be summed. In cases of ties, the sequential values equaling the number of ties will be summed and divided by the number of ties. For example, suppose values 7, 8, and 9 were all tied. The same value would be used in slots 7, 8, and 9, which is $(7 + 8 + 9)/3 = 8$.

TABLE 3 Data for Example 2

Region A (n_A)	Region B (n_B)
11.3	12.5
15.2	10.6
19.0	10.3
8.2	11.0
6.8	17.0
11.3	18.1
16.0	13.6
23.0	19.7
19.1	
10.6	

Step 4.   State the decision rule. Reject H_0 if:
$t_c < M_{(\alpha/2)}$

 or $t_c > M_{(1-\alpha/2)}$

where

$(n_A = 10)$

$(n_B = 8)$

$M_{(\alpha/2;n_A,n_B)} = M_{(0.05/2,\,10,8)} = 18$ from Table A.6, using $n_1 = n_A$ and
$\qquad\qquad n_2 = n_B$.

$M_{1-\alpha/2} = n_A n_B - M_{(\alpha/2;n_A,n_B)} = 10 \cdot 8 - 18 = 62$. So, if t_c is less than 18
$\qquad$ or greater than 62, we reject H_0 at $\alpha = 0.05$ (Fig. 3).

Step 5.   Compute the test statistic. First find $\sum_{i=1}^{n} R_A$ by ranking both
A and B (Table 4).

Step 6.   Because 39.5 is contained in the interval 18 to 62, one cannot
reject H_0 at $\alpha = 0.05$ (Fig. 4).

Let us now compute $M_{1-\alpha}$ and M_α to demonstrate both an upper and a
lower tail test. Set $\alpha = 0.05$.

 1.   Upper tail test
$\qquad H_0 : x_A \leq x_B$

$\qquad H_A : x_A > x_B$

$\qquad M_{1-\alpha} = n_A n_B - M_{(\alpha;n_A,n_B)} \leftarrow$, where $M_{(0.05;10,8)} = 21$, from Table A.6

$\qquad\quad = 10 \cdot 8 - 21$

$\qquad\quad = 80 - 21 = 59$

$\qquad M_{1-\alpha} = 59$

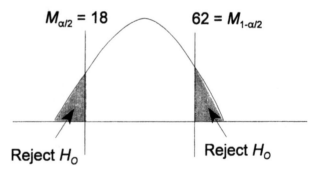

FIGURE 3   Example 2, step 4.

TABLE 4   Rank Values of A and B

X_A values	X_A rank values		X_B values	X_B rank values	
6.8	1				
8.2	2				
			10.3	3	
10.6	4.5		10.6	4.5	$(4+5) \div 2 = 4.5$
			11.0	6	
11.3	7.5	$(7+8) \div 2 = 7.5$			
11.3	7.5				
			12.5	9	
			13.6	10	
15.2	11				
16.0	12				
			17.0	13	
			18.1	14	
19.0	15				
19.1	16				
			19.7	17	
23.0	18				

$$\sum_{i=1}^{10} R_A = 94.5 \qquad n_A = 10 \qquad\qquad\qquad n_B = 8$$

$$t_c = \sum_{i=1}^{n} R_A - \frac{n_A(n_A+1)}{2} = 94.5 - \frac{10(10+1)}{2}$$

$$t_c = 39.5$$

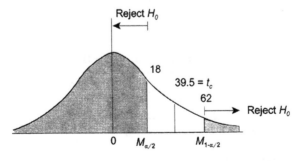

FIGURE 4   Example 2, step 6.

So, if $t_c > 59$, reject H_0 at $\alpha = 0.05$.

2. Lower tail test

$$H_0 : x_A \geq x_B$$

$$H_A : x_A < x_B$$

$$M_\alpha = M_{(\alpha; n_A, n_B)} = M_{(0.05; 10,8)} = 21, \text{ from Table A.6}$$

So, if $t_c < 21$, reject H_0 at $\alpha = 0.05$.

A. Comments

There is an adjustment component to be used with data that contain significant tied values, but a number of authors point out that the adjustment has little effect unless the proportion of tied values is large [40,41,44].

In cases where the sample size (n_1 or n_2) is greater than 20, the Mann–Whitney tables cannot be used. A large sample approximation must be used in its place [Eq. (4)].

$$Z_c = \frac{t_c - n_A n_B / 2}{\sqrt{n_A n_B (n_A + n_B + 1)/12}} \tag{4}$$

where

$$t_c = \sum_{i=1}^{n} R_i - \frac{n_A(n_A + 1)}{2}$$

The Z_C calculated value, then, is compared with the Z table values found in Table A.1, the normal distribution. The procedure is as previously shown except that Z is substituted for the M values.

B. Computer Program

The Mann–Whitney U-test is a standard routine in most statistical software packages. Table 5 is a Mini Tab® version of this.

TABLE 5 Mann–Whitney Test and C1: Region A, Region B

Region A	$n = 10$	Median $= 13.250$
Region B	$n = 8$	Median $= 13.050$
Point estimate for ETA1 − ETA2 is	-0.200	
95.4 percent CI for ETA1 − ETA2 is $(-5.400, 5.399)$		
W $= 94.5$		
Cannot reject at alpha $= 0.05$		

III. INTERVAL SCALE: TWO INDEPENDENT SAMPLES

The researcher has two options that work well when testing interval data: the Mann–Whitney U-test, as previously discussed, and the Moses test [40]. The Mann–Whitney U-test is applicable for median comparisons and, in this researcher's experience, is a powerful option. The Moses test, on the other hand, compares on the basis of σ (variability) or standard deviation equivalence. And it is important to remember that the Moses test is *not* applicable to nominal or ordinal data, only to interval data. I recommend that researchers use both of these tests to obtain intuitive experience and knowledge about which better describes their data. It is critical, however, that this endeavor be used not for "data mining" but for learning.

Because the Moses test does not assume equality in location parameters, it has wider application than other nonparametric tests. Also, it is useful when one wishes to focus on variability. The Moses test requirements are that:

1. Data collected are from two independent populations, A and B.
2. Data from each population are collected randomly.
3. Population distributions are interval data, having the same shape.

Both two-tail and one-tail tests can be conducted, and both approaches require that the x_A and x_B samples both be divided into several equal-size subsamples. The sum of the squared deviation values is then found for each subsample set. The number of values, k, in each subsample should be close to but not more than 10. The Mann–Whitney U procedure is then applied to these values for the results.

The six-step procedure can be used for this test.

Step 1.   Formulate the hypothesis.

Two tail	Upper tail	Lower tail
$H_0: \sigma_A = \sigma_B$	$H_0: \sigma_A \leq \sigma_B$	$H_0: \sigma_A \geq \sigma_B$
$H_A: \sigma_A \neq \sigma_B$	$H_A: \sigma_A > \sigma_B$	$H_A: \sigma_A < \sigma_B$

Step 2.   Select the α level.

Step 3.   Write out the test statistic.

$$t_c = \sum_{i=1}^{S_A} R_i - \frac{S_A(S_A + 1)}{2} \qquad (5)$$

where S_A = number of subgroups in group A
$\sum_{i=1}^{S_A} R_i$ = sum of the ranks assigned to the sums of squares values computed for the S_A subgroups

Step 4. Make the decision rule.

Two tail*	Upper tail	Lower tail
Reject H_0, when	Reject H_0, if	Reject H_0, if
$t_c < M_{(\alpha/2, S_A, S_B)}$ or $t_c > M_{(1-\alpha/2)} =$ $S_A S_B - M_{(\alpha/2; S_A, S_B)}$	$t_c > M_{(1-\alpha)} =$ $S_A S_B - M_{(\alpha; S_A, S_B)}$	$t_c < M_{(\alpha)} = M_{(\alpha; S_A, S_B)}$

*Use the tabled Mann-Whitney value for M where $n_A = S_A$ and $n_B = S_B$ in Table A.6

Step 5. Compute statistic.
Step 6. Conclusion.

Example 3: In the pharmaceutical arena, a quality control technician measured the dissolution rates of 50-mg tablets produced by two different facilities.

The technician wanted to know whether they differed in variability when dissolved in a solution at pH 5.2 held at 37°C in a water bath. Table 6 presents the dissolution rates in minutes of the tablets randomly sampled from each tablet press.

TABLE 6 Dissolution Rates in Minutes

n	Facility A	Facility B
1	2.6	3.2
2	2.9	3.2
3	3.1	3.0
4	2.7	3.1
5	2.7	2.9
6	3.2	3.4
7	3.3	2.7
8	2.7	3.7
9	2.5	
10	3.3	
11	3.4	
12	2.5	

Step 1. Formulate the hypothesis.The researcher will use a two-tail test to detect a difference.

$H_0 : \sigma_A = \sigma_B$ The variability of rates of dissolution of tables is the same for facility A and facility B.

$H_A : \sigma_A \neq \sigma_B$ There is a significant difference between the facilities in variability of dissolution rate.

Step 2. The researcher will use $\alpha = 0.05$, or $\alpha/2 = 0.025$.

Step 3. The test statistic is:

$$t_c = \sum_{i=1}^{S_A} R_i - \frac{S_A(S_A + 1)}{2}$$

Step 4. In this experimental statistical procedure, it is better, but not absolutely necessary, to keep S_A and S_B equal in size. Here S_A = number of subgroups in population A, and S_B = number of subgroups in population B. Let us use $k = 4$ samples per subgroup for a total of $S_A = 3$ ($n_A = 3$ for Table A.6) subgroups and $S_B = 2$ ($n_B = 2$ for Table A.6) subgroups. If $S_B = 9$, instead of 8, the researcher would merely drop one x_B value by random selection.

$M_{(\alpha/2; S_A, S_B)} = M_{(\alpha/2; n_1, n_2)},$ for using Table A.6, $= M_{(0.05/2; 3,2)} = 0$

$M_{(1-\alpha/2)} = S_A S_B - M_{(\alpha/2; S_A, S_B)} = 3 \cdot 2 - 0 = 6$

If t_c is < 0 or > 6, the researcher will reject H_0 at $\alpha = 0.05$ (Fig. 5).

Step 5. Perform analysis. First, randomly sample values, k, for each S group. Then find the means of the subgroups to find the sum of squares.

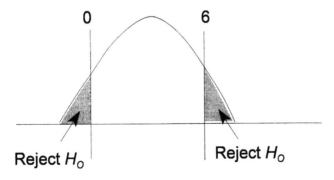

FIGURE 5   Example 3, step 4.

Sub sample	x_A				$\bar{x}_A$	Sum of squares(SS) = $(SS_{x_A}) =$ $\sum(x_{A_i} - \bar{x}_A)^2$
1	3.2	2.5	3.1	2.7	2.88	$(3.2 - 2.88)^2+$ $(2.5 - 2.88)^2+$ $(3.1 - 2.88)^2+$ $(2.7 - 2.88)^2 = 0.33$
2	2.9	3.3	2.7	3.4	3.10	$(2.9 - 3.10)^2$ $+ \ldots +$ $(3.4 - 3.10)^2 = 0.33$
3	2.7	3.3	2.5	2.6	2.78	$= 0.39$

Sub sample	x_B				$\bar{x}_B$	Sum of squares(SS) = $(SS_{x_B}) =$ $\sum(x_{B_i} - \bar{x}_B)^2$
1	3.0	3.1	2.7	3.2	3.00	$= 0.14$
2	3.4	2.9	3.7	3.2	3.30	$= 0.34$

Next, rank the sums of squares of x_A and x_B, SS_{x_A} and SS_{x_B}, and sum the ranks for $SS_{x_A} (= \sum r_i)$.

Sum of squares SS_{x_A}	R_i	Sum of squares SS_{x_B}	R_i
0.33	2.5	0.14	1
0.33	2.5	0.34	4
0.39	5		
	$\sum R_i = 10$		

Next, compute t_c:

$$t_c = \sum_{i=1}^{S_A} R_i - \frac{S_A(S_A + 1)}{2}$$

$$t_c = 10 - 3(4)/2$$

$$t_c = 10 - 6$$

$$t_c = 4$$

Step 6.   Because $t_c \not< 0$ and $\not> 6$, we cannot reject H_0 at $\alpha = 0.05$. There is no significant difference in the variability of the dissolution rates of the 50-mg tables from facilities A and B.

A.   Comments

1. When interval data are used and the researcher wants to evaluate differences in the medians, she or he should use the Mann–Whitney *U*-test directly.
2. However, if the researcher desires to evaluate variability — dispersion — differences, the Moses test should be used.
3. In cases of ties for the Moses test, as with the Mann–Whitney *U*-test, they will generally will not have undue influence, so a correction factor is not really necessary.

IV.   NOMINAL SCALE: TWO-SAMPLE RELATED OR PAIRED DATA

The McNemar statistic is probably the most useful for evaluating count or category data for two related samples. There are many times in research when paired data fall into one of two categories — for example, yes/no, 0/1, survived/did not survive, positive/negative, reacted/did not react, or before/after.

Recall that the objective in paired studies is to reduce variability among the test objects or items to increase the statistical power and efficiency of the evaluation. The pairing is done for variables such as weight, height, organ function, microbial species strain, or lot numbers to decrease the random variability in the data. Also, a paired test can be constructed where individual subjects are both the control and the test object. Caution should be used with this strategy, however, to ensure that environmental or historical changes that may affect the "external validity" of the study are controlled and accounted for. This type of error can creep in when a change over time occurs, for example, between conditions for the baseline and test procedures that is not directly related to the test proposition but biases the data.

The McNemar test requires that the researcher employ two matched groups and measure two outcome responses.

A.   Assumptions

1. The data consist of *n* pairs of test items, such as pairs of subjects. The paired items must be related or similar in a way relevant to the test proposition.
2. The measurement scale is nominal.

3. The matched pairs are independent of other pairs. When each subject is his or her own control, the subjects must be independent of one another.

The McNemar test is exclusively a two-tail test (Table 7). The basic model of the McNemar test is that of comparing two groups (x_A and x_B) under two conditions (0 and 1) to measure proportions of items or subjects with the test characteristics of interest. Here P_1 is the proportion of test items with the characteristics of interest under one condition and P_2 is the proportion of test items with the characteristics of interest under the other condition.

The McNemar test formula is:

$$Z_C = \frac{B - C}{\sqrt{B + C}} \tag{6}$$

where

$B + C \geq 10$ for normal distribution to apply

$$P_1 = \frac{A + B}{N}$$

$$P_2 = \frac{A + C}{N}$$

$$P_1 - P_2 = \frac{A + B}{N} - \frac{A + C}{N} = \frac{B - C}{N} \quad \text{or the proportion difference}$$

The six-step procedure can easily be applied to this test procedure.

TABLE 7　McNemar Test

		Classification of x_A				
		$x_A = 0$		$x_A = 1$		Total
Classification of x_B	$x_B = 0$	$x_A = 0$ $x_B = 0$	A	$x_A = 1$ $x_B = 0$	B	$A + B$
	$x_B = 1$	$x_A = 0$ $x_B = 1$	C	$x_A = 1$ $x_B = 1$	D	$C + D$
	Total	$A + C$		$B + D$		N

$N =$ total number of matched pairs (each $x_A x_B$ pair is matched).
$A =$ condition 0 for x_A and x_B.
$B =$ condition 1 for x_A and 0 for x_B.
$C =$ condition 0 for x_A and 1 for x_B.
$D =$ condition 1 for x_A and x_B.

TABLE 8   Step 4, Test Statistic Table

	Condition 1		Total
Condition 2	A	B	A + B
	C	D	C + D
Total	A + C	B + D	N

Step 1.   State hypothesis in a two-tail format.
  $H_0 : P_1 = P_2$ Treatment condition has no effect.
  $H_A : P_1 \neq P_2$ Treatment condition has an effect.
Step 2.   Specify α level.
Step 3.   Write test statistic.

$$Z_C = \frac{B - C}{\sqrt{B + C}} \quad \text{for normal distribution}$$

Step 4.   Write out the test statistic (Table 8).
Step 5.   The null hypothesis is rejected if $Z_c > Z_{\alpha/2}$ (Table A.1 normal distribution).
Step 6.   State the conclusion.

Example 4:   A researcher admits 40 individuals into a skin irritation study. The subjects begin the study by having their hands scored visually by a dermatologist, where no irritation $= 0$ and irritation $= 1$. Each subject performs five applications of a skin-conditioning lotion product and is then evaluated for beneficial change in skin condition. In this study, the subjects serve as their own controls (Table 9).

Step 1.   Formulate hypothesis.

  H_0: Before product application $=$ after product application.
  H_A: Before product application $\neq$ after product application.

Step 2.   Specify α. Let us set α at 0.05.
Step 3.   Write out the test statistic.

$$Z_c = \frac{B - C}{\sqrt{B + C}}$$

TABLE 9 Skin Irritation Study with 40 Subjects

			Before product application			
			Irritated		Not irritated	
After product application	Irritated	12	A	2	B	14 A + B
	Not irritated	23	C	3	D	26 C + D
		35	A + C	5	B + C	40

A = number of subjects admitted into the study with irritated hands that were still irritated after the study.

B = number of subjects admitted into the study with nonirritated hands that became irritated after the treatment.

C = number of subjects with irritated hands upon entering the study that improved with treatment

D = number of subjects admitted into the study with nonirritated hands that did not become irritated in the study.

Step 4. Decision rule.

If $|Z_c| > Z_t$, reject H_0 at $\alpha = 0.05$.

If $|Z_c| > Z_{t(0.05/2)} = 1.96$ (from normal Z table), reject H_0 at $\alpha = 0.05$.

Step 5. Compute statistic.

$$Z_c = \frac{B - C}{\sqrt{B + C}} = \frac{2 - 23}{\sqrt{2 + 23}} = \frac{-21}{5} = -4.20$$

Step 6. Because $|Z_c| = |4.20| > 1.96$, reject H_0 at $\alpha = 0.05$. There is a difference between treatments (pretreatment/posttreatment). The negative value here shows that the hands improved with use of the lotion.

V. ORDINAL SCALE: TWO-SAMPLE RELATED OR PAIRED DATA

The *sign test* for two paired samples is particularly useful when the measurement data are ordinal scale. Within each pair of data, the researcher can determine only which datum is larger than another that is ranked. If the measurement scale is interval, the researcher is advised to use the Wilcoxon matched-pair test.

The sign test for two paired samples is applicable for two-tail or one-tail evaluations. The assumptions for the sign test include:

1. The data consist of n pairs of measurements, x_A and x_B. Each $x_A x_B$ pair is matched according to influencing variables such as lot number, age, weight, or sex.
2. The n pairs of $x_A x_B$ measurements are independent of one another.
3. The measurement scale is ordinal.
4. The data distribution is continuous.

The concept of the sign test is very simple, consisting of working only with $+$ and $-$ signs. Given that the null hypothesis is true, there should be as many $+$ signs as there are $-$ signs for the sample differences.

In performing this test, the six-step procedure is amenable.

Step 1. Specify hypothesis.
Two-tail

H_0: $p(+) = p(-)$ Proportion of $+$ signs is equivalent to that of $-$ signs.

H_A: $p(+) \neq p(-)$ Proportion of $+$ signs is not equivalent to that of $-$ signs.

Upper tail

H_0: $p(+) \leq p(-)$

H_A: $p(+) > p(-)$ Proportion of $+$ signs is larger than proportion of $-$ signs.

Lower tail

H_0: $p(+) \geq p(-)$

H_A: $p(+) < p(-)$ Proportion of $+$ signs is less than proportion of $-$ signs.

Step 2. Specify α level.
Step 3. Write out test formula. The sign test is a special case of the binomial test from elementary statistics. The significance test is dependent upon the formula.

$$P(T \leq t \mid n, p) \tag{7}$$

or $P(T \leq t \mid n, 0.50)$ since P generally will be 0.50
where P = probability of event (generally 0.50)
T = the random variable (the number of $+$ signs of interest under H_0)
t = the critical value of T from the binomial table (Table G)
t_c = the observed number of $+$ outcomes from the sample set
n = sample size

Note: Ties are dropped from the evaluation; an n is dropped by 1 for each tied pair.

Step 4.   Decision rule.

Two tail	Upper tail	Lower tail
Reject H_0, when	Reject H_0, if	Reject H_0, if
$P(T \leqslant t)\|n, 0.50) \leqslant \alpha/2$ or	$P(T \geqslant n - t)\|n, 0.50) \leqslant \alpha$	$P(T \leqslant t)\|n, 0.50) \leqslant \alpha$
$P(T \geqslant n - t)\|n, 0.50) \leqslant \alpha/2$		

Step 5.   Perform calculations.
Step 6.   Conclusion.

Example 5:   In a preference evaluation of alcohol lotion hand cleansers, participants received two formula types, A and B. The investigator wanted to know whether formula A is perceived as "cooler to the touch" than formula B. One type was applied to the back of one hand randomly selected and the other to the back of the other hand, simultaneously by two technicians. Subjects responded which product felt cooler, that on the left or right hand. The study was double-blinded and not decoded until the evaluation was finished. Ties were dropped from the study.
The data was coded:

+, if the subject preferred formula A
−, if the subject preferred formula B

Data results										
Subject	1	2	3	4	5	6	7	8	9	10
	+	+	+	−	+	+	−	−	+	+

We use the six-step procedure:

Step 1.   State hypothesis.
   Upper tail
      H_0: $p(+) \leq p(-)$, or product A perceived as no cooler than B
      H_A: $p(+) > p(-)$, or product A perceived as cooler than B
Step 2.   Set α level. Let us specify α as 0.10 for this one-tail test.
Step 3.   Write out the test formula.
   t_c = number of + signs for this test
Step 4.   Decision rule. We must find the critical value for the sign test from the binomial table (Table A.7), $P(T \geq n - t \mid n, 0.50) \leq \alpha$, where $n = 10$, and $p = 0.5$ at $\alpha = 0.10$. From Table G, the binomial

distribution table, $t = r = 3$ at $\alpha \approx 0.1172$, and $n-t = 10-3 = 7$. If the number of $+$ outcomes is seven or greater, the H_0 hypothesis is rejected at $\alpha = 0.1172$, so $P(T \geq 7 \mid 10, 0.5) \leq 0.1172$.

You will note that the value of α is 0.1172. Because the binomial table deals with discrete t values (the r values, in the binomial tables), 1, 2, 3 ... r, the α level is not specifically 0.05, 0.10, etc. Hence, the researcher must select the value closest to the specified α level and formulate the decision rule.

Note: If this had been a two-tail test at $\alpha = 0.10$, $\alpha/2 = 0.05$, then

$$P(T \leq t \mid 10, 0.50) \leq 0.05 \approx P(T \leq 2 \mid 10, 0.50) \leq 0.0439 \text{ and}$$

$$P(T \geq n - t \mid 10, 0.50) \leq 0.05 \approx P(T \geq 8 \mid 10, 0.50) \leq 0.0439.$$

If $t_c \geq 8$ or $t_c \leq 2$, the H_0 hypothesis is rejected at $\alpha = 0.0439 + 0.0439 = 0.0878$.
If this had been a lower tail test at $\alpha = 0.10$, then

$$P(T \leq t \mid 10, 0.50) \leq 0.10 = P(T \leq 3 \mid 10, 0.50) \leq 0.1172.$$

Step 5. Calculate the test statistic.
$t_c =$ the number of $+$ signs, which is 7
Step 6. Conclusion. We conclude that, given we have seven $+$ signs for this test, H_0 is rejected at $\alpha = 0.1172$. There is strong evidence that product A "feels" cooler than product B.

The sign test can be used on "stronger" data, too. Suppose the investigator matched pairs of subjects in terms of blood serum levels of penicillin (mg/dL) following use of penicillin tablets, A and B, of the same strength. The collected data are presented in Table 10.

The researcher would conduct the evaluation using the six-step procedure, as before. The numerical data are easily reexpressed in the $+/-$ format, where $+$ denotes a subject using tablet A who showed a higher serum level of penicillin than the matched subjects who used tablet B.

TABLE 10 Example 5 Data

n	1	2	3	4	5	6	7	8	9	10	11
Tablet A ($+$)	53	59	38	49	52	96	49	79	48	72	57
Tablet B ($-$)	21	28	39	51	53	92	53	85	55	65	63
Higher value $+$ or $-$	$+$	$+$	$-$	$-$	$-$	$+$	$-$	$-$	$-$	$+$	$-$

Here $t_c = 4 =$ number of $+$ signs.

TABLE 11 Sign Test for Median: Numeric

		SIGN TEST OF MEDIAN = 0.00000 VERSUS NOT = 0.00000				
	N	BELOW	EQUAL	ABOVE	P	MEDIAN
C1 MTB >	11	7	0	4	0.5488	−1.000

The sign test for ordinal data is simple to use. Although this test is often considered a "quick and dirty" one, this researcher has found it exceptionally useful as long as a meaningful construction of test pairs is conscientiously performed.

Many computer software packages have this routine. Table 11 shows the MiniTab® version with the numerical data. First, subtract sample group B from sample group A.

VI. INTERVAL SCALE: TWO-SAMPLE RELATED OR PAIRED DATA

The Wilcoxon matched-pairs signed-ranks statistic is a very useful and popular nonparametric statistic for evaluating two related or paired samples when the collected data are interval scale. As with the two-sample matched-pair t-test of parametric statistics, the Wilcoxon test converts the two samples, x_A and x_B, to one sample, which we label "D" for difference.

$$D_i = x_{A_i} - x_{Bi} \quad \text{for } i = 1, 2, \ldots n \tag{8}$$

The test is then performed on these sample value differences.

A. Assumptions

1. The data consist of n values of D_i, where $D_i = x_{A_i} - x_{B_i}$. Each pair of measurements, x_{A_i} and x_{B_i}, is taken on the same subject (e.g., before/after, pre/post) or on subjects that have been paired meaningfully with respect to important but nonmeasured variables (e.g., sex, weight, organ function).
2. The sampling of each pair, x_{A_i} and x_{B_i}, is random.
3. The differences (D_i) between each pair represent a continuous random variable instead of discrete variables. This, in theory, is a variable that potentially has an infinite number of trailing values to the right of a decimal point (e.g., 1.379000...). The level of a drug measured from the blood exemplifies a continuous scale. However, the

assumption of differences representing a continuous variable is often violated with little practical effect. For example, the number of bacteria or viruses remaining on the hands after an antimicrobial treatment regimen is discrete. That is, 0.031 of a bacterium is meaningless. Yet, numbers of bacteria or viruses can be treated as a continuous variable with no harm because one is usually dealing with large numbers of discrete values that approximate a continuous distribution.

4. Each D_i is independent of all other D_is.
5. The D_is are at least interval scale.
6. The D_is have a symmetrical distribution. That is, the data to the left and right of a constant, usually the median (or mean), mirror each other. With absolute symmetry of distribution, as we recall from parametric statistics, the median equals the mean value. That is, they are the same value.

The Wilcoxon matched-pairs test can be used for both two-tail and one-tail tests and the test procedure is straightforward.

First, the signed value difference, D_i, of each x_A and x_B data set is obtained.

$$D_i = X_{A_i} - X_{B_i}$$

Second, the absolute values, $|D_i|$, are ranked from smallest to largest. Finally, the original signs from $D_i = X_{A_i} - X_{B_i}$ are reinstated, and the positive ranks $(R+)$ and the negative ranks $(R-)$ are summed. Depending upon the direction, upper or lower tail, one merely sums the $R+$ or $R-$ values to derive the W_C value and compares that value with the Wilcoxon table value, W_t (d in Table A.8), for a specific significance level. The Wilcoxon Table A.8 has one- and two-tail options and requires the n value (number of D_i values) and the d value (corresponding to the desired α value), which is compared with the W_C value (the sum of the $R+$ or $R-$ values). The tabled values can be used for a number of D_i values up to $n = 25$. For n larger than 25, a correction factor can be used to enable one to use the normal distribution.

The correction factor is:

$$Z_C = \frac{W_C - [n(n+1)]/4}{\sqrt{n(n+1)(2n+1)/24}} \tag{9}$$

where $n =$ number of D_i values
   $W_C =$ sum of ranks of the negative or positive R values, depending on direction of the test

B. Ties

There are two types of ties. The first occurs when specific x_A, x_B values to be paired are equal so the D_i is 0. All pairs of $x_{A_i} = x_{B_i}$ are dropped from the analysis, and n is reduced 1 for each pair dropped. In the other case, two or more D_is in the same sample group are equal. These ties receive the average rank value. This researcher has not found the tie correction formulas to be of much practical value.

Step 1. Specify hypothesis.

Two tail	Upper tail	Lower tail
$H_0: x_A - x_B = 0$ or $x_A = x_B$	$H_0: x_A \leqslant x_B$	$H_0: x_A \geqslant x_B$
$H_A: x_A - x_B \neq 0$ or $x_A \neq x_B$	$H_A: x_A > x_B$	$H_A: x_A < x_B$

Step 2. Specify the α level. Use $\alpha/2$ for two-tail tests for a specific level of α, as always, and α for single-tail tests.

Step 3. Write out the test statistic to use. For small sample sizes ($n \leq 25$, which is the number of D_i values), the Wilcoxon table (Table A.8) can be used directly, using merely the sum of the ranks of W_C+ or W_C- values, depending on the direction of the test. For larger samples, the correction factor must be used. That is:

$$Z_C = \frac{W_C - [n(n-1)]/4}{\sqrt{n(n+1)(2n+1)/24}} \qquad (9)$$

Step 4. Specify the decision rule.

Two tail	Upper tail	Lower tail
The test is dependent on the sum of the ranks (W_C), + or −, using whichever is the smaller. If W_C is equal to or less than the d tabled value at α, reject H_0 at α	The test uses the sum of the ranks of the negative values, W_C-. If W_C- is equal to or smaller than the d tabled value at α, reject H_0.	The test uses the sum of the ranks (W_C) of the positive values, W_C+. If W_C is equal to or smaller than the d tabled value at the desired α, reject H_0.

Step 5. Perform the calculation.
Step 6. Formulate the conclusion.

Example 6:   A researcher in a skin care laboratory wants to evaluate a dermatological lotion's ability to reduce atopic dermatitis of the hands associated with standard work-related tasks of healthcare workers (e.g., skin exposure to heat and cold, to skin cleansers, to wearing surgical or examination gloves over periods of time, and to repeated washing). Prior to the use of the test lotion, the researcher used a Visioscan device to measure scaliness of the skin of the hands of 10 randomly selected healthcare workers. This represented the baseline measurement (x_A). After a 24-hour period of treatment during which the test dermatological lotion was used three times, the skin on the hands of the subjects was again measured (x_B) for degree of scaliness. The study was an in-use study in which healthcare workers went about their usual activities in a normal manner.

On the basis of the before-and-after Visioscan data (Table 12), the researcher wants to know whether the treatment was effective in reducing skin scaliness at an $\alpha = 0.05$ level of confidence.

The six-step procedure will work well here.

Step 1.   Formulate hypothesis. The researcher wants to determine whether the lotion treatment reduced skin scaliness. For that to occur, the x_B values must be significantly lower than the x_A values. Hence, this is an upper tail test ($H_A: x_A > x_B$ or $x_A - x_B > 0$).

$H_0: x_A \leq x_B$

$H_A: x_A > x_B$ The treatment reduces the scaliness of the skin.
For purposes of this analysis, the hypotheses are restated as:

$H_0: D_i \leq 0$

$H_A: D_i > 0$ Difference greater than zero (upper tail)

Step 2.   Specify α. Let us set α at 0.05.

TABLE 12   Visioscan Data for Degree of Skin Scaliness, Processed for a Wilcoxon Analysis

Subject	1	2	3	4	5	6	7	8	9	10
Baseline 0 (pretreatment) (x_A)	54	57	85	81	69	72	83	58	75	87
24 hours (posttreatment) (x_B)	41	53	63	81	73	69	75	54	69	70
Difference (D_i)	13	4	22	0	−4	3	8	4	6	17
Rank ($|D_i|$)	7	3	9	Omit	3	1	6	3	5	8
Signed rank (R)	+7	+3	+9	N/A	−3	+1	+6	+3	+5	+8

This is a one-tail test, an upper tail test. We sum the R^- values to calculate W_C, (sum value of the R^- values) which is expected to be small, if H_0 is to be rejected.

Step 3.   Decision rule. The tabled value of W_t is found from Table A.8 (the Wilcoxon table) for $n = 9$ (one pair value was lost due to a tie) and a one-tail $\alpha = 0.05$. For this table, as with the sign test, the α value (α'' for two tail-tests and α' for one-tail tests) is not precisely 0.001, 0.01, 0.025, 0.05, or 0.10, so the researcher uses the tabled α value closest to the specified α value. In this case, with $n = 9$ and $\alpha' = 0.05$, the tabled value is $d = W_t = 9$ at $\alpha = 0.049$. Hence, we reject H_0 if W_C, the sum of the ranked negative values $(R-)$, is less than or equal to 9 at $\alpha = 0.049$.

Step 4.   Choose the test statistic. Because this is an upper tail test, we sum the negative rank values $(R-)$ and compare the result (W_C) with $W_t = 9$. If $R - (W_C) \leq 9$, reject H_0 at $\alpha = 0.049$.

Step 5.   Perform analysis. The sum of the negative rank values $(R-)$ is 3.

Step 6.   Conclusion. Because the sum of the negative rank values, $W_C = 3$, is less than the tabled value of 9, we reject at $\alpha = 0.05$ the H_0 hypothesis that the treatment does not significantly reduce skin scaliness. The actual p value of a $W_C = 3$ is $p < 0.006$.

C. Comments

Suppose this had been a two-tail test at $\alpha = 0.05$:

$H_0 : x_A = x_B$

$H_A : x_A \neq x_B$

The sum of negative or positive R values, whichever R_i is smaller, must be less than or equal to 7 at $\alpha'' = 0.055$ (Table H). The sum of $R- = 3$, so we reject H_0 at $\alpha = 0.055$, with a p value less than 0.012.

Suppose the test was a lower tail test.

$H_0 : x_A \geq x_B$

$H_A : x_A < x_B$

In this case, we use the sum of the positive ranks. If the sum of the positive ranks is ≤ 9 with an n of 9, we reject H_0 at $\alpha = 0.049$.

$$W_C - R+ = 7 + 3 + 9 + 1 + 6 + 3 + 5 + 8 = 42$$

$$W_C = 42 > W_t = 9, \text{ so we cannot reject } H_0 \text{ at } \alpha = 0.049$$

TABLE 13   Stem-and-Leaf Display of the D_i Using MiniTab

	Stem-and-leaf of differences	"D" N = 10
1	−0	4
5	0	0344
5	0	68
3	1	3
2	1	7
1	2	2

D. Remarks

It is a good idea to perform EDA procedures on the data, D_i, because we assume symmetry. In this D_i data set, the values are skewed to the right or higher values, which can be seen in both the stem-and-leaf display (Table 13) and the letter-value display (Table 14). It is important that the researcher sees this and uses his or her field experience, more than statistical ability, to judge its validity.

The MiniTab® software computer program for the Wilcoxon matched-pair test is used (Table 15). Some manual adjustment may be necessary when applying this computerized analysis because it sums only the $R+$ values.

VII. NOMINAL SCALE: MULTIPLE INDEPENDENT SAMPLES $(n > 2)$

The chi square (χ^2) test for independence—goodness of fit—is one of if not the most useful of all the statistical tests for this category. All chi square tests and their derivatives are based on the work of Karl Pearson in the early 1900s [42,45]. These tests consist of generating expected frequencies and comparing observed frequencies with them. The goodness of fit is then determined

TABLE 14   Letter-Value display of the D_i Using MiniTab®

	DEPTH	LOWER		UPPER	MID	SPREAD
N=	10					
M	5.5		5.000		5.000	
H	3.0	3.000		13.000	8.000	10.000
E	2.0	0.000		17.000	8.500	17.000
	1	−4.000		22.000	9.000	26.000

TABLE 15   Wilcoxon Matched-Pair Test

WILCOXON SIGNED RANK TEST: DIFFERENCE				
TEST OF MEDIAN − 0.000000 VERSUS MEDIAN NOT = 0.000000				
	N	N FOR TEST	WILCOXON STATISTIC	P	ESTIMATED MEDIAN
DIFFERENCE	10	9	42.0	0.024	6.500

on the basis of how closely those data match the expected results as a function of the chi square distribution.

In a research situation, one question that arises frequently is, "are the data related—associated?" That is, if one variable changes, does another variable also change in a consistent, predictable manner?

One particular recent application of this test by this author was in a preliminary evaluation of the effectiveness of ozone used as a hand disinfectant in an automated hand-cleansing system. It is well known that ozone is a powerful oxidizing agent and, therefore, a useful disinfectant, but when it is delivered through water its disinfectant characteristics are altered. Even so, it was worth evaluating. A study was constructed to determine whether incremental changes in ozone concentrations were related to changes in numbers of viable microorganisms collected from the hands. The chi square test was used to evaluate the data.

The chi square test for independence is a contingency table that measures row–column association. The different rows usually represent samples from different test populations (e.g., product A, B, C) and the columns different categories of classification of the data from the samples (e.g., time 1, 2, 3, or concentration 1, 2, 3). A row–column dependence (i.e., the data are associated) is construed as functional dependence or association. Similarly, if the observations from a single sample are classified into rows and columns on the basis of two different criteria, a row–column association or dependence can be determined.

A. Assumptions

1. The data are randomly sampled.
2. Each data point consists of one value corresponding to one column level and one row level.
3. The data are nominal (note, though, that interval and ordinal data can be reduced to nominal scale).

The chi square test uses a row by column ($r \times c$) contingency table (Table 16).

TABLE 16   Chi Square Table

	Column level				
	1	2	...	c	Total
1	n_{11}	n_{12}	...	n_{1c}	$n_{1.}$
2	n_{21}	n_{22}	...	n_{2c}	$n_{2.}$
Row level .	.	.	...	.	.
.	.	.	...	.	.
.	.	.	...	.	.
r	n_{r1}	n_{r2}	...	n_{rc}	$n_{r.}$
Total	$n_{.1}$	$n_{.2}$	...	$n_{.c}$	$n_{..}$

Two frequency values are measured: (1) the observed frequency and (2) the expected frequency. The observed data are the cell ($r \times c$) entries, usually labeled $O_{ij} = n_{ij}$. The observed cell frequency represents the joint occurrence of the ith row component and the jth column component. To obtain the expected frequency of each cell (E_{ij}), two basic statistical laws of probability are used. Recall from elementary statistics that if two events (components) are independent, the probability of their joint occurrence is the product of their individual probabilities. In addition, if the two events (components) are independent, the probability of including a subject in a specific n_{ij} cell is equal to counting it in the ith row times the jth column. To obtain a specific E_{ij}, the researcher divides this product by the total sample size ($n_{..}$). The computational formula to use is $E_{ij} = n_{i.} n_{.j} / n_{..}$.

From the observed cell frequencies O_{ij} and the corresponding E_{ij}, we are interested in the magnitude of difference between them. That is, we want to know whether the difference between them is large enough to dismiss random chance.

This is done by calculation of the chi square test statistic:

$$\chi_c^2 = \sum_{i=1}^{r} \sum_{j=1}^{c} \left[\frac{(O_{ij} - E_{ij})^2}{E_{ij}} \right] \tag{10}$$

The chi square distribution has $(r-1)(c-1)$ degrees of freedom. If $\chi_c^2 > \chi_t^2$, the H_0 hypothesis is rejected.

The χ^2 statistic is distributed as a χ^2 distribution (given H_0 is true) only if the expected frequencies (E_{ij}) are large. Just how large is a debated issue. Some statisticians specify that each E_{ij} should be at least 10. However, Cochran [9] argued that an E_{ij} could be as low as 1 provided 20% or fewer of the cells have expected frequencies less than 5. This researcher has found that adjacent rows and/or columns can be combined to achieve a higher frequency per cell.

The χ^2 test is easily completed with the six-step procedure.

Step 1. Formulate the hypothesis.
H_0: Components A and B are independent.
H_A: Components A and B are not independent.
Step 2. Specify α.
Step 3. Write out the test statistic.

$$\chi_c^2 = \sum_{i=1}^{r} \sum_{j=1}^{c} \left[\frac{(O_{ij} - E_{ij})^2}{E_{ij}} \right]$$

Step 4. Formulate the decision rule. If χ_c^2 computed $> \chi_t^2$ tabled, reject H_0 at α.
Step 5. Compute statistic.
Step 6. Conclusion.

Example 7: A researcher wanted to determine whether increasing the amount of ozone (O_3) delivered through water at a flow rate of 3.3 gallons per minute (for a 60-second wash cycle) is associated with $\log_{10}$ reductions in numbers of *Escherichia coli*. Five levels of ozone were used, with 10 replicates per level, and microbial $\log_{10}$ reductions observed were categorized into four levels (Table 17).

Let us analyze the experiment using the six-step procedure.

Step 1. Formulate hypothesis.
H_0: The ozone levels and microbial $\log_{10}$ reductions are independent
H_A: The ozone levels and microbial $\log_{10}$ reductions are not independent

TABLE 17   Observed Data

Log$_{10}$ reduction	Ozone level (ppm)					
	0.5	0.8	1.0	1.3	1.6	Total ($n_{\cdot j}$)
0–1	8	2	1	1	0	12
1–2	1	6	3	1	1	12
2–3	1	2	4	6	3	16
3–4	0	0	2	2	6	10
Total $n_{j\cdot}$	10	10	10	10	10	$n_{\cdot\cdot} = 50$

Step 2. Specify α. Because this is a pilot study and the client was interested in developing an ozone technology, the α was set higher, $\alpha = 0.10$.

Step 3. Write out the test statistic.

$$\chi_c^2 = \sum_{i=1}^{r}\sum_{j=1}^{c}\left[\frac{(O_{ij}-E_{ij})^2}{E_{ij}}\right]$$

Step 4. Decision rule.
If $\chi_c^2 > \chi_t^2$, reject H_0.
$$\chi_t^2 = \chi_{1-\alpha[(r-1)(c-1)]}^2 = \chi_{1-0.10[(4-1)(5-1)]}^2 = \chi_{0.90(12)}^2 = 18.55$$
So, if $\chi_c^2 > 18.55$, reject H_0 at $\alpha = 0.10$.

Step 5. Compute statistic. From the observed frequency table (Table 17), we compute an expected E_{ij} table (each $E_{ij} = n_i n_j / n_{..}$) (Table 18). Then by using both tables 17 and 18, we calculated χ_c^2.

$$
\begin{aligned}
\chi_c^2 = &\left[\frac{(8-2.4)^2}{2.4}+\frac{(2-2.4)^2}{2.4}+\frac{(1-2.4)^2}{2.4}+\frac{(1-2.4)^2}{2.4}+\frac{(0-2.4)^2}{2.4}\right.\\
&+\frac{(1-2.4)^2}{2.4}+\frac{(6-2.4)^2}{2.4}+\frac{(3-2.4)^2}{2.4}+\frac{(1-2.4)^2}{2.4}+\frac{(1-2.4)^2}{2.4}\\
&+\frac{(1-3.2)^2}{3.2}+\frac{(2-3.2)^2}{3.2}+\frac{(4-3.2)^2}{3.2}+\frac{(6-3.2)^2}{3.2}+\frac{(3-3.2)^2}{3.2}\\
&\left.+\frac{(0-2)^2}{2}+\frac{(0-2)^2}{2}+\frac{(2-2)^2}{2}+\frac{(2-2)^2}{2}+\frac{(6-2)^2}{2}\right]\\
= &\ 41.79
\end{aligned}
$$

TABLE 18 Expected E_{ij} Table

Log$_{10}$ reduction	Ozone (ppm)					
	0.5	0.8	1.0	1.3	1.6	Total ($n_{.j}$)
0–1	2.4	2.4	2.4	2.4	2.4	12.0
1–2	2.4	2.4	2.4	2.4	2.4	12.0
2–3	3.2	3.2	3.2	3.2	3.2	16.0
3–4	2.0	2.0	2.0	2.0	2.0	10.0
Total $n_{i.}$	10.0	10.0	10.0	10.0	10.0	$n_{..} = 50.0$

Note: $n_{11} = 10 \cdot 12 / 50 = 2.4$.

TABLE 19 Tabulated Statistics: Log_{10} Reduction, Ozone Level (ppm)

ROWS: LOG_{10} REPLICATES   COLUMNS: OZONE LEVEL

	0.5	0.8	1.0	1.3	1.6	ALL
1	8	2	1	1	0	12
	2.40	2.40	2.40	2.40	2.40	12.00
	3.61	−0.26	−0.90	−0.90	−1.55	—
2	1	6	3	1	1	12
	2.40	2.40	2.40	2.40	2.40	12.00
	−0.90	2.32	0.39	−0.90	−0.90	—
3	1	2	4	6	3	16
	3.20	3.20	3.20	3.20	3.20	16.00
	−1.23	−0.67	0.45	1.57	−0.11	—
4	0	0	2	2	6	10
	2.00	2.00	2.00	2.00	2.00	10.00
	−1.41	−1.41	0.00	0.00	2.83	—
ALL	10	10	10	10	10	50
	10.00	10.00	10.00	10.00	10.00	50.00
	—	—	—	—	—	—

CHI-SQUARE = 41.792, DF = 12, P-VALUE = 0.000 20
CELLS WITH EXPECTED COUNTS LESS THAN 5.0

Step 6.   Conclusion. Because $\chi_c^2(41.79) > \chi_t^2(18.55)$, the H_0 hypothesis of independence is rejected at $\alpha = 0.10$. We cannot conclude that ozone levels and log_{10} reductions in bacteria are independent of each other. There is evidence that this form of ozone delivery is worth pursuing. In fact, the evidence is very strong. At an α level of 0.005, the H_0 is still rejected ($\chi_{0.995}^2 = 28.30$).

Notice that none of the expected cell frequencies (E_{ij}) exceeded 5. Because this was a pilot study, it was used only as an orienting tool, leading to further research and refinements.

Table 19 provides a MiniTab® computer software application of this χ^2 analysis.

VIII. ORDINAL OR INTERVAL SCALE: MULTIPLE INDEPENDENT SAMPLES ($n > 2$)

The Kruskal–Wallis test is a nonparametric version of the one-factor analysis of variance and is probably the nonparametric test most widely used for comparing more than two samples [44]. It can be used, too, when only two samples are compared and, in that application, is equivalent to the Mann–Whitney U-test for two independent samples.

The data used by the Kruskal–Wallis test consist of randomly sampled treatment groups, which may differ in size but must comprise data at least of ordinal (rank) scale. The data are arranged into k columns and then ranked in ascending order. In cases of ties, the tied observations are assigned the average ranks of those ties based on the rank value that would be assigned if no ties existed. If the H_0 hypothesis is true, the k column sums of ranks will be equivalent.

A. Assumptions

1. The collected data consist of k random samples of size $n_1, n_2, \ldots n_k$. The sample sizes do not need to be equal.
2. The sample sets are independent.
3. The observations are independent within samples.
4. The variables of interest are continuous or approximate a continuous distribution.
5. The measurement scale is at least ordinal.
6. The populations are identical (i.e., the population distributions) except possibly in location (e.g., median) for at least one population.

The test statistic is:

$$t_c = \frac{12}{N(N+1)} \sum_{i=1}^{k} \frac{1}{n_i} \left[R_i - \frac{n_i(N+1)}{2} \right]^2 \tag{11}$$

which is computationally equivalent to an easier hand-computed formula:

$$t_c = \frac{12}{N(N+1)} \sum_{i=1}^{k} \frac{R_i^2}{n_i} - 3(N+1) \tag{12}$$

where $N = \sum_{i=1}^{k} n_i$ (total number of observations in the k samples)

R_i = sum of the ranks of the ith sample
n_i = sample size of the ith sample

In situations in which each sample size is less than 5 observations with a k of 3, the t_c (test statistic computed) is compared in Table A.9, critical values of the Kruskal–Wallis test statistic. When the number of samples and/or observations per sample exceeds these, use Table J, the χ^2 table with $k - 1$ degrees of freedom. Kruskal [48] demonstrated that, for large values of n_i and k, the t_c approximates the χ^2 distribution with $k - 1$ degrees of freedom.

B. Correction for Ties

If there are many ties (say, one fourth of the values or more), the test can be made more powerful by an adjustment, which is:

$$t_{c(\text{adjusted})} = \frac{t_c}{1 - \sum_{i=1}^{k} T/(N^3 - N)} \tag{13}$$

where $T = t^3 - t$ for each group of sample data
$\qquad t =$ the number of tied observations in a group of tied scores
$\qquad N =$ the $\sum_{i=1}^{k} n_i$ values

The effect of the tie adjustment is to inflate the test statistic's computed value. Hence, if t_c is significant at the computed (nonadjusted) value, there is no need to make a tie adjustment.

The six-step procedure can easily be used in computing the Kruskal–Wallis test.

Step 1. State the hypothesis.
$\qquad H_0$: The k populations are equivalent.
$\qquad H_A$: At least one of the k populations is different in its median value.
Step 2. Specify α.
Step 3. Decision rule. There are two versions.
  1. If $k = 3$ and each sample n is less than or equal to 5, use Table A.9, Kruskal–Wallis, to find the critical value. If $t_c >$ the tabled critical value at α, reject H_0. If there are many ties (one fourth or more of the sample) and t_c is not significant (i.e., greater than the critical value), apply the adjustment formula [Eq. (13)].

If $t_{c(\text{adjusted})} >$ critical value at α, reject H_0.

  2. If $k > 3$ and/or the n_i values are > 5, use Table A.10, χ^2 table, with $k - 1$ degrees of freedom. If $t_c > \chi^2_{t(\alpha, k-1)}$, reject H_0. If there are many ties (one fourth or more of the sample) and t_c is not significant, again, apply the adjustment formula [Eq. (13)].

If $t_{c(\text{adjusted})} > \chi^2_{t(\alpha, k-1)}$, reject H_0 at α.

Step 4.   Write out the test statistic. Use

$$t_c = \frac{12}{N(N+1)} \sum_{i=1}^{k} \frac{R_i^2}{n_i} - 3(N+1)$$

If a significant number of ties exist, use the correction factor.

Step 5.   Compute statistic.
Step 6.   Conclusion.

Example 8:   Three different antimicrobial wound dressings were se-lected to use in a simulated wound care model. The model substrate was a fresh, degermed pig skin, incubated at 35–37°C, with 3-cm incisions made and inoculated with 10^8 colony-forming units (CFU) of *Staphylococcus epi-dermidis* bacteria in a mix of bovine blood serum. The three wound dres-sings—A = 25% chlorhexidine gluconate, B = silver halide, and C = zinc oxide—were applied, and one inoculated wound was left untreated to pro-vide a baseline value. Each pigskin was placed in a sealed container with dis-tilled water to provide moisture and incubated for 24 hours. Sampling was performed using the cup scrub procedure. The $\log_{10}$ reductions recorded are presented in Table 20.

The investigator wants to know whether there was a significant differ-ence between wound antimicrobial products in terms of bacterial $\log_{10}$ re-ductions.

Step 1.   Formulate hypothesis.
H_0:   group A = group B = group C in $\log_{10}$ reductions.
H_A: At least one group differs from the other two.
Step 2.   Set α. The investigator will use $\alpha = 0.10$.

TABLE 20   Log$_{10}$ Reductions

$A = 1$	R_1	$B = 2$	R_2	$C = 3$	R_3
3.10	6.5	5.13	12.0	2.73	1.5
5.70	13.0	4.57	9.0	3.51	8.0
4.91	10.0	3.01	4.5	3.01	4.5
3.10	6.5	2.98	3.0	2.73	1.5
5.01	11.0				
	$\sum R_1 = 47$		$\sum R_2 = 28.5$		$\sum R_3 = 15.5$
	$n_1 = 5$		$n_2 = 4$		$n_3 = 4$

A, B, C = wound dressing types; R_i = rank of values in each wound dressing group.

Step 3.   Write the test statistic to be used.

$$t_c = \frac{12}{N(N+1)} \sum_{i=1}^{3} \frac{R_i^2}{n_i} - 3(N+1)$$

Step 4.   Decision rule. If $t_c >$ critical value, reject H_0. From the Kruskal–Wallis table (Table A.9), for $n_1 = 5, n_2 = n_3 = 4$, and $\alpha = 0.10$, the critical value is 4.6187. So if $t_c > 4.6187$, reject H_0 at $\alpha = 0.10$. Because nearly one half of the data are ties, if t_c is not significant, we will also use the adjustment formula.

$$t_{c(\text{adjusted})} = \frac{t_c}{1 - \sum T/(N^3 - N)}$$

Step 5.   Compute statistic.

$$t_c = \frac{12}{N(N+1)} \sum_{i=1}^{3} \frac{R_i^2}{n_i} - 3(N+1)$$

$$t_c = \frac{12}{13(14)} \left[\frac{47^2}{5} + \frac{28.5^2}{4} + \frac{15.5^2}{4} \right] - 3(14) = 4.4786$$

Because t_c is not significant, we will use the correction factor adjustment for ties,

$$t_{c(\text{adjusted})} = \frac{t_c}{1 - \sum T/(N^3 - N)}$$

where $T = t^3 - t$ for each group of sample data
$\quad\quad\quad t = $ number of ties
$\quad\quad\quad T_1 = 2^3 - 2 = 6$
$\quad\quad\quad T_2 = 0$
$\quad\quad\quad T_3 = 2^3 - 2 = 6$

$$= \frac{4.4786}{1 - [(6+0+6)/(13^3 - 13)]} = 4.5033$$

Step 6.   Conclusion. Because $t_{c(\text{adjusted})} = 4.5033 \not> 4.61876$, one cannot reject H_0 at $\alpha = 0.10$. But this is so close that for $\alpha = 0.15$, the H_0 hypothesis would be rejected.

The Kruskal–Wallis statistic can be particularly valuable in subjective ranking of scores (ordinal data). For example, in skin irritation studies, the score that one can get may range between 0 and 5, 0 representing no irritation and 5 representing severe. Suppose three products are evaluated and the following irritation scores result.

Product 1	Product 2	Product 3
0	1	4
0	1	4
1	1	3
2	3	2
1	2	0
1	2	1
1	0	5
3	1	
	1	

This evaluation is performed in exactly the same way as the previous one, with the tie adjustment formula applied.

C. Multiple Contrasts

In nonparametric statistics, as in parametric statistics, if a difference is detected when evaluating more than two sample groups, one cannot know where it lies—between what samples—without performing a multiple contrast procedure. The Kruskal–Wallis multiple comparison, like the parametric ANOVA contrast, provides a $1-\alpha$ confidence level for the family of contrasts performed.

The procedure is straightforward. First, one computes the sum-of-rank means, $\bar{R}_j$. Next, a value of α is selected that is generally larger than the customary $\alpha = 0.05$—e.g., 0.15, 0.20, or even 0.25, depending on the number of groups, k. The larger the k value, the more difficult it is to detect differences. From a practical standpoint, try to limit k to 3 or at most 4. The next step is to find, in the normal distribution table (Table A.1), the value of Z that has $\alpha/k(k-1)$ area to its right and compare the possible $n(n+1)/2$ contrast pairs $\bar{R}_i - \bar{R}_j|$ with the test inequalities.

use:

$$\sqrt{\frac{N(N+1)}{12}\left(\frac{1}{n_i}+\frac{1}{n_j}\right)} \quad \text{for uneven sample sizes} \tag{14}$$

use:

$$\sqrt{\frac{K(N+1)}{6}} \quad \text{for even sample sizes} \tag{15}$$

The entire contrast procedure is:

$$\text{If } |\bar{R}_i - \bar{R}_j| > Z_{\alpha/k(k-1)}\sqrt{\frac{N(N+1)}{12}\left(\frac{1}{n_i}+\frac{1}{n_j}\right)}, \text{ reject } H_0 \tag{16}$$

because a significant difference exists between $|\bar{R}_i - \bar{R}_j|$ at α.

Example 8 (continued): Let us use the data from Example 8 even though no significant difference between the groups was detected. This is only a demonstration of the computation of the multiple comparison. Let us set $\alpha = 0.15$.

$$\bar{R}_1 = \frac{47.0}{5} = 9.40$$

$$\bar{R}_2 = \frac{28.5}{4} = 7.13$$

$$\bar{R}_3 = \frac{15.5}{4} = 3.88$$

$$\frac{n(n-1)}{2} = 3 \text{ contrasts possible, which are } (\bar{R}_1\bar{R}_2), (\bar{R}_1\bar{R}_3), (\bar{R}_2\bar{R}_3)$$

First contrast:

$$|\bar{R}_1 - \bar{R}_2| = |9.40 - 7.13| \leq Z_{0.15/3(2)} = Z_{0.025}\sqrt{\frac{13(14)}{12}\left(\frac{1}{5}+\frac{1}{4}\right)}$$

$$= 2.27 \leq Z_{0.025}(2.6125)$$

The Z value is found in Table A.1, where $0.5 - 0.025 \approx 0.4750$, providing a tabled value of $1.96 = Z$. Hence,

$$2.27 \leq 1.96(2.6125) = 5.1205$$

Therefore, no difference exists at $\alpha = 0.15$.
    Second contrast:

$$|\bar{R}_1 - \bar{R}_3| = |9.40 - 3.88|$$

Hence, $5.52 > 5.1205$, so a significant difference exists at $\alpha = 0.15$.
    Third contrast:

$$|\bar{R}_2 - \bar{R}_3| = |7.13 - 3.88|$$

$$= 3.25 \leq (1.96)\sqrt{\frac{13(14)}{12}\left(\frac{1}{4}+\frac{1}{4}\right)}$$

$$= 3.25 \leq (1.96)2.7538 = 3.25 \leq 5.3974$$

Again, there is no significant difference at $\alpha = 0.15$.

TABLE 21   Kruskal–Wallis Comparisons

Kruskal–Wallis: Multiple Comparisons
Kruskal–Wallis Test on the Data

Group	N	Median	Average rank	Z
A	5	4.910	9.4	1.76
B	4	3.790	7.1	0.08
C	4	2.870	3.9	−1.93
Overall	13		7.0	

$H = 4.48$ $Df = 2$ $P = 0.107$
$H = 4.52$ $Df = 2$ $P = 0.105$ (adjusted for ties)
*Note: One or more small samples.

Kruskal–Wallis: All Pairwise Comparisons

Comparisons:	3
Ties:	3
Family alpha:	0.1
Bonferroni individual alpha:	0.033
Bonferroni Z-value (2-sided):	2.128

Standardized Absolute Mean Rank Difference
| Rbar (I) − Rbar (J) |/Stdev
Rows: Group I= $1, \ldots, N$
Columns: Group J= $1, \ldots, N$
1.   Table of Z-values

A	0.00000	*	*
B	0.87072	0.00000	*
C	2.11486	1.18019	0

Adjusted for Ties in the Data
1.   Table of Z-values

A	0.00000	*	*
B	0.87443	0.00000	*
C	2.12363	1.18509	0

2.   Table of P-values

A	1.00000	*	*

MiniTab®also provides the test (Table 21).

IX.   NOMINAL SCALE: MULTIPLE RELATED SAMPLES ($n > 2$)

Cochran's test for related observations is a useful test when the outcome can be presented in 0/1 format, a binomial outcome. The 0/1 arrangement can represent lived/died, success/failure, true/false, pass/not pass, etc. Recall from our previous sections that nominal data were analyzed using a 2×2 contingency table or an $r \times c$ contingency table. However, these tests are intended for independent samples. It is often possible and usually preferable to block groups across the treatments so that the power of the statistic can be increased. This frequently can be accomplished by applying all k treatments to the same related block but randomizing the k treatments within the block.

Take, for example, a preliminary skin reaction test where $0 =$ no reaction, and $1 =$ reaction. Suppose there are $k = 4$ products, 3 test and 1 control, and that each subject is a complete block, measuring all four treatments. Because the study is of nominal scale (0/1), Cochran's test for related samples is ideal.

Cochran's test for related samples requires that all k treatments be applied to each of the b blocks and the resultant data be categorized as 0/1 results. The result is a $k \times l$ table in which the row totals are identified as B_j and the column totals as the ks (Table 22). The χ^2 distribution is used with $\chi^2_{(\alpha, l-1)}$. That is, there are $l - 1$ degrees of freedom.

A. Assumptions

1. The blocks are randomly selected.
2. The data are nominal.

TABLE 22 $K \times L$ Table

		Treatments				
		1	2	$\cdots$	l	Row total x_{lk}
Blocks	1	x_{11}	x_{12}	$\cdots$	x_{1l}	B_1
						$B_i =$ block totals, $i = 1,2,\ldots,k$
	2	x_{21}	x_{22}	$\cdots$	x_{2l}	B_2
						$R_j =$ Column totals, $j = 1,2,\ldots,l$
	·	·	·	·	·	·
	·	·	·	·	·	·
	·	·	·	·	·	·
	k	x_{k1}	x_{k2}		x_{kl}	B_k
	Column total	C_1	C_2		C_l	$N =$ grand total

3. The samples are randomized within the block (e.g., sites on a single subject are randomly assigned to products).
4. The data results can be organized as 0/1.

The test hypothesis is a two-tail one.

H_0: The l treatments are equivalent.
H_A: There is a difference between at least two of the l treatments.

The test statistic is:

$$t_c = \frac{l(l-1)\sum_{j=1}^{l} C_j^2 - (l-1)N^2}{lN - \sum_{i=1}^{k} B_i^2} \tag{17}$$

where: l = number of columns or treatments
C_j = treatment totals for each jth column
N = number of rows times number of columns.
B_i = block total for each ith block

This test can easily be adapted into the six-step procedure.

Step 1. Formulate the hypothesis.
H_0: The C treatments are equal
H_A: The C treatments are not equal
Step 2. Select α. This will be a χ^2 distribution with $l-1$ degrees of freedom at α.
Step 3. Write out the test statistic to be used:

$$t_c = \frac{l(l-1)\sum_{j=1}^{l} C_j^2 - (l-1)N^2}{lN - \sum_{i=1}^{k} B_i^2}$$

Step 4. Decision rule.
If $t_c > \chi^2_{\alpha(l-1)}$, reject the H_0 hypothesis at α.
Step 5. Perform computation.
Step 6. Conclusion.

Example 9: In a primary skin irritation/sensitization study, five test products were applied to the backs of selected human subjects every other day for 21 days. A 7-day rest period was then observed so that, if the immune system was undergoing sensitization, it would have enough time to develop hypersensitivity. Following that, the five products were reintroduced to the back for 24 h. A reaction is designated 1 and no reaction 0. The investigator wants to know whether the test products differ at $\alpha = 0.05$. The results are presented in Table 23.

TABLE 23 Data

	Product					
	1	2	3	4	5	Total
Subject (block)						
1	0	0	0	0	0	0
2	1	1	1	1	0	4
3	1	0	0	0	0	1
4	0	0	0	0	0	0
5	1	0	1	1	0	3
6	1	0	0	0	0	1
7	1	0	0	0	0	1
8	1	1	0	1	1	4
9	0	0	0	0	0	0
10	1	0	1	1	0	3
Total treatments	7	2	3	4	1	17

Step 1. Formulate hypothesis.

H_0: Product 1 = product 2 = product 3 = product 4 = product 5

H_A: At least one product is different from the others in irritation

Step 2. Specify α. $\alpha = 0.05$.

Step 3. Write out the test statistic.

$$t_c = \frac{l(l-1)\sum\limits_{j=1}^{l} C_j^2 - (l-1)N^2}{lN - \sum\limits_{i=1}^{k} B_i^2}$$

Step 4. Specify decision rule.

If $t_c > \chi^2_{0.05(5-1)} = 9.488$, reject H_0 at $\alpha = 0.05$.

Step 5. Perform computation.

$$t_c = \frac{l(l-1)\sum\limits_{j=1}^{l} C_j^2 - (l-1)N^2}{lN - \sum\limits_{i=1}^{k} B_i^2}$$

$$t_c = \frac{5(5-1)[7^2 + 2^2 + 3^2 + 4^2 + 1^2] - (5-1)17^2}{5(17) - [0^2 + 4^2 + 1^2 + 0^2 + 3^2 + 1^2 + 1^2 + 4^2 + 0^2 + 3^2]}$$

$$= \frac{424}{32} = 13.25$$

Step 6. Conclusion. Because $t_c = 13.25 > \chi^2 = 9.488$), one rejects the H_0 hypothesis at $\alpha = 0.05$. The products do differ in irritation potential.

B. Multiple Comparisons

If the H_0 hypothesis is rejected, pairwise comparisons can be performed using the McNemar test, which is a variation on the sign test. Recall that the McNemar test is a two-sample test for related samples. The test is used as a pairwise test, so P tests must be computed for each pair compared. For demonstration purposes, suppose a researcher wanted to compare product 1 with product 5 and product 4 with product 5. (1 = reaction, 0 = no reaction) Product 1 versus 5. Let $x_A = 1$, $x_B = 5$, and let $\alpha = 0.05$.

		Product 1		Total
	Reaction	0	1	
Product 5	0	3	6	9
	1	0	1	1
	Total	3	7	10

If $|Z_c| = Z_t$, reject H_0 at α.
For $\alpha = 0.05$, $0.05/2 = 0.025$, $0.500 - 0.025 = 0.4750$. From table A, Z table, $Z_t = 1.96$.
So, if $|Z_c| > 1.96$, reject H_0.

$$Z_c = \frac{B - C}{\sqrt{B + C}} \quad \text{where} \quad \begin{array}{cc} A & B \\ C & D \end{array}$$

$$Z_c = \frac{6 - 0}{\sqrt{6 + 0}} = 2.4495$$

Because $Z_c = 2.4495 > Z_t = 1.96$, products 1 and 5 differ at $\alpha = 0.05$.
Product 4 versus 5. Let $x_A = 4$, $x_B = 5$, and let $\alpha = 0.05$.

		Product 4		Total
	Reaction	0	1	
Product 5	0	6	3	9
	1	0	1	1
	Total	6	4	10

If $|Z_c| > 1.96$, reject H_0.

$$Z_c = \frac{B - C}{\sqrt{B + C}} \qquad \text{where} \qquad \begin{matrix} A & B \\ C & D \end{matrix}$$

$$= \frac{3 - 0}{\sqrt{3 + 0}} = 1.7321$$

Because $Z_c = 1.7321 < Z_t = 1.96$, one cannot reject H_0 at $\alpha = 0.05$.

The researcher can continue to compare pairs of products in this manner.

X. ORDINAL SCALE: MULTIPLE RELATED SAMPLES (> 2)

Another very useful test in multiple sample comparisons, but with ordinal data, is the Friedman test. This test is a nonparametric statistical analog of the randomized complete block ANOVA model discussed in Chap. 5. The Friedman test is an extension of the Wilcoxon signed-ranks test for two samples, and when the number of samples is 2, it is essentially that test. The test is particularly useful in situations where the attributes of multiple products, services, or sensory experiences are ranked subjectively. For example, in a subjective preference test, a group of panelists (professional or naive) may be asked to rank mildness, sudsing, feel, fragrance, roughness, etc. of several different products. The Friedman test, which uses blocks (panelists in this case), is generally more powerful than the Kruskal–Wallis test, which is not blocked. This author has used this test for many years and finds it both powerful and robust.

The data display is like that of Cochran's test for nominal data (Table 24).

TABLE 24   Friedman Test

		Treatment				
		1	2	...	I	Row total
Blocks	1	x_{11}	x_{12}	...	x_{1I}	B_1
	2	x_{21}	x_{22}	...	x_{2I}	B_2
	.	.	.	.	.	.
	.	.	.	.	.	.
	.	.	.	.	.	.
	k	x_{k1}	x_{k2}		x_{kI}	B_k
	Column total	C_1	C_2		C_I	$N =$ grand total

A. Assumptions

1. The data consist of k mutually independent blocks of size l.
2. The data are blocked in meaningful ways (e.g., weight, height, sex, or same subject).
3. The data are continuous or, if discrete, can be treated as continuous (i.e., integer ranks).
4. No significant interaction between blocks and treatments is present.
5. Scale is at least ordinal (observations within blocks can be ranks, i.e., 1, 2, ..., l).

The test hypothesis is two-tail:

H_0: The populations are equivalent.
H_A: At least one population group differs from the other l groups.

B. Procedure

If the data collected are interval data, the first procedure is to rank them within blocks as though they were ordinal.

		Group			
		1	2	3	4
Values	Block 1	10.3	9.5	66.1	75.9
	Block 2	15.3	14.9	13.0	16.0
Ranked values by blocks	Block 1	2	1	3	4
	Block 2	3	2	1	4

If the data collected are already in ranks, this step is not necessary. Note that, in the Kruskal–Wallis test, the ranking is performed per treatment group, but the ranking for the Friedman test is done within the blocks, across groups.

If the H_0 hypothesis is true for the Friedman test, the ranks between the blocks will be random, none significantly larger or smaller than the others. If the H_0 hypothesis is rejected, it will be due to nonrandom order of the blocks.

After each block has been ranked, the next step is to obtain the rank-sums of the columns (C_is). If the H_0 hypothesis is true, the C_is will be nearly the same value.

The test statistic is:

$$\chi_c^2 = \frac{12}{lk(l+1)} \sum_{j=1}^{l} C_j^2 - 3k(l+1)$$

where l = number of treatments
           k = number of blocks
           C_j = sum of the jth treatment

If $\chi_c^2 \geq \chi_t^2 = \chi_{\alpha(l-1)}^2$ reject H_0 at α.

Note: When l and k are small ($l = 3$ or $4, k = 2, \ldots, 9$), one can use Friedman's test exact tables (Table A.11) to find χ_t^2. In using this table, l = number of treatments, k = number of blocks. Otherwise, use the chi square tables (Table A.10) with $l - 1$ degrees of freedom.

C. Ties

From a theoretical perspective, ties within blocks should not occur, but they do. Ties are handled, as always, by summing the ties (nontied ranks) in each block and dividing by the number of ties.

When a significant number of ties occur, about one fourth of the blocks or more, the test statistic should be adjusted and the χ_c^2 values should be expressed as $\chi_{c(MOD)}^2$

$$\chi_{c(MOD)}^2 = \frac{\chi_c^2}{1 - \sum_{i=1}^{k} T_i / lk(l^2 - 1)} \tag{18}$$

where: $T_i = \sum t_i^2 - \sum t_i$, when t_i is the number of observations tied in the ith block

     l = number of treatments
     k = number of blocks

The entire procedure can again be handled efficiently using the six-step procedure.

Step 1.   Formulate the test hypothesis, which will be a two-tail test.
     H_0: The groups are equal.
     H_A: The groups are not equal.
Step 2.   Set α.
Step 3.   Write out the test statistic.
Step 4.   Present decision rule using Friedman exact tables (Table A.11) if l and k are small; otherwise use the chi square table (Table A.10). If there are significant ties, these will affect
Step 5.   Perform statistical analysis.
Step 6.   Conclusion.

Example 10: A researcher wants to evaluate three skin-conditioning products for user perceptions of their moisturizing abilities. That is, the user participants rank the products in terms of how well they feel their skin has been moisturized. Ten panelists are recruited and randomly provided one of the products for use, then the second and the third. Before application of a test product, subjects are to apply an alcohol product to remove excess skin lipids from the skin so that each product can be applied with a minimum bias. Rankings were 1 = best, 2 = second best, and 3 = least good. The researcher set $\alpha = 0.10$. The results are presented in Table 25.

Step 1. Formulate hypothesis.
H_0: Product 1 = product 2 = product 3, in subjective perception
H_A: At least one product is different from the others
Step 2. Specify α. $\alpha = 0.10$.
Step 3. Write out the test statistic.

$$\chi_c^2 = \frac{12}{lK(l-1)} \sum_{j=1}^{l} c_j^2 - 3K(l+1)$$

Because there are significant ties in the data, χ_c^2 is adjusted by computing:

$$\chi_{c(MOD)}^2 = \frac{\chi_c^2}{1 - \sum_{j=1}^{k} T_i/K(l^2-1)}$$

Step 4. Specify decision rule. We must use the chi square table because K is greater than 9. If $\chi_{c(MOD)}^2 \geq \chi_t^2 = \chi_{t(a,l-1)}^2 = \chi_{t(0.10,3.1)}^2 = 4.605$, reject H_0 at $\alpha = 0.10$.

TABLE 25 Example Data

Panelist	Product 1	Product 2	Product 3
1	3.0	1	2.0
2	3.0	1	2.0
3	2.5	1	2.5
4	2.0	1	3.0
5	2.0	1	3.0
6	2.5	1	2.5
7	2.0	1	3.0
8	1.5	1.5	3.0
9	2.5	1	2.5
10	2.0	1	3.0
	$C_1 = 23.0$	$C_2 = 10.5$	$C_3 = 26.5$

TABLE 26   Friedman Test: MiniTab® Version

Friedman Test for Rank by Product Blocks by Panelist				
S = 14.15 Df = 2 P = 0.001				
S = 15.72 Df = 2 P = 0.000 (Adjusted for Ties)				
Product		N	Est Median	Sum of Ranks
1		10	2.1667	23.0
2		10	1.0000	10.5
3		10	2.5833	26.5
Grand Median = 1.9167				

Step 5.   Perform computation.

$$\chi_c^2 = \frac{12}{3(10)(3+1)}[23.0^2 + 10.5^2 + 26.5^2] - 3(10)(3+1)$$

$$\chi_c^2 = 134.15 - 120.00$$

$$\chi_c^2 = 14.15$$

Because there were a number of ties, the adjustment process will be used.

$$\chi_c^2 = \frac{\chi_c^2}{1 - \sum T_i/3(10)(3^2 - 1)}$$

There are four ties of two values:

$$T_i = (2^3 - 2) + (2^3 - 2) + (2^3 - 2) + (2^3 - 2) = 24$$

$$\chi_{c(\text{MOD})}^2 = \frac{14.15}{1 - [24/3(10)(9 - 1)]}$$

$$\chi_{c(\text{MOD})}^2 = 15.722$$

Step 6.   Conclusion.   Because $\chi_{c(\text{MOD})}^2 = 15.722 > \chi_t^2 = 4.605$, the researcher rejects H_0 at $\alpha = 0.10$. The products differ in subjective preference at $\alpha = 0.10$.

A MiniTab® version of this test is shown in Table 26.

D. Multiple Contrasts

Given that the H_0 hypothesis is rejected, the researcher will want to know which treatment groups differ. A very useful comparison of all possible contrasts, $l(l - 1)/2 = 3 \cdot 2/2 = 3$, can be made using the formula:

$$Z\sqrt{\frac{lk(l + 1)}{6}} \tag{19}$$

where Z corresponds to $\alpha/l(l - 1)$ in the normal Z tables (Table A.1). If $|C_i - C_j| \geq Z\sqrt{\frac{l(l+1)}{6}}$, reject H_0 at α.

Taking our example at $\alpha = 0.10$, $\alpha/l(l - 1) = 0.10/3(2) = 0.0167$. In the normal table, $0.5 - 0.0167 = 0.4833$, which provides a Z value of 2.13. So,

$$= Z\sqrt{\frac{l(l + 1)}{6}} = 2.13\sqrt{\frac{3(10)(3 + 1)}{6}} = 9.53$$

$$|C_1 - C_2| = |23.0 - 10.5| = 12.5 > 9.52 \qquad \text{Significant}$$

$$|C_1 - C_3| = |23.0 - 26.5| = 3.5 < 9.52 \qquad \text{Not Significant}$$

$$|C_2 - C_3| = |10.5 - 26.5| = 16 > 9.52 \qquad \text{Significant}$$

Hence, product 2 was ranked significantly higher than either product 1 or 3. Products 1 and 3 were not significantly different from each other at $\alpha = 0.10$.

XI. INTERVAL SCALE: MULTIPLE RELATED SAMPLES (> 2)

The nonparametric analog of the randomized complete block parametric statistic is the Quade test when using interval scale data. The Quade test, although less powerful than the parametric randomized complete block test, does not require a normal distribution [41,42]. Hence, in cases in which the distribution of interval data cannot be assured to be normal, the Quade test is the alternative. The Quade test is an extension of the Wilcoxon signed-ranks test. Although the Quade test will perform with ordinal "ranked" data, I have categorized it as an interval scale statistic because it has more theoretical assumptions than the Friedman test, so it is also more powerful. Yet this statement is not universally accepted. Some statisticians consider the Friedman and Quade tests to have about the same power. Some even suggest that the Friedman test, particularly when the number of treatment samples, l, is greater than six, is more powerful.

The Quade test is not as well known as the Kruskal–Wallis or Friedman test, but it is an extremely useful tool for the applied statistical researcher.

As with the last two tests discussed, the data display for the Quade test (interval data) is:

Blocks	Treatments			
	1	2	...	l
1	x_{11}	x_{12}	...	x_{1l}
2	x_{21}	x_{22}	...	x_{2l}
.	.	.		.
.	.	.		.
.	.	.		.
k	x_{k1}	x_{k2}		x_{kl}

A. Assumptions

1. The data consist of k mutually independent blocks of size l.
2. The data are blocked in meaningful ways (such as age, sex, weight, height, or same subject).
3. The data within each block can be ranked—data are at least ordinal. (This researcher prefers to use this test with interval data. It is suggested that, if the data are ordinal, the Friedman test be used.)
4. The sample range within each block can be determined. (There is a smallest and largest number in each block; the x values are not all equal.)
5. The blocks, themselves, must be rankable by range.
6. No significant interaction occurs between blocks and treatments.
7. The data are continuous.

The test hypothesis is a two-tail test.

H_0: The test populations are equivalent.
H_A: They differ in at least one.

Note: Ties do not adversely affect this test, so a correction factor is not necessary.

The F distribution table (Table A.3) is used in this test. The F_T value is $F_{\alpha[l-1;(l-1)(k-1)]}$. That is, the numerator degrees of freedom are $(l-1)$ and the denominator degrees of freedom are $(l-1)(k-1)$.

B. Procedure

Step 1. Let $R(x_{ij})$ be the rank from 1 to l of each block i. For example, in block (row) 1, the individual l treatments are ranked. A rank of 1 is provided to the smallest and a rank of l to the largest. Thus, step one is to rank all the observations, block by block, throughout the k blocks. In case of ties, the average rank is used, as before.

Step 2. Using the original x_{ij} values—not the ranks—determine the range of each block. The range in block $i = \text{MAX}(X_{ij}) - \text{MIN}(x_{ij})$. There will be k sample ranges, one for each block.

Step 3. Once the ranges are determined, rank the block ranges, assigning 1 to the smallest up to k for the largest. If ties occur, use the average rank. Let $R_1, R_2, \ldots R_k$ be the ranks assigned to the $1, 2, \ldots k$ blocks.

Step 4. Each block rank, R_i, is then multiplied by the difference between the rank within block i, $[R(x_{ij})]$, and the average rank within the blocks, $(l + 1)/2$, to get the value for S_{ij}, which represents the relative size of each observation within the block, adjusted to portray the relative significance of the block in which it appears. Each S_{ij} value $= R_i[R(x_{ij} - (l+1)/2]$. Each treatment group sum is denoted by $S_{ij} = \sum_{i=1}^{k} S_{ij}$.

The test statistic is similar to that in ANOVA.

$$\text{SS}_{\text{TOTAL}} = \sum_{i=1}^{k} \sum_{j=1}^{l} S_{ij}^2 \tag{20}$$

If there are no ties in SS_{TOTAL}, a simpler equation can be used:

$$\text{SS}_{\text{TOTAL}} = \frac{k(k + 1)(2k + 1)l(l + 1)(l - 1)}{72}$$

The treatment sum of squares is:

$$\text{SS}_{\text{TREATMENT}} = \frac{1}{k} \sum_{j=1}^{l} S_j^2 \tag{21}$$

The test statistic is:

$$F_C = \frac{(k - 1)\text{SS}_{\text{TREATMENT}}}{\text{SS}_{\text{TOTAL}} - \text{SS}_{\text{TREATMENT}}} \tag{22}$$

Note: If $\text{SS}_{\text{TOTAL}} - \text{SS}_{\text{TREATMENT}} = 0$, use that point "0" as if it were in the critical region and calculate the critical level or "p" value as $(1/l!)^{k-1}$, where $l!$ is l factorial or $l \cdot (l - 1) \cdot (l - 2) \cdots (l - l + 1)$ (e.g., $l = 5, l! = 5 \cdot 4 \cdot 3 \cdot 2 \cdot 1 = 120$).

The decision rule is, if $F_C > F_t = F_{\alpha[l-1;(l-1)(k-1)]}$, reject H_0 at α.

Again, the six-step procedure is easily adapted to this statistical analysis.

Step 1. Formulate hypothesis, which will always be for a two-tail test.
   H_0:   The groups are equal.
   H_A: The groups are not equal.
Step 2. Choose α.
Step 3. Write out the test statistic.

$$F_C = \frac{(k-1)SS_{\text{TREATMENT}}}{SS_{\text{TOTAL}} - SS_{\text{TREATMENT}}}$$

Step 4. Decision rule.
   If $F_C > F_t$, reject H_0 at α.
Step 5. Perform statistic.
Step 6. Conclusion.

Example 11: A researcher working with *Pseudomonas aeruginosa* tested the resistance to biofilm formation of several antimicrobial compounds applied to the surface of venous/arterial catheters. Three different sample configurations of catheter material were introduced into five bioreactors, each of which was considered a block for the analysis. After a 72-hour growth period in a continuous-flow nutrient system, the catheter materials were removed, and the microorganism/biofilm levels were enumerated in terms of $\log_{10}$ colony-forming units. The researcher wanted to know whether there was a significant difference in microbial adhesion among the products.

		Test catheter		
		1	2	3
Reactors (blocks)	1	5.03	3.57	4.90
	2	3.25	2.17	3.10
	3	7.56	5.16	6.12
	4	4.92	3.12	4.92
	5	6.53	4.23	5.99

The collected data were tabulated, as shown here. Because the study was a small pilot study with few replicate blocks and the blocks varied so much, a nonparametric model was selected.

Step 1. Formulate hypothesis.
   H_0:   Catheter material $1 = 2 = 3$ in microbial adherence
   H_A: At least one catheter material is different
Step 2. Specify α. Because this was a small study, α was selected as 0.10.

Step 3. Write out the test statistic. The test statistic to be used is:

$$F_C = \frac{(k-1)SS_{\text{TREATMENT}}}{SS_{\text{TOTAL}} - SS_{\text{TREATMENT}}}$$

Step 4. Present decision rule.

If $F_C > F_t$, reject H_0 at $\alpha = 0.10$.
$F_t = F_{t\alpha[l-1;(l-1)(k-1)]}$, where numerator degrees of freedom $= l - 1 = 2$, denominator degrees of freedom $= (l-1)(k-1) - (3-1)(5-1) = 8$, and $\alpha = 0.10$.

$F_{t[0.10(2,8)]} = 3.11$. Therefore, if $F_C > F_t = 3.11$, reject H_0 at $\alpha = 0.10$.

Step 5. Perform computation (the collected results are reconstructed here).

		Test catheter		
		1	2	3
Reactors (reactor)	1	5.03 (3)	3.57 (1)	4.90 (2)	$R(X_{13})$
	2	3.25 (3)	2.17 (1)	3.10 (2)
	3	7.56 (3)	5.16 (1)	6.12 (2)
	4	4.92 (2.5)	3.12 (1)	4.92 (2.5)
	5	6.53 (3)	4.23 (1)	5.99 (2)

1. First rank blocks in $1, 2, 3, \ldots$ order.
2. Next, determine range of actual values, from high value to low value.

   Block $1: 5.03 - 3.57 = 1.46$ $4: 4.92 - 3.12 = 1.80$
                 $2: 3.25 - 2.17 = 1.08$ $5: 6.53 - 4.23 = 2.30$
                 $3: 7.56 - 5.16 = 2.40$

3. Next, rank the blocks.
4. Determine $S_{ij} = R_i[R(x_{ij}) - \frac{l+1}{2}]$ for each x_{ij}

$$S_{11} = 2\left(3 - \frac{3+1}{2}\right) = 2$$

$$S_{12} = 2(1-2) = -2$$

$$S_{13} = 2(2-2) = 0$$

$$S_{21} = 1(3-2) = 1$$

$$S_{22} = 1(1 - 2) = -1$$

$$S_{23} = 1(2 - 2) = 0$$

$$S_{31} = 5(3 - 2) = 5$$

$$S_{32} = 5(1 - 2) = -5$$

$$S_{33} = 5(2 - 2) = 0$$

$$S_{41} = 3(2.5 - 2) = 1.5$$

$$S_{42} = 3(1 - 2) + -3$$

$$S_{43} = 3(2.5 - 2) = 1.5$$

$$S_{51} = 4(3 - 2) = 4$$

$$S_{52} = 4(1 - 2) = -4$$

$$S_{53} = 4(2 - 2) = 0$$

Block	Sample block range	Block rank (R_i)	Catheter		
			1	2	3
1	1.46	2	2	-2	0
2	1.08	1	1	-1	0
3	2.40	5	5	-5	0
4	1.80	3	1.5	-3	1.5
5	2.30	4	4	-4	0
			$S_1 = 13.5$	$S_2 = -15.0$	$S_3 = 1.5$

5. Determine SS_{TOTAL}

$$SS_{TOTAL} = \sum_{i=1}^{k} \sum_{j=1}^{l} S_{ij}^2$$

$$= 2^2 + (-2)^2 + 0^2 + 1^2 + (-1)^2 + 0^2$$
$$+ 5^2 + (-5)^2 + 0^2 + 1.5^2 + (-3)^2 + 1.5^2$$

$$+ 4^2 + (-4)^2 + 0^2$$
$$= 105.50$$

$$SS_{TOTAL} = 105.50$$

$$SS_{TREATMENT} = \frac{1}{k} \sum_{j=1}^{l} S_{ij}^2 = \frac{1}{5}[13.5^2 + (-15)^2 + 1.5^2] = 81.90$$

$$SS_{TREATMENT} = 81.90$$

Next, Compute F_C:

$$F_C = \frac{(k-1)SS_{TREATMENT}}{SS_{TOTAL} - SS_{TREATMENT}} = \frac{(5-1)81.90}{105.50 - 81.90} = 13.88$$

$$F_C = 13.88$$

Step 6. Conclusion. Because $F_C = 13.88 > F_T = 3.11$, the H_0 hypothesis is rejected at $\alpha = 0.10$. Performance of one catheter is different from the others.

C. Multiple Contrasts

As before, multiple contrasts are conducted only when H_0 is rejected. The computation formula is for all possible $l(l-1)/2$ contrast combinations. If $|S_i - S_j|$ is greater than

$$t_{\alpha/2} \sqrt{\frac{2k(SS_{TOTAL} - SS_{TREATMENT})}{(l-1)(k-1)}} \tag{23}$$

conclude that the difference is significant at α.

Let us contrast the catheter products.

$$\sqrt{\frac{2k(SS_{TOTAL} - SS_{TREATMENT})}{(l-1)(k-1)}} = \sqrt{\frac{2(5)(105.5 - 81.90)}{2(4)}} = 5.4314$$

$t_{0.10/2}$ with $(l-1)(k-1)$ df $= t_{(0.05,8)} = 1.86$. (table B, Student's T table)

So,

$$t_{\alpha/2} \sqrt{\frac{2k(SS_{TOTAL} - SS_{TREATMENT})}{(l-1)(k-1)}} = 1.86(5.4314) = 10.10$$

Catheter product contrasts:

$$1 \text{ vs. } 2 = |13.5 - (-15)| = 28.5 > 10.10 \qquad \text{Significant}$$
$$1 \text{ vs. } 3 = |13.5 - 1.5| = 12 > 10.10 \qquad \text{Significant}$$
$$2 \text{ vs. } 3 = |-15 - 1.5| = 16.5 > 10.10 \qquad \text{Significant}$$

Each of the catheter products is significantly different from the others at $\alpha = 0.10$.

XII. SIMPLE LINEAR REGRESSION WITH NONPARAMETRIC STATISTICS

Regression analysis, as we have seen, is a very widely used and valuable procedure in applied research. In Chap. 11, we discussed parametric regression methods. The methods of regression require that the data meet fairly rigid restrictions. When those restrictions cannot be met, and many times they cannot, nonparametric methods offer a valuable alternative.

Recall that in simple linear regression, there are two variables, the independent variable x and the dependent or response variable y. The regression parameters b_0 and b_1 are determined from the x, y data set providing the simple linear regression equation:

$$y = b_0 + b_1 x$$

There are several nonparametric methods that use standard parametric procedures, the least squares approach, for determining both b_0 and b_1. This researcher recommends using not those methods but, instead, a method developed by Mood and Brown [43].

A. Mood–Brown Regression Method (with Paulson Modification)

This method is fairly involved, but for small samples it is easily accomplished using pen and paper. For larger data sets, a software statistical program, such as MiniTab®, is useful.

The y values are first portioned into two sets: (1) those having x values to the left of the median of x, that is, specifically less than or equal to the median of x, and (2) those having x values greater than the x value median. The predicted values of b_0 and b_1 are the values that present a line in which the median of the deviations around the regression line is 0 in both of the data sets. Predicting 0 is not always possible, but one wants to be as close to it as possible.

B. Mood-Brown Determinants of b_0 and b_1

Step 1.   Linearize the data, and prepare a scattergram of the sample data. It is recommended that EDA be performed on any data intended for regression. If the assumptions of parametric regression cannot be assured, use the nonparametric statistic.

Step 2.   Draw a vertical line through the x median. If one or more points fall on the x median, shift the line to the left or right such that the numbers of points to the left and right of the x median are equal or as equal as possible.

Step 3.   Determine the medians of x and those of y for the two subgroups, left and right. [There will be one pair of (x, y) medians for the left group, called (x_1, y_1), and one pair of (x, y) medians for the right group, called x_2, y_2.]

Step 4.   For the first group of data [the (x, y) values with the x_1 values less than or equal to the x median], plot the point representing the (x, y) median intercept. Do the same for the second (x_2, y_2) group of data. There will be two points when this is completed, represented by (x_1, y_1) and (x_2, y_2).

Step 5.   Draw a line connecting the two points. This is the first estimate of the regression line.

Step 6.   If the median of the vertical deviation of points from this line is not 0 for both groups, shift the regression line to a new position until you find where the deviation of each group is 0.

Step 7.   The value of b_0 is the point where the y intercept is crossed when $x = 0$, based on the scribed regression line.

$$b_1 = \frac{y_1 - y_2}{x_1 - x_2} \tag{24}$$

C. Mood-Brown Assumptions

1.   The data collected are interval scale.
2.   The data collected are continuous.
3.   The (x, y) values are associated.
4.   Generally, the x values are selected, not randomly determined.

Let us work an example (Example 12).

Example 12:   In a pilot evaluation, a researcher wanted to know the rate of bacterial reductions and the expected number of bacteria on a death curve (regression slope). *Streptococcus pyogenes* were used with a baseline (initial) population of 1.72×10^8 CFU/mL. Five time intervals were used: 0, 30, 60, 90, and 120 seconds. The colony-forming unit counts were as follows:

x = time (seconds)	y = microbial population (CFU/mL)
0	1.72×10^8
30	2.58×10^7
60	1.56×10^6
90	2.73×10^5
120	1.43×10^4

Because the data were not linear, the researcher performed a $\log_{10}$ transformation on the y values, termed y'.

x = time (seconds)	y' = microbial population ($\log_{10} y$)
0	8.24
30	7.41
60	6.19
90	5.44
120	4.16

Please note, also, that when using nonparametric regression, the data size, n, is usually small. Otherwise, a parametric model would probably be used. In this researcher's opinion, it is easiest to plot the data points by means of a computer printout. Figure 6 is the MiniTab® version.

The actual x median is 60 (solid line), but because it cuts a value (6.19) in half, the line is moved slightly left or right. We will move it right (dashed line).

The (x_1, y_1) median values of the three data points to the left of the median ($x = 60$) are (30, 7.41). The (x_2, y_2) median values of the two observations to the right of 60 are $x_2 = (90 + 120)/2 = 105$ and for y_2 are $(5.44 + 4.16)/2 = 4.80$.

$$x_2, y_2 = (105, 4.80)$$

A regression line is drawn through (x_1, y_1) and $(x_2, y_2) = (30, 7.41)$ and $(105, 4.80)$. Now, using the algebraic formula for the slope:

$$\text{Slope } b_1 = m = \frac{y_2 - y_1}{x_2 - x_1} = \frac{4.80 - 7.41}{105 - 30} = -0.0348$$

the slope, b_1, is estimated.

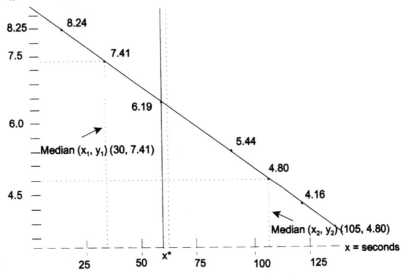

FIGURE 6   Annotated MiniTab® printout.

So, $b_1 = -0.0348$, which means that for every 1-second exposure, the microbial population decreases by 0.0348 log.

D. Paulson Modification

Instead of trying to draw and, from the drawing, find the differences between the y values and the $\hat{y}$ predicted values, use the function $y = mx + b$ to determine the regression line. Because the function is linear, use (x_1, y_1) or (x_2, y_2)—it does not matter which—and solve for $b_0 = y$ intercept.

$y = mx + b$,   where $y = y_2$ and $x = x_2$

$y_2 = 4.80$, $x_2 = 105$, $m = -0.0348$

$4.80 = -0.0348(105) + b_0$,   solve for b_0

$b_0 = 4.80 + 3.654 = 8.45$

So the entire regression equation is, by the Paulson modification.

Then construct a regression function:

$$\hat{y} = b_0 + b_1 x = 8.45 - 0.0348x$$

Next compute $\hat{y}$ for each x, and subtract $\hat{y}$ from y_ϵ.

x	y	$\hat{y}$	$\epsilon = y - \hat{y}$
0	8.24	8.45	−0.23
30	7.41	7.41	0.00
60	6.19	6.36	−0.17
90	5.44	5.32	0.12
120	4.16	4.27	−0.11
			$\sum \epsilon = -0.39$

Here $\sum \epsilon = -0.39$—notice that the error magnitudes oscillate around the regression line midpoint of 60, so the slope b_1 is fine, but the b_0 estimate can probably be improved. So, we will "tweak" b_0 in order to reduce $\sum \epsilon$.

Let $b_0 = 8.35$, and see what happens; $\hat{y} = 8.35 - 0.0348x$ and recalculate the $\hat{y}$ value as well as on a new $\sum \epsilon$.

x	y	$\hat{y}$	$\epsilon = y - \hat{y}$
0	8.24	8.35	−0.11
30	7.41	7.31	0.10
60	6.19	6.26	−0.07
90	5.44	5.22	0.22
120	4.16	4.17	−0.01
			$\sum \epsilon = 0.13$

Because $\sum \epsilon = 0.13$, the error is positive, so we will tweak b_0 again by increasing it a couple of points and see what happens.

Let us set b_0 at 8.38; $\hat{y} = 8.38 - 0.0348x$ and again recalculate the $\hat{y}$ value and $\sum \epsilon$.

x	y	$\hat{y}$	$\epsilon = y - \hat{y}$
0	8.24	8.38	−0.14
30	7.41	7.34	0.07
60	6.19	6.29	−0.10
90	5.44	5.25	0.19
120	4.16	4.20	−0.04
			$\sum \epsilon = -0.02$

Here $\sum \epsilon = -0.02$, which is very good for practical purposes. The regression at a cumulated error term of -0.02 is, for this researcher, good enough.

The regression formula via this nonparametric procedure is:

$$\hat{y} = b_0 + b_1 x$$

$$\hat{y} = 8.38 - 0.0348(x)$$

If the data had originally provided negative errors for the data to the left of the $x = 60$ median and positive for the data to the right of the $x = 60$ median, the $\hat{y}$ values in $b_1 = m = (y_1 - y_2)/(x_1 - x_2) = \Delta y/\Delta x$ would have been iteratively changed by decreasing the $\hat{y}$ values to reduce the slope. This would be done until all the errors to the left and right of the $x = 60$ median were equally positive and negative. If further corrections were then needed, it would be done at b_0, as the example portrayed (Fig. 7).

E. Suggestions

1. If the study is controlled in the sense that the x_i values are pre-determined, be sure the range of x_i values extends as far as possible. That is, the span from the lowest to the highest values

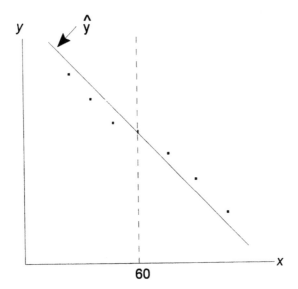

FIGURE 7   Further corrections.

should be as great as is practical. This will provide value in two ways. It will enable the estimates of the regression parameters, b_0 and b_1, to be more accurate and precise. Second, it will enable the researcher to better determine whether the regression function is, in fact, linear. If it is not, the researcher will need to linearize the data set by one of the transformations discussed previously in the EDA section (Chap. 3) and the regression section (Chap. 11).

2. Be sure to replicate each of the x_i values. A minimum of two or, better yet, three replicates per x_i value is preferred. If one's budget is extremely tight, skimp on replicating the middle x_i values, not the outside high and low data sets. For example, Fig. 8 portrays this strategy in that the outside values have 3 replicates each, the next values 2 each, and the inside two 1 each.

3. It is also important to perform true replicates. All too often, applied researchers think replication is merely multiple measurements of the same x_i condition (e.g., same subject, same lot, same experiment). This is appropriate only if the researcher is measuring "observation" error (repeated measurement), measuring the precision of the experimental process itself. But most researchers are interested in the induction process. They want to make a generalized claim about the experiment conducted, using specific conditions. That requires actual replication, which is essentially performing a single experiment "n" times.

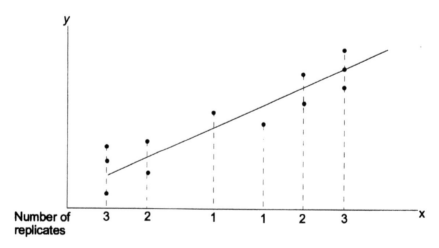

FIGURE 8 "Skimping" strategy.

XIII. HYPOTHESIS TESTING FOR b_0 AND b_1

Several authors suggest using the Brown and Mood procedure for hypothesis testing of both b_0 and b_1 once these estimates have been determined [41,42,44].

> $H_0: b_0 = b_0'$
> $H_A: b_0 \neq b_0'$, where b_0' is 0 or some fixed value for the y coordinate intercept when $x = 0$

and

> $H_0: b_1 = b_1'$
> $H_A: b_1 \neq b_1'$, where b_i' is 0 or some other fixed value for regression slope

The procedure is applicable from our previous calculations of b_0 and b_1.

One merely looks at the last (final) regression function drawn and counts the y_i values above the final regression line ($\hat{y}$) in the first (left of the vertical x median line) group of data separated by the vertical x_{median} line. [Recall that we moved the vertical median line to the right of $x_{median} = 60$ because 60 has a value. We showed this with a theoretical dashed line (Fig. 9) It serves no purpose other than to include $x_{median} = 60$ in the left side data.] Call this value n_1. Do the same with the values to the right of the center line, which are above.

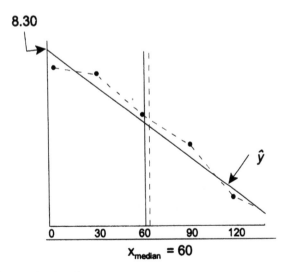

FIGURE 9   Regression function.

There is only one value y greater than the $\hat{y}$ in the first group to the left of the vertical line x_{median}, so $n_1 = 1$. For the values above $\hat{y}$ in the second group, there is also one value, so $n_2 = 1$.

Note: This can also be determined by residuals (ϵ).

	x	y	$\hat{y}$	$\epsilon = y - \hat{y}$		
Data group to	0	8.24	8.38	−0.14		Count the number of positive
the left of	30	7.41	7.34	0.07	n_1	values of ϵ left of and including
median	60	6.19	6.29	−0.10		$x_{med} = 60$, which is 1.
						$n_1 = 1$.
	90	5.44	5.25	0.19		For the second group, count
Data group to						the number of positive ϵ values
the right					n_2	to the right of the vertical median
of median						line. There is also 1 positive value
	120	4.16	4.20	−0.04		in this group, so $n_2 = 1$.

The n_1 and n_2 have binomial distributions with the indicator value of 0.5, and the test statistic is:

$$\chi_c^2 = \frac{8}{n}\left[\left(n_1 - \frac{n}{4}\right)^2 + \left(n_2 - \frac{n}{4}\right)^2\right] \tag{25}$$

where: n = number of (x,y) coordinate values

n_1 = number of positive values, $y_i > \hat{y}$, in the left one half data group

n_2 = number of positive values, $y_i > \hat{y}$, in the right one half data group, which is distributed as a chi square (χ^2) distribution with 2 degrees of freedom: $\chi_{t(\alpha,2)}^2$

If $\chi_c^2 > \chi_t^2$, reject H_0 at α.

Let us work an example, specifying $b_0' = 8.38$ and $b_1' = -0.0348$. This works well using the six-step procedure.

Step 1. Formulate the hypothesis.
$H_0: b_0 = 8.38$ and $b_1 = -0.0348$
$H_A: b_0 \neq 8.38$ and $b_1 \neq -0.0348$

Step 2. Set α. Let $\alpha = 0.10$. But this time we will also determine the p value. That is, given the H_0 hypothesis is true, with the χ_C^2 value we will compute, how likely is its probability?

Step 3. Write out the test statistic to be used.

$$\chi_c^2 = \frac{8}{n}\left[\left(n_1 - \frac{n}{4}\right)^2 + \left(n_2 - \frac{n}{4}\right)^2\right]$$

Step 4. Decision rule.

If $\chi_c^2 > \chi_t^2$ (where $\chi_{t(0.10,2)}^2 = 4.605$), from table J, reject H_0.

Step 5. Perform calculation.

$$\chi_c^2 = \frac{8}{5}\left[\left(1 - \frac{5}{4}\right)^2 + \left(1 - \frac{5}{4}\right)^2\right]$$

$$\chi_c^2 = 0.20 < \chi_t^2 = (4.605)$$

Step 6. Conclusion. Because $\chi_c^2 < \chi_t^2$, one cannot reject H_0 at $\alpha = 0.10$. b_0 is not significantly different from 8.38, and b_1 is not significantly different from -0.0348.

A. Evaluating Two Regression Slopes (B_1) for Parallelism

There are times when a researcher will want to compare two regression slopes (b_1) for equivalence. For example, if two moisturizing products are evaluated in terms of the rate of moisturizing, two antimicrobial products are evaluated for rate of bacterial inactivation, or two drugs are evaluated for rate of absorption by the liver, this procedure can be useful.

In this investigator's opinion, it is extremely useful to evaluate the b_1 values of multiple test groups—with small samples—using nonparametric procedures. In fact, when large sample sizes are used, the math becomes a real burden.

There are a number of procedures applicable for regression slope evaluations. One devised by Hollander [48] is particularly useful, using a modification of the Wilcoxon matched-pair signed-ranks test discussed earlier in this chapter.

B. Assumptions

1. Both regression functions are linear and can be adequately described by:
    $$\hat{y}_A = b_{0_A} + b_{1_A} \quad \text{for population A}$$
    and
    $$\hat{y}_B = b_{0_B} + b_{1_B} \quad \text{for population B}$$

2. Each y value (response or dependent variable) is measured without bias for each x point set. The x values for both models are "pre-set," not random variables, themselves.
3. The ϵ values $(y - \hat{y})$ are random errors for each population and are independent of one another.

C. Hypothesis Testing

We will concern ourselves with testing only two different sample sets, which can be written as:

Population A: $\hat{y}_{ia} = b_{0a} + b_{0a}x_{ia} + e_{ia}$

Population B: $\hat{y}_{ib} = b_{0b} + b_{0b}x_{ib} + e_{ib}$

Both two-tail and one-tail tests can be performed:

Two tail	Lower tail	Upper tail
$H_0: \beta_{1a} = \beta_{1b}$	$H_0: \beta_{1a} \geq \beta_{1b}$	$H_0: \beta_{1a} \leq \beta_{1b}$
$H_A: \beta_{1a} \neq \beta_{1b}$	$H_A: \beta_{1a} < \beta_{1b}$	$H_A: \beta_{1a} > \beta_{1b}$

D. Equal and Even Sample Sizes

This procedure requires that the numbers of observations for populations A and B be equal, $n_a = n_b$, and that they be even in number. If they are not, one evens and equalizes them by random removal of (x, y) pair values until $n_a = n_b$ and n_a and n_b are even (divisible by 2 with no remainder).

E. Procedure

1. The two sample populations, equal in size and even in number, are arranged in ascending order based on the x_i values. That is, $x_1 \leq x_2 \leq x_3 \cdots \leq x_n$. There will be two groups, A and B.
2. Divide each group in two based on the x_i values. The total sample size of each x data group will be $2n$. Pair the x_i values as x_i, x_{i+n}, e.g., $i = 1, 2, \ldots, n$. For example, if you have 16 values of x_{ia}, they are separated into two groups of 8. The pairing will be (based on original order)

$$x_i, x_{i+n} \quad = x_1, x_{1+8=9} \quad x_1 x_9$$
$$= x_2, x_{2+8=10} \quad x_2 x_{10}$$
$$\cdots \qquad\qquad \cdots$$
$$= x_n, x_{n+8} \qquad x_n x_{n+n}$$

3. Compute the n slope estimated for group A, then group B.

$$S_{A_i} = \frac{y_{(i+n)} - y_i}{x_{(i+n)} - x_i} \tag{26}$$

where A = group A, $i = 1, 2, \ldots, n,$

$$S_{B_i} = \frac{y_{(i+n)} - y_i}{x_{(i+n)} - x_i} \tag{27}$$

where B= group B, $i = 1, 2, \ldots, n.$

4. Randomly pair the S_{A_i}s and S_{B_i}s so that each S_{A_i} is paired with each S_{B_i}.
5. Compute the n difference.

$$D_i = S_{A_i} - S_{B_i} \tag{28}$$

6. The n differences are:

$$D_1, D_2, \ldots, D_n$$

7. The procedure from here on is identical to the Wilcoxon signed-rank test. The absolute values of the differences, $|D_i|$, are ranked from smallest to largest. Ties among D_is are assigned the mean of the n tied values, as always.
8. Each of the resulting ranks is assigned the sign (plus/minus) of the difference for which the absolute value yields that rank.
9. Compute the R_i:

$R+ = $ sum of ranks positive

$R- = $ sum of ranks negative

The test statistic is exactly as previously presented. The process will be presented in the six-step procedure.

Step 1. Specify hypothesis.

Two tail	Lower tail	Upper tail
$H_0 : \beta_{1a} = \beta_{1b}$	$H_0 : \beta_{1a} \geqslant \beta_{1b}$	$H_0 : \beta_{1a} \leqslant \beta_{1b}$
$H_A : \beta_{1a} \neq \beta_{1b}$	$H_A : \beta_{1a} < \beta_{1b}$	$H_A : \beta_{1a} > \beta_{1b}$

Step 2.   Select α. Use $\alpha/2$ for two-tail tests at α.

Step 3.   Write out the test statistic directly off the Wilcoxon table (Table A.8) Tables H and A in Appendix.

$$Z_c = \frac{R - [n(n+1)]/4}{\sqrt{n(n+1)(2n+1)/24}} \tag{29}$$

where R = sum of squares, as used according to step 4; it will be either $R+$ or $R-$, depending upon which tail test is chosen

$R+$ = sum of positive rank values

$R-$ = sum of negative rank values

Step 4.   Specify decision rule.*

Wilcoxon Table

Two-tail test	Upper tail test	Lower tail test
The test depends upon the sum of the ranks, $R+$ or $R,-$ whichever is smaller. If $R-/+$ is equal to or less than the tabled d value value, reject H_0 at α.	This test uses the sum of the ranks of negative values $(R-)$. If $R-$ is smaller than or equal to d tabled (Wilcoxon table, Table H in Appendix), reject H_0 at α.	This test uses the sum of the ranks of positive values $(R+)$. If $R+$ is smaller than or equal to d tabled (Table H in Appendix), reject H_0 at α.

Step 5.   Perform calculations.

Step 6.   Conclusion.

Example 13: A researcher performs a pilot study to determine whether the lethality rates of two hard-surface disinfectants are equivalent (parallel). The two products are:

Product A $= 0.5\%$ PCMX

Product B $= 0.5\%$ triclosan

---

*Note: In using the Wilcoxon table (Table H in Appendix), the d value is the $R+$ or $R-$ value and the number of D_i pairs is n.

The exposure times are 0 (baseline control), 15 seconds, 30 seconds, 60 seconds, 90 seconds, and 120 seconds. The results are microbial counts, in $\log_{10}$ scale to linearize the data, as follows:

	Product A		Product B
	Microbial counts		**Microbial Counts**
x (seconds)	y (log)	x (seconds)	y (log)
0	8.01	0	9.15
15	7.49	15	8.23
30	6.38	30	7.15
60	5.43	60	6.23
90	3.23	75	5.89
120	2.15	90	4.16
		105	3.27
		120	2.70

Prior to performing any statistics, it is wise to plot both data sets. They are presented in Figs. 10 and 11 in MiniTab® computer software output. Note that I removed product B readings at 75 and 105 seconds to equalize n_A and n_B. The observations are also even in number, $n_A = n_B = 6$. The plotted data for both products look linear, so we will go ahead with the comparison, using the six-step procedure.

Step 1. Formulate hypothesis for comparing the two slopes (b_1).
  H_0: Product A = product B in rates of microbial reduction
  H_A: Product A $\neq$ product B in rates of microbial reduction
Step 2. Select α. For this pilot study, set $\alpha = 0.10$.
Step 3. Because $n < 25$, we can use Wilcoxon Table H directly for this evaluation.
Step 4. Decision rule. Looking at Table H for the Wilcoxon test, n (number of D_is) = 3; for a two-tail test $0.10/2 = 0.05 = \alpha$. There is no corresponding value, so we will use $\alpha = 0.25$ because it is the best we can do. We will take the smaller of the two R values, $R+$ or $R-$, which corresponds to d on the table, and use $\alpha = 0.25$. We will reject H_0 if the smaller sum of the ranks (either $R+$ or $R-$) is less than or equal to 1 at $\alpha = 0.25$.

So, if "R smaller" ≤ 1, reject H_0 at $0.25 = \alpha$. The sample size is too small to be useful for anything but an extreme difference.

Step 5. Perform computation.

590   **Chapter 12**

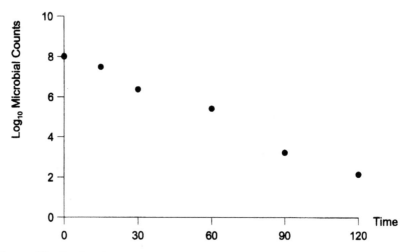

FIGURE 10   Product A.

Product A	Product B
$x_1 x_4 = x_0 x_{60}$	$x_1 x_4 = x_0 x_{60}$
$x_2 x_5 = x_{15} x_{90}$	$x_2 x_5 = x_{15} x_{90}$
$x_3 x_6 = x_{30} x_{120}$	$x_3 x_6 = x_{30} x_{120}$
$S_{A_1} = \frac{y_4 - y_1}{x_4 - x_1} = \frac{y_{60} - y_0}{x_{60} - x_0} = \frac{5.43 - 8.01}{60 - 0} = -0.043$	$S_{B_1} = \frac{y_4 - y_1}{x_4 - x_1} = \frac{y_{60} - y_0}{x_{60} - x_0} = \frac{6.23 - 9.15}{60 - 0} = -0.049$
$S_{A_2} = \frac{y_{90} - y_{15}}{x_{90} - x_{15}} = \frac{3.23 - 7.49}{90 - 15} = -0.057$	$S_{B_2} = \frac{y_{90} - y_{15}}{x_{90} - x_{15}} = \frac{4.16 - 8.23}{90 - 15} = -0.054$
$S_{A_3} = \frac{y_{120} - y_{30}}{x_{120} - x_{30}} = \frac{2.15 - 6.38}{120 - 30} = -0.047$	$S_{B_3} = \frac{y_{120} - y_{30}}{x_{120} - x_{30}} = \frac{2.70 - 7.15}{120 - 30} = -0.049$

A. First, pair the two data sets.
B. Then randomly pair the S_{A_i} and S_{B_i} values, and rank.

Randomly pair S_{A_i} and S_{B_i} values

	Difference	D_i	Rank (ascending order)
$S_{A_3} S_{B_1} =$	$\|-0.047 - (-0.049)\| = 0.002(+)$		1
$S_{A_1} S_{B_3} =$	$\|-0.043 - (-0.049)\| = 0.006(+)$		3
$S_{A_2} S_{B_3} =$	$\|-0.057 - (-0.054)\| = 0.003(-)$		2

$R+ = 1 + 3 = 4$
$R- = 2$

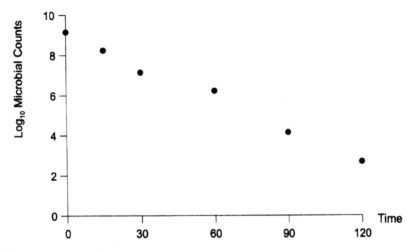

FIGURE 11   Product B.

Step 6.   Conclusion. Because $R-$ was the smaller of $R+$ and $R-$ and it was 2, we cannot reject H_0 at $\alpha = 0.25$.

or via p value notation:

$P(d \leq 2)\,|H_0$ true$) \leq 0.25$

We cannot conclude that the slopes are different at $\alpha = 0.25$.
Note that for one-tail tests:

Upper tail	Lower tail
H_0: $B_{A_1} \leqslant B_{B_1}$	H_0: $B_{A_1} \geqslant B_{B_1}$
H_A: $B_{A_1} > B_{B_1}$	H_A: $B_{A_1} < B_{B_1}$
If the sum of the ranks of the $R-$ values $\leqslant 1$, reject H_0 at $\alpha = 0.125$.	If the sum of the ranks of the $R+$ values $\leqslant 1$, reject H_0 at $\alpha = 0.125$.
Because $R- = 2 > 1$, we cannot reject H_0 at $\alpha = 0.125$.	Because $R+ = 4 > 1$, we cannot reject H_0 at $\alpha = 0.125$.

Note: Remember $-0.47 > -0.49$, so greater here really means less antimicrobial activity.

From these tests, the researcher will get the feeling that the B_{A_1} and B_{B_2} group rates of inactivation are probably the same.

F. Nonparametric Linear Regression (Monotonic Regression)

Monotonic regression can be used with data that increase or decrease non-linearly [42, 43]. Figure 12 shows all examples of monotonically decreasing or increasing data. Figure 13 presents some examples of nonmonotonic curves.

Monotonic functions are as follows:

1. As x increases, y increases at an increasing or decreasing rate.
2. or, as x increases, y decreases at a decreasing or increasing rate.

These functions are fairly easy to linearize, but there are times one does not wish to transform the data to linearize them. Perhaps one is not comfortable with changing a scale and expecting repeated testing to model the proposed transformation.

G. Assumptions

1. The data consist of determined (set) x values, and the corresponding y values are dependent upon the x values.
2. The individual ϵ (error) values are independent random variables.
3. The regression function is monotonic.

There are two things we can do:

1. A point estimate (an estimate of a y given an x value)
2. An estimate of the regression function $y = b_0 + b_1 x$

H. Estimate of *y* at Specific *x*

The process can be ordered by distinct steps:

1. Obtain the ranks of the x and y values. For ties, take the average, as usual.
2. Determine the regression parameters via ranks.

Regression form: $y = b_0 + b_1 x$

$$b_1 = \frac{\sum_{i=1}^{n} R(x_i)R(y_i) - n(n+1)^2/4}{\sum_{i=1}^{n} [R(x_i)]^2 - n(n+1)^2/4} \qquad (30)$$

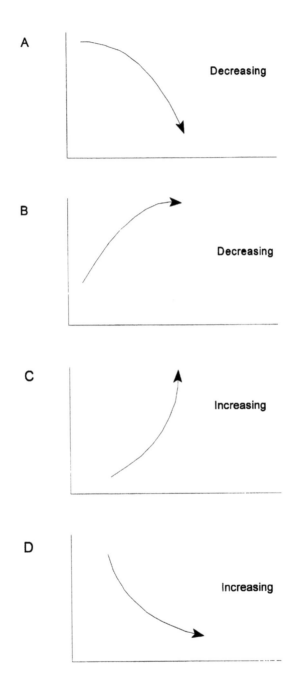

FIGURE 12 Examples of monotonic regression curves.

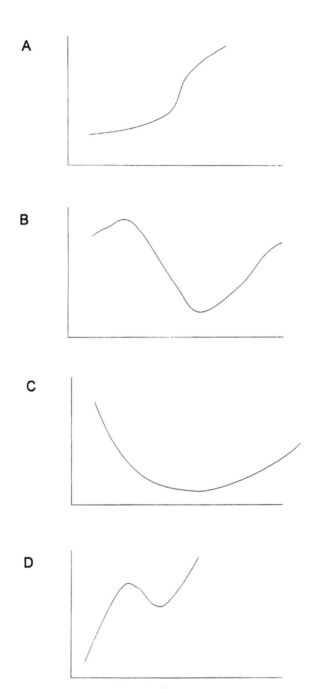

FIGURE 13   Examples of nonmonotonic curves.

where
$$R(x_i) = \text{rank of } x_i \text{ values}$$
$$R(y_i) = \text{rank of } y_i \text{ values}$$

$$b_0 = \frac{(1 - b_1)(n + 1)}{2} \qquad (31)$$

Let $x_e = x$ estimate.

3. Obtain the rank of a specific x_e.
   a. If x_e is one of the x values already observed, let $R(x_e) = $ that specific x value rank.
   b. If x_e is between two adjacent x_i values, where $x_i < x_e < x_j$, interpolate to get its rank $R(x_e)$ using the formula:

$$R(x_e) = R(x_i) + \frac{x_e - x_i}{x_j - x_i}\left[R(x_j) - R(x_i)\right] \qquad (32)$$

   $R(x_e)$ may not be an integer, and that is all right. If (x_e) is larger than the largest x_j, do not extrapolate. The test cannot be used for *extrapolation*.

4. Next, replace x in the equation $\hat{y} = b_0 + b_1 x$ with $R(x_e)$ to predict $E[R(y_e)]$.

$$E[R(y_e)] = R(\hat{y}_e) = b_0 + b_1 R(x_e)$$

5. Then convert $R(\hat{y}_e)$ into $E(y_e)$ applying the following rules:

   a. If $R(y_e)$ equals the rank of one of the y_i observations, $R(y_i)$, then the estimate of $E(y_e)$ will equal that observation, y_i.
   b. If $R(y_e)$ lies between the ranks of two adjacent values y_i and y_j, that is, $R(y_i) < R(y_e) < R(y_j)$, interpolate using the formula:

$$E(y_e) = y_i + \frac{R(y_e) - R(y_i)}{R(y_j) - R(y_i)}(y_j - y_i) \qquad (33)$$

   c. If $R(y_e)$ is greater than the largest observed rank of y, let $R(y_e)$ be equal to the largest observed y. If $R(y_e)$ is less than the smallest observed rank y, let $R(y_e)$ be equal to the smallest observed y.

Example 14: An experimenter performed a study with one hard-surface disinfectant and the microorganism, *Bacillus subtilis*, a spore-forming bacterial species, to determine the rate of inactivation (to be discussed in the next section) and the expected lethality after a 4.5-minute exposure. The following data were collected in log_{10} scale.

x = time (minutes)	$y = log_{10}$ microbial counts
0	9.18
1	8.37
2	7.81
3	6.72
4	4.11
5	1.92
6	0.51

As always, it is a good idea to plot the data (Fig. 14). The researcher concludes that the data are monotonic and wants to know what the log_{10} microbial population is at time 4.5 minutes.

x = time (minutes)	$y = log_{10}$ microbial counts	$R(x)$	$R(y)$
0	9.18	1	7
1	8.37	2	6
2	7.81	3	5
3	6.72	4	4
4	4.11	5	3
5	1.92	6	2
6	0.51	7	1
		$\Sigma\ R(x) = 28$	$\Sigma\ R(y) = 28$

Step 1. Obtain the ranks of x and y values.
Step 2. Determine the regression parameter via ranks.

Log$_{10}$ microbial counts

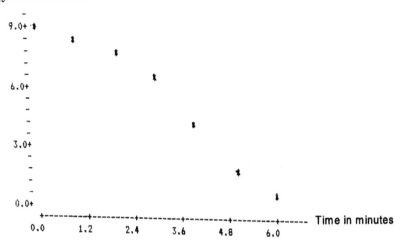

FIGURE 14   MiniTab$^{®}$ plot of data.

Regression form: $\hat{y} = b_0 + b_1 x$

$$b_1 = \frac{\sum\limits_{i=1}^{n} R(x_i)R(y_i) - n(n+1)^2/4}{\sum\limits_{i=1}^{n}[R(x_i)]^2 - n(n+1)^2/4}$$

$$b_1 = \frac{[(1\cdot7)+(2\cdot6)+(3\cdot5)+(4\cdot4)+(5\cdot3)+(6\cdot2)+(7\cdot1)]-7(7+1)^2/4}{[1^2+2^2+3^2+4^2+5^2+6^2+7^2]-7(7+1)^2/4}$$

$$b_1 = \frac{84-112}{140-112} = -1.0$$

$$b_0 = (1-b_1)\left(\frac{n+1}{2}\right) = 1-(-1)\left(\frac{8}{2}\right) = 8.0$$

Step 3.   Let $x_e = x_{\text{estimate}} = 4.5$
$x_i < x_e < x_j = 4 < 4.5 < 5$

$$R(x_e) = R(x_i) + \frac{x_e - x_i}{x_j - x_i}[R(x_j) - R(x_i)]$$

$$= 5 + \frac{4.5-4}{5-4}[6-5] = 5.5$$

Step 4. Next, replace x in the equation $\hat{y} = b_0 + b_1 x$ with $R(x_e) = 5.5$
to predict $\hat{y} = E(y_e)$.
$$\hat{y} = b_0 + b_1(R(x_e)) = 8 - 1(5.5) = 2.5$$

The rank of $y_e = 2.5$

Step 5. Convert $R(\hat{y}_e) = \hat{y}$ into $E[(y_e)]$
$$R(y_i) < R(y_e) < R(y_j)$$

   2   2.5   3

$$E(y_e) = y_i + \frac{R(y_e) - R(y_i)}{R(y_j) - R(y_i)}(y_j - y_i)$$

where

$$R(y_e) = 2, \quad R(y_j) = 3, \quad R(y_e) = 2.5, \quad y_i = 1.92, \quad \text{and} \quad y_j = 4.11$$

$$E(y_e) = 1.92 + \frac{2.5 - 2}{3 - 2}(4.11 - 1.92) = 3.015$$

$$E(y_e) = 3.015$$

So, when $x = 4.5$, $\hat{y} = 3.015$ logs. Look back at the plot and notice
how close 3.015 appears to be. This is a very useful method.

I. Estimate of the Regression Function *y* on *x*

Step 1. Obtain the end points of the regression function curve by using
the smallest $x_{(1)}$ and the largest $x_{(n)}$ observations in the previous procedure. Plug $R(x_1)$ and $R(x_2)$ into the formula:

$$R(\hat{y}) = b_0 + b_1(Rx) \tag{34}$$

Step 2. For each rank of y, $R(y_i)$, estimate the rank of x_i, $R(x_e)$, from
$R(\hat{y}) = b_0 + b_1 x_1$, which is

$$R(x_e) = \frac{[R(y_i) - b_0]}{b_1} \quad i = 1, 2, \ldots, n \tag{35}$$

Step 3. Convert each $R(x_i)$ to an estimate of x_e such that
a.   If $R(x_e)$ equals the rank of some observation, $R(x_i)$, then x_e equals
that value.

b. If $R(x_e)$ lies between the ranks of two adjacent observations, x_i and x_j, where $x_i < x_j$, then interpolate to get x_e:

$$x_e = x_i + \frac{R(x_e) - R(x_i)}{R(x_j) - R(x_i)} (x_j - x_i) \tag{36}$$

c. If $R(x_e)$ is less than the smallest observed rank of x or larger than the largest observed rank, no estimate for x_e can be found.

Step 4. Plot each of the points found in step 3 on graph paper (or plot as a computer printout). Do not forget to plot the two end points with $E(y)$ for x_1 and x_n.

Step 5. Connect the points with straight lines that, cumulatively, are what make up the regression function $\hat{y} = b_0 + b_1 x$.

Now, continuing with our previews example:

Step 1. Obtain the end points of the regression curve by using the smallest x_1 and largest x_n to obtain the expected values of on x_1 and on x_n.

$\hat{y} = b_0 + b_1 x$

$\hat{y} = 8 - 1(x)$

$x_1 = 0 \neq R(x_1) = 1$

$x_n = x_7 = 6 \neq R(x_7) = 7$

$R(\hat{y}) = b_0 + b_1 R(x_1) \qquad x_i = 0, \quad R(x_i) = 1$

$R(\hat{y}) = 8 - 1(1)$

$R(\hat{y}) = 7, R(x_1)$

$R(\hat{y}) = 8 - 1(6)$

$R(\hat{y}) = 2, R(x_7)$

So, $x_1 = 0, \quad R(x_1) = 1, \quad R(y) = 7$
$\ x_7 = 6, \quad R(x_7) = 6, \quad R(y) = 2.$

Step 2. For each rank of y, $R(y_i)$, find the estimate, $R(x_e)$.

$$R(x_i) = \frac{R(y_i) - b_0}{b_1}$$

Let us reconstruct our table.

n	x = time (minutes)	y = log$_{10}$ microbial counts	R(x)	R(y)	R(x$_e$)	x$_e$
1	0	9.18	1	7	1	0
2	1	8.37	2	6	2	1
3	2	7.81	3	5	3	2
4	3	6.72	4	4	4	3
5	4	4.11	5	3	5	4
6	5	1.92	6	2	6	5
7	6	0.51	7	1	7	6

$$R(x_{1_e}) = \frac{7-8}{-1} = 1$$

$$R(x_{2_e}) = \frac{6-8}{-1} = 2$$

$$R(x_{3_e}) = \frac{5-8}{-1} = 3$$

$$R(x_{4_e}) = \frac{4-8}{-1} = 4$$

$$R(x_{5_e}) = \frac{3-8}{-1} = 5$$

$$R(x_{6_e}) = \frac{2-8}{-1} = 6$$

$$R(x_{7_e}) = \frac{1-8}{-1} = 7$$

Step 3.   Convert each $R(x_i)$ to an estimate of x_i.

$R(x_1) = x_1 = 0,$ $x_1 = 0,$ $x_1 = 0$

$R(x_2) = x_2 = 1,$ $x_2 = 1,$ $x_2 = 1$

$R(x_3) = x_3 = 2,$ $x_3 = 2,$ $x_3 = 2$

$R(x_4) = x_4 = 3,$ $x_4 = 3,$ $x_4 = 3$

$R(x_5) = x_5 = 4,$ $x_5 = 4,$ $x_5 = 4$

$R(x_6) = x_6 = 5,$ $x_6 = 5,$ $x_6 = 5$

$R(x_7) = x_7 = 6,$ $x_7 = 6,$ $x_7 = 6$

Step 4.   Plot the points x_e, y and
Step 5.   Correct them with a line (Fig. 15).

x_e	$y = \log_{10}$ microbial counts
0	9.18
1	8.37
2	7.81
3	6.72
4	4.11
5	1.92
6	0.51

Notice that this procedure will always predict y on any x and interpolate between $(y_i - y_j)/(x_i - x_j)$ points. It is very useful in some exploratory phases.

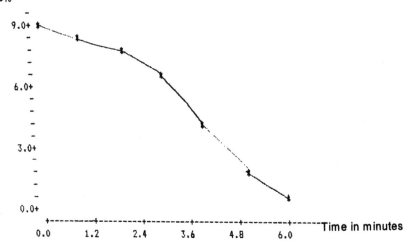

FIGURE 15   MiniTab® plot.

XIV. NONPARAMETRIC CORRELATION

Recall that, in parametric regression analysis, we worked with the correlation coefficient, r, and with r^2, the coefficient of determination. A useful and very well known nonparametric correlation coefficient test involves the Spearman rank correlation coefficient. Correlation, as you recall, is the measure of association between variables (x, y). A correlation of 1 is a perfect fit, and a correlation of 0 is total randomness. In nonparametric statistics, we do not use the 0–1 scale but only whether the correlation is significant or not significant at a specific α. There is not a useful r^2 value equivalent in nonparametrics, and the range of $r = -1$ to 1 is difficult to interpret directly.

A. Assumptions

1. The data consist of any (x, y) pair of data.
2. The data can be ranked from smallest to largest.
3. The data are at least of ordinal or interval scale.
4. Both two-tail and one-tail tests can be applied.

The Spearman test statistic is:

$$r_c = 1 - \frac{6 \sum_{i=1}^{n} d_i^2}{n(n^2 - 1)} \tag{37}$$

where:

$$\sum_{i=1}^{n} d_i^2 = \sum_{i=1}^{n} [R(x_i) - R(y_i)]^2 \tag{38}$$

The r_c values will always be from -1 to 1. The entire analysis can be approached via the six-step procedure.

Two tail	Upper tail	Lower tail
H_0 : x and y are independent	H_0: x and y are independent	H_0: x and y are independent
H_A: x and y are associated	H_A: x and y are positively associated (as x increases, y increases)	H_A: x and y are negatively associated (as x increases, y decreases)

Step 1. Formulate hypothesis.
Step 2. Set α.

Step 3.   Write out the test statistic.

$$r_c = 1 - \frac{6 \sum\limits_{i=1}^{n} d_i^2}{n(n^2 - 1)}$$

Step 4.   Decision rule.

Two tail	Upper tail	Lower tail
If $|r_c| > r_{t(\alpha/2,n)}$, reject H_0 at level α.	If $r_c > r_{t(\alpha,n)}$, reject H_0 at level α.	If $r_c < -r_{t(\alpha,n)}$, reject H_0 at level α.

Note: For sample pairs from 4 to 30, use the Spearman rank table (Table A.15). For larger sample sizes, use the Z table (normal distribution, Table A.1) where:

$$Z_c = r_c \sqrt{n - 1}, \tag{39}$$

Step 5.   Perform calculations.
Step 6.   Conclusion.

Example 15:   Let us use the regression data from Example 14.

x minutes	y $\log_{10}$ microbial counts
0	9.18
1	8.37
2	7.81
3	6.72
4	4.11
5	1.92
6	0.51

Step 1.   Determine hypothesis. Two-tail:
  H_0: x and y are independent.
  H_A: x and y are associated.
Step 2.   Determine α. Let us set $\alpha = 0.05$.

Step 3. Write out the test statistic. Because $n = 7$, we will use the Spearman rank table (Table A.15). The formula is:

x	y	R(x_i)	R(y)	$d_i = R(x_i) - R(y_i)$	d^2
0	9.18	1	7	−6	36
1	8.37	2	6	−4	16
2	7.81	3	5	−2	4
3	6.72	4	4	0	0
4	4.11	5	3	2	4
5	1.92	6	2	4	16
6	0.51	7	1	6	36
					$\Sigma d_i^2 = 112.0$

$$r_c = 1 - \frac{6 \sum_{i=1}^{n} d_i^2}{n(n^2 - 1)}$$

Step 4. Decision rule.

If $|r_c| > r_{t(\alpha/2,n)}$, reject H_0 at α.

$r_{t(\alpha/2,n)} = r_{(0.05/2,7)} = 0.7450$

So, if $|r|_c > 0.7450$, reject H_0 at α.

Step 5. Perform computation.

Upper tail	Lower tail
H_0: x and y are independent	H_0: x and y are independent
H_A: x and y are positively correlated	H_A: x and y are negatively correlated
If $r_c > r_{t(\alpha,n)}$, reject H_0 at α.	If $r_c < -r_{t(\alpha,n)}$, reject H_0 at α.
$r_{0.05,7} = 0.6786$	$r_{0.05,7} = 0.6786$
Because $-1 < 0.6786$, we cannot reject H_0 at $\alpha = 0.05$. The x and y variables are not positively correlated at H_0 at $\alpha = 0.05$.	Because $-1 < -0.6786$, reject H_0 at $\alpha = 0.05$. The x and y variables are negatively correlated at H_0 at $\alpha = 0.05$. Actually, it is a perfect correlation.

$$r_c = 1 - \frac{6(112)}{7(7^2 - 1)} = 1 - \frac{672}{336} = -1 \quad \text{and} \quad |r_c| = 1$$

$|r_c| > 0.745$

Step 6. Conclusion. Because $|r_c| = 1 > 0.745$, we reject H_0 at $\alpha = 0.05$. Actually, the data are perfectly negatively correlated.

Note: Let us do an upper and a lower tail test at $\alpha = 0.05$.

B. Ties

If ties occur, as always, assign them the average value. If ties are excessive (over one fourth of the values of x or y), and usually they are not for regression, the following correction factor formula should be used.

$$r'_c = \frac{\sum x^2 + \sum y^2 - \sum d_i^2}{2\sqrt{\sum x^2 \sum y^2}} \tag{40}$$

where:

$$x^2 = \frac{n^3 - n}{12} - \sum t_x \tag{41}$$

and

$$t_x = \text{ties of } x = \frac{t_x^3 - t_x}{12}$$

$$y^2 = \frac{n^3 - n}{12} - \sum t_y, \quad \text{where } t_y = \frac{t_y^3 - t_y}{12} \tag{42}$$

XV. CONCLUSION

The researcher now has a broad array of nonparametric tools to meet research needs. Nearly every method we explored previously using parametric statistics can now be accomplished using nonparametric methods. Familiarity is important, and that will come through application, practice, and experience.

13

Introduction to Research Synthesis and
Meta-Analysis and Concluding Remarks

I. RESEARCH SYNTHESIS AND META-ANALYSIS

Research synthesis, or "meta-analysis," comprises a family of statistical methods used to evaluate and compare multiple research studies using their conclusive data as the raw data. In short, in meta-analysis, one is interested in evaluating the treatment effects of a product or process across multiple studies [49–53].

For example, in the evaluation of the efficacy of a surgical preparation product, multiple studies may have been conducted, some displaying favorable results and some unfavorable. How does one evaluate the efficacy of the product when the study outcomes conflict? The answer is meta-analysis. The data used for meta-analysis are the results from the various studies completed in the past [50]. A prime use of meta-analysis is in the evaluation of data compiled through literature review. In the past, researchers reviewed the literature and formed their own subjective opinion concerning the meaning of experimental data. This subjective approach is increasingly being abandoned in favor of meta-analysis statistical tests [51].

Meta-analysis is especially valuable for the field researcher, but to apply it, expertise in the field of study is necessary to determining which studies to include. For example, if a drug should be used for 5 days in treatment, one would avoid including studies in which the drug was used, inappropriately, for 1 or 2 days.

It is useful to have acceptance criteria as well as rejection criteria clearly spelled out before a meta-analysis of data from the literature is performed. It is also valuable to include studies that evaluate the product or process under a wide range of conditions. For example, selecting studies to encompass both sexes, different ages, different test methods, different races, different geophysical areas, etc., will make the meta-analysis results broader in scope and the conclusions more robust.

The literature contains reference to a variety of statistical methods applicable to meta-analysis. In this book, we will explicate only one. As a start to application of meta-analysis, this researcher suggests using the inverse chi square (χ^2) method [50]. Given k independent studies and the p values for each study, $p_1, \ldots, p_k$, this procedure combines the p values. The method is based on the uniform distribution (U) of success/failure. If U is a uniform distribution, then $-2\ell np_i$ has a chi square distribution with $2k$ degrees of freedom.

$$\text{We reject } H_0 \quad \text{if } P = -2\sum_{i=1}^{k} \ell np_i > \chi^2_{t(\alpha,2k)}.$$

This statistic, I believe, as do others, is more robust and powerful than the inverse normal method or the logit method [50,51].

The six-step procedure can be adapted for application to meta-analysis.

Step 1. Formulate hypothesis.
H_0: The combined studies show product/process not effective.
H_A: Combined studies show product/process effective.
Step 2. Set α.
Step 3. The test statistic is:

$$P = -2\sum_{i=1}^{k} \ell np_i$$

where ℓn = natural (or Naperian) logarithm (base e)
          p_i = the p value for each study result, $p_i, \ldots, p_k$
Step 4. Decision rule.
    If $P_c > \chi^2_{t(\alpha,2k)}$, reject H_0.
Step 5. Perform computation.
Step 6. Conclusion.

Example 1:   A researcher was interested in evaluating the positive results of using an alcohol gel product for sanitizing the hands of students in various schools across the country. Students were selected randomly to use the product, ad libitum, or to not. In several studies, two indices were evaluated over the course of several months. The first was the incidence of

Staphylococcus aureus cultured from the hands, and the second, the days students were absent from school because of "colds or flu." The studies were conducted by different researchers using different methods in six different school districts across the country. Generally, the *t*-test was used to analyze the data.

A = frequency of *S. aureus* on hands of product users compared with those of nonusers

B = study of absenteeism, users versus nonusers

The data from the multiple studies, processed for meta-analysis, were as follows.

SCHOOL DISTRICT	Calculated value Student's *t* test	Student's *t* P value	$\ell n\, P$
1	$A_t = 2.78$	.0029	−5.8430
	$B_t = 2.59$	.0100	−4.6052
2	$A_t = 2.807$	.005	−5.2983
	$B_t = 1.33$	.1100	−2.2073
3	$A_t = 2.12$	0.025	−3.6889
	$B_t = 0.686$	0.5392	−0.6176
4	A_t = (not given)	.0312	−3.4673
	B_t = (not given)	0.0310	−3.4738
5	A_t = (not given)	.0500	−2.9957
	B_t = (not given)	.0200	−3.9120
6	$A_t = 0.701$	.2510	−1.3823
	$B_t = 1.323$	.0998	−2.3046
			$\Sigma \ell n\, p = -39.7960$

Step 1. Formulate hypothesis.
H_0: The school studies showed that the product was not effective.
H_A: The school studies showed that the product was effective.
Step 2. Set α. Let $\alpha = 0.05$.
Step 3. The test statistic to be used is:

$$P = -2 \sum_{i=1}^{k} \ell n\, p$$

Step 4. Decision rule.

If $P_c > \chi^2_{t(0.05,12)} = 21.03$, reject H_0 at $\alpha = 0.05$.

Step 5. Perform computation.

$$P_c = -2 \sum \ell n \, p_i = -2(-39.7960)$$

$$P_c = 79.5920$$

Step 6. Conclusion. Because $P_c = 79.59 > \chi_t^2 = 21.03$, we reject the H_0 hypothesis at $\alpha = 0.05$. There is good reason to believe the product is effective, although, obviously, there is much potential for confounding here. But all in all, the data point to beneficial effects.

In conclusion, meta-analysis is a very useful tool. It has been my experience that this inverse χ^2 test is very useful and manageable without making many assumptions about the data that cannot be met.

II. CONCLUDING REMARKS

Over these 13 chapters, we have covered many useful statistical methods. A researcher who has an intimate understanding of his or her data should benefit enormously from the information presented in this text. Obviously, not all needs of the researcher in all circumstances could be addressed, but the background presented here can be used by the researcher as a springboard to enhance his or her investigational ability and, therefore, effectiveness. As I stated at the book's beginning, statistics is a method of communicating. That is what I hope we have done over the course of this work. I would be interested in your comments and applications.

Appendix : Tables of Mathematical Values

TABLE A.1 Z-Table (Normal Curve Areas [Entries in the Body of the Table Give the Area Under the Standard Normal Curve from 0 to z])

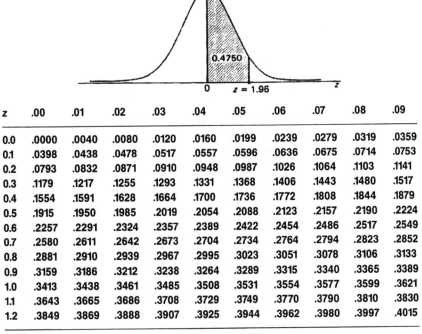

z	.00	.01	.02	.03	.04	.05	.06	.07	.08	.09
0.0	.0000	.0040	.0080	.0120	.0160	.0199	.0239	.0279	.0319	.0359
0.1	.0398	.0438	.0478	.0517	.0557	.0596	.0636	.0675	.0714	.0753
0.2	.0793	.0832	.0871	.0910	.0948	.0987	.1026	.1064	.1103	.1141
0.3	.1179	.1217	.1255	.1293	.1331	.1368	.1406	.1443	.1480	.1517
0.4	.1554	.1591	.1628	.1664	.1700	.1736	.1772	.1808	.1844	.1879
0.5	.1915	.1950	.1985	.2019	.2054	.2088	.2123	.2157	.2190	.2224
0.6	.2257	.2291	.2324	.2357	.2389	.2422	.2454	.2486	.2517	.2549
0.7	.2580	.2611	.2642	.2673	.2704	.2734	.2764	.2794	.2823	.2852
0.8	.2881	.2910	.2939	.2967	.2995	.3023	.3051	.3078	.3106	.3133
0.9	.3159	.3186	.3212	.3238	.3264	.3289	.3315	.3340	.3365	.3389
1.0	.3413	.3438	.3461	.3485	.3508	.3531	.3554	.3577	.3599	.3621
1.1	.3643	.3665	.3686	.3708	.3729	.3749	.3770	.3790	.3810	.3830
1.2	.3849	.3869	.3888	.3907	.3925	.3944	.3962	.3980	.3997	.4015

(Continued)

TABLE A.1 (Continued)

z	.00	.01	.02	.03	.04	.05	.06	.07	.08	.09
1.3	.4032	.4049	.4066	.4082	.4099	.4115	.4131	.4147	.4162	.4177
1.4	.4192	.4207	.4222	.4236	.4251	.4265	.4279	.4292	.4306	.4319
1.5	.4332	.4345	.4357	.4370	.4382	.4394	.4406	.4418	.4429	.4441
1.6	.4452	.4463	.4474	.4484	.4495	.4505	.4515	.4525	.4535	.4545
1.7	.4554	.4564	.4573	.4582	.4591	.4599	.4608	.4616	.4625	.4633
1.8	.4641	.4649	.4656	.4664	.4671	.4678	.4686	.4693	.4699	.4706
1.9	.4713	.4719	.4726	.4732	.4738	.4744	.4750	.4756	.4761	.4767
2.0	.4772	.4778	.4783	.4788	.4793	.4798	.4803	.4808	.4812	.4817
2.1	.4821	.4826	.4830	.4834	.4838	.4842	.4846	.4850	.4854	.4857
2.2	.4861	.4864	.4868	.4871	.4875	.4878	.4881	.4884	.4887	.4890
2.3	.4893	.4896	.4898	.4901	.4904	.4906	.4909	.4911	.4913	.4916
2.4	.4918	.4920	.4922	.4925	.4927	.4929	.4931	.4932	.4934	.4936
2.5	.4938	.4940	.4941	.4943	.4945	.4946	.4948	.4949	.4951	.4952
2.6	.4953	.4955	.4956	.4957	.4959	.4960	.4961	.4962	.4963	.4964
2.7	.4965	.4966	.4967	.4968	.4969	.4970	.4971	.4972	.4973	.4974
2.8	.4974	.4975	.4976	.4977	.4977	.4978	.4979	.4979	.4980	.4981
2.9	.4981	.4982	.4982	.4983	.4984	.4984	.4985	.4985	.4986	.4986
3.0	.4987	.4987	.4987	.4988	.4988	.4989	.4989	.4989	.4990	.4990

Source: Freund JE, Williams FJ. Elementary Business Statistics; The Modern Approach. 2nd ed. 1972; reprinted by permission of Prentice-Hall, Inc., Englewood Cliffs, NJ.

TABLE A.2 Student's t Table (Percentage Points of the t Distribution)

v \ α	.40	.25	.10	.05	.025	.01	.005	.0025	.001	.0005
1	.325	1.000	3.078	6.314	12.706	31.821	63.657	127.32	318.31	636.62
2	.289	.816	1.886	2.920	4.303	6.965	9.925	14.089	23.326	31.598
3	.277	.765	1.638	2.353	3.182	4.541	5.841	7.453	10.213	12.924
4	.271	.741	1.533	2.132	2.776	3.747	4.604	5.598	7.173	8.610
5	.267	.727	1.476	2.015	2.571	3.365	4.032	4.773	5.893	6.869
6	.265	.727	1.440	1.943	2.447	3.143	3.707	4.317	5.208	5.959
7	.263	.711	1.415	1.895	2.365	2.998	3.499	4.019	4.785	5.408
8	.262	.706	1.397	1.860	2.306	2.896	3.355	3.833	4.501	5.041
9	.261	.703	1.383	1.833	2.262	2.821	3.250	3.690	4.297	4.781
10	.260	.700	1.372	1.812	2.228	2.764	3.169	3.581	4.144	4.587
11	.260	.697	1.363	1.796	2.201	2.718	3.106	3.497	4.025	4.437
12	.259	.695	1.356	1.782	2.179	2.681	3.055	3.428	3.930	4.318
13	.259	.694	1.350	1.771	2.160	2.650	3.012	3.372	3.852	4.221

v = degrees of freedom

(Continued)

TABLE A.2 (Continued)

ν \ α	.40	.25	.10	.05	.025	.01	.005	.0025	.001	.0005
14	.258	.692	1.345	1.761	2.145	2.624	2.977	3.326	3.787	4.140
15	.258	.691	1.341	1.753	2.131	2.602	2.947	3.286	3.733	4.073
16	.258	.690	1.337	1.746	2.120	2.583	2.921	3.252	3.686	4.015
17	.257	.689	1.333	1.740	2.110	2.567	2.898	3.222	3.646	3.965
18	.257	.688	1.330	1.734	2.101	2.552	2.878	3.197	3.610	3.922
19	.257	.688	1.328	1.729	2.093	2.539	2.861	3.174	3.579	3.883
20	.257	.687	1.325	1.725	2.086	2.528	2.845	3.153	3.552	3.850
21	.257	.686	1.323	1.721	2.080	2.518	2.831	3.135	3.527	3.819
22	.256	.686	1.321	1.717	2.074	2.508	2.819	3.119	3.505	3.792
23	.256	.685	1.319	1.714	2.069	2.500	2.807	3.104	3.485	3.767
24	.256	.685	1.318	1.711	2.064	2.492	2.797	3.091	3.467	3.745
25	.256	.684	1.316	1.708	2.060	2.485	2.787	3.078	3.450	3.725
26	.256	.684	1.315	1.706	2.056	2.479	2.779	3.067	3.435	3.707
27	.256	.684	1.314	1.703	2.052	2.473	2.771	3.057	3.421	3.690
28	.256	.683	1.313	1.701	2.048	2.467	2.763	3.047	3.408	3.674
29	.256	.683	1.311	1.699	2.045	2.462	2.756	3.038	3.396	3.659
30	.256	.683	1.310	1.697	2.042	2.457	2.750	3.030	3.385	3.646
40	.255	.681	1.303	1.684	2.021	2.423	2.704	2.971	3.307	3.551
60	.254	.679	1.296	1.671	2.000	2.390	2.660	2.915	3.232	3.460
120	.254	.677	1.289	1.658	1.980	2.358	2.617	2.860	3.160	3.373
∞	.253	.674	1.282	1.645	1.960	2.326	2.576	2.807	3.090	3.291

ν = degrees of freedom.
Source: Pearson Es, Hartley HO. Biometrika Tables for Statisticians. Vol 1, 3rd ed.: Cambridge: Cambridge University Press, 1966.

TABLE A.3 F Distribution Tables

$F_{0.25}(v_1, v_2)$

v_2 \ v_1	1	2	3	4	5	6	7	8	9	10	12	15	20	24	30	40	60	120	∞
1	5.83	7.50	8.20	8.58	8.82	8.98	9.10	9.19	9.26	9.32	9.41	9.49	9.58	9.63	9.67	9.71	9.76	9.80	9.85
2	2.57	3.00	3.15	3.23	3.28	3.31	3.34	3.35	3.37	3.38	3.39	3.41	3.43	3.43	3.44	3.45	3.46	3.47	3.48
3	2.02	2.28	2.36	2.39	2.41	2.42	2.43	2.44	2.44	2.44	2.45	2.46	2.46	2.46	2.47	2.47	2.47	2.47	2.47
4	1.81	2.00	2.05	2.06	2.07	2.08	2.08	2.08	2.08	2.08	2.08	2.08	2.08	2.08	2.08	2.08	2.08	2.08	2.08
5	1.69	1.85	1.88	1.89	1.89	1.89	1.89	1.89	1.89	1.89	1.89	1.89	1.88	1.88	1.88	1.88	1.87	1.87	1.87
6	1.62	1.76	1.78	1.79	1.79	1.78	1.78	1.78	1.77	1.77	1.77	1.76	1.76	1.75	1.75	1.75	1.74	1.74	1.74
7	1.57	1.70	1.72	1.72	1.71	1.71	1.70	1.70	1.70	1.69	1.68	1.68	1.67	1.67	1.66	1.66	1.65	1.65	1.65
8	1.54	1.66	1.67	1.66	1.66	1.65	1.64	1.64	1.63	1.63	1.62	1.62	1.61	1.60	1.60	1.59	1.59	1.58	1.58
9	1.51	1.62	1.63	1.63	1.62	1.61	1.60	1.60	1.59	1.59	1.58	1.57	1.56	1.56	1.55	1.54	1.54	1.53	1.53
10	1.49	1.60	1.60	1.59	1.59	1.58	1.57	1.56	1.56	1.55	1.54	1.53	1.52	1.52	1.51	1.51	1.50	1.49	1.48
11	1.47	1.58	1.58	1.57	1.56	1.55	1.54	1.53	1.53	1.52	1.51	1.50	1.49	1.49	1.48	1.47	1.47	1.46	1.45
12	1.46	1.56	1.56	1.55	1.54	1.53	1.52	1.51	1.51	1.50	1.49	1.48	1.47	1.46	1.45	1.45	1.44	1.43	1.42
13	1.45	1.55	1.55	1.53	1.52	1.51	1.50	1.49	1.49	1.48	1.47	1.46	1.45	1.44	1.43	1.42	1.42	1.41	1.40
14	1.44	1.53	1.53	1.52	1.51	1.50	1.49	1.48	1.47	1.46	1.45	1.44	1.43	1.42	1.41	1.41	1.40	1.39	1.38
15	1.43	1.52	1.52	1.51	1.49	1.48	1.47	1.46	1.46	1.45	1.44	1.43	1.41	1.41	1.40	1.39	1.38	1.37	1.36
16	1.42	1.51	1.51	1.50	1.48	1.47	1.46	1.45	1.44	1.44	1.43	1.41	1.40	1.39	1.38	1.37	1.36	1.35	1.34
17	1.42	1.51	1.50	1.49	1.47	1.46	1.45	1.44	1.43	1.43	1.41	1.40	1.39	1.38	1.37	1.36	1.35	1.34	1.33
18	1.41	1.50	1.49	1.48	1.46	1.45	1.44	1.43	1.42	1.42	1.40	1.39	1.38	1.37	1.36	1.35	1.34	1.33	1.32
19	1.41	1.49	1.49	1.47	1.46	1.44	1.43	1.42	1.41	1.41	1.40	1.38	1.37	1.36	1.35	1.34	1.33	1.32	1.30
20	1.40	1.49	1.48	1.47	1.45	1.44	1.43	1.42	1.41	1.40	1.39	1.37	1.36	1.35	1.34	1.33	1.32	1.31	1.29
21	1.40	1.48	1.48	1.46	1.44	1.43	1.42	1.41	1.40	1.39	1.38	1.37	1.35	1.34	1.33	1.32	1.31	1.30	1.28
22	1.40	1.48	1.47	1.45	1.44	1.42	1.41	1.40	1.39	1.39	1.37	1.36	1.34	1.33	1.32	1.31	1.30	1.29	1.28
23	1.39	1.47	1.47	1.45	1.43	1.42	1.41	1.40	1.39	1.38	1.37	1.35	1.34	1.33	1.32	1.31	1.30	1.28	1.27
24	1.39	1.47	1.46	1.44	1.43	1.41	1.40	1.39	1.38	1.38	1.36	1.35	1.33	1.32	1.31	1.30	1.29	1.28	1.26
25	1.39	1.47	1.46	1.44	1.42	1.41	1.40	1.39	1.38	1.37	1.36	1.34	1.33	1.32	1.31	1.29	1.28	1.27	1.25

Degrees of Freedom for the Numerator (V_1)

Degrees Freedom Denominator V_2

	1	2	3	4	5	6	7	8	9	10	12	15	20	24	30	40	60	120	∞
26	1.38	1.46	1.45	1.44	1.42	1.41	1.39	1.38	1.37	1.37	1.35	1.34	1.32	1.31	1.30	1.29	1.28	1.26	1.25
27	1.38	1.46	1.45	1.43	1.42	1.40	1.39	1.38	1.37	1.36	1.35	1.33	1.32	1.31	1.30	1.28	1.27	1.26	1.24
28	1.38	1.46	1.45	1.43	1.41	1.40	1.39	1.38	1.37	1.36	1.34	1.33	1.31	1.31	1.29	1.28	1.27	1.25	1.24
29	1.38	1.45	1.45	1.43	1.41	1.40	1.38	1.37	1.37	1.35	1.34	1.32	1.31	1.30	1.29	1.27	1.26	1.25	1.23
30	1.38	1.45	1.44	1.42	1.41	1.39	1.38	1.37	1.36	1.35	1.34	1.32	1.30	1.29	1.28	1.27	1.26	1.24	1.23
40	1.36	1.44	1.42	1.40	1.39	1.37	1.36	1.35	1.34	1.33	1.31	1.30	1.28	1.26	1.25	1.24	1.22	1.21	1.19
60	1.35	1.42	1.41	1.38	1.37	1.35	1.33	1.32	1.31	1.30	1.29	1.27	1.25	1.24	1.22	1.21	1.19	1.17	1.15
120	1.34	1.40	1.39	1.37	1.35	1.33	1.31	1.30	1.29	1.28	1.26	1.24	1.22	1.21	1.19	1.18	1.16	1.13	1.10
∞	1.32	1.39	1.37	1.35	1.33	1.31	1.29	1.28	1.27	1.25	1.24	1.22	1.19	1.18	1.16	1.14	1.12	1.08	1.00

$F_{0.10}$ (v_1, v_2) Degrees of Freedom for the Numerator (V_1)

v_2	1	2	3	4	5	6	7	8	9	10	12	15	20	24	30	40	60	120	∞
1	39.86	49.50	53.59	55.83	57.24	58.20	58.91	59.44	59.86	60.19	60.71	61.22	61.74	62.00	62.26	62.53	62.79	63.06	63.33
2	8.53	9.00	9.16	9.24	9.29	9.33	9.35	9.37	9.38	9.39	9.41	9.42	9.44	9.45	9.46	9.47	9.47	9.48	9.49
3	5.54	5.46	5.39	5.34	5.31	5.28	5.27	5.25	5.24	5.23	5.22	5.20	5.18	5.18	5.17	5.16	5.15	5.14	5.13
4	4.54	4.32	4.19	4.11	4.05	4.01	3.98	3.95	3.94	3.92	3.90	3.87	3.84	3.83	3.82	3.80	3.79	3.78	3.76
5	4.06	3.78	3.62	3.52	3.45	3.40	3.37	3.34	3.32	3.30	3.27	3.24	3.21	3.19	3.17	3.16	3.14	3.12	3.10
6	3.78	3.46	3.29	3.18	3.11	3.05	3.01	2.98	2.96	2.94	2.90	2.87	2.84	2.82	2.80	2.78	2.76	2.74	2.72
7	3.59	3.26	3.07	2.96	2.88	2.83	2.78	2.75	2.72	2.70	2.67	2.63	2.59	2.58	2.56	2.54	2.51	2.49	2.47
8	3.46	3.11	2.92	2.81	2.73	2.67	2.62	2.59	2.56	2.54	2.50	2.46	2.42	2.40	2.38	2.36	2.34	2.32	2.29
9	3.36	3.01	2.81	2.69	2.61	2.55	2.51	2.47	2.44	2.42	2.38	2.34	2.30	2.28	2.25	2.23	2.21	2.18	2.16
10	3.29	2.92	2.73	2.61	2.52	2.46	2.41	2.38	2.35	2.32	2.28	2.24	2.20	2.18	2.16	2.13	2.11	2.08	2.06
11	3.23	2.86	2.66	2.54	2.45	2.39	2.34	2.30	2.27	2.25	2.21	2.17	2.12	2.10	2.08	2.05	2.03	2.00	1.97
12	3.18	2.81	2.61	2.48	2.39	2.33	2.28	2.24	2.21	2.19	2.15	2.10	2.06	2.04	2.01	1.99	1.96	1.93	1.90
13	3.14	2.76	2.56	2.43	2.35	2.28	2.23	2.20	2.16	2.14	2.10	2.05	2.01	1.98	1.96	1.93	1.90	1.88	1.85
14	3.10	2.73	2.52	2.39	2.31	2.24	2.19	2.15	2.12	2.10	2.05	2.01	1.96	1.94	1.91	1.89	1.86	1.83	1.80
15	3.07	2.70	2.49	2.36	2.27	2.21	2.16	2.12	2.09	2.06	2.02	1.97	1.92	1.90	1.87	1.85	1.82	1.79	1.76
16	3.05	2.67	2.46	2.33	2.24	2.18	2.13	2.09	2.06	2.03	1.99	1.94	1.89	1.87	1.84	1.81	1.78	1.75	1.72

(Continued)

TABLE A.3 (Continued)

$F_{0.10}(v_1, v_2)$ Degrees of Freedom for the Numerator (V_1)

v_2 \ v_1	1	2	3	4	5	6	7	8	9	10	12	15	20	24	30	40	60	120	∞
17	3.03	2.64	2.44	2.31	2.22	2.15	2.10	2.06	2.03	2.00	1.96	1.91	1.86	1.84	1.81	1.78	1.75	1.72	1.69
18	3.01	2.62	2.42	2.29	2.20	2.13	2.08	2.04	2.00	1.98	1.93	1.89	1.84	1.81	1.78	1.75	1.72	1.69	1.66
19	2.99	2.61	2.40	2.27	2.18	2.11	2.06	2.02	1.98	1.96	1.91	1.86	1.81	1.79	1.76	1.73	1.70	1.67	1.63
20	2.97	2.59	2.38	2.25	2.16	2.09	2.04	2.00	1.96	1.94	1.89	1.84	1.79	1.77	1.74	1.71	1.68	1.64	1.61
21	2.96	2.57	2.36	2.23	2.14	2.08	2.02	1.98	1.95	1.92	1.87	1.83	1.78	1.75	1.72	1.69	1.66	1.62	1.59
22	2.95	2.56	2.35	2.22	2.13	2.06	2.01	1.97	1.93	1.90	1.86	1.81	1.76	1.73	1.70	1.67	1.64	1.60	1.57
23	2.94	2.55	2.34	2.21	2.11	2.05	1.99	1.96	1.92	1.89	1.84	1.80	1.74	1.72	1.69	1.66	1.62	1.59	1.55
24	2.93	2.54	2.33	2.19	2.10	2.04	1.98	1.94	1.91	1.88	1.83	1.78	1.73	1.70	1.67	1.64	1.61	1.57	1.53
25	2.92	2.53	2.32	2.18	2.09	2.02	1.97	1.93	1.89	1.87	1.82	1.77	1.72	1.69	1.66	1.63	1.59	1.56	1.52
26	2.91	2.52	2.31	2.17	2.08	2.01	1.96	1.92	1.88	1.86	1.81	1.76	1.71	1.68	1.65	1.61	1.58	1.54	1.50
27	2.90	2.51	2.30	2.17	2.07	2.00	1.95	1.91	1.87	1.85	1.80	1.75	1.70	1.67	1.64	1.60	1.57	1.53	1.49
28	2.89	2.50	2.29	2.16	2.06	2.00	1.94	1.90	1.87	1.84	1.79	1.74	1.69	1.66	1.63	1.59	1.56	1.52	1.48
29	2.89	2.50	2.28	2.15	2.06	1.99	1.93	1.89	1.86	1.83	1.78	1.73	1.68	1.65	1.62	1.58	1.55	1.51	1.47
30	2.88	2.49	2.28	2.14	2.03	1.98	1.93	1.88	1.85	1.82	1.77	1.72	1.67	1.64	1.61	1.57	1.54	1.50	1.46
40	2.84	2.44	2.23	2.09	2.00	1.93	1.87	1.83	1.79	1.76	1.71	1.66	1.61	1.57	1.54	1.51	1.47	1.42	1.38
60	2.79	2.39	2.18	2.04	1.95	1.87	1.82	1.77	1.74	1.71	1.66	1.60	1.54	1.51	1.48	1.44	1.40	1.35	1.29
120	2.75	2.35	2.13	1.99	1.90	1.82	1.77	1.72	1.68	1.65	1.60	1.55	1.48	1.45	1.41	1.37	1.32	1.26	1.19
∞	2.71	2.30	2.08	1.94	1.85	1.77	1.72	1.67	1.63	1.60	1.55	1.49	1.42	1.38	1.34	1.30	1.24	1.17	1.00

Degrees Freedom Denominator ($V2$)

$F_{0.05}(v_1, v_2)$ Degrees of Freedom for the Numerator (V_1)

v_2 \ v_1	1	2	3	4	5	6	7	8	9	10	12	15	20	24	30	40	60	120	∞
1	161.4	199.5	215.7	224.6	230.2	234.0	236.8	238.9	240.5	241.9	243.9	245.9	248.0	249.1	250.1	251.1	252.2	253.3	254.3
2	18.51	19.00	19.16	19.25	19.30	19.33	19.35	19.37	19.38	19.40	19.41	19.43	19.45	19.45	19.46	19.47	19.48	19.49	19.50
3	10.13	9.55	9.28	9.12	9.01	8.94	8.89	8.85	8.81	8.79	8.74	8.70	8.66	8.64	8.62	8.59	8.57	8.55	8.53

4	5.63	5.66	5.69	5.72	5.75	5.77	5.80	5.86	5.91	5.96	6.00	6.04	6.09	6.16	6.26	6.39	6.59	6.94	7.71
5	4.36	4.40	4.43	4.46	4.50	4.53	4.56	4.62	4.68	4.74	4.77	4.82	4.88	4.95	5.05	5.19	5.41	5.79	6.61
6	3.67	3.70	3.74	3.77	3.81	3.84	3.87	3.94	4.00	4.06	4.10	4.15	4.21	4.28	4.39	4.53	4.76	5.14	5.99
7	3.23	3.27	3.30	3.34	3.38	3.41	3.44	3.51	3.57	3.64	3.68	3.73	3.79	3.87	3.97	4.12	4.35	4.74	5.59
8	2.93	2.97	3.01	3.04	3.08	3.12	3.15	3.22	3.28	3.35	3.39	3.44	3.50	3.58	3.69	3.84	4.07	4.46	5.32
9	2.71	2.75	2.79	2.83	2.86	2.90	2.94	3.01	3.07	3.14	3.18	3.23	3.29	3.37	3.48	3.63	3.86	4.26	5.12
10	2.54	2.58	2.62	2.66	2.70	2.74	2.77	2.85	2.91	2.98	3.02	3.07	3.14	3.22	3.33	3.48	3.71	4.10	4.96
11	2.40	2.45	2.49	2.53	2.57	2.61	2.65	2.72	2.79	2.85	2.90	2.95	3.01	3.09	3.20	3.36	3.59	3.98	4.84
12	2.30	2.34	2.38	2.43	2.47	2.51	2.54	2.62	2.69	2.75	2.80	2.85	2.91	3.00	3.11	3.26	3.49	3.89	4.75
13	2.21	2.25	2.30	2.34	2.38	2.42	2.46	2.53	2.60	2.67	2.71	2.77	2.83	2.92	3.03	3.18	3.41	3.81	4.67
14	2.13	2.18	2.22	2.27	2.31	2.35	2.39	2.46	2.53	2.60	2.65	2.70	2.76	2.85	2.96	3.11	3.34	3.74	4.60
15	2.07	2.11	2.16	2.20	2.25	2.29	2.33	2.40	2.48	2.54	2.59	2.64	2.71	2.79	2.90	3.06	3.29	3.68	4.54
16	2.01	2.06	2.11	2.15	2.19	2.24	2.28	2.35	2.42	2.49	2.54	2.59	2.66	2.74	2.85	3.01	3.24	3.63	4.49
17	1.96	2.01	2.06	2.10	2.15	2.19	2.23	2.31	2.38	2.45	2.49	2.55	2.61	2.70	2.81	2.96	3.20	3.59	4.45
18	1.92	1.97	2.02	2.06	2.11	2.15	2.19	2.27	2.34	2.41	2.46	2.51	2.58	2.66	2.77	2.93	3.16	3.55	4.41
19	1.88	1.93	1.98	2.03	2.07	2.11	2.16	2.23	2.31	2.38	2.42	2.48	2.54	2.63	2.74	2.90	3.13	3.52	4.38
20	1.84	1.90	1.95	1.99	2.04	2.08	2.12	2.20	2.28	2.35	2.39	2.45	2.51	2.60	2.71	2.87	3.10	3.49	4.35
21	1.81	1.87	1.92	1.96	2.01	2.05	2.10	2.18	2.25	2.32	2.37	2.42	2.49	2.57	2.68	2.84	3.07	3.47	4.32
22	1.78	1.84	1.89	1.94	1.98	2.03	2.07	2.15	2.23	2.30	2.34	2.40	2.46	2.55	2.66	2.82	3.05	3.44	4.30
23	1.76	1.81	1.86	1.91	1.96	2.01	2.05	2.13	2.20	2.27	2.32	2.37	2.44	2.53	2.64	2.80	3.03	3.42	4.28
24	1.73	1.79	1.84	1.89	1.94	1.98	2.03	2.11	2.18	2.25	2.30	2.36	2.42	2.51	2.62	2.78	3.01	3.40	4.26
25	1.71	1.77	1.82	1.87	1.92	1.96	2.01	2.09	2.16	2.24	2.28	2.34	2.40	2.49	2.60	2.76	2.99	3.39	4.24
26	1.69	1.75	1.80	1.85	1.90	1.95	1.99	2.07	2.15	2.22	2.27	2.32	2.39	2.47	2.59	2.74	2.98	3.37	4.23
27	1.67	1.73	1.79	1.84	1.88	1.93	1.97	2.06	2.13	2.20	2.25	2.31	2.37	2.46	2.57	2.73	2.96	3.35	4.21
28	1.65	1.71	1.77	1.82	1.87	1.91	1.96	2.04	2.12	2.19	2.24	2.29	2.36	2.45	2.56	2.71	2.95	3.34	4.20
29	1.64	1.70	1.75	1.81	1.85	1.90	1.94	2.03	2.10	2.18	2.22	2.28	2.35	2.43	2.55	2.70	2.93	3.33	4.18
30	1.62	1.68	1.74	1.79	1.84	1.89	1.93	2.01	2.09	2.16	2.21	2.27	2.33	2.42	2.53	2.69	2.92	3.32	4.17

(Continued)

TABLE A.3 (Continued)

$F_{0.10}(V_1, V_2)$ Degrees of Freedom for the Numerator (V_1)

V_2	1	2	3	4	5	6	7	8	9	10	12	15	20	24	30	40	60	120	∞
40	4.08	3.23	2.84	2.61	2.45	2.34	2.25	2.18	2.12	2.08	2.00	1.92	1.84	1.79	1.74	1.69	1.64	1.58	1.51
60	4.00	3.15	2.76	2.53	2.37	2.25	2.17	2.10	2.04	1.99	1.92	1.84	1.75	1.70	1.65	1.59	1.53	1.47	1.39
120	3.92	3.07	2.68	2.45	2.29	2.17	2.09	2.02	1.96	1.91	1.83	1.75	1.66	1.61	1.55	1.55	1.43	1.35	1.25
∞	3.84	3.00	2.60	2.37	2.21	2.10	2.01	1.94	1.88	1.83	1.75	1.67	1.57	1.52	1.46	1.39	1.32	1.22	1.00

$F_{0.025}(V_1, V_2)$ Degrees of Freedom for the Numerator (V_1)

V_2	1	2	3	4	5	6	7	8	9	10	12	15	20	24	30	40	60	120	∞
1	647.8	799.5	864.2	899.6	921.8	937.1	948.2	956.7	963.3	968.6	976.7	984.9	993.1	997.2	1001	1006	1010	1014	1018
2	38.51	39.00	39.17	39.25	39.30	39.33	39.36	39.37	39.39	39.40	39.41	39.43	39.45	39.46	39.46	39.47	39.48	39.49	39.50
3	17.44	16.04	15.44	15.10	14.88	14.73	14.62	14.54	14.47	14.42	14.34	14.25	14.17	14.12	14.08	14.04	13.99	13.95	13.90
4	12.22	10.65	9.98	9.60	9.36	9.20	9.07	8.98	8.90	8.84	8.75	8.66	8.56	8.51	8.46	8.41	8.36	8.31	8.26
5	10.01	8.43	7.76	7.39	7.15	6.98	6.85	6.76	6.68	6.62	6.52	6.43	6.33	6.28	6.23	6.18	6.12	6.07	6.02
6	8.81	7.26	6.60	6.23	5.99	5.82	5.70	5.60	5.52	5.46	5.37	5.27	5.17	5.12	5.07	5.01	4.96	4.90	4.85
7	8.07	6.54	5.89	5.52	5.29	5.12	4.99	4.90	4.82	4.76	4.67	4.57	4.47	4.42	4.36	4.31	4.25	4.20	4.14
8	7.57	6.06	5.42	5.05	4.82	4.65	4.53	4.43	4.36	4.30	4.20	4.10	4.00	3.95	3.89	3.84	3.78	3.73	3.67
9	7.21	5.71	5.08	4.72	4.48	4.32	4.20	4.10	4.03	3.96	3.87	3.77	3.67	3.61	3.56	3.51	3.45	3.39	3.33
10	6.94	5.46	4.83	4.47	4.24	4.07	3.95	3.85	3.78	3.72	3.62	3.52	3.42	3.37	3.31	3.26	3.20	3.14	3.08
11	6.72	5.26	4.63	4.28	4.04	3.88	3.76	3.66	3.59	3.53	3.43	3.33	3.23	3.17	3.12	3.06	3.00	2.94	2.88
12	6.55	5.10	4.47	4.12	3.89	3.73	3.61	3.51	3.44	3.37	3.28	3.18	3.07	3.02	2.96	2.91	2.85	2.79	2.72
13	6.41	4.97	4.35	4.00	3.77	3.60	3.48	3.39	3.31	3.25	3.15	3.05	2.95	2.89	2.84	2.78	2.72	2.66	2.60
14	6.30	4.86	4.24	3.89	3.66	3.50	3.38	3.29	3.21	3.15	3.05	2.95	2.84	2.79	2.73	2.67	2.61	2.55	2.49
15	6.20	4.77	4.15	3.80	3.58	3.41	3.29	3.20	3.12	3.06	2.96	2.86	2.76	2.70	2.64	2.59	2.52	2.46	2.40
16	6.12	4.69	4.08	3.73	3.50	3.34	3.22	3.12	3.05	2.99	2.89	2.79	2.68	2.63	2.57	2.51	2.45	2.38	2.32
17	6.04	4.62	4.01	3.66	3.44	3.28	3.16	3.06	2.98	2.92	2.82	2.72	2.62	2.56	2.50	2.44	2.38	2.32	2.25

Degrees Freedom Denominator V_2

v_2	1	2	3	4	5	6	7	8	9	10	12	15	20	24	30	40	60	120	∞
18	5.98	4.56	3.95	3.61	3.38	3.22	3.10	3.01	2.93	2.87	2.77	2.67	2.56	2.50	2.44	2.38	2.32	2.26	2.19
19	5.92	4.51	3.90	3.56	3.33	3.17	3.05	2.96	2.88	2.82	2.72	2.62	2.51	2.45	2.39	2.33	2.27	2.20	2.13
20	5.87	4.46	3.86	3.51	3.29	3.13	3.01	2.91	2.84	2.77	2.68	2.57	2.46	2.41	2.35	2.29	2.22	2.16	2.09
21	5.83	4.42	3.82	3.48	3.25	3.09	2.97	2.87	2.80	2.73	2.64	2.53	2.42	2.37	2.31	2.25	2.18	2.11	2.04
22	5.79	4.38	3.78	3.44	3.22	3.05	2.93	2.84	2.76	2.70	2.60	2.50	2.39	2.33	2.27	2.21	2.14	2.08	2.00
23	5.75	4.35	3.75	3.41	3.18	3.02	2.90	2.81	2.73	2.67	2.57	2.47	2.36	2.30	2.24	2.18	2.11	2.04	1.97
24	5.72	4.32	3.72	3.38	3.15	2.99	2.87	2.78	2.70	2.64	2.54	2.44	2.33	2.27	2.21	2.15	2.08	2.01	1.94
25	5.69	4.29	3.69	3.35	3.13	2.97	2.85	2.75	2.68	2.61	2.51	2.41	2.30	2.24	2.18	2.12	2.05	1.98	1.91
26	5.66	4.27	3.67	3.33	3.10	2.94	2.82	2.73	2.65	2.59	2.49	2.39	2.28	2.22	2.16	2.09	2.03	1.95	1.88
27	5.63	4.24	3.65	3.31	3.08	2.92	2.80	2.71	2.63	2.57	2.47	2.36	2.25	2.19	2.13	2.07	2.00	1.93	1.85
28	5.61	4.22	3.63	3.29	3.06	2.90	2.78	2.69	2.61	2.55	2.45	2.34	2.23	2.17	2.11	2.05	1.98	1.91	1.83
29	5.59	4.20	1.61	3.27	3.04	2.88	2.76	2.67	2.59	2.53	2.43	2.32	2.21	2.15	2.09	2.03	1.96	1.89	1.81
30	5.57	4.18	3.59	3.25	3.03	2.87	2.75	2.65	2.57	2.51	2.41	2.31	2.20	2.14	2.07	2.01	1.94	1.87	1.79
40	5.42	4.05	3.46	3.13	2.90	2.74	2.62	2.53	2.45	2.39	2.29	2.18	2.07	2.01	1.94	1.88	1.80	1.72	1.64
60	5.29	3.93	3.34	3.01	2.79	2.63	2.51	2.41	2.33	2.27	2.17	2.06	1.94	1.88	1.82	1.74	1.67	1.58	1.48
120	5.15	3.80	3.23	2.89	2.67	2.52	2.39	2.30	2.22	2.16	2.05	1.94	1.82	1.76	1.69	1.61	1.53	1.43	1.31
∞	5.02	3.69	3.12	2.79	2.57	2.41	2.29	2.19	2.11	2.05	1.94	1.83	1.71	1.64	1.57	1.48	1.39	1.27	1.00

$F_{0.01}(v_1, v_2)$ Degrees of Freedom for the Numerator (V_1)

v_2	1	2	3	4	5	6	7	8	9	10	12	15	20	24	30	40	60	120	∞
1	4052	4999.5	5403	5625	5764	5859	5928	5982	6022	6056	6106	6157	6209	6235	6261	6287	6313	6339	6366
2	98.50	99.00	99.17	99.25	99.30	99.33	99.36	99.37	99.39	99.40	99.42	99.43	99.45	99.46	99.47	99.47	99.48	99.49	99.50
3	34.12	30.82	29.46	28.71	28.24	27.91	27.67	27.49	27.35	27.23	27.05	26.87	26.69	26.60	26.50	26.41	26.32	26.22	26.13
4	21.20	18.00	16.69	15.98	15.52	15.21	14.98	14.80	14.66	14.55	14.37	14.20	14.02	13.93	13.84	13.75	13.65	13.56	13.46
5	16.26	13.27	12.06	11.39	10.97	10.67	10.46	10.29	10.16	10.05	9.89	9.72	9.55	9.47	9.38	9.29	9.20	9.11	9.02
6	13.75	10.92	9.78	9.15	8.75	8.47	8.26	8.10	7.98	7.87	7.72	7.56	7.40	7.31	7.23	7.14	7.06	6.97	6.88
7	12.25	9.55	8.45	7.85	7.46	7.19	6.99	6.84	6.72	6.62	6.47	6.31	6.16	6.07	5.99	5.91	5.82	5.74	5.65

(Continued)

TABLE A.3 (Continued)

$F_{0.01}(v_1, v_2)$ Degrees of Freedom for the Numerator (V_1)

v_2	1	2	3	4	5	6	7	8	9	10	12	15	20	24	30	40	60	120	∞
8	11.26	8.65	7.59	7.01	6.63	6.37	6.18	6.03	5.91	5.81	5.67	5.52	5.36	5.28	5.20	5.12	5.03	4.95	4.86
9	10.56	8.02	6.99	6.42	6.06	5.80	5.61	5.47	5.35	5.26	5.11	4.96	4.81	4.73	4.65	4.57	4.48	4.40	4.31
10	10.04	7.56	6.55	5.99	5.64	5.39	5.20	5.06	4.94	4.85	4.71	4.56	4.41	4.33	4.25	4.17	4.08	4.00	3.91
11	9.65	7.21	6.22	5.67	5.32	5.07	4.89	4.74	4.63	4.54	4.40	4.25	4.10	4.02	3.94	3.86	3.78	3.69	3.60
12	9.33	6.93	5.95	5.41	5.06	4.82	4.64	4.50	4.39	4.30	4.16	4.01	3.86	3.78	3.70	3.62	3.54	3.45	3.36
13	9.07	6.70	5.74	5.21	4.86	4.62	4.44	4.30	4.19	4.10	3.96	3.82	3.66	3.59	3.51	3.43	3.34	3.25	3.17
14	8.86	6.51	5.56	5.04	4.69	4.46	4.28	4.14	4.03	3.94	3.80	3.66	3.51	3.43	3.35	3.27	3.18	3.09	3.00
15	8.68	6.36	5.42	4.89	4.56	4.32	4.14	4.00	3.89	3.80	3.67	3.52	3.37	3.29	3.21	3.13	3.05	2.96	2.87
16	8.53	6.23	5.29	4.77	4.44	4.20	4.03	3.89	3.78	3.69	3.55	3.41	3.26	3.18	3.10	3.02	2.93	2.84	2.75
17	8.40	6.11	5.18	4.67	4.34	4.10	3.93	3.79	3.68	3.59	3.46	3.31	3.16	3.08	3.00	2.92	2.83	2.75	2.65
18	8.29	6.01	5.09	4.58	4.25	4.01	3.84	3.71	3.60	3.51	3.37	3.23	3.08	3.00	2.92	2.84	2.75	2.66	2.57
19	8.18	5.93	5.01	4.50	4.17	3.94	3.77	3.63	3.52	3.43	3.30	3.15	3.00	2.92	2.84	2.76	2.67	2.58	2.49
20	8.10	5.85	4.94	4.43	4.10	3.87	3.70	3.56	3.46	3.37	3.23	3.09	2.94	2.86	2.78	2.69	2.61	2.52	2.42
21	8.02	5.78	4.87	4.37	4.04	3.81	3.64	3.51	3.40	3.31	3.17	3.03	2.88	2.80	2.72	2.64	2.55	2.46	2.36
22	7.95	5.72	4.82	4.31	3.99	3.76	3.59	3.45	3.35	3.26	3.12	2.98	2.83	2.75	2.67	2.58	2.50	2.40	2.31
23	7.88	5.66	4.76	4.26	3.94	3.71	3.54	3.41	3.30	3.21	3.07	2.93	2.78	2.70	2.62	2.54	2.45	2.35	2.26
24	7.82	5.61	4.72	4.22	3.90	3.67	3.50	3.36	3.26	3.17	3.03	2.89	2.74	2.66	2.58	2.49	2.40	2.31	2.21
25	7.77	5.57	4.68	4.18	3.85	3.63	3.46	3.32	3.22	3.13	2.99	2.85	2.70	2.62	2.54	2.45	2.36	2.27	2.17
26	7.72	5.53	4.64	4.14	3.82	3.59	3.42	3.29	3.18	3.09	2.96	2.81	2.66	2.58	2.50	2.42	2.33	2.23	2.13
27	7.68	5.49	4.60	4.11	3.78	3.56	3.39	3.26	3.15	3.06	2.93	2.78	2.63	2.55	2.47	2.38	2.29	2.20	2.10
28	7.64	5.45	4.57	4.07	3.75	3.53	3.36	3.23	3.12	3.03	2.90	2.75	2.60	2.52	2.44	2.35	2.26	2.17	2.06
29	7.60	5.42	4.54	4.04	3.73	3.50	3.33	3.20	3.09	3.00	2.87	2.73	2.57	2.49	2.41	2.33	2.23	2.14	2.03
30	7.56	5.39	4.51	4.02	3.70	3.47	3.30	3.17	3.07	2.98	2.84	2.70	2.55	2.47	2.39	2.30	2.21	2.11	2.01
40	7.31	5.18	4.31	3.83	3.51	3.29	3.12	2.99	2.89	2.80	2.66	2.52	2.37	2.29	2.20	2.11	2.02	1.92	1.80
60	7.08	4.98	4.13	3.65	3.34	3.12	2.95	2.82	2.72	2.63	2.50	2.35	2.20	2.12	2.03	1.94	1.84	1.73	1.60
120	6.85	4.79	3.95	3.48	3.17	2.96	2.79	2.66	2.56	2.47	2.34	2.19	2.03	1.95	1.86	1.76	1.66	1.53	1.38
∞	6.63	4.61	3.78	3.32	3.02	2.80	2.64	2.51	2.41	2.32	2.18	2.04	1.88	1.79	1.70	1.59	1.47	1.32	1.00

Degrees Freedom Denominator V_2

TABLE **A.4**   Power Tables (Fixed Effects)

A.4.1. Power and sample size in analysis of variance; $V_1 = 1$.
A.4.2. Power and sample size in analysis of variance; $V_1 = 2$.
A.4.3. Power and sample size in analysis of variance; $V_1 = 3$.
A.4.4. Power and sample size in analysis of variance; $V_1 = 4$.
A.4.5. Power and sample size in analysis of variance; $V_1 = 5$.
A.4.6. Power and sample size in analysis of variance; $V_1 = 6$.
A.4.7. Power and sample size in analysis of variance; $V_1 = 7$.
A.4.8. Power and sample size in analysis of variance; $V_1 = 8$.

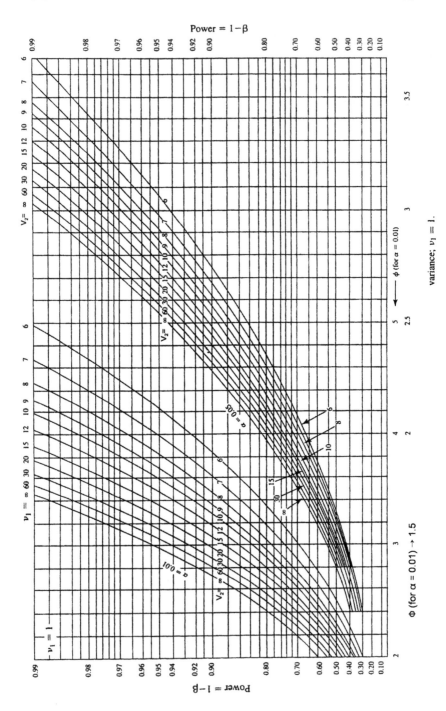

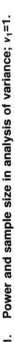

A.4.1.   Power and sample size in analysis of variance; ν_1=1.

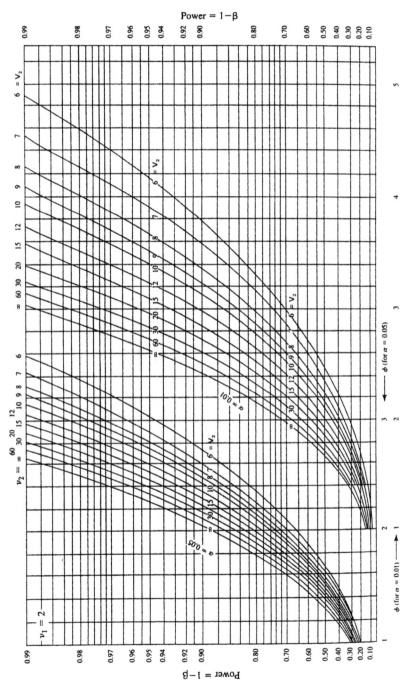

A.4.2.   Power and sample size in analysis of variance; $v_1 = 2$.

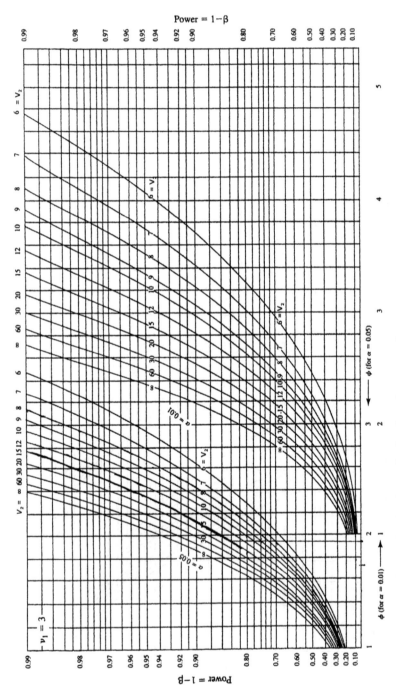

A.4.3. Power and sample size in analysis of variance; v_1=3.

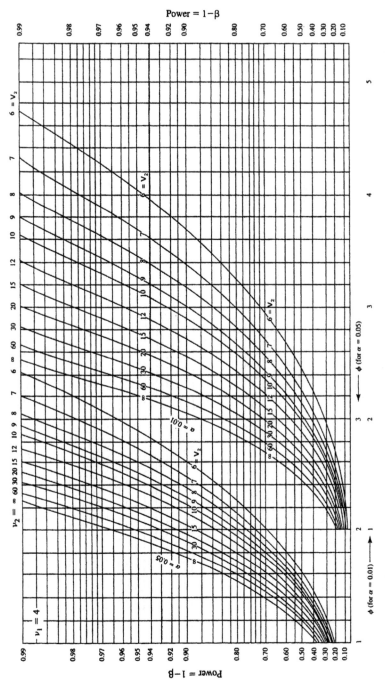

A.4.4.   Power and sample size in analysis of variance; v_1=4.

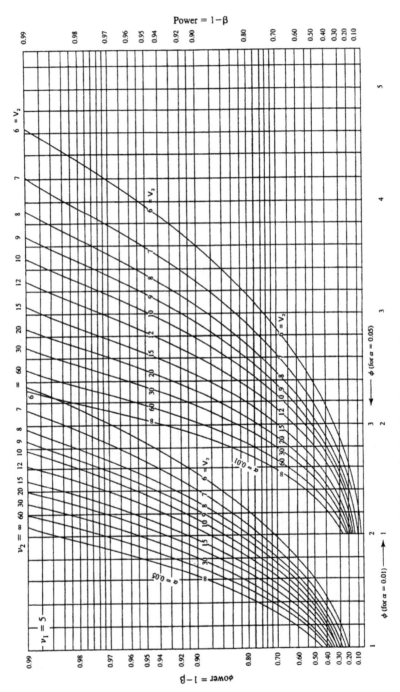

A.4.5. Power and sample size in analysis of variance; v_1=5.

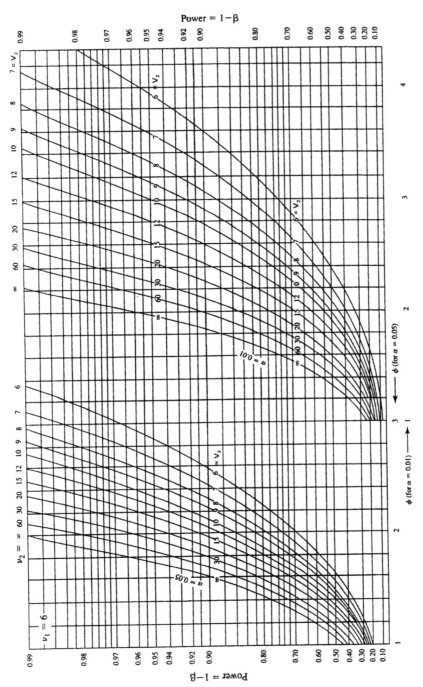

A.4.6. Power and sample size in analysis of variance; $v_1=6$.

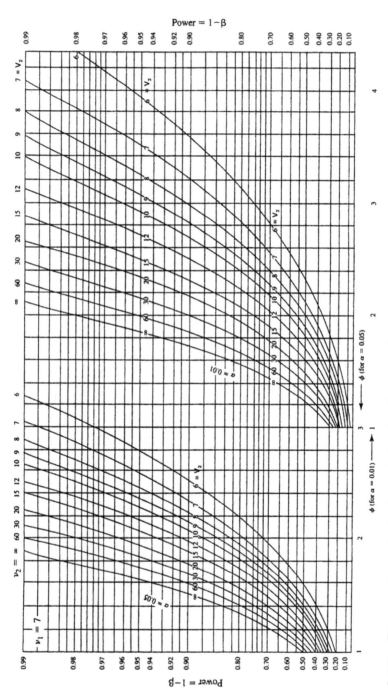

A.4.7.   Power and sample size in analysis of variance; $v_1=7$.

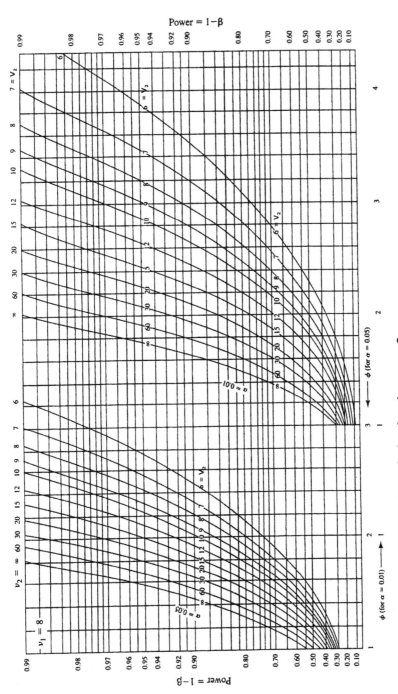

A.4.8. Power and sample size in analysis of variance; $v_1=8$.

TABLE A.5   Significant Ranges for Duncan's Multiple Range Test

$$r_{0.01}(p, f)$$

f	p											
	2	3	4	5	6	7	8	9	10	20	50	100
1	90.0	90.0	90.0	90.0	90.0	90.0	90.0	90.0	90.0	90.0	90.0	90.0
2	14.0	14.0	14.0	14.0	14.0	14.0	14.0	14.0	14.0	14.0	14.0	14.0
3	8.26	8.5	8.6	8.7	8.8	8.9	8.9	9.0	9.0	9.3	9.3	9.3
4	6.51	6.8	6.9	7.0	7.1	7.1	7.2	7.2	7.3	7.5	7.5	7.5
5	5.70	5.96	6.11	6.18	6.26	6.33	6.40	6.44	6.5	6.8	6.8	6.8
6	5.24	5.51	5.65	5.73	5.81	5.88	5.95	6.00	6.0	6.3	6.3	6.3
7	4.95	5.22	5.37	5.45	5.53	5.61	5.69	5.73	5.8	6.0	6.0	6.0
8	4.74	5.00	5.14	5.23	5.32	5.40	5.47	5.51	5.5	5.8	5.8	5.8
9	4.60	4.86	4.99	5.08	5.17	5.25	5.32	5.36	5.4	5.7	5.7	5.7
10	4.48	4.73	4.88	4.96	3.06	5.13	5.20	5.24	5.28	5.55	5.55	5.55
11	4.39	4.63	4.77	4.86	4.94	5.01	5.06	5.12	5.15	5.39	5.39	5.39
12	4.32	4.55	4.68	4.76	4.84	4.92	4.96	5.02	5.07	5.26	5.26	5.26
13	4.26	4.48	4.62	4.69	4.74	4.84	4.88	4.94	4.98	5.15	5.15	5.15
14	4.21	4.42	4.55	4.63	4.70	4.78	4.83	4.87	4.91	5.07	5.07	5.07
15	4.17	4.37	4.50	4.58	4.64	4.72	4.77	4.81	4.84	5.00	5.00	5.00
16	4.13	4.34	4.45	4.54	4.60	4.67	4.72	4.76	4.79	4.94	4.94	4.94
17	4.10	4.30	4.41	4.50	4.56	4.63	4.68	4.73	4.75	4.89	4.89	4.89
18	4.07	4.27	4.38	4.46	4.53	4.59	4.64	4.68	4.71	4.85	4.85	4.85
19	4.05	4.24	4.35	4.43	4.50	4.56	4.61	4.64	4.67	4.82	4.82	4.82
20	4.02	4.22	4.33	4.40	4.47	4.53	4.58	4.61	4.65	4.79	4.79	4.79
30	3.89	4.06	4.16	4.22	4.32	4.36	4.41	4.45	4.48	4.65	4.71	4.71
40	3.82	3.99	4.10	4.17	4.24	4.30	4.34	4.37	4.41	4.59	4.69	4.69
60	3.76	3.92	4.03	4.12	4.17	4.23	4.27	4.31	4.34	4.53	4.66	4.66
100	3.71	3.86	3.98	4.06	4.11	4.17	4.21	4.25	4.29	4.48	4.64	4.65
∞	3.64	3.80	3.90	3.98	4.04	4.09	4.14	4.17	4.20	4.41	4.60	4.68

$$r_{0.05}(p, f)$$

f	p											
	2	3	4	5	6	7	8	9	10	20	50	100
1	18.0	18.0	18.0	18.0	18.0	18.0	18.0	18.0	18.0	18.0	18.0	18.0
2	6.09	6.09	6.09	6.09	6.09	6.09	6.09	6.09	6.09	6.09	6.09	6.09
3	4.50	4.50	4.50	4.50	4.50	4.50	4.50	4.50	4.50	4.50	4.50	4.50
4	3.93	4.01	4.02	4.02	4.02	4.02	4.02	4.02	4.02	4.02	4.02	4.02
5	3.64	3.74	3.79	3.83	3.83	3.83	3.83	3.83	3.83	3.83	3.83	3.83
6	3.46	3.58	3.64	3.68	3.68	3.68	3.68	3.68	3.68	3.68	3.68	3.68

(Continued)

TABLE A.5 (Continued)

$$r_{0.05}(p, f)$$

f	2	3	4	5	6	7	8	9	10	20	50	100
						p						
7	3.35	3.47	3.54	3.58	3.60	3.61	3.61	3.61	3.61	3.61	3.61	3.61
8	3.26	3.39	3.47	3.52	3.55	3.56	3.56	3.56	3.56	3.56	3.56	3.56
9	3.20	3.34	3.41	3.47	3.50	3.52	3.52	3.52	3.52	3.52	3.52	3.52
10	3.15	3.30	3.37	3.43	3.46	3.47	3.47	3.47	3.47	3.48	3.48	3.48
11	3.11	3.27	3.35	3.39	3.43	3.44	3.45	3.46	3.46	3.48	3.48	3.48
12	3.08	3.23	3.33	3.36	3.40	3.42	3.44	3.44	3.46	3.48	3.48	3.48
13	3.06	3.21	3.30	3.35	3.38	3.41	3.42	3.44	3.45	3.47	3.47	3.47
14	3.03	3.18	3.27	3.33	3.37	3.39	3.41	3.42	3.44	3.47	3.47	3.47
15	3.01	3.16	3.25	3.31	3.36	3.38	3.40	3.42	3.43	3.47	3.47	3.47
16	3.00	3.15	3.23	3.30	3.34	3.37	3.39	3.41	3.43	3.47	3.47	3.47
17	2.98	3.13	3.22	3.28	3.33	3.36	3.38	3.40	3.42	3.47	3.47	3.47
18	2.97	3.12	3.21	3.27	3.32	3.35	3.37	3.39	3.41	3.47	3.47	3.47
19	2.96	3.11	3.19	3.26	3.31	3.35	3.37	3.39	3.41	3.47	3.47	3.47
20	2.95	3.10	3.18	3.25	3.30	3.34	3.36	3.38	3.40	3.47	3.47	3.47
30	2.89	3.04	3.12	3.20	3.25	3.29	3.32	3.35	3.37	3.47	3.47	3.47
40	2.86	3.01	3.10	3.17	3.22	3.27	3.30	3.33	3.35	3.47	3.47	3.47
60	2.83	2.98	3.08	3.14	3.20	3.24	3.28	3.31	3.33	3.47	3.48	3.48
100	2.80	2.95	3.05	3.12	3.18	3.22	3.26	3.29	3.32	3.47	3.53	3.53
∞	2.77	2.92	3.02	3.09	3.15	3.19	3.23	3.26	3.29	3.47	3.61	3.67

f = degrees of freedom.
Source: Adapted from Duncan DB. Biometrics 1(1):1–42, 1995.

TABLE A.6 Quantiles of the Mann–Whitney Test Statistic

n_1	p	$n_2=2$	3	4	5	6	7	8	9	10	11	12	13	14	15	16	17	18	19	20
	.001	0	0	0	0	0	0	0	0	0	0	0	0	0	0	0	0	0	0	0
	.005	0	0	0	0	0	0	0	0	0	0	0	0	0	0	0	0	0	1	1
2	.01	0	0	0	0	0	0	0	0	0	0	0	1	1	1	1	1	1	2	2
	.025	0	0	0	0	0	0	1	1	1	1	2	2	2	2	2	3	3	3	3
	.05	0	0	0	1	1	1	2	2	2	2	3	3	4	4	4	4	5	5	5
	.10	0	1	1	2	2	2	3	3	4	4	5	5	5	6	6	7	7	8	8
	.001	0	0	0	0	0	0	0	0	0	0	0	0	0	0	0	1	1	1	1
	.005	0	0	0	0	0	0	0	1	1	1	2	2	2	3	3	3	3	4	4

(Continued)

TABLE A.6 Continued

3	.01	0	0	0	0	0	1	1	2	2	2	3	3	3	4	4	5	5	5	6
	.025	0	0	0	1	2	2	3	3	4	4	5	5	6	6	7	7	8	8	9
	.05	0	1	1	2	3	3	4	5	5	6	6	7	8	8	9	10	10	11	12
	.10	1	2	2	3	4	5	6	6	7	8	9	10	11	11	12	13	14	15	16
	.001	0	0	0	0	0	0	0	0	1	1	1	2	2	2	3	3	4	4	4
	.005	0	0	0	0	1	1	2	2	3	3	4	4	5	6	6	7	7	8	9
4	.01	0	0	0	1	2	2	3	4	4	5	6	6	7	9	8	9	10	10	11
	.025	0	0	1	2	3	4	5	5	6	7	8	9	10	11	12	12	13	14	15
	.05	0	1	2	3	4	5	6	7	8	9	10	11	12	13	15	16	17	18	19
	.10	1	2	4	5	6	7	8	10	11	12	13	14	16	17	18	19	21	22	23
	.001	0	0	0	0	0	0	1	2	2	3	3	4	4	5	6	6	7	8	8
	.005	0	0	0	1	2	2	3	4	5	6	7	8	8	9	10	11	12	13	14
5	.01	0	0	1	2	3	4	5	6	7	8	9	10	11	12	13	14	15	16	17
	.025	0	1	2	3	4	6	7	8	9	10	12	13	14	15	16	18	19	20	21
	.05	1	2	3	5	6	7	9	10	12	13	14	16	17	19	20	21	23	24	26
	.10	2	3	5	6	8	9	11	13	14	16	18	19	21	23	24	26	28	29	31
	.001	0	0	0	0	0	0	2	3	4	5	5	6	7	8	9	10	11	12	13
	.005	0	0	1	2	3	4	5	6	7	8	10	11	12	13	14	16	17	18	19
6	.01	0	0	2	3	4	5	7	8	9	10	12	13	14	16	17	19	20	21	23
	.025	0	2	3	4	6	7	9	11	12	14	15	17	18	20	22	23	25	26	28
	.05	1	3	4	6	8	9	11	13	15	17	18	20	22	24	26	27	29	31	33
	.10	2	4	6	8	10	12	14	16	18	20	22	24	26	28	30	32	35	37	39
	.001	0	0	0	0	1	2	3	4	6	7	8	9	10	11	12	14	15	16	17
	.005	0	0	1	2	4	5	7	8	10	11	13	14	16	17	19	20	22	23	25
7	.01	0	1	2	4	5	7	8	10	12	13	15	17	18	20	22	24	25	27	29
	.025	0	2	4	6	7	9	11	13	15	17	19	21	23	25	27	29	31	33	35
	.05	1	3	5	7	9	12	14	16	18	20	22	25	27	29	31	34	36	38	40
	.10	2	5	7	9	12	14	17	19	22	24	27	29	32	34	37	39	42	44	47
	.001	0	0	0	1	2	3	5	6	7	9	10	12	13	15	16	18	19	21	22
	.005	0	0	2	3	5	7	8	10	12	14	16	18	19	21	23	25	27	29	31
8	.01	0	1	3	5	7	8	10	12	14	16	18	21	23	25	27	29	31	33	35
	.025	1	3	5	7	9	11	14	16	18	20	23	25	27	30	32	35	37	39	42

(Continued)

TABLE A.6 Continued

n_1	p	$n_2=2$	3	4	5	6	7	8	9	10	11	12	13	14	15	16	17	18	19	20
	.05	2	4	6	9	11	14	16	19	21	24	27	29	32	34	37	40	42	45	48
	.10	3	6	8	11	14	17	20	23	25	28	31	34	37	40	43	46	49	52	55
	.001	0	0	0	2	3	4	6	8	9	11	13	15	16	18	20	22	24	26	27
	.005	0	1	2	4	6	8	10	12	14	17	19	21	23	25	28	30	32	34	37
9	.01	0	2	4	6	8	10	12	15	17	19	22	24	27	29	32	34	37	39	41
	.025	1	3	5	8	11	13	16	18	21	24	27	29	32	35	38	40	43	46	49
	.05	2	5	7	10	13	16	19	22	25	28	31	34	37	40	43	46	49	52	55
	.10	3	6	10	13	16	19	23	26	29	32	36	39	42	46	49	53	56	59	63
	.001	0	0	1	2	4	6	7	9	11	13	15	18	20	22	24	26	28	30	33
	.005	0	1	3	5	7	10	12	14	17	19	22	25	27	30	32	35	38	40	43
10	.01	0	2	4	7	9	12	14	17	20	23	25	28	31	34	37	39	42	45	48
	.025	1	4	6	9	12	15	18	21	24	27	30	34	37	40	43	46	49	53	56
	.05	2	5	8	12	15	18	21	25	28	32	35	38	42	45	49	52	56	59	63
	.10	4	7	11	14	18	22	25	29	33	37	40	44	48	52	55	59	63	67	71
	.001	0	0	1	3	5	7	9	11	13	16	18	21	23	25	28	30	33	35	38
	.005	0	1	3	6	8	11	14	17	19	22	25	28	31	34	37	40	43	46	49
11	.01	0	2	5	8	10	13	16	19	23	26	29	32	35	38	42	45	48	51	54
	.025	1	4	7	10	14	17	20	24	27	31	34	38	41	45	48	52	56	59	63
	.05	2	6	9	13	17	20	24	28	32	35	39	43	47	51	55	58	62	66	70
	.10	4	8	12	16	20	24	28	32	37	41	45	49	53	58	62	66	70	74	79
	.001	0	0	1	3	5	8	10	13	15	18	21	24	26	29	32	35	38	41	43
	.005	0	2	4	7	10	13	16	19	22	25	28	32	35	38	42	45	48	52	55
12	.01	0	3	6	9	12	15	18	22	25	29	32	36	39	43	47	50	54	57	61
	.025	2	5	8	12	15	19	23	27	30	34	38	42	46	50	54	58	62	66	70
	.05	3	6	10	14	18	22	27	31	35	39	43	48	52	56	61	65	69	73	78
	.10	5	9	13	18	22	27	31	36	40	45	50	54	59	64	68	73	78	82	87
	.001	0	0	2	4	6	9	12	15	18	21	24	27	30	33	36	39	43	46	49
	.005	0	2	4	8	11	14	18	21	25	28	32	35	39	43	46	50	54	58	61
13	.01	1	3	6	10	13	17	21	24	28	32	36	40	44	48	52	56	60	64	68
	.025	2	5	9	13	17	21	25	29	34	38	42	46	51	55	60	64	68	73	77
	.05	3	7	11	16	20	25	29	34	38	43	48	52	57	62	66	71	76	81	85
	.10	5	10	14	19	24	29	34	39	44	49	54	59	64	69	75	80	85	90	95
	.001	0	0	2	4	7	10	13	16	20	23	26	30	33	37	40	44	47	51	55
	.005	0	2	5	8	12	16	19	23	27	31	35	39	43	47	51	55	59	64	68
14	.01	1	3	7	11	14	18	23	27	31	35	39	44	48	52	57	61	66	70	74
	.025	2	6	10	14	18	23	27	32	37	41	46	51	56	60	65	70	75	79	84
	.05	4	8	12	17	22	27	32	37	42	47	52	57	62	67	72	78	83	88	93
	.10	5	11	16	21	26	32	37	42	48	53	59	64	70	75	81	86	92	98	103
	.001	0	0	2	5	8	11	15	18	22	25	29	33	37	41	44	48	52	56	60
	.005	0	3	6	9	13	17	21	25	30	34	38	43	47	52	56	61	65	70	74

(Continued)

TABLE A.6   Continued

n_1	p	$n_2=2$	3	4	5	6	7	8	9	10	11	12	13	14	15	16	17	18	19	20
15	.01	I	4	8	12	16	20	25	29	34	38	43	48	52	57	62	67	71	76	81
	.025	2	6	11	15	20	25	30	35	40	45	50	55	60	65	71	76	81	86	91
	.05	4	8	13	19	24	29	34	40	45	51	56	62	67	73	78	84	89	95	101
	.10	6	11	17	23	28	34	40	46	52	58	64	69	75	81	87	93	99	105	111
	.001	0	0	3	6	9	12	16	20	24	28	32	36	40	44	49	53	57	61	66
	.005	0	3	6	10	14	19	23	28	32	37	42	46	51	56	61	66	71	75	80
16	.01	I	4	8	13	17	22	27	32	37	42	47	52	57	62	67	72	77	83	88
	.025	2	7	12	16	22	27	32	38	43	48	54	60	65	71	76	82	87	93	99
	.05	4	9	15	20	26	31	37	43	49	55	61	66	72	78	84	90	96	102	108
	.10	6	12	18	24	30	37	43	49	55	62	68	75	81	87	94	100	107	113	120
	.001	0	1	3	6	10	14	18	22	26	30	35	39	44	48	53	58	62	67	71
	.005	0	3	7	11	16	20	25	30	35	40	45	50	55	61	66	71	76	82	87
17	.01	1	5	9	14	19	24	29	34	39	45	50	56	61	67	72	78	83	89	94
	.025	3	7	12	18	23	29	35	40	46	52	58	64	70	76	82	88	94	100	106
	.05	4	10	16	21	27	34	40	46	52	58	65	71	78	84	90	97	103	110	116
	.10	7	13	19	26	32	39	46	53	59	66	73	80	86	93	100	107	114	121	128
	.001	0	1	4	7	11	15	19	24	28	33	38	43	47	52	57	62	67	72	77
	.005	0	3	7	12	17	22	27	32	38	43	48	54	59	65	71	76	82	88	93
18	.01	1	5	10	15	20	25	31	37	42	48	54	60	66	71	77	83	89	95	101
	.025	3	8	13	19	25	31	37	43	49	56	62	68	75	81	87	94	100	107	113
	.05	5	10	17	23	29	36	42	49	56	62	69	76	83	89	96	103	110	117	124
	.10	7	14	21	28	35	42	49	56	63	70	78	85	92	99	107	114	121	129	136
	.001	0	1	4	8	12	16	21	26	30	35	41	46	51	56	61	67	72	78	83
	.005	1	4	8	13	18	23	29	34	40	46	52	58	64	70	75	82	88	94	100
19	.01	2	5	10	16	21	27	33	39	45	51	57	64	70	76	83	89	95	102	108
	.025	3	8	14	20	26	33	39	46	53	59	66	73	79	86	93	100	107	114	120
	.05	5	11	18	24	31	38	45	52	59	66	73	81	88	95	102	110	117	124	131
	.10	8	15	22	29	37	44	52	59	67	74	82	90	98	105	113	121	129	136	144
	.001	0	1	4	8	13	17	22	27	33	38	43	49	55	60	66	71	77	83	89
	.005	1	4	9	14	19	25	31	37	43	49	55	61	68	74	80	87	93	100	106
20	.01	2	6	11	17	23	29	35	41	48	54	61	68	74	81	88	94	101	108	115
	.025	3	9	15	21	28	35	42	49	56	63	70	77	84	91	99	106	113	120	128
	.05	5	12	19	26	33	40	48	55	63	70	78	85	93	101	108	116	124	131	139
	.10	8	16	23	31	39	47	55	63	71	79	87	95	103	111	120	128	136	144	152

TABLE A.7 Binomial Probability Distribution

$$P(r \mid n, P) = \binom{n}{r} p^r q^{n-r}$$

n=1

r \ p	.01	.02	.03	.04	.05	.06	.07	.08	.09	.10
0	.9900	.9800	.9700	.9600	.9500	.9400	.9300	.9200	.9100	.9000
1	.0100	.0200	.0300	.0400	.0500	.0600	.0700	.0800	.0900	.1000
	.11	.12	.13	.14	.15	.16	.17	.18	.19	.20
0	.8900	.8800	.8700	.8600	.8500	.8400	.8300	.8200	.8100	.8000
1	.1100	.1200	.1300	.1400	.1500	.1600	.1700	.1800	.1900	.2000
	.21	.22	.23	.24	.25	.26	.27	.28	.29	.30
0	.7900	.7800	.7700	.7600	.7500	.7400	.7300	.7200	.7100	.7000
1	.2100	.2200	.2300	.2400	.2500	.2600	.2700	.2800	.2900	.3000
	.31	.32	.33	.34	.35	.36	.37	.38	.39	.40
0	.6900	.6800	.6700	.6600	.6500	.6400	.6300	.6200	.6100	.6000
	.3100	.3200	.3300	.3400	.3500	.3600	.3700	.3800	.3900	.4000
	.41	.42	.43	.44	.45	.46	.47	.48	.49	.50
0	.5900	.5800	.5700	.5600	.5500	.5400	.5300	.5200	.5100	.5000
1	.4100	.4200	.4300	.4400	.4500	.4600	.4700	.4800	.4900	.5000

n = 2

	.01	.02	.03	.04	.05	.06	.07	.08	.09	.10
0	.9801	.9604	.9409	.9216	.9025	.8836	.8649	.8464	.8281	.8100
1	.0198	.0392	.0582	.0768	.0950	.1128	.1302	.1472	.1638	.1800
2	.0001	.0004	.0009	.0016	.0025	.0036	.0049	.0064	.0081	.0100
	.11	.12	.13	.14	.15	.16	.17	.18	.19	.20
0	.7921	.7744	.7569	.7396	.7225	.7056	.6889	.6724	.6561	.6400
1	.1958	.2112	.2262	.2408	.2550	.2688	.2822	.2952	.3078	.3200
2	.0121	.0144	.0169	.0196	.0225	.0256	.0289	.0324	.0361	.0400
	.21	.22	.23	.24	.25	.26	.27	.28	.29	.30
0.	.6241	.6084	.5929	.5776	.5625	.5476	.5329	.5184	.5041	.4900
1.	.3318	.3432	.3542	.3648	.3750	.3848	.3942	.4032	.4118	.4200
2	.0441	.0484	.0529	.0576	.0625	.0676	.0729	.0784	.0841	.0900
	.31	.32	.33	.34	.35	.36	.37	.38	.39	.40
0	.4761	.4624	.4489	.4356	.4225	.4096	.3969	.3844	.3721	.3600
1	.4278	.4352	.4422	.4488	.4550	.4608	.4662	.4712	.4758	.4800
2	.0961	.1024	.1089	.1156	.1225	.1296	.1369	.1444	.1521	.1600
	.41	.42	.43	.44	.45	.46	.47	.48	.49	.50
0	.3481	.3364	.3249	.3136	.3025	.2916	.2809	.2704	.2601	.2500
1	.4838	.4872	.4902	.4928	.4950	.4968	.4982	.4992	.4998	.5000
2	.1681	.1764	.1849	.1936	.2025	.2116	.2209	.2304	.2401	.2500

(Continued)

TABLE A.7 (Continued)

r \ p	.01	.02	.03	.04	.05	.06	.07	.08	.09	.10

n=3

r	.01	.02	.03	.04	.05	.06	.07	.08	.09	.10
0	.9704	.9412	.9127	.8847	.8574	.8306	.8044	.7787	.7536	.7290
1	.0294	.0576	.0847	.1106	.1354	.1590	.1816	.2031	.2236	.2430
2	.0003	.0012	.0026	.0046	.0071	.0102	.0137	.0177	.0221	.0270
3	.0000	.0000	.0000	.0001	.0001	.0002	.0003	.0005	.0007	.0010
	.11	.12	.13	.14	.15	.16	.17	.18	.19	.20
0	.7050	.6815	.6585	.6361	.6141	.5927	.5718	.5514	.5314	.5120
1	.2614	.2788	.2952	.3106	.3251	.3387	.3513	.3631	.3740	.3840
2	.0323	.0380	.0441	.0506	.0574	.0645	.0720	.0797	.0877	.0960
3	.0013	.0017	.0022	.0027	.0034	.0041	.0049	.0058	.0069	.0080
	.21	.22	.23	.24	.25	.26	.27	.28	.29	.30
0	.4930	.4746	.4565	.4390	.4219	.4052	.3890	.3732	.3579	.3430
1	.3932	.4015	.4091	.4159	.4219	.4271	.4316	.4355	.4386	.4410
2	.1045	.1133	.1222	.1313	.1406	.1501	.1597	.1693	.1791	.1890
3	.0093	.0106	.0122	.0138	.0156	.0176	.0197	.0220	.0244	.0270
	.31	.32	.33	.34	.35	.36	.37	.38	.39	.40
0	.3285	.3144	.3008	.2875	.2746	.2621	.2500	.2383	.2270	.2160
1	.4428	.4439	.4444	.4443	.4436	.4424	.4406	.4382	.4354	.4320
2	.1989	.2089	.2189	.2289	.2389	.2488	.2587	.2686	.2783	.2880
3	.0298	.0328	.0359	.0393	.0429	.0467	.0507	.0549	.0593	.0640
	.41	.42	.43	.44	.45	.46	.47	.48	.49	.50
0	.2054	.1951	.1852	.1756	.1664	.1575	.1489	.1406	.1327	.1250
1	.4282	.4239	.4191	.4140	.4084	.4024	.3961	.3894	.3823	.3750
2	.2975	.3069	.3162	.3252	.3341	.3428	.3512	.3594	.3674	.3750
3	.0689	.0741	.0795	.0852	.0911	.0973	.1038	.1106	.1176	.1250

n = 4

r	.01	.02	.03	.04	.05	.06	.07	.08	.09	.10
0	.9606	.9224	.8853	.8493	.8145	.7807	.7481	.7164	.6857	.6561
1	.0388	.0753	.1095	.1416	.1715	.1993	.2252	.2492	.2713	.2916
2	.0006	.0023	.0051	.0088	.0135	.0191	.0254	.0325	.0402	.0486
3	.0000	.0000	.0001	.0002	.0005	.0008	.0013	.0019	.0027	.0036
4	.0000	.0000	.0000	.0000	.0000	.0000	.0000	.0000	.0001	.0001
	.11	.12	.13	.14	.15	.16	.17	.18	.19	.20
0	.6274	.5997	.5729	.5470	.5220	.4979	.4746	.4521	.4305	.4096
1	.3102	.3271	.3424	.3562	.3685	.3793	.3888	.3970	.4039	.4096
2	.0575	.0669	.0767	.0870	.0975	.1084	.1195	.1307	.1421	.1536

(Continued)

Appendix

TABLE A.7 (Continued)

					n=4					
r \ p	.11	.12	.13	.14	.15	.16	.17	.18	.19	.20
3	.0047	.0061	.0076	.0094	.0115	.0138	.0163	.0191	.0222	.0256
4	.0001	.0002	.0003	.0004	.0005	.0007	.0008	.0010	.0013	.0016
	.21	.22	.23	.24	.25	.26	.27	.28	.29	.30
0	.3895	.3702	.3515	.3336	.3164	.2999	.2840	.2687	.2541	.2401
1	.4142	.4176	.4200	.4214	.4219	.4214	.4201	.4180	.4152	.4116
2	.1651	.1767	.1882	.1996	.2109	.2221	.2331	.2439	.2544	.2646
3	.0293	.0332	.0375	.0420	.0469	.0520	.0575	.0632	.0693	.0756
4	.0019	.0023	.0028	.0033	.0039	.0046	.0053	.0061	.0071	.0081
	.31	..32	.33	.34	.35	.36	.37	.38	.39	.40
0	.2267	.2138	.2015	.1897	.1785	.1678	.1575	.1478	.1385	.1296
1	.4074	.4025	.3970	.3910	.3845	.3775	.3701	.3623	.3541	.3456
2	.2745	.2841	.2933	.3021	.3105	.3185	.3260	.3330	.3396	.3456
3	.0822	.0891	.0963	.1038	.1115	.1194	.1276	.1361	.1447	.1536
4	.0092	.0105	.0119	.0134	.0150	.0168	.0187	.0209	.0231	.0256
	.41	.42	.43	.44	.45	.46	.47	.48	.49	.50
0	.1212	.1132	.1056	.0983	.0915	.0850	.0789	.0731	.0677	.0625
1	.3368	.3278	.3185	.3091	.2995	.2897	.2799	.2700	.2600	.2500
2	.3511	.3560	.3604	.3643	.3675	.3702	.3723	.3738	.3747	.3750
3	.1627	.1719	.1813	.1908	.2005	.2102	.2201	.2300	.2400	.2500
4	.0283	.0311	.0342	.0375	.0410	.0448	.0488	.0531	.0576	.0625

					n = 5					
	.01	.02	.03	.04	.05	.06	.07	.08	.09	.10
0	.9510	.9039	.8587	.8154	.7738	.7339	.6957	.6591	.6240	.5905
1	.0480	.0922	.1328	.1699	.2036	.2342	.2618	.2866	.3086	.3280
2	.0010	.0038	.0082	.0142	.0214	.0299	.0394	.0498	.0610	.0729
3	.0000	.0001	.0003	.0006	.0011	.0019	.0030	.0043	.0060	.0081
4	.0000	.0000	.0000	.0000	.0000	.0001	.0001	.0002	.0003	.0004
	.11	.12	.13	.14	.15	.16	.17	.18	.19	.20
0	.5584	.5277	.4984	.4704	.4437	.4182	.3939	.3707	.3487	.3277
1	.3451	.3598	.3724	.3829	.3915	.3983	.4034	.4069	.4089	.4096
2	.0853	.0981	.1113	.1247	.1382	.1517	.1652	.1786	.1919	.2048
3	.0105	.0134	.0166	.0203	.0244	.0289	.0338	.0392	.0450	.0512
4	.0007	.0009	.0012	.0017	.0022	.0028	.0035	.0043	.0053	.0064
5	.0000	.0000	.0000	.0001	.0001	.0001	.0001	.0002	.0002	.0003
	.21	.22	.23	.24	.25	.26	.27	.28	.29	.30
0	.3077	.2887	.2707	.2536	.2373	.2219	.2073	.1935	.1804	.1681
1	.4090	.4072	.4043	.4003	.3955	.3898	.3834	.3762	.3685	.3602

(Continued)

TABLE A.7 (Continued)

n=5

r \ p	.21	.22	.23	.24	.25	.26	.27	.28	.29	.30
2	.2174	.2297	.2415	.2529	.2637	.2739	.2836	.2926	.3010	.3087
3	.0578	.0648	.0721	.0798	.0879	.0962	.1049	.1138	.1229	.1323
4	.0077	.0091	.0108	.0126	.0146	.0169	.0194	.0221	.0251	.0284
5	.0004	.0005	.0006	.0008	.0010	.0012	.0014	.0017	.0021	.0024
	.31	.32	.33	.34	.35	.36	.37	.38	.39	.40
0	.1564	.1454	.1350	.1252	.1160	1074	.0992	.0916	.0845	.0778
1	.3513	.3421	.3325	.3226	.3124	.3020	.2914	.2808	.2700	.2592
2	.3157	.3220	.3275	.3323	.3364	.3397	.3423	.3441	.3452	.3456
3	.1418	.1515	.1613	.1712	.1811	.1911	.2010	.2109	.2207	.2304
4	.0319	.0357	.0397	.0441	.0488	.0537	.0590	.0646	.0706	.0768
5	.0029	.0034	.0039	.0045	.0053	.0060	.0069	.0079	.0090	.0102
	.41	.42	.43	.44	.45	.46	.47	.48	.49	.50
0	.0715	.0656	.0602	.0551	.0503	.0459	.0418	.0380	.0345	.0312
1	.2484	.2376	.2270	.2164	.2059	.1956	.1854	.1755	.1657	.1562
2	.3452	.3442	.3424	.3400	.3369	.3332	.3289	.3240	.3185	.3125
3	.2399	.2492	.2583	.2671	.2757	.2838	.2916	.2990	.3060	.3125
4	.0834	.0902	.0974	.1049	.1128	.1209	.1293	.1380	.1470	.1562
5	.0116	.0131	.0147	.0165	.0185	.0206	.0229	.0255	.0282	.0312

n = 6

r	.01	.02	.03	.04	.05	.06	.07	.08	.09	.10
0	.9415	.8858	.8330	.7828	.7351	.6899	.6470	.6064	.5679	.5314
1	.0571	.1085	.1546	.1957	.2321	.2642	.2922	.3164	.3370	.3543
2	.0014	.0055	.0120	.0204	.0305	.0422	.0550	.0688	.0833	.0984
3	.0000	.0002	.0005	.0011	.0021	.0036	.0055	.0080	.0110	.0146
4	.0000	.0000	.0000	.0000	.0001	.0002	.0003	.0005	.0008	.0012
5	.0000	.0000	.0000	.0000	.0000	.0000	.0000	.0000	.0000	.0001
	.11	.12	.13	.14	.15	.16	.17	.18	.19	.20
0	.4970	.4644	.4336	.4046	.3771	.3513	.3269	.3040	.2824	.2621
1	.3685	.3800	.3888	.3952	.3993	.4015	.4018	.4004	.3975	.3932
2	.1139	.1295	.1452	.1608	.1762	.1912	.2057	.2197	.2331	.2458
3	.0188	.0236	.0289	.0349	.0415	.0486	.0562	.0643	.0729	.0819
4	.0017	.0024	.0032	.0043	.0055	.0069	.0086	.0106	.0128	.0154
5	.0001	.0001	.0002	.0003	.0004	.0005	.0007	.0009	.0012	.0015
6	.0000	.0000	.0000	.0000	.0000	.0000	.0000	.0000	.0000	.0001
	.21	.22	.23	.24	.25	.26	.27	.28	.29	.30
0	.2431	.2552	.2084	.1927	.1780	.1642	.1513	.1393	.1281	.1176
1	.3877	.3811	.3735	.3651	.3560	.3462	.3358	.3251	.3139	.3025

(Continued)

TABLE A.7 (Continued)

n=6

r\p	.21	.22	.23	.24	.25	.26	.27	.28	.29	.30
2	.2577	.2687	.2789	.2882	.2966	.3041	.3105	.3160	.3206	.3241
3	.0913	.1011	.1111	.1214	.1318	.1424	.1531	.1639	.1746	.1852
4	.0182	.0214	.0249	.0287	.0330	.0375	.0425	.0478	.0535	.0595
5	.0019	.0024	.0030	.0036	.0044	.0053	.0063	.0074	.0087	.0102
6	.0001	.0001	.0001	.0002	.0002	.0003	.0004	.0005	.0006	.0007
	.31	.32	.33	.34	.35	.36	.37	.38	.39	.40
0	.1079	.0989	.0905	.0827	.0754	.0687	.0625	.0568	.0515	.0467
1	.2909	.2792	.2673	.2555	.2437	.2319	.2203	.2089	.1976	.1866
2	.3267	.3284	.3292	.3290	.3280	.3261	.3235	.3201	.3159	.3110
3	.1957	.2061	.2162	.2260	.2355	.2446	.2533	.2616	.2693	.2765
4	.0660	.0727	.0799	.0873	.0951	.1032	.1116	.1202	.1291	.1382
5	.0119	.0137	.0157	.0180	.0205	.0232	.0262	.0295	.0330	.0369
6	.0009	.0011	.0013	.0015	.0018	.0022	.0026	.0030	.0035	.0041
	.41	.42	.43	.44	.45	.46	.47	.48	.49	.50
0	.0422	.0381	.0343	.0308	.0277	.0248	.0222	.0198	.0176	.0156
1	.1759	.1654	.1552	.1454	.1359	.1267	.1179	.1095	.1014	.0938
2	.3055	.2994	.2928	.2856	.2780	.2699	.2615	.2527	.2436	.2344
3	.2831	.2891	.2945	.2992	.3032	.3065	.3091	.3110	.3121	.3125
4	.1475	.1570	.1666	.1763	.1861	.1958	.2056	.2153	.2249	.2344
5	.0410	.0455	.0503	.0554	.0609	.0667	.0729	.0795	.0864	.0938
6	.0048	.0055	.0063	.0073	.0083	.0095	.0108	.0122	.0138	.0156

n = 7

	.01	.02	.03	.04	.05	.06	.07	.08	.09	.10
0	.9321	.8681	.8080	.7514	.6983	.6485	.6017	.5578	.5168	.4783
1	.0659	.1240	.1749	.2192	.2573	.2897	.3170	.3396	.3578	.3720
2	.0020	.0076	.0162	.0274	.0406	.0555	.0716	.0886	.1061	.1240
3	.0000	.0003	.0008	.0019	.0036	.0059	.0090	.0128	.0175	.0230
4	.0000	.0000	.0000	.0001	.0002	.0004	.0007	.0011	.0017	.0026
5	.0000	.0000	.0000	.0000	.0000	.0000	.0000	.0001	.0001	.0002
	.11	.12	.13	.14	.15	.16	.17	.18	.19	.20
0	.4423	.4087	.3773	.3479	.3206	.2951	.2714	.2493	.2288	.2097
1	.3827	.3901	.3946	.3965	.3960	.3935	.3891	.3830	.3756	.3670
2	.1419	.1596	.1769	.1936	.2097	.2248	.2391	.2523	.2643	.2753
3	.0292	.0363	.0441	.0525	.0617	.0714	.0816	.0923	.1033	.1147
4	.0036	.0049	.0066	.0086	.0109	.0136	.0167	.0203	.0242	.0287
5	.0003	.0004	.0006	.0008	.0012	.0016	.0021	.0027	.0034	.0043
6	.0000	.0000	.0000	.0000	.0001	.0001	.0001	.0002	.0003	.0004

(Continued)

TABLE A.7   (Continued)

r \ p	.21	.22	.23	.24	.25	.26	.27	.28	.29	.30
					n=7					
0	.1920	.1757	.1605	.1465	.1335	.1215	.1105	.1003	.0910	.0824
1	.3573	.3468	.3356	.3237	.3115	.2989	.2860	.2731	.2600	.2471
2	.2850	.2935	.3007	.3067	.3115	.3150	.3174	.3186	.3186	.3177
3	.1263	.1379	.1497	.1614	.1730	.1845	.1956	.2065	.2169	.2269
4	.0336	.0389	.0447	.0510	.0577	.0648	.0724	.0803	.0886	.0972
5	.0054	.0066	.0080	.0097	.0115	.0137	.0161	.0187	.0217	.0250
6	.0005	.0006	.0008	.0010	.0013	.0016	.0020	.0024	.0030	.0036
7	.0000	.0000	.0000	.0000	.0001	.0001	.0001	.0001	.0002	.0002
	.31	.32	.33	.34	.35	.36	.37	.38	.39	.40
0	.0745	.0672	.0606	.0546	.0490	.0440	.0394	.0352	.0314	.0280
1	.2342	.2215	.2090	.1967	.1848	.1732	.1619	.1511	.1407	.1306
2	.3156	.3127	.3088	.3040	.2985	.2922	.2853	.2778	.2698	.2613
3	.2363	.2452	.2535	.2610	.2679	.2740	.2793	.2838	.2875	.2903
4	.1062	.1154	.1248	.1345	.1442	.1541	.1640	.1739	.1838	.1935
5	.0286	.0326	.0369	.0416	.0466	.0520	.0578	.0640	.0705	.0774
6	.0043	.0051	.0061	.0071	.0084	.0098	.0113	.0131	.0150	.0172
7	.0003	.0003	.0004	.0005	.0006	.0008	.0009	.0011	.0014	.0016
	.41	.42	.43	.44	.45	.46	.47	.48	.49	.50
0	.0249	.0221	.0195	.0173	.0152	.0134	.0117	.0103	.0090	.0078
1	.1211	.1119	.1032	.0950	.0872	.0798	.0729	.0664	.0604	.0547
2	.2524	.2431	.2336	.2239	.2140	.2040	.1940	.1840	.1740	.1641
3	.2923	.2934	.2937	.2932	.2918	.2897	.2867	.2830	.2786	.2734
4	.2031	.2125	.2216	.2304	.2388	.2468	.2543	.2612	.2676	.2734
5	.0847	.0923	.1003	.1086	.1172	.1261	.1353	.1447	.1543	.1641
6	.0196	.0223	.0252	.0284	.0320	.0358	.0400	.0445	.0494	.0547
7	.0019	.0023	.0027	.0032	.0037	.0044	.0051	.0059	.0068	.0078

	.01	.02	.03	.04	.05	.06	.07	.08	.09	.10
					n = 8					
0	.9227	.8508	.7837	.7214	.6634	.6096	.5596	.5132	.4703	.4305
1	.0746	.1389	.1939	.2405	.2793	.3113	.3370	.3570	.3721	.3826
2	.0026	.0099	.0210	.0351	.0515	.0695	.0888	.1087	.1288	.1488
3	.0001	.0004	.0013	.0029	.0054	.0089	.0134	.0189	.0255	.0331
4	.0000	.0000	.0001	.0002	.0004	.0007	.0013	.0021	.0031	.0046
5	.0000	.0000	.0000	.0000	.0000	.0000	0001	.0001	.0002	.0004
	.11	.12	.13	.14	.15	.16	.17	.18	.19	.20
0	.3937	.3596	.3282	.2992	.2725	.2479	.2252	.2044	.1853	1678
1	.3892	.3923	.3923	.3897	.3847	.3777	.3691	.3590	.3477	.3355

(Continued)

Appendix

641

TABLE A.7   (Continued)

r \ p	.11	.12	.13	.14	n=8 .15	.16	.17	.18	.19	.20
2	.1684	.1872	.2052	.2220	.2376	.2518	.2646	.2758	.2855	.2936
3	.0416	.0511	.0613	.0723	.0839	.0959	.1084	.1211	.1339	.1468
4	.0064	.0087	.0115	.0147	.0185	.0228	.0277	.0332	.0393	.0459
5	.0006	.0009	.0014	.0019	.0026	.0035	.0045	.0058	.0074	.0092
6	.0000	.0001	.0001	.0002	.0002	.0003	.0005	.0006	.0009	.0011
7	.0000	.0000	.0000	.0000	.0000	.0000	.0000	.0000	.0001	.0001
	.21	.22	.23	.24	.25	.26	.27	.28	.29	.30
0	.1517	.1370	.1236	.1113	.1001	.0899	.0806	.0722	.0646	.0576
1	.3226	.3092	.2953	.2812	.2670	.2527	.2386	.2247	.2110	.1977
2	.3002	.3052	.3087	.3108	.3115	.3108	.3089	.3058	.3017	.2965
3	.1596	.1722	.1844	.1963	.2076	.2184	.2285	.2379	.2464	.2541
4	.0530	.0607	.0689	.0775	.0865	.0959	.1056	.1156	.1258	.1361
5	.0113	.0137	.0165	.0196	.0231	.0270	.0313	.0360	.0411	.0467
6	.0015	.0019	.0025	.0031	.0038	.0047	.0058	.0070	.0084	.0100
7	.0001	.0002	.0002	.0003	.0004	.0005	.0006	.0008	.0010	.0012
8	.0000	.0000	.0000	.0000	.0000	.0000	.0000	.0000	.0001	.0001
	.31	.32	.33	.34	.35	.36	.37	.38	.39	.40
0	.0514	.0457	.0406	.0360	.0319	.0281	.0248	.0218	.0192	.0168
1	.1847	.1721	.1600	.1484	.1373	.1267	.1166	.1071	.0981	.0896
2	.2904	.2835	.2758	.2675	.2587	.2494	.2397	.2297	.2194	.2090
3	.2609	.2668	.2717	.2756	.2786	.2805	.2815	.2815	.2806	.2787
4	.1465	.1569	.1673	.1775	.1875	.1973	.2067	.2157	.2242	.2322
5	.0527	.0591	.0659	.0732	.0808	.0888	.0971	.1058	.1147	.1239
6	.0118	.0139	.0162	.0188	.0217	.0250	.0285	.0324	.0367	.0413
7	.0015	.0019	.0023	.0028	.0033	.0040	.0048	.0057	.0067	.0079
8	.0001	.0001	.0001	.0002	.0002	.0003	.0004	.0004	.0005	.0007
	.41	.42	.43	.44	.45	.46	.47	.48	.49	.50
0	.0147	.0128	.0111	.0097	.0084	.0072	.0062	.0053	.0046	.0039
1	.0816	.0742	.0672	.0608	.0548	.0493	.0442	.0395	.0352	.0312
2	.1985	.1880	.1776	.1672	.1569	.1469	.1371	.1275	.1183	.1094
3	.2759	.2723	.2679	.2627	.2568	.2503	.2431	.2355	.2273	.2188
4	.2397	.2465	.2526	.2580	.2627	.2665	.2695	.2717	.2730	.2734
5	.1332	.1428	.1525	.1622	.1719	.1816	.1912	.2006	.2098	.2188
6	.0463	.0517	.0575	.0637	.0703	.0774	.0848	.0926	.1008	.1094
7	.0092	.0107	.0124	.0143	.0164	.0188	.0215	.0244	.0277	.0312
8	.0008	.0010	.0012	.0014	.0017	.0020	.0024	.0028	.0033	.0039

(Continued)

TABLE A.7   (Continued)

					n=9					
r\p	.01	.02	.03	.04	.05	.06	.07	.08	.09	.10
0	.9135	.8337	.7602	.6925	.6302	.5730	.5204	.4722	.4279	.3874
1	.0830	.1531	.2116	.2597	.2985	.3292	.3525	.3695	.3809	.3874
2	.0034	.0125	.0262	.0433	.0629	.0840	.1061	.1285	.1507	.1722
3	.0001	.0006	.0019	.0042	.0077	.0125	.0186	.0261	.0348	.0446
4	.0000	.0000	.0001	.0003	.0006	.0012	.0021	.0034	.0052	.0074
5	.0000	.0000	.0000	.0000	.0000	.0001	.0002	.0003	.0005	.0008
6	.0000	.0000	.0000	.0000	.0000	.0000	.0000	.0000	.0000	.0001
	.11	.12	.13	.14	.15	.16	.17	.18	.19	.20
0	.3504	.3165	.2855	.2573	.2316	.2082	.1869	.1676	.1501	.1342
1	.3897	.3884	.3840	.3770	.3679	.3569	.3446	.3312	.3169	.3020
2	.1927	.2119	.2295	.2455	.2597	.2720	.2823	.2908	.2973	.3020
3	.0556	.0674	.0800	.0933	.1069	.1209	.1349	.1489	.1627	.1762
4	.0103	.0138	.0179	.0228	.0283	.0345	.0415	.0490	.0573	.0661
5	.0013	.0019	.0027	.0037	.0050	.0066	.0085	.0108	.0134	.0165
6	.0001	.0002	.0003	.0004	.0006	.0008	.0012	.0016	.0021	.0028
7	.0000	.0000	.0000	.0000	.0000	.0001	.0001	.0001	.0002	.0003
	.21	.22	.23	.24	.25	.26	.27	.28	.29	.30
0	.1199	.1069	.0952	.0846	.0751	.0665	.0589	.0520	.0458	.0404
1	.2867	.2713	.2558	.2404	.2253	.2104	.1960	.1820	.1685	.1556
2	.3049	.3061	.3056	.3037	.3003	.2957	.2899	.2831	.2754	.2668
3	.1891	.2014	.2130	.2238	.2336	.2424	.2502	.2569	.2624	.2668
4	.0754	.0852	.0954	.1060	.1168	.1278	.1388	.1499	.1608	.1715
5	.0200	.0240	.0285	.0335	.0389	.0449	.0513	.0583	.0657	.0735
6	.0036	.0045	.0057	.0070	.0087	.0105	.0127	.0151	.0179	.0210
7	.0004	.0005	.0007	.0010	.0012	.0016	.0020	.0025	.0031	.0039
8	.0000	.0000	.0001	.0001	.0001	.0001	.0002	.0002	.0003	.0004
	.31	.32	.33	.34	.35	.36	.37	.38	.39	.40
0	.0355	.0311	.0272	.0238	.0207	.0180	.0156	.0135	.0117	.0101
1	.1433	.1317	.1206	.1102	.1004	.0912	.0826	.0747	.0673	.0605
2	.2576	.2478	.2376	.2270	.2162	.2052	.1941	.1831	.1721	.1612
3	.2701	.2721	.2731	.2729	.2716	.2693	.2660	.2618	.2567	.2508
4	.1820	.1921	.2017	.2109	.2194	.2272	.2344	.2407	.2462	.2508
5	.0818	.0904	.0994	.1086	.1181	.1278	.1376	.1475	.1574	.1672
6	.0245	.0284	.0326	.0373	.0424	.0479	.0539	.0603	.0671	.0743
7	.0047	.0057	.0069	.0082	.0098	.0116	.0136	.0158	.0184	.0212
8	.0005	.0007	.0008	.0011	.0013	.0016	.0020	.0024	.0029	.0035
9	.0000	.0000	.0000	.0001	.0001	.0001	.0001	.0002	.0002	.0003

(Continued)

TABLE A.7 (Continued)

n=9

r \ p	.41	.42	.43	.44	.45	.46	.47	.48	.49	.50
0	.0087	.0074	.0064	.0054	.0046	.0039	.0033	.0028	.0023	.0020
1	.0542	.0484	.0431	.0383	.0339	.0299	.0263	.0231	.0202	.0176
2	.1506	.1402	.1301	.1204	.1110	.1020	.0934	.0853	.0776	.0703
3	.2442	.2369	.2291	.2207	.2119	.2027	.1933	.1837	.1739	.1641
4	.2545	.2573	.2592	.2601	.2600	.2590	.2571	.2543	.2506	.2461
5	.1769	.1863	.1955	.2044	.2128	.2207	.2280	.2347	.2408	.2461
6	.0819	.0900	.0983	.1070	.1160	.1253	.1348	.1445	.1542	.1641
7	.0244	.0279	.0318	.0360	.0407	.0458	.0512	.0571	.0635	.0703
8	.0042	.0051	.0060	.0071	.0083	.0097	.0114	.0132	.0153	.0176
9	.0003	.0004	.0005	.0006	.0008	.0009	.0011	.0014	.0016	.0020

n = 10

	.01	.02	.03	.04	.05	.06	.07	.08	.09	.10
0	.9044	.8171	.7374	.6648	.5987	.5386	.4840	.4344	.3894	.3487
1	.0914	.1667	.2281	.2770	.3151	.3438	.3643	.3777	.3851	.3874
2	.0042	.0153	.0317	.0519	.0746	.0988	.1234	.1478	.1714	.1937
3	.0001	.0008	.0026	.0058	.0105	.0168	.0248	.0343	.0452	.0574
4	.0000	.0000	.0001	.0004	.0010	.0019	.0033	.0052	.0078	.0112
5	.0000	.0000	.0000	.0000	.0001	.0001	.0003	.0005	.0009	.0015
6	.0000	.0000	.0000	.0000	.0000	.0000	.0000	.0000	.0001	.0001
	.11	.12	.13	.14	.15	.16	.17	.18	.19	.20
0	.3118	.2785	.2484	.2213	.1969	.1749	.1552	.1374	.1216	.1074
1	.3854	.3798	.3712	.3603	.3474	.3331	.3178	.3017	.2852	.2684
2	.2143	.2330	.2496	.2639	.2759	.2856	.2929	.2980	.3010	.3020
3	.0706	.0847	.0995	.1146	.1298	.1450	.1600	.1745	.1883	.2013
4	.0153	.0202	.0260	.0326	.0401	.0483	.0573	.0670	.0773	.0881
5	.0023	.0033	.0047	.0064	.0085	.0111	.0141	.0177	.0218	.0264
6	.0002	.0004	.0006	.0009	.0012	.0018	.0024	.0032	.0043	.0055
7	.0000	.0000	.0000	.0001	.0001	.0002	.0003	.0004	.0006	.0008
8	.0000	.0000	.0000	.0000	.0000	.0000	.0000	.0000	.0001	.0001
	.21	.22	.23	.24	.25	.26	.27	.28	.29	.30
0	.0947	.0834	.0733	.0643	.0563	.0492	.0430	.0374	.0326	.0282
1	.2517	.2351	.2188	.2030	.1877	.1730	.1590	.1456	.1330	.1211
2	.3011	.2984	.2942	.2885	.2816	.2735	.2646	.2548	.2444	.2335
3	.2134	.2244	.2343	.2429	.2503	.2563	.2609	.2642	.2662	.2668
4	.0993	.1108	.1225	.1343	.1460	.1576	.1689	.1798	.1903	.2001
5	.0317	.0375	.0439	.0509	.0584	.0664	.0750	.0839	.0933	.1029

(Continued)

TABLE A.7   (Continued)

					n=10					
r \ p	.21	.22	.23	.24	.25	.26	.27	.28	.29	.30
6	.0070	.0088	.0109	.0134	.0162	.0195	.0231	.0272	.0317	.0368
7	.0011	.0014	.0019	.0024	.0031	.0039	.0049	.0060	.0074	.0090
8	.0001	.0002	.0002	.0003	.0004	.0005	.0007	.0009	.0011	.0014
9	.0000	.0000	.0000	.0000	.0000	.0000	.0001	.0001	.0001	.0001
	.31	.32	.33	.34	.35	.36	.37	.38	.39	.40
0	.0245	.0211	.0182	.0157	.0135	.0115	.0098	.0084	.0071	.0060
1	.1099	.0995	.0898	.0808	.0725	.0649	.0578	.0514	.0456	.0403
2	.2222	.2107	.1990	.0873	.1757	.1642	.1529	.1419	.1312	.1209
3	.2662	.2644	.2614	.2573	.2522	.2462	.2394	.2319	.2237	.2150
4	.2093	.2177	.2253	.2320	.2377	.2424	.2461	.2487	.2503	.2508
5	.1128	.1229	.1332	.1434	.1536	.1636	.1734	.1829	.1920	.2007
6	.0422	.0482	.0547	.0616	.0689	.0767	.0849	.0934	.1023	.1115
7	.0108	.0130	.0154	.0181	.0212	.0247	.0285	.0327	.0374	.0425
8	.0018	.0023	.0028	.0035	.0043	.0052	.0063	.0075	.0090	.0106
9	.0002	.0002	.0003	.0004	.0005	.0006	.0008	.0010	.0013	.0016
10	.0000	.0000	.0000	.0000	.0000	.0000	.0000	.0001	.0001	.0001
	.41	.42	.43	.44	.45	.46	.47	.48	.49	.50
0	.0051	.0043	.0036	.0030	.0025	.0021	.0017	.0014	.0012	.0010
1	.0355	.0312	.0273	.0238	.0207	.0180	.0155	.0133	.0114	.0098
2	.1111	.1017	.0927	.0843	.0763	.0688	.0619	.0554	.0494	.0439
3	.2058	.1963	.1865	.1765	.1665	.1564	.1464	.1364	.1267	.1172
4	.2503	.2488	.2462	.2427	.2384	.2331	.2271	.2204	.2130	.2051
5	.2087	.2162	.2229	.2289	.2340	.2383	.2417	.2441	.2456	.2461
6	.1209	.1304	.1401	.1499	.1596	.1692	.1786	.1878	.1966	.2051
7	.0480	.0540	.0604	.0673	.0746	.0824	.0905	.0991	.1080	.1172
8	.0125	.0147	.0171	.0198	.0229	.0263	.0301	.0343	.0389	.0439
9	.0019	.0024	.0029	.0035	.0042	.0050	.0059	.0070	.0083	.0098
10	.0001	.0002	.0002	.0003	.0003	.0004	.0005	.0006	.0008	.0010

					n = 11					
	.01	.02	.03	.04	.05	.06	.07	.08	.09	.10
0	.8953	.8007	.7153	.6382	.5688	.5063	.4501	.3996	.3544	.3138
1	.0995	.1798	.2433	.2925	.3293	.3555	.3727	.3823	.3855	.3835
2	.0050	.0183	.0376	.0609	.0867	.1135	.1403	.1662	.1906	.2131
3	.0002	.0011	.0035	.0076	.0137	.0217	.0317	.0434	.0566	.0710
4	.0000	.0000	.0002	.0006	.0014	.0028	.0048	.0075	.0112	.0158
5	.0000	.0000	.0000	.0000	.0001	.0002	.0005	.0009	.0015	.0025
6	.0000	.0000	.0000	.0000	.0000	.0000	.0000	.0001	.0002	.0003

(Continued)

TABLE A.7 (Continued)

r \ p	.11	.12	.13	.14	.15	.16	.17	.18	.19	.20
					n=11					
0	.2775	.2451	.2161	.1903	.1673	.1469	.1288	.1127	.0985	.0859
1	.3773	.3676	.3552	.3408	.3248	.3078	.2901	.2721	.2541	.2362
2	.2332	.2507	.2654	.2774	.2866	.2932	.2971	.2987	.2980	.2953
3	.0865	.1025	.1190	.1355	.1517	.1675	.1826	.1967	.2097	.2215
4	.0214	.0280	.0356	.0441	.0536	.0638	.0748	.0864	.0984	.1107
5	.0037	.0053	.0074	.0101	.0132	.0170	.0214	.0265	.0323	.0388
6	.0005	.0007	.0011	.0016	.0023	.0032	.0044	.0058	.0076	.0097
7	.0000	.0001	.0001	.0002	.0003	.0004	.0006	.0009	.0013	.0017
8	.0000	.0000	.0000	.0000	.0000	.0000	.0001	.0001	.0001	.0002
	.21	.22	.23	.24	.25	.26	.27	.28	.29	.30
0	.0748	.0650	.0564	.0489	.0422	.0364	.0314	.0270	.0231	.0198
1	.2187	.2017	.1854	.1697	.1549	.1408	.1276	.1153	.1038	.0932
2	.2907	.2845	.2768	.2680	.2581	.2474	.2360	.2242	.2121	.1998
3	.2318	.2407	.2481	.2539	.2581	.2608	.2619	.2616	.2599	.2568
4	.1232	.1358	.1482	.1603	.1721	.1832	.1937	.2035	.2123	.2201
5	.0459	.0536	.0620	.0709	.0803	.0901	.1003	.1108	.1214	.1321
6	.0122	.0151	.0185	.0224	.0268	.0317	.0371	.0431	.0496	.0566
7	.0023	.0030	.0039	.0050	.0064	.0079	.0098	.0120	.0145	.0173
8	.0003	.0004	.0006	.0008	.0011	.0014	.0018	.0023	.0030	.0037
9	.0000	.0000	.0001	.0001	.0001	.0002	.0002	.0003	.0004	.0005
	.31	.32	.33	.34	.35	.36	.37	.38	.39	.40
0	.0169	.0144	.0122	.0104	.0088	.0074	.0062	.0052	.0044	.0036
1	.0834	.0744	.0662	.0587	.0518	.0457	.0401	.0351	.0306	.0266
2	.1874	.1751	.1630	.1511	.1395	.1284	.1177	.1075	.0978	.0887
3	.2526	.2472	.2408	.2335	.2254	.2167	.2074	.1977	.1876	.1774
4	.2269	.2326	.2372	.2406	.2428	.2438	.2436	.2423	.2399	.2365
5	.1427	.1533	.1636	.1735	.1830	.1920	.2003	.2079	.2148	.2207
6	.0641	.0721	.0806	.0894	.0985	.1080	.1176	.1274	.1373	.1471
7	.0206	.0242	.0283	.0329	.0379	.0434	.0494	.0558	.0627	.0701
8	.0046	.0057	.0070	.0085	.0102	.0122	.0145	.0171	.0200	.0234
9	.0007	.0009	.0011	.0015	.0018	.0023	.0028	.0035	.0043	.0052
10	.0001	.0001	.0001	.0001	.0002	.0003	.0003	.0004	.0005	.0007
	.41	.42	.43	.44	.45	.46	.47	.48	.49	.50
0	.0030	.0025	.0021	.0017	.0014	.0011	.0009	.0008	.0006	.0005
1	.0231	.0199	.0171	.0147	.0125	.0107	.0090	.0076	.0064	.0054
2	.0801	.0721	.0646	.0577	.0513	.0454	.0401	.0352	.0308	.0269
3	.1670	.1566	.1462	.1359	.1259	.1161	.1067	.0976	.0888	.0806
4	.2321	.2267	.2206	.2136	.2060	.1978	.1892	.1801	.1707	.1611

(Continued)

TABLE A.7 (Continued)

					n=11					
r\p	.41	.42	.43	.44	.45	.46	.47	.48	.49	.50
5	.2258	.2299	.2329	.2350	.2360	.2359	.2348	.2327	.2296	.2256
6	.1569	.1664	.1757	.1846	.1931	.2010	.2083	.2148	.2206	.2256
7	.0779	.0861	.0947	.1036	.1128	.1223	.1319	.1416	.1514	.1611
8	.0271	.0312	.0357	.0407	.0462	.0521	.0585	.0654	.0727	.0806
9	.0063	.0075	.0090	.0107	.0126	.0148	.0173	.0201	.0233	.0269
10	.0009	.0011	.0014	.0017	.0021	.0025	.0031	.0037	.0045	.0054
11	.0001	.0001	.0001	.0001	.0002	.0002	.0002	.0003	.0004	.0005

					n = 12					
	.01	.02	.03	.04	.05	.06	.07	.08	.09	.10
0	.8864	.7847	.6938	.6127	.5404	.4759	.4186	.3677	.3225	.2824
1	.1074	.1922	.2575	.3064	.3413	.3645	.3781	.3837	.3827	.3766
2	.0060	.0216	.0438	.0702	.0988	.1280	.1565	.1835	.2082	.2301
3	.0002	.0015	.0045	.0098	.0173	.0272	.0393	.0532	.0686	.0852
4	.0000	.0001	.0003	.0009	.0021	.0039	.0067	.0104	.0153	.0213
5	.0000	.0000	.0000	.0001	.0002	.0004	.0008	.0014	.0024	.0038
6	.0000	.0000	.0000	.0000	.0000	.0000	.0001	.0001	.0003	.0005
	.11	.12	.13	.14	.15	.16	.17	.18	.19	.20
0	.2470	.2157	.1880	.1637	.1422	.1234	.1069	.0924	.0798	.0687
1	.3663	.3529	.3372	.3197	.3012	.2821	.2627	.2434	.2245	.2062
2	.2490	.2647	.2771	.2863	.2924	.2955	.2960	.2939	.2897	.2835
3	.1026	.1203	.1380	.1553	.1720	.1876	.2021	.2151	.2265	.2362
4	.0285	.0369	.0464	.0569	.0683	.0804	.0931	.1062	.1195	.1329
5	.0056	.0081	.0111	.0148	.0193	.0245	.0305	.0373	.0449	.0532
6	.0008	.0013	.0019	.0028	.0040	.0054	.0073	.0096	.0123	.0155
7	.0001	.0001	.0002	.0004	.0006	.0009	.0013	.0018	.0025	.0033
8	.0000	.0000	.0000	.0000	.0001	.0001	.0002	.0002	.0004	.0005
9	.0000	.0000	.0000	.0000	.0000	.0000	.0000	.0000	.0000	.0001
	.21	.22	.23	.24	.25	.26	.27	.28	.29	.30
0	.0591	.0507	.0434	.0371	.0317	.0270	.0229	.0194	.0164	.0138
1	.1885	.1717	.1557	.1407	.1267	.1137	.1016	.0906	.0804	.0712
2	.2756	.2663	.2558	.2444	.2323	.2197	.2068	.1937	.1807	.1678
3	.2442	.2503	.2547	.2573	.2581	.2573	.2549	.2511	.2460	.2397
4	.1460	.1589	.1712	.1828	.1936	.2034	.2122	.2197	.2261	.2311
5	.0621	.0717	.0818	.0924	.1032	.1143	.1255	.1367	.1477	.1585
6	.0193	.0236	.0285	.0340	.0401	.0469	.0542	.0620	.0704	.0792
7	.0044	.0057	.0073	.0092	.0115	.0141	.0172	.0207	.0246	.0291

(Continued)

TABLE A.7 (Continued)

n=12

r \ p	.21	.22	.23	.24	.25	.26	.27	.28	.29	.30
8	.0007	.0010	.0014	.0018	.0024	.0031	.0040	.0050	.0063	.0078
9	.0001	.0001	.0002	.0003	.0004	.0005	.0007	.0009	.0011	.0015
10	.0000	.0000	.0000	.0000	.0000	.0001	.0001	.0001	.0001	.0002
	.31	.32	.33	.34	.35	.36	.37	.38	.39	.40
0	.0016	.0098	.0082	.0068	.0057	.0047	.0039	.0032	.0027	.0022
1	.0628	.0552	.0484	.0422	.0368	.0319	.0276	.0237	.0204	.0174
2	.1552	.1429	.1310	.1197	.1088	.0986	.0890	.0800	.0716	.0639
3	.2324	.2241	.2151	.2055	.1954	.1849	.1742	.1634	.1526	.1419
4	.2349	.2373	.2384	.2382	.2367	.2340	.2302	.2254	.2195	.2128
5	.1688	.1787	.1879	.1963	.2039	.2106	.2163	.2210	.2246	.2270
6	.0885	.0981	.1079	.1180	.1281	.1382	.1482	.1580	.1675	.1766
7	.0341	.0396	.0456	.0521	.0591	.0666	.0746	.0830	.0918	.1009
8	.0096	.0116	.0140	.0168	.0199	.0234	.0274	.0318	.0367	.0420
9	.0019	.0024	.0031	.0038	.0048	.0059	.0071	.0087	.0104	.0125
10	.0003	.0003	.0005	.0006	.0008	.0010	.0013	.0016	.0020	.0025
11	.0000	.0000	.0000	.0001	.0001	.0001	.0001	.0002	.0002	.0003
	.41	.42	.43	.44	.45	.46	.47	.48	.49	.50
0	.0018	.0014	.0012	.0010	.0008	.0006	.0005	.0004	.0003	.0002
1	.0148	.0126	.0106	.0090	.0075	.0063	.0052	.0043	.0036	.0029
2	.0567	.0502	.0442	.0388	.0339	.0294	.0255	.0220	.0189	.0161
3	.1314	.1211	.1111	.1015	.0923	.0836	.0754	.0676	.0604	.0537
4	.2054	.1973	.1886	.1794	.1700	.1602	.1504	.1405	.1306	.1208
5	.2284	.2285	.2276	.2256	.2225	.2184	.2134	.2075	.2008	.1934
6	.1851	.1931	.2003	.2068	.2124	.2171	.2208	.2234	.2250	.2256
7	.1103	.1198	.1295	.1393	.1498	.1585	.1678	.1768	.1853	.1934
8	.0479	.0542	.0611	.0684	.0762	.0844	.0930	.1020	.1113	.1208
9	.0148	.0175	.0205	.0239	.0277	.0319	.0367	.0418	.0475	.0537
10	.0031	.0038	.0046	.0056	.0068	.0082	.0098	.0116	.0137	.0161
11	.0004	.0005	.0006	.0008	.0010	.0013	.0016	.0019	.0024	.0029
12	.0000	.0000	.0000	.0001	.0001	.0001	.0001	.0001	.0002	.0002

n = 13

r	.01	.02	.03	.04	.05	.06	.07	.08	.09	.10
0	.8775	.7690	.6730	.5882	.5133	.4474	.3893	.3383	.2935	.2542
1	.1152	.2040	.2706	.3186	.3512	.3712	.3809	.3824	.3773	.3672
2	.0070	.0250	.0502	.0797	.1109	.1422	.1720	.1995	.2239	.2448
3	.0003	.0019	.0057	.0122	.0214	.0333	.0475	.0636	.0812	.0997
4	.0000	.0001	.0004	.0013	.0028	.0053	.0089	.0138	.0201	.0277
5	.0000	.0000	.0000	.0001	.0003	.0006	.0012	.0022	.0036	.0055
6	.0000	.0000	.0000	.0000	.0000	.0001	.0001	.0003	.0005	.0008
7	.0000	.0000	.0000	.0000	.0000	.0000	.0000	.0000	.0000	.0001

TABLE A.7   (Continued)

					n=12					
r \ p	.11	.12	.13	.14	.15	.16	.17	.18	.19	.20
0	.2198	.1898	.1636	.1408	.1209	.1037	.0887	.0758	.0646	.0550
1	.3532	.3364	.3178	.2979	.2774	.2567	.2362	.2163	.1970	.1787
2	.2619	.2753	.2849	.2910	.2937	.2934	.2903	.2848	.2773	.2680
3	.1187	.1376	.1561	.1737	.1900	.2049	.2180	.2293	.2385	.2457
4	.0367	.0469	.0583	.0707	.0838	.0976	.1116	.1258	.1399	.1535
5	.0082	.0115	.0157	.0207	.0266	.0335	.0412	.0497	.0591	.0691
6	.0013	.0021	.0031	.0045	.0063	.0085	.0112	.0145	.0185	.0230
7	.0002	.0003	.0005	.0007	.0011	.0016	.0023	.0032	.0043	.0058
8	.0000	.0000	.0001	.0001	.0001	.0002	.0004	.0005	.0008	.0011
9	.0000	.0000	.0000	.0000	.0000	.0000	.0000	.0001	.0001	.0001
	.21	.22	.23	.24	.25	.26	.27	.28	.29	.30
0	.0467	.0396	.0334	.0282	.0238	.0200	.0167	.0140	.0117	.0097
1	.1613	.1450	.1299	.1159	.1029	.0911	.0804	.0706	.0619	.0540
2	.2573	.2455	.2328	.2195	.2059	.1921	.1784	.1648	.1516	.1388
3	.2508	.2539	.2550	.2542	.2517	.2475	.2419	.2351	.2271	.2181
4	.1667	.1790	.1904	.2007	.2097	.2174	.2237	.2285	.2319	.2337
5	.0797	.0909	.1024	.1141	.1258	.1375	.1489	.1600	.1705	.1803
6	.0283	.0342	.0408	.0480	.0559	.0644	.0734	.0829	.0928	.1030
7	.0075	.0096	.0122	.0152	.0186	.0226	.0272	.0323	.0379	.0442
8	.0015	.0020	.0027	.0036	.0047	.0060	.0075	.0094	.0116	.0142
9	.0002	.0003	.0005	.0006	.0009	.0012	.0015	.0020	.0026	.0034
10	.0000	.0000	.0001	.0001	.0001	.0002	.0002	.0003	.0004	.0006
11	.0000	.0000	.0000	.0000	.0000	.0000	.0000	.0000	.0000	.0001
	.31	.32	.33	.34	.35	.36	.37	.38	.39	.40
0.	.0080	.0066	.0055	.0045	.0037	.0030	.0025	.0020	.0016	.0013
1	.0469	.0407	.0351	.0302	.0259	.0221	.0188	.0159	.0135	.0113
2	.1265	.1148	.1037	.0933	.0836	.0746	.0663	.0586	.0516	.0453
3	.2084	.1981	.1874	.1763	.1651	.1538	.1427	.1317	.1210	.1107
4	.2341	.2331	.2307	.2270	.2222	.2163	.2095	.2018	.1934	.1845
5	.1893	.1974	.2045	.2105	.2154	.2190	.2215	.2227	.2226	.2214
6	.1134	.1239	.1343	.1446	.1546	.1643	.1734	.1820	.1898	.1968
7	.0509	.0583	.0662	.0745	.0833	.0924	.1019	.1115	.1213	.1312
8	.0172	.0206	.0244	.0288	.0336	.0390	.0449	.0513	.0582	.0656
9	.0043	.0054	.0067	.0082	.0101	.0122	.0146	.0175	.0207	.0243
10	.0008	.0010	.0013	.0017	.0022	.0027	.0034	.0043	.0053	.0065
11	.0001	.0001	.0002	.0002	.0003	.0004	.0006	.0007	.0009	.0012
12	.0000	.0000	.0000	.0000	.0000	.0000	.0001	.0001	.0001	.0001

(Continued)

TABLE A.7 (Continued)

n=13

r\p	.41	.42	.43	.44	.45	.46	.47	.48	.49	.50
0	.0010	.0008	.0007	.0005	.0004	.0003	.0003	.0002	.0002	.0001
1	.0095	.0079	.0066	.0054	.0045	.0037	.0030	.0024	.0020	.0016
2	.0395	.0344	.0298	.0256	.0220	.0188	.0160	.0135	.0114	.0095
3	.1007	.0913	.0823	.0739	.0660	.0587	.0519	.0457	.0401	.0349
4	.1750	.1653	.1553	.1451	.1350	.1250	.1151	.1055	.0962	.0873
5	.2189	.2154	.2108	.2053	.1989	.1917	.1838	.1753	.1664	.1571
6	.2029	.2080	.2121	.2151	.2169	.2177	.2173	.2158	.2131	.2095
7	.1410	.1506	.1600	.1690	.1775	.1854	.1927	.1992	.2048	.2095
8	.0735	.0818	.0905	.0996	.1089	.1185	.1282	.1379	.1476	.1571
9	.0284	.0329	.0379	.0435	.0495	.0561	.0631	.0707	.0788	.0873
10	.0079	.0095	.0114	.0137	.0162	.0191	.0224	.0261	.0303	.0349
11	.0015	.0019	.0024	.0029	.0036	.0044	.0054	.0066	.0079	.0095
12	.0002	.0002	.0003	.0004	.0005	.0006	.0008	.0010	.0013	.0016
13	.0000	.0000	.0000	.0000	.0000	.0000	.0001	.0001	.0001	.0001

n = 14

	.01	.02	.03	.04	.05	.06	.07	.08	.09	.10
0	.8687	.7536	.6528	.5647	.4877	.4205	.3620	.3112	.2670	.2288
1	.1229	.2153	.2827	.3294	.3593	.3758	.3815	.3788	.3698	.3559
2	.0081	.0286	.0568	.0892	.1229	.1559	.1867	.2141	.2377	.2570
3	.0003	.0023	.0070	.0149	.0259	.0398	.0562	.0745	.0940	.1142
4	.0000	.0001	.0006	.0017	.0037	.0070	.0116	.0178	.0256	.0349
5	.0000	.0000	.0000	.0001	.0004	.0009	.0018	.0031	.0051	.0078
6	.0000	.0000	.0000	.0000	.0000	.0001	.0002	.0004	.0008	.0013
7	.0000	.0000	.0000	.0000	.0000	.0000	.0000	.0000	.0001	.0002

	.11	.12	.13	.14	.15	.16	.17	.18	.19	.20
0	.1956	.1670	.1423	.1211	.1028	.0871	.0736	.0621	.0523	.0440
1	.3385	.3188	.2977	.2759	.2539	.2322	.2112	.1910	.1719	.1539
2	.2720	.2826	.2892	.2919	.2912	.2875	.2811	.2725	.2620	.2501
3	.1345	.1542	.1728	.1901	.2056	.2190	.2303	.2393	.2459	.2501
4	.0457	.0578	.0710	.0851	.0998	.1147	.1297	.1444	.1586	.1720
5	.0113	.0158	.0212	.0277	.0352	.0437	.0531	.0634	.0744	.0860
6	.0021	.0032	.0048	.0068	.0093	.0125	.0163	.0209	.0262	.0322
7	.003	.0005	.0008	.0013	.0019	.0027	.0038	.0052	.0070	.0092
8	.0000	.0001	.0001	.0002	.0003	.0005	.0007	.0010	.0014	.0020
9	.0000	.0000	.0000	.0000	.0000	.0001	.0001	.0001	.0002	.0003

(Continued)

TABLE A.7 (Continued)

					n=14					
r\p	.21	.22	.23	.24	.25	.26	.27	.28	.29	.30
0	.0369	.0309	.0258	.0214	.0178	.0148	.0122	.0101	.0083	.0068
1	.1372	.1218	.1077	.0948	.0832	.0726	.0632	.0548	.0473	.0407
2	.2371	.2234	.2091	.1946	.1802	.1659	.1519	.1385	.1256	.1134
3	.2521	.2520	.2499	.2459	.2402	.2331	.2248	.2154	.2052	.1943
4	.1843	.1955	.2052	.2135	.2202	.2252	.2286	.2304	.2305	.2290
5	.0980	.1103	.1226	.1348	.1468	.1583	.1691	.1792	.1883	.1963
6	.0391	.0466	.0549	.0639	.0734	.0834	.0938	.1045	.1153	.1262
7	.0119	.0150	.0188	.0231	.0280	.0335	.0397	.0464	.0538	.0618
8	.0028	.0037	.0049	.0064	.0082	.0103	.0128	.0158	.0192	.0232
9	.0005	.0007	.0010	.0013	.0018	.0024	.0032	.0041	.0052	.0066
10	.0001	.0001	.0001	.0002	.0003	.0004	.0006	.0008	.0011	.0014
11	.0000	.0000	.0000	.0000	.0000	.0001	.0001	.0001	.0002	.0002
	.31	.32	.33	.34	.35	.36	.37	.38	.39	.40
0	.0055	.0045	.0037	.0030	.0024	.0019	.0016	.0012	.0010	.0008
1	.0349	.0298	.0253	.0215	.0181	.0152	.0128	.0106	.0088	.0073
2	.1018	.0911	.0811	.0719	.0634	.0557	.0487	.0424	.0367	.0317
3	.1830	.1715	.1598	.1481	.1366	.1253	.1144	.1039	.0940	.0845
4	.2261	.2219	.2164	.2098	.2022	.1938	.1848	.1752	.1652	.1549
5	.2032	.2088	.2132	.2161	.2178	.2181	.2170	.2147	.2112	.2066
6	.1369	.1474	.1575	.1670	.1759	.1840	.1912	.1974	.2026	.2066
7	.0703	.0793	.0886	.0983	.1082	.1183	.1283	.1383	.1480	.1574
8	.0276	.0326	.0382	.0443	.0510	.0582	.0659	.0742	.0828	.0918
9	.0083	.0102	.0125	.0152	.0183	.0218	.0258	.0303	.0353	.0408
10	.0019	.0024	.0031	.0039	.0049	.0061	.0076	.0093	.0113	.0136
11	.0003	.0004	.0006	.0007	.0010	.0013	.0016	.0021	.0026	.0033
12	.0000	.0000	.0001	.0001	.0001	.0002	.0002	.0003	.0004	.0005
13	.0000	.0000	.0000	.0000	.0000	.0000	.0000	.0000	.0000	.0001
	.41	.42	.43	.44	.45	.46	.47	.48	.49	.50
0	.0006	.0005	.0004	.0003	.0002	.0002	.0001	.0001	.0001	.0001
1	.0060	.0049	.0040	.0033	.0027	.0021	.0017	.0014	.0011	.0009
2	.0272	.0233	.0198	.0168	.0141	.0118	.0099	.0082	.0068	.0056
3	.0757	.0674	.0597	.0527	.0462	.0403	.0350	.0303	.0260	.0222
4	.1446	.1342	.1239	.1138	.1040	.0945	.0854	.0768	.0687	.0611
5	.2009	.1943	.1869	.1788	.1701	.1610	.1515	.1418	.1320	.1222
6	.2094	.2111	.2115	.2108	.2088	.2057	.2015	.1963	.1902	.1833
7	.1663	.1747	.1824	.1892	.1952	.2003	.2043	.2071	.2089	.2095
8	.1011	.1107	.1204	.1301	.1398	.1493	.1585	.1673	.1756	.1833
9	.0469	.0534	.0605	.0682	.0762	.0848	.0937	.1030	.1125	.1222
10	.0163	.0193	.0228	.0268	.0312	.0361	.0415	.0475	.0540	.0611

(Continued)

TABLE A.7 (Continued)

n=14

r \ p	.41	.42	.43	.44	.45	.46	.47	.48	.49	.50
11	.0041	.0051	.0063	.0076	.0093	.0112	.0134	.0160	.0189	.0222
12	.0007	.0009	.0012	.0015	.0019	.0024	.0030	.0037	.0045	.0056
13	.0001	.0001	.0001	.0002	.0002	.0003	.0004	.0005	.0007	.0009
14	.0000	.0000	.0000	.0000	.0000	.0000	.0000	.0000	.0000	.0001

n = 15

	.01	.02	.03	.04	.05	.06	.07	.08	.09	.10
0	.8601	.7386	.6333	.5421	.4633	.3953	.3367	.2863	.2430	.2059
1	.1303	.2261	.2938	.3388	.3658	.3785	.3801	.3734	.3605	.3432
2	.0092	.0323	.0636	.0988	.1348	.1691	.2003	.2273	.2496	.2669
3	.0004	.0029	.0085	.0178	.0307	.0468	.0653	.0857	.1070	.1285
4	.0000	.0002	.0008	.0022	.0049	.0090	.0148	.0223	.0317	.0428
5	.0000	.0000	.0001	.0002	.0006	.0013	.0024	.0043	.0069	.0105
6	.0000	.0000	.0000	.0000	.0000	.0001	.0003	.0006	.0011	.0019
7	.0000	.0000	.0000	.0000	.0000	.0000	.0000	.0001	.0001	.0003
	.11	.12	.13	.14	.15	.16	.17	.18	.19	.20
0	.1741	.1470	.1238	.1041	.0874	.0731	.0611	.0510	.0424	.0352
1	.3228	.3006	.2775	.2542	.2312	.2090	.1878	.1678	.1492	.1319
2	.2793	.2870	.2903	.2897	.2856	.2787	.2692	.2578	.2449	.2309
3	.1496	.1696	.1880	.2044	.2184	.2300	.2389	.2452	.2489	.2501
4	.0555	.0694	.0843	.0998	.1156	.1314	.1468	.1615	.1752	.1876
5	.0151	.0208	.0277	.0357	.0449	.0551	.0662	.0780	.0904	.1032
6	.0031	.0047	.0069	.0097	.0132	.0175	.0226	.0285	.0353	.0430
7	.0005	.0008	.0013	.0020	.0030	.0043	.0059	.0081	.0107	.0138
8	.0001	.0001	.0002	.0003	.0005	.0008	.0012	.0018	.0025	.0035
9	.0000	.0000	.0000	.0000	.0001	.0001	.0002	.0003	.0005	.0007
10	.0000	.0000	.0000	.0000	.0000	.0000	.0000	.0000	.0001	.0001
	.21	.22	.23	.24	.25	.26	.27	.28	.29	.30
0	.0291	.0241	.0198	.0163	.0134	.0109	.0089	.0072	.0059	.0047
1	.1162	.1018	.0889	.0772	.0668	.0576	.0494	.0423	.0360	.0305
2	.2162	.2010	.1858	.1707	.1559	.1416	.1280	.1150	.1029	.0916
3	.2490	.2457	.2405	.2336	.2252	.2156	.2051	.1939	.1812	.1700
4	.1986	.2079	.2155	.2213	.2252	.2273	.2276	.2262	.2231	.2186
5	.1161	.1290	.1416	.1537	.1651	.1757	.1852	.1935	.2005	.2061
6	.0514	.0606	.0705	.0809	.0917	.1029	.1142	.1254	.1365	.1472
7	.0176	.0220	.0271	.0329	.0393	.0465	.0543	.0627	.0717	.0811
8	.0047	.0062	.0081	.0104	.0131	.0163	.0201	.0244	.0293	.0348
9	.0010	.0014	.0019	.0025	.0034	.0045	.0058	.0074	.0093	.0116
10	.0002	.0002	.0003	.0005	.0007	.0009	.0013	.0017	.0023	.0030
11	.0000	.0000	.0000	.0001	.0001	.0002	.0002	.0003	.0004	.0006
12	.0000	.0000	.0000	.0000	.0000	.0000	.0000	.0000	.0001	.0001

TABLE A.7   (Continued)

					n=15					
r\p	.31	.32	.33	.34	.35	.36	.37	.38	.39	.40
0	.0038	.0031	.0025	.0020	.0016	.0012	.0010	.0008	.0006	.0005
1	.0258	.0217	.0182	.0152	.0126	.0104	.0086	.0071	.0058	.0047
2	.0811	.0715	.0627	.0547	.0476	.0411	.0354	.0303	.0259	.0219
3	.1579	.1457	.1338	.1222	.1110	.1002	.0901	.0805	.0716	.0634
4	.2128	.2057	.1977	.1888	.1792	.1692	.1587	.1481	.1374	.1268
5	.0210	.2130	.2142	.2140	.2123	.2093	.2051	.1997	.1933	.1859
6	.1575	.1671	.1759	.1837	.1906	.1963	.2008	.2040	.2059	.2066
7	.0910	.1011	.1114	.1217	.1319	.1419	.1516	.1608	.1693	.1771
8	.0409	.0476	.0549	.0627	.0710	.0798	.0890	.0985	.1082	.1181
9	.0143	.0174	.0210	.0251	.0298	.0349	.0407	.0470	.0538	.0612
10	.0038	.0049	.0062	.0078	.0096	.0118	.0143	.0173	.0206	.0245
11	.0008	.0011	.0014	.0018	.0024	.0030	.0038	.0048	.0060	.0074
12	.0001	.0002	.0002	.0003	.0004	.0006	.0007	.0010	.0013	.0016
13	.0000	.0000	.0000	.0000	.0001	.0001	.0001	.0001	.0002	.0003
	.41	.42	.43	.44	.45	.46	.47	.48	.49	.50
0	.0004	.0003	.0002	.0002	.0001	.0001	.0001	.0001	.0000	.0000
1	.0038	.0031	.0025	.0020	.0016	.0012	.0010	.0008	.0006	.0005
2	.0185	.0156	.0130	.0108	.0090	.0074	.0060	.0049	.0040	.0032
3	.0558	.0489	.0426	.0369	.0318	.0272	.0232	.0197	.0166	.0139
4	.1163	.1061	.0963	.0869	.0780	.0696	.0617	.0545	.0478	.0417
5	.1778	.1691	.1598	.1502	.1404	.1304	.1204	.1106	.1010	.0916
6	.2060	.2041	.2010	.1967	.1914	.1851	.1780	.1702	.1617	.1527
7	.1840	.1900	.1949	.1987	.2013	.2028	.2030	.2020	.1997	.1964
8	.1279	.1376	.1470	.1561	.1647	.1727	.1800	.1864	.1919	.1964
9	.0691	.0775	.0863	.0954	.1048	.1144	.1241	.1338	.1434	.1527
10	.0288	.0337	.0390	.0450	.0515	.0585	.0661	.0741	.0827	.0916
11	.0091	.0111	.0134	.0161	.0191	.0226	.0266	.0311	.0361	.0417
12	.0021	.0027	.0034	.0042	.0052	.0064	.0079	.0096	.0116	.0139
13	.0003	.0004	.0006	.0008	.0010	.0013	.0016	.0020	.0026	.0032
14	.0000	.0000	.0001	.0001	.0001	.0002	.0002	.0003	.0004	.0005

					n = 16					
	.01	.02	.03	.04	.05	.06	.07	.08	.09	.10
0	.8515	.7238	.6143	.5204	.4401	.3716	.3131	.2634	.2211	.1853
1	.1376	.2363	.3040	.3469	.3706	.3795	.3771	.3665	.3499	.3294
2	.0104	.0362	.0705	.1084	.1463	.1817	.2129	.2390	.2596	.2745
3	.0005	.0034	.0102	.0211	.0359	.0541	.0748	.0970	.1198	.1423
4	.0000	.0002	.0010	.0029	.0061	.0112	.0183	.0274	.0385	.0514
5	.0000	.0000	.0001	.0003	.0008	.0017	.0033	.0057	.0091	.0137

(Continued)

TABLE A.7   (Continued)

					n=16					
r\p	.01	.02	.03	.04	.05	.06	.07	.08	.09	.10
6	.0000	.0000	.0000	.0000	.0001	.0002	.0005	.0009	.0017	.0028
7	.0000	.0000	.0000	.0000	.0000	.0000	.0000	.0001	.0002	.0004
8	.0000	.0000	.0000	.0000	.0000	.0000	.0000	.0000	.0000	.0001
	.11	.12	.13	.14	.15	.16	.17	.18	.19	.20
0	.1550	.1293	.1077	.0895	.0743	.0614	.0507	.0418	.0343	.0281
1	.3065	.2822	.2575	.2332	.2097	.1873	.1662	.1468	.1289	.1126
2	.2841	.2886	.2886	.2847	.2775	.2675	.2554	.2416	.2267	.2111
3	.1638	.1837	.2013	.2163	.2285	.2378	.2441	.2475	.2482	.2463
4	.0658	.0814	.0977	.1144	.1311	.1472	.1625	.1766	.1892	.2001
5	.0195	.0266	.0351	.0447	.0555	.0673	.0799	.0930	.1065	.1201
6	.0044	.0067	.0096	.0133	.0180	.0235	.0300	.0374	.0458	.0550
7	.0008	.0013	.0020	.0031	.0045	.0064	.0088	.0117	.0153	.0197
8	.0001	.0002	.0003	.0006	.0009	.0014	.0020	.0029	.0041	.0055
9	.0000	.0000	.0000	.0001	.0001	.0002	.0004	.0006	.0008	.0012
10	.0000	.0000	.0000	.0000	.0000	.0000	.0001	.0001	.0001	.0002
	.21	.22	.23	.24	.25	.26	.27	.28	.29	.30
0	.0230	.0188	.0153	.0124	.0100	.0081	.0065	.0052	.0042	.0033
1	.0979	.0847	.0730	.0626	.0535	.0455	.0385	.0325	.0273	.0228
2	.1952	.1792	.1635	.1482	.1336	.1198	.1068	.0947	.0835	.0732
3	.2421	.2359	.2279	.2185	.2079	.1964	.1843	.1718	.1591	.1465
4	.2092	.2162	.2212	.2242	.2252	.2243	.2215	.2171	.2112	.2040
5	.1334	.1464	.1586	.1699	.1802	.1891	.1966	.2026	.2071	.2099
6	.0650	.0757	.0869	.0984	.1101	.1218	.1333	.1445	.1551	.1649
7	.0247	.0305	.0371	.0444	.0524	.0611	.0704	.0803	.0905	.1010
8	.0074	.0097	.0125	.0158	.0197	.0242	.0293	.0351	.0416	.0487
9	.0017	.0024	.0033	.0044	.0058	.0075	.0096	.0121	.0151	.0185
10	.0003	.0005	.0007	.0010	.0014	.0019	.0025	.0033	.0043	.0056
11	.0000	.0001	.0001	.0002	.0002	.0004	.0005	.0007	.0010	.0013
12	.0000	.0000	.0000	.0000	.0000	.0001	.0001	.0001	.0002	.0002
	.31	.32	.33	.34	.35	.36	.37	.38	.39	.40
0	.0026	.0021	.0016	.0013	.0010	.0008	.0006	.0005	.0004	.0003
1	.0190	.0157	.0130	.0107	.0087	.0071	.0058	.0047	.0038	.0030
2	.0639	.0555	.0480	.0413	.0353	.0301	.0255	.0215	.0180	.0150
3	.1341	.1220	.1103	.0992	.0888	.0790	.0699	.0615	.0538	.0468
4	.1958	.1865	.1766	.1662	.1553	.1444	.1333	.1224	.1118	.1014
5	.2111	.2107	.2088	.2054	.2008	.1949	.1879	.1801	.1715	.1623
6	.1739	.1818	.1885	.1940	.1982	.2010	.2024	.2024	.2010	.1983
7	.1116	.1222	.1326	.1428	.1524	.1615	.1698	.1772	.1836	.1889
8	.0564	.0647	.0735	.0827	.0923	.1022	.1122	.1222	.1320	.1417

(Continued)

TABLE A.7 (Continued)

n=16

r \ p	.31	.32	.33	.34	.35	.36	.37	.38	.39	.40
9	.0225	.0271	.0322	.0379	.0442	.1511	.0586	.0666	.0750	.0840
10	.0071	.0089	.0111	.0137	.0167	.0201	.0241	.0286	.0336	.0392
11	.0017	.0023	.0030	.0038	.0049	.0062	.0077	.0095	.0117	.0142
12	.0003	.0004	.0006	.0008	.0011	.0014	.0019	.0024	.0031	.0040
13	.0000	.0001	.0001	.0001	.0002	.0003	.0003	.0005	.0006	.0008
14	.0000	.0000	.0000	.0000	.0000	.0000	.0000	.0001	.0001	.0001
	.41	.42	.43	.44	.45	.46	.47	.48	.49	.50
0	.0002	.0002	.0001	.0001	.0001	.0001	.0000	.0000	.0000	.0000
1	.0024	.0019	.0015	.0012	.0009	.0007	.0005	.0004	.0003	.0002
2	.0125	.0103	.0085	.0069	.0056	.0046	.0037	.0029	.0023	.0018
3	.0405	.0349	.0299	.0254	.0215	.0181	.0151	.0126	.0104	.0085
4	.0915	.0821	.0732	.0649	.0572	.0501	.0436	.0378	.0325	.0278
5	.1526	.1426	.1325	.1224	.1123	.1024	.0929	.0837	.0749	.0667
6	.1944	.1894	.1833	.1762	.1684	.1600	.1510	.1416	.1319	.1222
7	.1930	.1959	.1975	.1978	.1969	.1947	.1912	.1867	.1811	.1746
8	.1509	.1596	.1676	.1749	.1812	.1865	.1908	.1939	.1958	.1964
9	.0932	.1027	.1124	.1221	.1318	.1413	.1504	.1591	.1672	.1746
10	.0453	.0521	.0594	.0672	.0755	.0842	.0934	.1028	.1124	.1222
11	.0172	.0206	.0244	.0288	.0337	.0391	.0452	.0518	.0589	.0667
12	.0050	.0062	.0077	.0094	.0115	.0139	.0167	.0199	.0236	.0278
13	.0011	.0014	.0018	.0023	.0029	.0036	.0046	.0057	.0070	.0085
14	.0002	.0002	.0003	.0004	.0005	.0007	.0009	.0011	.0014	.0018
15	.0000	.0000	.0000	.0000	.0001	.0001	.0001	.0001	.0002	.0002

n = 17

r	.01	.02	.03	.04	.05	.06	.07	.08	.09	.10
0	.8429	.7093	.5958	.4996	.4181	.3493	.2912	.2423	.2012	.1668
1	.1447	.2461	.3133	.3539	.3741	.3790	.3726	.3582	.3383	.3150
2	.0117	.0402	.0775	.1180	.1575	.1935	.2244	.2492	.2677	.2800
3	.0006	.0041	.0120	.0246	.0415	.0618	.0844	.1083	.1324	.1556
4	.0000	.0003	.0013	.0036	.0076	.0138	.0222	.0330	.0458	.0605
5	.0000	.0000	.0001	.0004	.0010	.0023	.0044	.0075	.0118	.0175
6	.0000	.0000	.0000	.0000	.0001	.0003	.0007	.0013	.0023	.0039
7	.0000	.0000	.0000	.0000	.0000	.0000	.0001	.0002	.0004	.0007
8	.0000	.0000	.0000	.0000	.0000	.0000	.0000	.0000	.0000	.0001

(Continued)

TABLE A.7 (Continued)

					n=17					
r\p	.11	.12	.13	.14	.15	.16	.17	.18	.19	.20
0	.1379	.1138	.0937	.0770	.0631	.0516	.0421	.0343	.0278	.0225
1	.2898	.2638	.2381	.2131	.1893	.1671	.1466	.1279	.1109	.0957
2	.2865	.2878	.2846	.2775	.2673	.2547	.2402	.2245	.2081	.1914
3	.1771	.1963	.2126	.2259	.2359	.2425	.2460	.2464	.2441	.2393
4	.0766	.0937	.1112	.1287	.1457	.1617	.1764	.1893	.2004	.2093
5	.0246	.0332	.0432	.0545	.0668	.0801	.0939	.1081	.1222	.1361
6	.0061	.0091	.0129	.0177	.0236	.0305	.0385	.0474	.0573	.0680
7	.0012	.0019	.0030	.0045	.0065	.0091	.0124	.0164	.0211	.0267
8	.0002	.0003	.0006	.0009	.0014	.0022	.0032	.0045	.0062	.0084
9	.0000	.0000	.0001	.0002	.0003	.0004	.0006	.0010	.0015	.0021
10	.0000	.0000	.0000	.0000	.0000	.0001	.0001	.0002	.0003	.0004
11	.0000	.0000	.0000	.0000	.0000	.0000	.0000	.0000	.0000	.0001
	.21	.22	.23	.24	.25	.26	.27	.28	.29	.30
0	.0182	.0146	.0118	.0094	.0075	.0060	.0047	.0038	.0030	.0023
1	.0822	.0702	.0597	.0505	.0426	.0357	.0299	.0248	.0206	.0169
2	.1747	.1584	.1427	.1277	.1136	.1005	.0883	.0772	.0672	.0581
3	.2322	.2234	.2131	.2016	.1893	.1765	.1634	.1502	.1372	.1245
4	.2161	.2205	.2228	.2228	.2209	.2170	.2115	.2044	.1961	.1868
5	.1493	.1617	.1730	.1830	.1914	.1982	.2033	.2067	.2083	.2081
6	.0794	.0912	.1034	.1156	.1276	.1393	.1504	.1608	.1701	.1784
7	.0332	.0404	.0485	.0573	.0668	.0769	.0874	.0982	.1092	.1201
8	.0110	.0143	.0181	.0226	.0279	.0338	.0404	.0478	.0558	.0644
9	.0029	.0040	.0054	.0071	.0093	.0119	.0150	.0186	.0228	.0276
10	.0006	.0009	.0013	.0018	.0025	.0033	.0044	.0058	.0074	.0095
11	.0001	.0002	.0002	.0004	.0005	.0007	.0010	.0014	.0019	.0026
12	.0000	.0000	.0000	.0001	.0001	.0001	.0002	.0003	.0004	.0006
13	.0000	.0000	.0000	.0000	.0000	.0000	.0000	.0000	.0001	.0001
	.31	.32	.33	.34	.35	.36	.37	.38	.39	.40
0	.0018	.0014	.0011	.0009	.0007	.0005	.0004	.0003	.0002	.0002
1	.0139	.0114	.0093	.0075	.0060	.0048	.0039	.0031	.0024	.0019
2	.0500	.0428	.0364	.0309	.0260	.0218	.0182	.0151	.0125	.0102
3	.1123	.1007	.0898	.0795	.0701	.0614	.0534	.0463	.0398	.0341
4	.1766	.1659	.1547	.1434	.1320	.1208	.1099	.0993	.0892	.0796
5	.2063	.2030	.1982	.1921	.1849	.1767	.1677	.1582	.1482	.1379
6	.1854	.1910	.1952	.1979	.1991	.1988	.1970	.1939	.1895	.1839
7	.1309	.1413	.1511	.1602	.1685	.1757	.1818	.1868	.1904	.1927
8	.0735	.0831	.0930	.1032	.1134	.1235	.1335	.1431	.1521	.1606
9	.0330	.0391	.0458	.0531	.0611	.0695	.0784	.0877	.0973	.1070

(Continued)

TABLE A.7 (Continued)

					n=17					
r\p	.31	.32	.33	.34	.35	.36	.37	.38	.39	.40
10	.0119	.0147	.0181	.0219	.0263	.0313	.0368	.0430	.0498	.0571
11	.0034	.0044	.0057	.0072	.0090	.0112	.0138	.0168	.0202	.0242
12	.0008	.0010	.0014	.0018	.0024	.0031	.0040	.0051	.0065	.0081
13	.0001	.0002	.0003	.0004	.0005	.0007	.0009	.0012	.0016	.0021
14	.0000	.0000	.0000	.0001	.0001	.0001	.0002	.0002	.0003	.0004
15	.0000	.0000	.0000	.0000	.0000	.0000	.0000	.0000	.0000	.0001
	.41	.42	.43	.44	.45	.46	.47	.48	.49	.50
0	.0001	.0001	.0001	.0001	.0000	.0000	.0000	.0000	.0000	.0000
1	.0015	.0012	.0009	.0007	.0005	.0004	.0003	.0002	.0002	.0001
2	.0084	.0068	.0055	.0044	.0035	.0028	.0022	.0017	.0013	.0010
3	.0290	.0246	.0207	.0173	.0144	.0119	.0097	.0079	.0064	.0052
4	.0706	.0622	.0546	.0475	.0411	.0354	.0302	.0257	.0217	.0182
5	.1276	.1172	.1070	.0971	.0875	.0784	.0697	.0616	.0541	.0472
6	.1773	.1697	.1614	.1525	.1432	.1335	.1237	.1138	.1040	.0944
7	.1936	.1932	.1914	.1883	.1841	.1787	.1723	.1650	.1570	.1484
8	.1682	.1748	.1805	.1850	.1883	.1903	.1910	.1904	.1886	.1855
9	.1169	.1266	.1361	.1453	.1540	.1621	.1694	.1758	.1812	.1855
10	.0650	.0733	.0822	.0914	.1008	.1105	.1202	.1298	.1393	.1484
11	.0287	.0338	.0394	.0457	.0525	.0599	.0678	.0763	.0851	.0944
12	.0100	.0122	.0149	.0179	.0215	.0255	.0301	.0352	.0409	.0472
13	.0027	.0034	.0043	.0054	.0068	.0084	.0103	.0125	.0151	.0182
14	.0005	.0007	.0009	.0012	.0016	.0020	.0026	.0033	.0041	.0052
15	.0001	.0001	.0001	.0002	.0003	.0003	.0005	.0006	.0008	.0010
16	.0000	.0000	.0000	.0000	.0000	.0000	.0001	.0001	.0001	.0001

					n = 18					
	.01	.02	.03	.04	.05	.06	.07	.08	.09	.10
0	.8345	.6951	.5780	.4796	.3972	.3283	.2708	.2229	.1831	.1501
1	.1517	.2554	.3217	.3597	.3763	.3772	.3669	.3489	.3260	.3002
2	.0130	.0443	.0846	.1274	.1683	.2047	.2348	.2579	.2741	.2835
3	.0007	.0048	.0140	.0283	.0473	.0697	.0942	.1196	.1446	.1680
4	.0000	.0004	.0016	.0044	.0093	.0167	.0266	.0390	.0536	.0700
5	.0000	.0000	.0001	.0005	.0014	.0030	.0056	.0095	.0148	.0218
6	.0000	.0000	.0000	.0000	.0002	.0004	.0009	.0018	.0032	.0052
7	.0000	.0000	.0000	.0000	.0000	.0000	.0001	.0003	.0005	.0010
8	.0000	.0000	.0000	.0000	.0000	.0000	.0000	.0000	.0001	.0002

(Continued)

TABLE A.7   (Continued)

					n=18					
r \ p	.11	.12	.13	.14	.15	.16	.17	.18	.19	.20
0	.1227	.1002	.0815	.0662	.0536	.0434	.0349	.0281	.0225	.0180
1	.2731	.2458	.2193	.1940	.1704	.1486	.1288	.1110	.0951	.0811
2	.2869	.2850	.2785	.2685	.2556	.2407	.2243	.2071	.1897	.1723
3	.1891	.2072	.2220	.2331	.2406	.2445	.2450	.2425	.2373	.2297
4	.0877	.1060	.1244	.1423	.1592	.1746	.1882	.1996	.2087	.2153
5	.0303	.0405	.0520	.0649	.0787	.0931	.1079	.1227	.1371	.1507
6	.0081	.0120	.0168	.0229	.0301	.0384	.0479	.0584	.0697	.0816
7	.0017	.0028	.0043	.0064	.0091	.0126	.0168	.0220	.0280	.0350
8	.0003	.0005	.0009	.0014	.0022	.0033	.0047	.0066	.0090	.0120
9	.0000	.0001	.0001	.0003	.0004	.0007	.0011	.0016	.0024	.0033
10	.0000	.0000	.0000	.0000	.0001	.0001	.0002	.0003	.0005	.0008
11	.0000	.0000	.0000	.0000	.0000	.0000	.0000	.0001	.0001	.0001
	.21	.22	.23	.24	.25	.26	.27	.28	.29	.30
0	.0144	.0114	.0091	.0072	.0056	.0044	.0035	.0027	.0021	.0016
1	.0687	.0580	.0487	.0407	.0338	.0280	.0231	.0189	.0155	.0126
2	.1553	.1390	.1236	.1092	.0958	.0836	.0725	.0626	.0537	.0458
3	.2202	.2091	.1969	.1839	.1704	.1567	.1431	.1298	.1169	.1046
4	.2195	.2212	.2205	.2177	.2130	.2065	.1985	.1892	.1790	.1681
5	.1634	.1747	.1845	.1925	.1988	.2031	.2055	.2061	.2048	.2017
6	.0941	.1067	.1194	.1317	.1436	.1546	.1647	.1736	.1812	.1873
7	.0429	.0516	.0611	.0713	.0820	.0931	.1044	.1157	.1269	.1376
8	.0157	.0200	.0251	.0310	.0376	.0450	.0531	.0619	.0713	.0811
9	.0046	.0063	.0083	.0109	.0139	.0176	.0218	.0267	.0323	.0386
10	.0011	.0016	.0022	.0031	.0042	.0056	.0073	.0094	.0119	.0149
11	.0002	.0003	.0005	.0007	.0010	.0014	.0020	.0026	.0035	.0046
12	.0000	.0001	.0001	.0001	.0002	.0003	.0004	.0006	.0008	.0012
13	.0000	.0000	.0000	.0000	.0000	.0000	.0001	.0001	.0002	.0002
	.31	.32	.33	.34	.35	.36	.37	.38	.39	.40
0	.0013	.0010	.0007	.0006	.0004	.0003	.0002	.0002	.0001	.0001
1	.0102	.0082	.0066	.0052	.0042	.0033	.0026	.0020	.0016	.0012
2	.0388	.0327	.0275	.0229	.0190	.0157	.0129	.0105	.0086	.0069
3	.0930	.0822	.0722	.0630	.0547	.0471	.0404	.0344	.0292	.0246
4	.1567	.1450	.1333	.1217	.1104	.0994	.0890	.0791	.0699	.0614
5	.1971	.1911	.1838	.1755	.1664	.1566	.1463	.1358	.1252	.1146
6	.1919	.1948	.1962	.1959	.1941	.1908	.1862	.1803	.1734	.1655
7	.1478	.1572	.1656	.1730	.1792	.1840	.1875	.1895	.1900	.1892
8	.0913	.1017	.1122	.1226	.1327	.1423	.1514	.1597	.1671	.1734
9	.0456	.0532	.0614	.0701	.0794	.0890	.0988	.1087	.1187	.1284
10	.0184	.0225	.0272	.0325	.0385	.0450	.0522	.0600	.0683	.0771

(Continued)

TABLE A.7   (Continued)

n=18

r \ p	.31	.32	.33	.34	.35	.36	.37	.38	.39	.40
11	.0060	.0077	.0097	.0122	.0151	.0184	.0223	.0267	.0318	.0374
12	.0016	.0021	.0028	.0037	.0047	.0060	.0076	.0096	.0118	.0145
13	.0003	.0005	.0006	.0009	.0012	.0016	.0021	.0027	.0035	.0045
14	.0001	.0001	.0001	.0002	.0002	.0003	.0004	.0006	.0008	.0011
15	.0000	.0000	.0000	.0000	.0000	.0000	.0001	.0001	.0001	.0002

r \ p	.41	.42	.43	.44	.45	.46	.47	.48	.49	.50
0	.0001	.0001	.0000	.0000	.0000	.0000	.0000	.0000	.0000	.0000
1	.0009	.0007	.0005	.0004	.0003	.0002	.0002	.0001	.0001	.0001
2	.0055	.0044	.0035	.0028	.0022	.0017	.0013	.0010	.0008	.0006
3	.0206	.0171	.0141	.0116	.0095	.0077	.0062	.0050	.0039	.0031
4	.0536	.0464	.0400	.0342	.0291	.0246	.0206	.0172	.0142	.0117
5	.1042	.0941	.0844	.0753	.0666	.0586	.0512	.0444	.0382	.0327
6	.1569	.1477	.1380	.1281	.1181	.1081	.0983	.0887	.0796	.0708
7	.1869	.1833	.1785	.1726	.1657	.1579	.1494	.1404	.1310	.1214
8	.1786	.1825	.1852	.1864	.1864	.1850	.1822	.1782	.1731	.1669
9	.1379	.1469	.1552	.1628	.1694	.1751	.1795	.1828	.1848	.1855
10	.0862	.0957	.1054	.1151	.1248	.1342	.1433	.1519	.1598	.1669
11	.0436	.0504	.0578	.0658	.0742	.0831	.0924	.1020	.1117	.1214
12	.0177	.0213	.0254	.0301	.0354	.0413	.0478	.1549	.0626	.0708
13	.0057	.0071	.0089	.0109	.0134	.0162	.0196	.0234	.0278	.0327
14	.0014	.0018	.0024	.0031	.0039	.0049	.0062	.0077	.0095	.0117
15	.0003	.0004	.0005	.0006	.0009	.0011	.0015	.0019	.0024	.0031
16	.0000	.0000	.0001	.0001	.0001	.0002	.0002	.0003	.0004	.0006
17	.0000	.0000	.0000	.0000	.0000	.0000	.0000	.0000	.0000	.0001

n = 19

r \ p	.01	.02	.03	.04	.05	.06	.07	.08	.09	.10
0	.8262	.6812	.5606	.4604	.3774	.3086	.2519	.2051	.1666	.1351
1	.1586	.2642	.3294	.3645	.3774	.3743	.3602	.3389	.3131	.2852
2	.0144	.0485	.0917	.1367	.1787	.2150	.2440	.2652	.2787	.2852
3	.0008	.0056	.0161	.0323	.0533	.0778	.1041	.1307	.1562	.1796
4	.0000	.0005	.0020	.0054	.0112	.0199	.0313	.0455	.0618	.0798
5	.0000	.0000	.0002	.0007	.0018	.0038	.0071	.0119	.0183	.0266
6	.0000	.0000	.0000	.0001	.0002	.0006	.0012	.0024	.0042	.0069
7	.0000	.0000	.0000	.0000	.0000	.0001	.0002	.0004	.0008	.0014
8	.0000	.0000	.0000	.0000	.0000	.0000	.0000	.0001	.0001	.0002

(Continued)

TABLE A.7 (Continued)

						n=19				
r	p	.11	.12	.13	.14	.15	.16	.17	.18	.19	.20
0		.1092	.0881	.0709	.0569	.0456	.0364	.0290	.0230	.0182	.0144
1		.2565	.2284	.2014	.1761	.1529	.1318	.1129	.0961	.0813	.0685
2		.2854	.2803	.2708	.2581	.2428	.2259	.2081	.1898	.1717	.1540
3		.1999	.2166	.2293	.2381	.2428	.2439	.2415	.2361	.2282	.2182
4		.0988	.1181	.1371	.1550	.1714	.1858	.1979	.2073	.2141	.2182
5		.0366	.0483	.0614	.0757	.0907	.1062	.1216	.1365	.1507	.1636
6		.0106	.0154	.0214	.0288	.0374	.0472	.0581	.0699	.0825	.0955
7		.0024	.0039	.0059	.0087	.0122	.0167	.0221	.0285	.0359	.0443
8		.0004	.0008	.0013	.0021	.0032	.0048	.0068	.0094	.0126	.0166
9		.0001	.0001	.0002	.0004	.0007	.0011	.0017	.0025	.0036	.0051
10		.0000	.0000	.0000	.0001	.0001	.0002	.0003	.0006	.0009	.0013
11		.0000	.0000	.0000	.0000	.0000	.0000	.0001	.0001	.0002	.0003
		.21	.22	.23	.24	.25	.26	.27	.28	.29	.30
0		.0113	.0089	.0070	.0054	.0042	.0033	.0025	.0019	.0015	.0011
1		.0573	.0477	.0396	.0326	.0268	.0219	.0178	.0144	.0116	.0093
2		.1371	.1212	.1064	.0927	.0803	.0692	.0592	.0503	.0426	.0358
3		.2065	.1937	.1800	.1659	.1517	.1377	.1240	.1109	.0985	.0869
4		.2196	.2185	.2151	.2096	.2023	.1935	.1835	.1726	.1610	.1491
5		.1751	.1849	.1928	.1986	.2023	.2040	.2036	.2013	.1973	.1916
6		.1086	.1217	.1343	.1463	.1574	.1672	.1757	.1827	.1880	.1916
7		.0536	.0637	.0745	.0858	.0974	.1091	.1207	.1320	.1426	.1525
8		.0214	.0270	.0334	.0406	.0487	.0575	.0670	.0770	.0874	.0981
9		.0069	.0093	.0122	.0157	.0198	.0247	.0303	.0366	.0436	.0514
10		.0018	.0026	.0036	.0050	.0066	.0087	.0112	.0142	.0178	.0220
11		.0004	.0006	.0009	.0013	.0018	.0025	.0034	.0045	.0060	.0077
12		.0001	.0001	.0002	.0003	.0004	.0006	.0008	.0012	.0016	.0022
13		.0000	.0000	.0000	.0000	.0001	.0001	.0002	.0002	.0004	.0005
14		.0000	.0000	.0000	.0000	.0000	.0000	.0000	.0000	.0001	.0001
		.31	.32	.33	.34	.35	.36	.37	.38	.39	.40
0		.0009	.0007	.0005	.0004	.0003	.0002	.0002	.0001	.0001	.0001
1		.0074	.0059	.0046	.0036	.0029	.0022	.0017	.0013	.0010	.0008
2		.0299	.0249	.0206	.0169	.0138	.0112	.0091	.0073	.0058	.0046
3		.0762	.0664	.0574	.0494	.0422	.0358	.0302	.0253	.0211	.0175
4		.1370	.1249	.1131	.1017	.0909	.0806	.0710	.0621	.0540	.0467
5		.1846	.1764	.1672	.1572	.1468	.1360	.1251	.1143	.1036	.0933
6		.1935	.1936	.1921	.1890	.1844	.1785	.1714	.1634	.1546	.1451
7		.1615	.1692	.1757	.1808	.1844	.1865	.1870	.1860	.1835	.1797
8		.1088	.1195	.1298	.1397	.1489	.1573	.1647	.1710	.1760	.1797

(Continued)

TABLE A.7 (Continued)

					n=19					
r \ p	.31	.32	.33	.34	.35	.36	.37	.38	.39	.40
9	.0597	.0687	.0782	.0880	.0980	.1082	.1182	.1281	.1375	.1464
10	.0268	.0323	.0385	.0453	.0528	.0608	.0694	.0785	.0879	.0976
11	.0099	.0124	.0155	.0191	.0233	.0280	.0334	.0394	.0460	.0532
12	.0030	.0039	.0051	.0066	.0083	.0105	.0131	.0161	.0196	.0237
13	.0007	.0010	.0014	.0018	.0024	.0032	.0041	.0053	.0067	.0085
14	.0001	.0002	.0003	.0004	.0006	.0008	.0010	.0014	.0018	.0024
15	.0000	.0000	.0000	.0001	.0001	.0001	.0002	.0003	.0004	.0005
16	.0000	.0000	.0000	.0000	.0000	.0000	.0000	.0000	.0001	.0001
	.41	.42	.43	.44	.45	.46	.47	.48	.49	.50
0	.0000	.0000	.0000	.0000	.0000	.0000	.0000	.0000	.0000	.0000
1	.0006	.0004	.0003	.0002	.0002	.0001	.0001	.0001	.0001	.0000
2	.0037	.0029	.0022	.0017	.0013	.0010	.0008	.0006	.0004	.0003
3	.0144	.0118	.0096	.0077	.0062	.0049	.0039	.0031	.0024	.0018
4	.0400	.0341	.0289	.0243	.0203	.0168	.0138	.0113	.0092	.0074
5	.0834	.0741	.0653	.0572	.0497	.0429	.0368	.0313	.0265	.0222
6	.1353	.1252	.1150	.1049	.0949	.0853	.0751	.0674	.0593	.0518
7	.1746	.1683	.1611	.1530	.1443	.1350	.1254	.1156	.1058	.0961
8	.1820	.1829	.1823	.1803	.1771	.1725	.1668	.1601	.1525	.1442
9	.1546	.1618	.1681	.1732	.1771	.1796	.1808	.1806	.1791	.1762
10	.1074	.1172	.1268	.1361	.1449	.1530	.1603	.1667	.1721	.1762
11	.0611	.0694	.0783	.0875	.0970	.1066	.1163	.1259	.1352	.1442
12	.0283	.0335	.0394	.0458	.0529	.0606	.0688	.0775	.0866	.0961
13	.0106	.0131	.0160	.0194	.0233	.0278	.0328	.0385	.0448	.0518
14	.0032	.0041	.0052	.0065	.0082	.0101	.0125	.0152	.0185	.0222
15	.0007	.0010	.0013	.0017	.0022	.0029	.0037	.0047	.0059	.0074
16	.0001	.0002	.0002	.0003	.0005	.0006	.0008	.0011	.0014	.0018
17	.0000	.0000	.0000	.0000	.0001	.0001	.0001	.0002	.0002	.0003

					n = 20					
	.01	.02	.03	.04	.05	.06	.07	.08	.09	.10
0	.8179	.6676	.5438	.4420	.3585	.2901	.2342	.1887	.1516	.1216
1	.1652	.2725	.3364	.3683	.3774	.3703	.3526	.3282	.3000	.2702
2	.0159	.0528	.0988	.1458	.1887	.2246	.2521	.2711	.2818	.2852
3	.0010	.0065	.0183	.0364	.0596	.0860	.1139	.1414	.1672	.1901
4	.0000	.0006	.0024	.0065	.0133	.0233	.0364	.0523	.0703	.0898
5	.0000	.0000	.0002	.0009	.0022	.0048	.0088	.0145	.0222	.0319
6	.0000	.0000	.0000	.0001	.0003	.0008	.0017	.0032	.0055	.0089

(Continued)

TABLE A.7 (Continued)

r \ p	.01	.02	.03	.04	.05	.06	.07	.08	.09	.10
					n=20					

r \ p	.01	.02	.03	.04	.05	.06	.07	.08	.09	.10
7	.0000	.0000	.0000	.0000	.0000	.0001	.0002	.0005	.0011	.0020
8	.0000	.0000	.0000	.0000	.0000	.0000	.0000	.0001	.0002	.0004
9	.0000	.0000	.0000	.0000	.0000	.0000	.0000	.0000	.0000	.0001
	.11	.12	.13	.14	.15	.16	.17	.18	.19	.20
0	.0972	.0776	.0617	.0490	.0388	.0306	.0241	.0189	.0148	.0115
1	.2403	.2115	.1844	.1595	.1368	.1165	.0986	.0829	.0693	.0576
2	.2822	.2740	.2618	.2466	.2293	.2109	.1919	.1730	.1545	.1369
3	.2093	.2242	.2347	.2409	.2428	.2410	.2358	.2278	.2175	.2054
4	.1099	.1299	.1491	.1666	.1821	.1951	.2053	.2125	.2168	.2182
5	.0435	.0567	.0713	.1868	.1028	.1189	.1345	.1493	.1627	.1746
6	.0134	.0193	.0266	.0353	.0454	.0566	.0689	.0819	.0954	.1091
7	.0033	.0053	.0080	.0115	.0160	.0216	.0282	.0360	.0448	.0545
8	.0007	.0012	.0019	.0030	.0046	.0067	.0094	.0128	.0171	.0222
9	.0001	.0002	.0004	.0007	.0011	.0017	.0026	.0038	.0053	.0074
10	.0000	.0000	.0001	.0001	.0002	.0004	.0006	.0009	.0014	.0020
11	.0000	.0000	.0000	.0000	.0000	.0001	.0001	.0002	.0003	.0005
12	.0000	.0000	.0000	.0000	.0000	.0000	.0000	.0000	.0001	.0001
	.21	.22	.23	.24	.25	.26	.27	.28	.29	.30
0	.0090	.0069	.0054	.0041	.0032	.0024	.0018	.0014	.0011	.0008
1	.0477	.0392	.0321	.0261	.0211	.0170	.0137	.0109	.0087	.0068
2	.1204	.1050	.0910	.0783	.0669	.0569	.0480	.0403	.0336	.0278
3	.1920	.1777	.1631	.1484	.1339	.1199	.1065	.0940	.0823	.0716
4	.2169	.2131	.2070	.1991	.1897	.1790	.1675	.1553	.1429	.1304
5	.1845	.1923	.1979	.2012	.2023	.2013	.1982	.1933	.1868	.1789
6	.1226	.1356	.1478	.1589	.1686	.1768	.1833	.1879	.1907	.1916
7	.0652	.0765	.0883	.1003	.1124	.1242	.1356	.1462	.1558	.1643
8	.0282	.0351	.0429	.0515	.0609	.0709	.0815	.0924	.1034	.1144
9	.0100	.0132	.0171	.0217	.0271	.0332	.0402	.0479	.0563	.0654
10	.0029	.0041	.0056	.0075	.0099	.0128	.0163	.0205	.0253	.0308
11	.0007	.0010	.0015	.0022	.0030	.0041	.0055	.0072	.0094	.0120
12	.0001	.0002	.0003	.0005	.0008	.0011	.0015	.0021	.0029	.0039
13	.0000	.0000	.0001	.0001	.0002	.0002	.0003	.0005	.0007	.0010
14	.0000	.0000	.0000	.0000	.0000	.0000	.0001	.0001	.0001	.0002
	.31	.32	.33	.34	.35	.36	.37	.38	.39	.40
0	.0006	.0004	.0003	.0002	.0002	.0001	.0001	.0001	.0001	.0000
1	.0054	.0042	.0033	.0025	.0020	.0015	.0011	.0009	.0007	.0005
2	.0229	.0188	.0153	.0124	.0100	.0080	.0064	.0050	.0040	.0031
3	.0619	.0531	.0453	.0383	.0323	.0270	.0224	.0185	.0152	.0123

(Continued)

TABLE A.7   (Continued)

					n=20					
r \ p	.31	.32	.33	.34	.35	.36	.37	.38	.39	.40
4	.1181	.1062	.0947	.0839	.0738	.0645	.0559	.0482	.0412	.0350
5	.1698	.1599	.1493	.1384	.1272	.1161	.1051	.0945	.0843	.0746
6	.1907	.1881	.1839	.1782	.1712	.1632	.1543	.1447	.1347	.1244
7	.1714	.1770	.1811	.1836	.1844	.1836	.1812	.1774	.1722	.1659
8	.1251	.1354	.1450	.1537	.1614	.1678	.1730	.1767	.1790	.1797
9	.0750	.0849	.0952	.1056	.1158	.1259	.1354	.1444	.1526	.1597
10	.0370	.0440	.0516	.0598	.0686	.0779	.0875	.0974	.1073	.1171
11	.0151	.0188	.0231	.0280	.0336	.0398	.0467	.0542	.0624	.0710
12	.0051	.0066	.0085	.0108	.0136	.0168	.0206	.0249	.0299	.0355
13	.0014	.0019	.0026	.0034	.0045	.0058	.0074	.0094	.0118	.0146
14	.0003	.0005	.0006	.0009	.0012	.0016	.0022	.0029	.0038	.0049
15	.0001	.0001	.0001	.0002	.0003	.0004	.0005	.0007	.0010	.0013
16	.0000	.0000	.0000	.0000	.0000	.0001	.0001	.0001	.0002	.0003
	.41	.42	.43	.44	.45	.46	.47	.48	.49	.50
0	.0000	.0000	.0000	.0000	.0000	.0000	.0000	.0000	.0000	.0000
1	.0004	.0003	.0002	.0001	.0001	.0001	.0001	.0000	.0000	.0000
2	.0024	.0018	.0014	.0011	.0008	.0006	.0005	.0003	.0002	.0002
3	.0100	.0080	.0064	.0051	.0040	.0031	.0024	.0019	.0014	.0011
4	.0295	.0247	.0206	.0170	.0139	.0113	.0092	.0074	.0059	.0046
5	.0656	.0573	.0496	.0427	.0365	.0309	.0260	.0217	.0180	.0148
6	.1140	.1037	.0936	.0839	.0746	.0658	.0577	.0501	.0432	.0370
7	.1585	.1502	.1413	.1318	.1221	.1122	.1023	.0925	.0830	.0739
8	.1790	.1768	.1732	.1683	.1623	.1553	.1474	.1388	.1296	.1201
9	.1658	.1707	.1742	.1763	.1771	.1763	.1742	.1708	.1661	.1602
10	.1268	.1359	.1446	.1524	.1593	.1652	.1700	.1734	.1755	.1762
11	.0801	.0895	.0991	.1089	.1185	.1280	.1370	.1455	.1533	.1602
12	.0417	.0486	.0561	.0642	.0727	.0818	.0911	.1007	.1105	.1201
13	.0178	.0217	.0260	.0310	.0366	.0429	.0497	.0572	.0653	.0739
14	.0062	.0078	.0098	.0122	.0150	.0183	.0221	.0264	.0314	.0370
15	.0017	.0023	.0030	.0038	.0049	.0062	.0078	.0098	.0121	.0148
16	.0004	.0005	.0007	.0009	.0013	.0017	.0022	.0028	.0036	.0046
17	.0001	.0001	.0001	.0002	.0002	.0003	.0005	.0006	.0008	.0011
18	.0000	.0000	.0000	.0000	.0000	.0000	.0001	.0001	.0001	.0002

(Continued)

TABLE A.7   (Continued)

					n=25					
r\p	.01	.02	.03	.04	.05	.06	.07	.08	.09	.10
0	.7778	.6035	.4670	.3604	.2774	.2129	.1630	.1244	.0946	.0718
1	.1964	.3079	.3611	.3754	.3650	.3398	.3066	.2704	.2340	.1994
2	.0238	.0754	.1340	.1877	.2305	.2602	.2770	.2821	.2777	.2659
3	.0018	.0118	.0318	.0600	.0930	.1273	.1598	.1881	.2106	.2265
4	.0001	.0013	.0054	.0137	.0269	.0447	.0662	.0899	.1145	.1384
5	.0000	.0001	.0007	.0024	.0060	.0120	.0209	.0329	.0476	.0646
6	.0000	.0000	.0001	.0003	.0010	.0026	.0052	.0095	.0157	.0239
7	.0000	.0000	.0000	.0000	.0001	.0004	.0011	.0022	.0042	.0072
8	.0000	.0000	.0000	.0000	.0000	.0001	.0002	.0004	.0009	.0018
9	0	.0000	.0000	.0000	.0000	.0000	.0000	.0001	.0002	.0004
10	0	.0000	.0000	.0000	.0000	.0000	.0000	.0000	.0000	.0001
	.11	.12	.13	.14	.15	.16	.17	.18	.19	.20
0	.0543	.0409	.0308	.0230	.0172	.0128	.0095	.0070	.0052	.0038
1	.1678	.1395	.1149	.0938	.0759	.0609	.0486	.0384	.0302	.0236
2	.2488	.2283	.2060	.1832	.1607	.1392	.1193	.1012	.0851	.0708
3	.2358	.2387	.2360	.2286	.2174	.2033	.1874	.1704	.1530	.1358
4	.1603	.1790	.1940	.2047	.2110	.2130	.2111	.2057	.1974	.1867
5	.0832	.1025	.1217	.1399	.1564	.1704	.1816	.1897	.1945	.1960
6	.0343	.0466	.0606	.0759	.0920	.1082	.1240	.1388	.1520	.1633
7	.0115	.0173	.0246	.0336	.0441	.0559	.0689	.0827	.0968	.1108
8	.0032	.0053	.0083	.0123	.0175	.0240	.0318	.0408	.0511	.0623
9	.0007	.0014	.0023	.0038	.0058	.0086	.0123	.0169	.0226	.0294
10	.0001	.0003	.0006	.0010	.0016	.0026	.0040	.0059	.0085	.0118
11	.0000	.0001	.0001	.0002	.0004	.0007	.0011	.0018	.0027	.0040
12	.0000	.0000	.0000	.0000	.0001	.0002	.0003	.0005	.0007	.0012
13	.0000	.0000	.0000	.0000	.0000	.0000	.0001	.0001	.0002	.0003
14	.0000	.0000	.0000	.0000	.0000	.0000	.0000	.0000	.0000	.0001
	.21	.22	.23	.24	.25	.26	.27	.28	.29	.30
0	.0028	.0020	.0015	.0010	.0008	.0005	.0004	.0003	.0002	.0001
1	.0183	.0141	.0109	.0083	.0063	.0047	.0035	.0026	.0020	.0014
2	.0585	.0479	.0389	.0314	.0251	.0199	.0157	.0123	.0096	.0074
3	.1192	.1035	.0891	.0759	.0641	.0537	.0446	.0367	.0300	.0243
4	.1742	.1606	.1463	.1318	.1175	.1037	.0906	.0785	.0673	.0572
5	.1945	.1903	.1836	.1749	.1645	.1531	.1408	.1282	.1155	.1030
6	.1724	.1789	.1828	.1841	.1828	.1793	.1736	.1661	.1572	.1472
7	.1244	.1369	.1482	.1578	.1654	.1709	.1743	.1754	.1743	.1712
8	.0744	.0869	.0996	.1121	.1241	.1351	.1450	.1535	.1602	.1651
9	.0373	.0463	.0562	.0669	.0781	.0897	.1013	.1127	.1236	.1336
10	.0159	.0209	.0269	.0338	.0417	.0504	.0600	.0701	.0808	.0916

(Continued)

TABLE A.7 (Continued)

					n=25					
r \ p	.21	.22	.23	.24	.25	.26	.27	.28	.29	.50
11	.0058	.0080	.0109	.0145	.0189	.0242	.0302	.0372	.0450	.0536
12	.0018	.0026	.0038	.0054	.0074	.0099	.0130	.0169	.0214	.0268
13	.0005	.0007	.0011	.0017	.0025	.0035	.0048	.0066	.0088	.0115
14	.0001	.0002	.0003	.0005	.0007	.0010	.0015	.0022	.0031	.0042
15	.0000	.0000	.0001	.0001	.0002	.0003	.0004	.0006	.0009	.0013
16	.0000	.0000	.0000	.0000	.0000	0001	.0001	.0002	.0002	.0004
17	.0000	.0000	.0000	.0000	.0000	.0000	.0000	.0000	.0001	.0001
	.31	.32	.33	.34	.35	.36	.37	.38	.39	.40
0	.0001	.0001	.0000	.0000	.0000	.0000	.0000	.0000	.0000	.0000
1	.0011	.0008	.0006	.0004	.0003	.0002	.0001	.0001	.0001	.0000
2	.0057	.0043	.0033	.0025	.0018	.0014	.0010	.0007	.0005	.0004
3	.0195	.0156	.0123	.0097	.0076	.0058	.0045	.0034	.0026	.0019
4	.0482	.0403	.0334	.0274	.0224	.0181	.0145	.0115	.0091	.0071
5	.0910	.0797	.0691	.0594	.0506	.0427	.0357	.0297	.0244	.0199
6	.1363	.1250	.1134	.1020	.0908	.0801	.0700	.0606	.0520	.0442
7	.1662	.1596	.1516	.1426	.1327	.1222	.1115	.1008	.0902	.0800
8	.1680	.1690	.1681	.1652	.1607	.1547	.1474	.1390	.1298	.1200
9	.1426	.1502	.1563	.1608	.1635	.1644	.1635	.1609	.1567	.1511
10	.1025	.1131	.1232	.1325	.1409	.1479	.1536	.1578	.1603	.1612
11	.0628	.0726	.0828	.0931	.1034	.1135	.1230	.1319	.1398	.1465
12	.0329	.0399	.0476	.0560	.0650	.0745	.0843	.0943	.1043	.1140
13	.0148	.0188	.0234	.0288	.0350	.0419	.0495	.0578	.0667	.0760
14	.0057	.0076	.0099	.0127	.0161	.0202	.0249	.0304	.0365	.0434
15	.0019	.0026	.0036	.0048	.0064	.0083	.0107	.0136	.0171	.0212
16	.0005	.0008	.0011	.0015	.0021	.0029	.0039	.0052	.0068	.0088
17	.0001	.0002	.0003	.0004	.0006	.0009	.0012	.0017	.0023	.0031
18	.0000	.0000	.0001	.0001	.0001	.0002	.0003	.0005	.0007	.0009
19	.0000	.0000	.0000	.0000	.0000	.0000	.0001	.0001	.0002	.0002
	.41	.42	.43	.44	.45	.46	.47	.48	.49	.50
0	.0000	.0000	.0000	.0000	.0000	.0000	.0000	.0000	.0000	.0000
1	.0000	.0000	.0000	.0000	.0000	.0000	.0000	.0000	.0000	.0000
2	.0003	.0002	.0001	.0001	.0001	.0000	.0000	.0000	.0000	.0000
3	.0014	.0011	.0008	.0006	.0004	.0003	.0002	.0001	.0001	.0001
4	.0055	.0042	.0032	.0024	.0018	.0014	.0010	.0007	.0005	.0004
5	.0161	.0129	.0102	.0081	.0063	.0049	.0037	.0028	.0021	.0016
6	.0372	.0311	.0257	.0211	.0172	.0138	.0110	.0087	.0068	.0053
7	.0703	.0611	.0527	.0450	.0381	.0319	.0265	.0218	.0178	.0143
8	.1099	.0996	.0895	.0796	.0701	.0612	.0529	.0453	.0384	.0322

(Continued)

TABLE A.7   (Continued)

					n=25					
r \ p	.41	.42	.43	.44	.45	.46	.47	.48	.49	.50
9	.1442	.1363	.1275	.1181	.1084	.0985	.0886	.0790	.0697	.0609
10	.1603	.1579	.1539	.1485	.1419	.1342	.1257	.1166	.1071	.0974
11	.1519	.1559	.1583	.1591	.1583	.1559	.1521	.1468	.1404	.1328
12	.1232	.1317	.1393	.1458	.1511	.1550	.1573	.1581	.1573	.1550
13	.0856	.0954	.1051	.1146	.1236	.1320	.1395	.1460	.1512	.1550
14	.0510	.0592	.0680	.0772	.0867	.0964	.1060	.1155	.1245	.1328
15	.0260	.0314	.0376	.0445	.0520	.0602	.0690	.0782	.0877	.0974
16	.0113	.0142	.0177	.0218	.0266	.0321	.0382	.0451	.0527	.0609
17	.0042	.0055	.0071	.0091	.0115	.0145	.0179	.0220	.0268	.0322
18	.0013	.0018	.0024	.0032	.0042	.0055	.0071	.0090	.0114	.0143
19	.0003	.0005	.0007	.0009	.0013	.0017	.0023	.0031	.0040	.0053
20	.0001	.0001	.0001	.0002	.0003	.0004	.0006	.0009	.0012	.0016
21	.0000	.0000	.0000	.0000	.0001	.0001	.0001	.0002	.0003	.0004
22	.0000	.0000	.0000	.0000	.0000	.0000	.0000	.0000	.0000	.0001

TABLE A.8 Wilcoxon Table (d-Factors for Wilcoxon Signed-Rank Test and Confidence Intervals for the Median (α' = One-Sided Significance Level, α'' = Two-Sided Significance Level)

n	d	Confidence coefficient	α''	α'	n	d	Confidence coefficient	α''	α''
3	1	.750	.250	.125	14	13	.991	.009	.004
4	1	.875	.125	.063		14	.989	.011	.005
5	1	.938	.062	.031		22	.951	.049	.025
	2	.875	.125	.063		23	.942	.058	.029
6	1	.969	.031	.016		26	.909	.091	.045
	2	.937	.063	.031		27	.896	.104	.052
	3	.906	.094	.047	15	16	.992	.008	.004
	4	.844	.156	.078		17	.990	.010	.005
7	1	.984	.016	.008		26	.952	.048	.024
	2	.969	.031	.016		27	.945	.055	.028
	4	.922	.078	.039		31	.905	.095	.047
	5	.891	.109	.055		32	.893	.107	.054
8	1	.992	.008	.004	16	20	.991	.009	.005
	2	.984	.016	.008		21	.989	.011	.006
	4	.961	.039	.020		30	.956	.044	.022
	5	.945	.055	.027		31	.949	.051	.025
	6	.922	.078	.039		36	.907	.093	.047
	7	.891	.109	.055		37	.895	.105	.052
9	2	.992	.008	.004	17	24	.991	.009	.005
	3	.988	.012	.006		25	.989	.011	.006
	6	.961	.039	.020		35	.955	.045	.022
	7	.945	.055	.027		36	.949	.051	.025
	9	.902	.098	.049		42	.902	.098	.049
	10	.871	.129	.065		43	.891	.109	.054
10	4	.990	.010	.005	18	28	.991	.009	.005
	5	.986	.014	.007		29	.990	.010	.005
	9	.951	.049	.024		41	.952	.048	.024
	10	.936	.064	.032		42	.946	.054	.027
	11	.916	.084	.042		48	.901	.099	.049
	12	.895	.105	.053		49	.892	.108	.054
11	6	.990	.010	.005	19	33	.991	.009	.005
	7	.986	.014	.007		34	.989	.011	.005
	11	.958	.042	.021		47	.951	.049	.025
	12	.946	.054	.027		48	.945	.055	.027
	14	.917	.083	.042		54	.904	.096	.048
	15	.898	.102	.051		55	.896	.104	.052

(Continued)

TABLE A.8   (Continued)

n	d	Confidence coefficient	α''	α'	n	d	Confidence coefficient	α''	α'
12	8	.991	.009	.005	20	38	.991	.009	.005
	9	.988	.012	.006		39	.989	.011	.005
	14	.958	.042	.021		53	.952	.048	.024
	15	.948	.052	.026		54	.947	.053	.027
	18	.908	.092	.046		61	.903	.097	.049
	19	.890	.110	.055		62	.895	.105	.053
13	10	.992	.008	.004	21	43	.991	.009	.005
	11	.990	.010	.005		44	.990	.010	.005
	18	.952	.048	.024		59	.954	.046	.023
	19	.943	.057	.029		60	.950	.050	.025
	22	.906	.094	.047		68	.904	.096	.048
	23	.890	.110	.055		69	.897	.103	.052
22	49	.991	.009	.005	24	62	.990	.010	.005
	50	.990	.010	.005		63	.989	.011	.005
	66	.954	.046	.023		82	.951	.049	.025
	67	.950	.050	.025		83	.947	.053	.026
	76	.902	.098	.049		92	.905	.095	.048
	77	.895	.105	.053		93	.899	.101	.051
23	55	.991	.009	.005	25	69	.990	.010	.005
	56	.990	.010	.005		70	.989	.011	.005
	74	.952	.048	.024		90	.952	.048	.024
	75	.948	.052	.026		91	.948	.052	.026
	84	.902	.098	.049		101	.904	.096	.048
	85	.895	.105	.052		102	.899	.101	.051

Source: Wilcoxon F, Katti S, Wilcox RA. Critical Values and Probability Levels for the Wilcoxon Rank Sum Test and the Wilcoxon Signed Rank Test. Pearl River, NY: American Cyanamid Co., 1949; used by permission of American Cyanamid Company.

TABLE A.9   Critical Values of the Kruskal–Wallis Test

n_1	n_2	n_3	Critical value	α	n_1	n_2	n_3	Critical value	α
Sample sizes					Sample sizes				

n_1	n_2	n_3	Critical value	α	n_1	n_2	n_3	Critical value	α
2	1	1	2.7000	0.500				4.7000	0.101
2	2	1	3.6000	0.200	4	4	1	6.6667	0.010
2	2	2	4.5714	0.067				6.1667	0.022
			3.7143	0.200				4.9667	0.048
3	1	1	3.2000	0.300				4.8667	0.054
3	2	1	4.2857	0.100				4.1667	0.082
			3.8571	0.133				4.0667	0.102
3	2	2	5.3572	0.029	4	4	2	7.0364	0.006
			4.7143	0.048				6.8727	0.011
			4.5000	0.067				5.4545	0.046
			4.4643	0.105				5.2364	0.052
3	3	1	5.1429	0.043				4.5545	0.098
			4.5714	0.100				4.4455	0.103
			4.0000	0.129	4	4	3	7.1439	0.010
3	3	2	6.2500	0.011				7.1364	0.011
			5.3611	0.032				5.5985	0.049
			5.1389	0.061				5.5758	0.051
			4.5556	0.100				4.5455	0.099
			4.2500	0.121				4.4773	0.102
3	3	3	7.2000	0.004	4	4	4	7.6538	0.008
			6.4889	0.011				7.5385	0.011
			5.6889	0.029				5.6923	0.049
			5.6000	0.050				5.6538	0.054
			5.0667	0.086				4.6539	0.097
			4.6222	0.100				4.5001	0.104
4	1	1	3.5714	0.200	5	1	1	3.8571	0.143
4	2	1	4.8214	0.057	5	2	1	5.2500	0.036
			4.5000	0.076				5.0000	0.048
			4.0179	0.114				4.4500	0.071
4	2	2	6.0000	0.014				4.2000	0.095
			5.3333	0.033				4.0500	0.119
			5.1250	0.052	5	2	2	6.5333	0.008
			4.4583	0.100				6.1333	0.013
			4.1667	0.105				5.1600	0.034
4	3	1	5.8333	0.021				5.0400	0.056
			5.2083	0.050				4.3733	0.090
			5.0000	0.057				4.2933	0.122
			4.0556	0.093	5	3	1	6.4000	0.012
			3.8889	0.129				4.9600	0.048

(Continued)

TABLE A.9   (Continued)

n_1	n_2	n_3	Critical value	α	n_1	n_2	n_3	Critical value	α
Sample sizes					Sample sizes				
4	3	2	6.4444	0.008				4.8711	0.052
			6.3000	0.011				4.0178	0.095
			5.4444	0.046				3.8400	0.123
			5.4000	0.051	5	3	2	6.9091	0.009
			4.5111	0.098				6.8218	0.010
			4.4444	0.102				5.2509	0.049
4	3	3	6.7455	0.010				5.1055	0.052
			6.7091	0.013				4.6509	0.091
			5.7909	0.046				4.4945	0.101
			5.7273	0.050	5	3	3	7.0788	0.009
			4.7091	0.092				6.9818	0.011
5	3	3	5.6485	0.049	5	5	1	6.8364	0.011
			5.5152	0.051				5.1273	0.046
			4.5333	0.097				4.9091	0.053
			4.4121	0.109				4.1091	0.086
5	4	1	6.9545	0.008				4.0364	0.105
			6.8400	0.011	5	5	2	7.3385	0.010
			4.9855	0.044				7.2692	0.010
			4.8600	0.056				5.3385	0.047
			3.9873	0.098				5.2462	0.051
			3.9600	0.102				4.6231	0.097
5	4	2	7.2045	0.009				4.5077	0.100
			7.1182	0.010	5	5	3	7.5780	0.010
			5.2727	0.049				7.5429	0.010
			5.2682	0.050				5.7055	0.046
			4.5409	0.098				5.6264	0.051
			4.5182	0.101				4.5451	0.100
5	4	3	7.4449	0.010				4.5363	0.102
			7.3949	0.011	5	5	4	7.8229	0.010
			5.6564	0.049				7.7914	0.010
			5.6308	0.050				5.6657	0.049
			4.5487	0.099				5.6429	0.050
			4.5231	0.103				4.5229	0.099
5	4	4	7.7604	0.009				4.5200	0.101
			7.7440	0.011	5	5	5	8.0000	0.009
			5.6571	0.049				7.9800	0.010
			5.6176	0.050				5.7800	0.049
			4.6187	0.100				5.6600	0.051
			4.5527	0.102				4.5600	0.100
5	5	1	7.3091	0.009				4.5000	0.102

Source: Kruskal WH, Wallis WA. Use of ranks in one-criterion analysis of variance. *J Am Stat Assoc* 47:583–621, 1952. Addendum. Ibid 48:907–911, 1953.

TABLE A.10   Chi Square Table

df	$1-\alpha=\chi^2_{0.005}$	$\chi^2_{0.025}$	$\chi^2_{0.05}$	$\alpha=0.10$ $\chi^2_{0.90}$	0.05 $\chi^2_{0.95}$	0.025 $\chi^2_{0.975}$	0.01 $\chi^2_{0.99}$	0.005 $\chi^2_{0.995}$
1	0.0000393	0.000982	0.00393	2.706	3.841	5.024	6.635	7.879
2	0.0100	0.0506	0.103	4.605	5.991	7.378	9.210	10.597
3	0.0717	0.216	0.352	6.251	7.815	9.348	11.345	12.838
4	0.207	0.484	0.711	7.779	9.488	11.143	13.277	14.860
5	0.412	0.831	1.145	9.236	11.070	12.832	15.086	16.750
6	0.676	1.237	1.635	10.645	12.592	14.449	16.812	18.548
7	0.989	1.690	2.167	12.017	14.067	16.013	18.475	20.278
8	1.344	2.180	2.733	13.362	15.507	17.535	20.090	21.955
9	1.735	2.700	3.325	14.684	16.919	19.023	21.666	23.589
10	2.156	3.247	3.940	15.987	18.307	20.483	23.209	25.188
11	2.603	3.816	4.575	17.275	19.675	21.920	24.725	26.757
12	3.074	4.404	5.226	18.549	21.026	23.336	26.217	28.300
13	3.565	5.009	5.892	19.812	22.362	24.736	27.688	29.819
14	4.075	5.629	6.571	21.064	23.685	26.119	29.141	31.319
15	4.601	6.262	7.261	22.307	24.996	27.488	30.578	32.801
16	5.142	6.908	7.962	23.542	26.296	28.845	32.000	34.267
17	5.697	7.564	8.672	24.769	27.587	30.191	33.409	35.718
18	6.265	8.231	9.390	25.989	28.869	31.526	34.805	37.156
19	6.844	8.907	10.117	27.204	30.144	32.852	36.191	38.582
20	7.434	9.591	10.851	28.412	31.410	34.170	37.566	39.997
21	8.034	10.283	11.591	29.615	32.671	35.479	38.932	41.401
22	8.643	10.982	12.338	30.813	33.924	36.781	40.289	42.796
23	9.260	11.688	13.091	32.007	35.172	38.076	41.638	44.181
24	9.886	12.401	13.848	33.196	36.415	39.364	42.980	45.558
25	10.520	13.120	14.611	34.382	37.652	40.646	44.314	46.928
26	11.160	13.844	15.379	35.563	38.885	41.923	45.642	48.290
27	11.808	14.573	16.151	36.741	40.113	43.194	46.963	49.645
28	12.461	15.308	16.928	37.916	41.337	44.461	48.278	50.993
29	13.121	16.047	17.708	39.087	42.557	45.722	49.588	52.336
30	13.787	16.791	18.493	40.256	43.773	46.979	50.892	53.672
35	17.192	20.569	22.465	46.059	49.802	53.203	57.342	60.275
40	20.707	24.433	26.509	51.805	55.758	59.342	63.691	66.766
45	24.311	28.366	30.612	57.505	61.656	65.410	69.957	73.166
50	27.991	32.357	34.764	63.167	67.505	71.420	76.154	79.490
60	35.535	40.482	43.188	74.397	79.082	83.298	88.379	91.952
70	43.275	48.758	51.739	85.527	90.531	95.023	100.425	104.215
80	51.172	57.153	60.391	96.578	101.879	106.629	112.329	116.321
90	59.196	65.647	69.126	107.565	113.145	118.136	124.116	128.299
100	67.328	74.222	77.929	118.498	124.342	129.561	135.807	140.169

Source: Adapted from: Hald A, Sinkbaek SA. A table of percentage points of the χ^2 distribution. Skand Aktuarietidskr 33:168–175, 1950.

TABLE A.11   Friedman ANOVA Table [Exact distribution of χ_r^2 for Tables with Two to Nine Sets of Three Ranks ($l = 3$; $k = 2, 3, 4, 5, 6, 7, 8, 9$] p is the probability of obtaining a value of χ_r^2 as great as or greater than the corresponding value of χ_r^2

k = 2		k = 3		k = 4		k = 5	
χ_r^2	p	χ_r^2	p	χ_r^2	p	χ_r^2	p
0	1.000	0.000	1.000	0.0	1.000	0.0	1.000
1	0.833	0.667	0.944	0.5	0.931	0.4	0.954
3	0.500	2.000	0.528	1.5	0.653	1.2	0.691
4	0.167	2.667	0.361	2.0	0.431	1.6	0.522
		4.667	0.194	3.5	0.273	2.8	0.367
		6.000	0.028	4.5	0.125	3.6	0.182
				6.0	0.069	4.8	0.124
				6.5	0.042	5.2	0.093
				8.0	0.0046	6.4	0.039
						7.6	0.024
						8.4	0.0085
						10.0	0.00077

k = 6		k = 7		k = 8		k = 9	
χ_r^2	p	χ_r^2	p	χ_r^2	p	χ_r^2	p
0.00	1.000	0.000	1.000	0.00	1.000	0.000	1.000
0.33	0.956	0.286	0.964	0.25	0.967	0.222	0.971
1.00	0.740	0.857	0.768	0.75	0.794	0.667	0.814
1.33	0.570	1.143	0.620	1.00	0.654	0.889	0.865
2.33	0.430	2.000	0.486	1.75	0.531	1.556	0.569
3.00	0.252	2.571	0.305	2.25	0.355	2.000	0.398
4.00	0.184	3.429	0.237	3.00	0.285	2.667	0.328
4.33	0.142	3.714	0.192	3.25	0.236	2.889	0.278
5.33	0.072	4.571	0.112	4.00	0.149	3.556	0.187
6.33	0.052	5.429	0.085	4.75	0.120	4.222	0.154
7.00	0.029	6.000	0.052	5.25	0.079	4.667	0.107
8.33	0.012	7.143	0.027	6.25	0.047	5.556	0.069
9.00	0.0081	7.714	0.021	6.75	0.038	6.000	0.057
9.33	0.0055	8.000	0.016	7.00	0.030	6.222	0.048
10.33	0.0017	8.857	0.0084	7.75	0.018	6.889	0.031
12.00	0.00013	10.286	0.0036	9.00	0.0099	8.000	0.019
		10.571	0.0027	9.25	0.0080	8.222	0.016
		11.143	0.0012	9.75	0.0048	8.667	0.010
		12.286	0.00032	10.75	0.0024	9.556	0.0060
		14.000	0.000021	12.00	0.0011	10.667	0.0035
				12.25	0.00086	10.889	0.0029

(Continued)

Table A.11   (Continued)

n = 6		n = 7		n = 8		n = 9	
χ_r^2	p	χ_r^2	p	χ_r^2	p	χ_r^2	p
				13.00	0.00026	11.556	0.0013
				14.25	0.000061	12.667	0.00066
				16.00	0.0000036	13.556	0.00035
						14.000	0.00020
						14.222	0.000097
						14.889	0.000054
						16.222	0.000011
						18.000	0.0000006

$l = 4;\ k = 2, 3, 4$

k = 2		k = 3				k = 4	
χ_r^2	p	χ_r^2	p	χ_r^2	p	χ_r^2	p
0.0	1.000	0.2	1.000	0.0	1.000	5.7	0.141
0.6	0.958	0.6	0.958	0.3	0.992	6.0	0.105
1.2	0.834	1.0	0.910	0.6	0.928	6.3	0.094
1.8	0.792	1.8	0.727	0.9	0.900	6.6	0.077
2.4	0.625	2.2	0.608	1.2	0.800	6.9	0.068
3.0	0.542	2.6	0.524	1.5	0.754	7.2	0.054
3.6	0.458	3.4	0.446	1.8	0.677	7.5	0.052
4.2	0.375	3.8	0.342	2.1	0.649	7.8	0.036
4.8	0.208	4.2	0.300	2.4	0.524	8.1	0.033
5.4	0.167	5.0	0.207	2.7	0.508	8.4	0.019
6.0	0.042	5.4	0.175	3.0	0.432	8.7	0.014
		5.8	0.148	3.3	0.389	9.3	0.012
		6.6	0.075	3.6	0.355	9.6	0.0069
		7.0	0.054	3.9	0.324	9.9	0.0062
		7.4	0.033	4.5	0.242	10.2	0.0027
		8.2	0.017	4.8	0.200	10.8	0.0016
		9.0	0.0017	5.1	0.190	11.1	0.00094
				5.4	0.158	12.0	0.000072

Source: Friedman M. The use of ranks to avoid the assumption of normality implicit in the analysis of variance. J Am Stat Assoc 32:675–701, 1937.

TABLE A.12 Studentized Range Table

$q_{0.05}(p, f)$

f \ p	2	3	4	5	6	7	8	9	10	11	12	13	14	15	16	17	18	19	20
1	18.1	26.7	32.8	37.2	40.5	43.1	45.4	47.3	49.1	50.6	51.9	53.2	54.3	55.4	56.3	57.2	58.0	58.8	59.6
2	6.09	8.28	9.80	10.89	11.73	12.43	13.03	13.54	13.99	14.39	14.75	15.08	15.38	15.65	15.91	16.14	16.36	16.57	16.77
3	4.50	5.88	6.83	7.51	8.04	8.47	8.85	9.18	9.46	9.72	9.95	10.16	10.35	10.52	10.69	10.84	10.98	11.12	11.24
4	3.93	5.00	5.76	6.31	6.73	7.06	7.35	7.60	7.83	8.03	8.21	8.37	8.52	8.67	8.80	8.92	9.03	9.14	9.24
5	3.64	4.60	5.22	5.67	6.03	6.33	6.58	6.80	6.99	7.17	7.32	7.47	7.60	7.72	7.83	7.93	8.03	8.12	8.21
6	3.46	4.34	4.90	5.31	5.63	5.89	6.12	6.32	6.49	6.65	6.79	6.92	7.04	7.14	7.24	7.34	7.43	7.51	7.59
7	3.34	4.16	4.68	5.06	5.35	5.59	5.80	5.99	6.15	6.29	6.42	6.54	6.65	6.75	6.84	6.93	7.01	7.08	7.16
8	3.26	4.04	4.53	4.89	5.17	5.40	5.60	5.77	5.92	6.05	6.18	6.29	6.39	6.48	6.57	6.65	6.73	6.80	6.87
9	3.20	3.95	4.42	4.76	5.02	5.24	5.43	5.60	5.74	5.87	5.98	6.09	6.19	6.28	6.36	6.44	6.51	6.58	6.65
10	3.15	3.88	4.33	4.66	4.91	5.12	5.30	5.46	5.60	5.72	5.83	5.93	6.03	6.12	6.20	6.27	6.34	6.41	6.47
11	3.11	3.82	4.26	4.58	4.82	5.03	5.20	5.35	5.49	5.61	5.71	5.81	5.90	5.98	6.06	6.14	6.20	6.27	6.33
12	3.08	3.77	4.20	4.51	4.75	4.95	5.12	5.27	5.40	5.51	5.61	5.71	5.80	5.88	5.95	6.02	6.09	6.15	6.21
13	3.06	3.73	4.15	4.46	4.69	4.88	5.05	5.19	5.32	5.43	5.53	5.63	5.71	5.79	5.86	5.93	6.00	6.06	6.11
14	3.03	3.70	4.11	4.41	4.64	4.83	4.99	5.13	5.25	5.36	5.46	5.56	5.64	5.72	5.79	5.86	5.92	5.98	6.03
15	3.01	3.67	4.08	4.37	4.59	4.78	4.94	5.08	5.20	5.31	5.40	5.49	5.57	5.65	5.72	5.79	5.85	5.91	5.96
16	3.00	3.65	4.05	4.34	4.56	4.74	4.90	5.03	5.15	5.26	5.35	5.44	5.52	5.59	5.66	5.73	5.79	5.84	5.90
17	2.98	3.62	4.02	4.31	4.52	4.70	4.86	4.99	5.11	5.21	5.31	5.39	5.47	5.55	5.61	5.68	5.74	5.79	5.84
18	2.97	3.61	4.00	4.28	4.49	4.67	4.83	4.96	5.07	5.17	5.27	5.35	5.43	5.50	5.57	5.63	5.69	5.74	5.79
19	2.96	3.59	3.98	4.26	4.47	4.64	4.79	4.92	5.04	5.14	5.23	5.32	5.39	5.46	5.53	5.59	5.65	5.70	5.75
20	2.95	3.58	3.96	4.24	4.45	4.62	4.77	4.90	5.01	5.11	5.20	5.28	5.36	5.43	5.50	5.56	5.61	5.66	5.71

(Continued)

TABLE A.12 (Continued)

$q_{0.05}(p, f)$

f \ p	2	3	4	5	6	7	8	9	10	11	12	13	14	15	16	17	18	19	20
24	2.92	3.53	3.90	4.17	4.37	4.54	4.68	4.81	4.92	5.01	5.10	5.18	5.25	5.32	5.38	5.44	5.50	5.55	5.59
30	2.89	3.48	3.84	4.11	4.30	4.46	4.60	4.72	4.83	4.92	5.00	5.08	5.15	5.21	5.27	5.33	5.38	5.43	5.48
40	2.86	3.44	3.79	4.04	4.23	4.39	4.52	4.63	4.74	4.82	4.90	4.98	5.05	5.11	5.17	5.22	5.27	5.32	5.36
60	2.83	3.40	3.74	3.98	4.16	4.31	4.44	4.55	4.65	4.73	4.81	4.88	4.94	5.00	5.06	5.11	5.15	5.20	5.24
120	2.80	3.36	3.69	3.92	4.10	4.24	4.36	4.47	4.56	4.64	4.71	4.78	4.84	4.90	4.95	5.00	5.04	5.09	5.13
∞	2.77	3.32	3.63	3.86	4.03	4.17	4.29	4.39	4.47	4.55	4.62	4.68	4.74	4.80	4.84	4.89	4.93	4.97	5.01

$q_{0.01}(p, f)$

f \ p	2	3	4	5	6	7	8	9	10	11	12	13	14	15	16	17	18	19	20
1	90.0	135	164	186	202	216	227	237	246	253	260	266	272	277	282	286	290	294	298
2	14.0	19.0	22.3	24.7	26.6	28.2	29.5	30.7	31.7	32.6	33.4	34.1	34.8	35.4	36.0	36.5	37.0	37.5	37.9
3	8.26	10.6	12.2	13.3	14.2	15.0	15.6	16.2	16.7	17.1	17.5	17.9	18.2	18.5	18.8	19.1	19.3	19.5	19.8
4	6.51	8.12	9.17	9.96	10.6	11.1	11.5	11.9	12.3	12.6	12.8	13.1	13.3	13.5	13.7	13.9	14.1	14.2	14.4
5	5.70	6.97	7.80	8.42	8.91	9.32	9.67	9.97	10.24	10.48	10.70	10.89	11.08	11.24	11.40	11.55	11.68	11.81	11.93
6	5.24	6.33	7.03	7.56	7.97	8.32	8.61	8.87	9.10	9.30	9.49	9.65	9.81	9.95	10.08	10.21	10.32	10.43	10.54
7	4.95	5.92	6.54	7.01	7.37	7.68	7.94	8.17	8.37	8.55	8.71	8.86	9.00	9.12	9.24	9.35	9.46	9.55	9.65
8	4.74	5.63	6.20	6.63	6.96	7.24	7.47	7.68	7.87	8.03	8.18	8.31	8.44	8.55	8.66	8.76	8.85	8.94	9.03
9	4.60	5.43	5.96	6.35	6.66	6.91	7.13	7.32	7.49	7.65	7.78	7.91	8.03	8.13	8.23	8.32	8.41	8.49	8.57
10	4.48	5.27	5.77	6.14	6.43	6.67	6.87	7.05	7.21	7.36	7.48	7.60	7.71	7.81	7.91	7.99	8.07	8.15	8.22

(Continued)

TABLE A.12 (Continued)

$$q_{0.01}(p, f)$$

$f \backslash p$	2	3	4	5	6	7	8	9	10	11	12	13	14	15	16	17	18	19	20
11	4.39	5.14	5.62	5.97	6.25	6.48	6.67	6.84	6.99	7.13	7.25	7.36	7.46	7.56	7.65	7.73	7.81	7.88	7.95
12	4.32	5.04	5.50	5.84	6.10	6.32	6.51	6.67	6.81	6.94	7.16	7.17	7.26	7.36	7.44	7.52	7.59	7.66	7.73
13	4.26	4.96	5.40	5.73	5.98	6.19	6.37	6.53	6.67	6.79	6.90	7.01	7.10	7.19	7.27	7.34	7.42	7.48	7.55
14	4.21	4.89	5.32	5.63	5.88	6.08	6.26	6.41	6.54	6.66	6.77	6.87	6.96	7.05	7.12	7.20	7.27	7.33	7.39
15	4.17	4.83	5.25	5.56	5.80	5.99	6.16	6.31	6.44	6.55	6.66	6.76	6.84	6.93	7.00	7.07	7.14	7.20	7.26
16	4.13	4.78	5.19	5.49	5.72	5.92	6.08	6.22	6.35	6.46	6.56	6.66	6.74	6.82	6.90	6.97	7.03	7.09	7.15
17	4.10	4.74	5.14	5.43	5.66	5.85	6.01	6.15	6.27	6.38	6.48	6.57	6.66	6.73	6.80	6.87	6.94	7.00	7.05
18	4.07	4.70	5.09	5.38	5.60	5.79	5.94	6.08	6.20	6.31	6.41	6.50	6.58	6.65	6.72	6.79	6.85	6.91	6.96
19	4.05	4.67	5.05	5.33	5.55	5.73	5.89	6.02	6.14	6.25	6.34	6.43	6.51	6.58	6.65	6.72	6.78	6.84	6.89
20	4.02	4.64	5.02	5.29	5.51	5.69	5.84	5.97	6.09	6.19	6.29	6.37	6.45	6.52	6.59	6.65	6.71	6.76	6.82
24	3.96	4.54	4.91	5.17	5.37	5.54	5.69	5.81	5.92.	6.02	6.11	6.19	6.26	6.33	6.39	6.45	6.51	6.56	6.61
30	3.89	4.45	4.80	5.05	5.24	5.40	5.54	5.65.	5.76	5.85	5.93	6.01	6.08	6.14	6.20	6.26	6.31	6.36	6.41
40	3.82	4.37	4.70	4.93	5.11	5.27	5.39	5.50	5.60	5.69	5.77	5.84	5.90	5.96	6.02	6.07	6.12	6.17	6.21
60	3.76	4.28	4.60	4.82	4.99	5.13	5.25	5.36	5.45	5.53	5.60	5.67	5.73	5.79	5.84	5.89	5.93	5.98	6.02
120	3.70	4.20	4.50	4.71	4.87	5.01	5.12	5.21	5.30	5.38	5.44	5.51	5.56	5.61	5.66	5.71	5.75	5.79	5.83
∞	3.64	4.12	4.40	4.60	4.76	4.88	4.99	5.08	5.16	5.23	5.29	5.35	5.40	5.45	5.49	5.54	5.57	5.61	5.65

f = degrees of freedom.

Source: Adapted from May JM. Extended and corrected tables of the upper percentage points of the studentized range. *Biometrika* 39:192–193, 1952.

TABLE A.13   Critical Values for Dunnett's Test (Treatments vs. Control)

$$d_{0.05}(a-1,f)$$

Two-Sided Comparisons

$a-1 =$ Number of Treatment Means (excluding control)

f	1	2	3	4	5	6	7	8	9
5	2.57	3.03	3.29	3.48	3.62	3.73	3.82	3.90	3.97
6	2.45	2.86	3.10	3.26	3.39	3.49	3.57	3.64	3.71
7	2.36	2.75	2.97	3.12	3.24	3.33	3.41	3.47	3.53
8	2.31	2.67	2.88	3.02	3.13	3.22	3.29	3.35	3.41
9	2.26	2.61	2.81	2.95	3.05	3.14	3.20	3.26	3.32
10	2.23	2.57	2.76	2.89	2.99	3.07	3.14	3.19	3.24
11	2.20	2.53	2.72	2.84	2.94	3.02	3.08	3.14	3.19
12	2.18	2.50	2.68	2.81	2.90	2.98	3.04	3.09	3.14
13	2.16	2.48	2.65	2.78	2.87	2.94	3.00	3.06	3.10
14	2.14	2.46	2.63	2.75	2.84	2.91	2.97	3.02	3.07
15	2.13	2.44	2.61	2.73	2.82	2.89	2.95	3.00	3.04
16	2.12	2.42	2.59	2.71	2.80	2.87	2.92	2.97	3.02
17	2.11	2.41	2.58	2.69	2.78	2.85	2.90	2.95	3.00
18	2.10	2.40	2.56	2.68	2.76	2.83	2.89	2.94	2.98
19	2.09	2.39	2.55	2.66	2.75	2.81	2.87	2.92	2.96
20	2.09	2.38	2.54	2.65	2.73	2.80	2.86	2.90	2.95
24	2.06	2.35	2.51	2.61	2.70	2.76	2.81	2.86	2.90
30	2.04	2.32	2.47	2.58	2.66	2.72	2.77	2.82	2.86
40	2.02	2.29	2.44	2.54	2.62	2.68	2.73	2.77	2.81
60	2.00	2.27	2.41	2.51	2.58	2.64	2.69	2.73	2.77
120	1.98	2.24	2.38	2.47	2.55	2.60	2.65	2.69	2.73
∞	1.96	2.21	2.35	2.44	2.51	2.57	2.61	2.65	2.69

$$d_{0.01}(a-1,f)$$

Two-Sided Comparisons

$a-1 =$ Number of Treatment Means (excluding control)

f	1	2	3	4	5	6	7	8	9
5	4.03	4.63	4.98	5.22	5.41	5.56	5.69	5.80	5.89
6	3.71	4.21	4.51	4.71	4.87	5.00	5.10	5.20	5.28
7	3.50	3.95	4.21	4.39	4.53	4.64	4.74	4.82	4.89
8	3.36	3.77	4.00	4.17	4.29	4.40	4.48	4.56	4.62
9	3.25	3.63	3.85	4.01	4.12	4.22	4.30	4.37	4.43
10	3.17	3.53	3.74	3.88	3.99	4.08	4.16	4.22	4.28
11	3.11	3.45	3.65	3.79	3.89	3.98	4.05	4.11	4.16
12	3.05	3.39	3.58	3.71	3.81	3.89	3.96	4.02	4.07
13	3.01	3.33	3.52	3.65	3.74	3.82	3.89	3.94	3.99

(Continued)

TABLE A.13 (Continued)

14	2.98	3.29	3.47	3.59	3.69	3.76	3.83	3.88	3.93
15	2.95	3.25	3.43	3.55	3.64	3.71	3.78	3.83	3.88
16	2.92	3.22	3.39	3.51	3.60	3.67	3.73	3.78	3.83
17	2.90	3.19	3.36	3.47	3.56	3.63	3.69	3.74	3.79
18	2.88	3.17	3.33	3.44	3.53	3.60	3.66	3.71	3.75
19	2.86	3.15	3.31	3.42	3.50	3.57	3.63	3.68	3.72
20	2.85	3.13	3.29	3.40	3.48	3.55	3.60	3.65	3.69
24	2.80	3.07	3.22	3.32	3.40	3.47	3.52	3.57	3.61
30	2.75	3.01	3.15	3.25	3.33	3.39	3.44	3.49	3.52
40	2.70	2.95	3.09	3.19	3.26	3.32	3.37	3.41	3.44
60	2.66	2.90	3.03	3.12	3.19	3.25	3.29	3.33	3.37
120	2.62	2.85	2.97	3.06	3.12	3.18	3.22	3.26	3.29
∞	2.58	2.79	2.92	3.00	3.06	3.11	3.15	3.19	3.22

$$d_{0.05}(a-1, f)$$
One-Sided Comparisons
$a-1$ = Number of Treatment Means (excluding control)

f	1	2	3	4	5	6	7	8	9
5	2.02	2.44	2.68	2.85	2.98	3.08	3.16	3.24	3.30
6	1.94	2.34	2.56	2.71	2.83	2.92	3.00	3.07	3.12
7	1.89	2.27	2.48	2.62	2.73	2.82	2.89	2.95	3.01
8	1.86	2.22	2.42	2.55	2.66	2.74	2.81	2.87	2.92
9	1.83	2.18	2.37	2.50	2.60	2.68	2.75	2.81	2.86
10	1.81	2.15	2.34	2.47	2.56	2.64	2.70	2.76	2.81
11	1.80	2.13	2.31	2.44	2.53	2.60	2.67	2.72	2.77
12	1.78	2.11	2.29	2.41	2.50	2.58	2.64	2.69	2.74
13	1.77	2.09	2.27	2.39	2.48	2.55	2.61	2.66	2.71
14	1.76	2.08	2.25	2.37	2.46	2.53	2.59	2.64	2.69
15	1.75	2.07	2.24	2.36	2.44	2.51	2.57	2.62	2.67
16	1.75	2.06	2.23	2.34	2.43	2.50	2.56	2.61	2.65
17	1.74	2.05	2.22	2.33	2.42	2.49	2.54	2.59	2.64
18	1.73	2.04	2.21	2.32	2.41	2.48	2.53	2.58	2.62
19	1.73	2.03	2.20	2.31	2.40	2.47	2.52	2.57	2.61
20	1.72	2.03	2.19	2.30	2.39	2.46	2.51	2.56	2.60
24	1.71	2.01	2.17	2.28	2.36	2.43	2.48	2.53	2.57
30	1.70	1.99	2.15	2.25	2.33	2.40	2.45	2.50	2.54
40	1.68	1.97	2.13	2.23	2.31	2.37	2.42	2.47	2.51
60	1.67	1.95	2.10	2.21	2.28	2.35	2.39	2.44	2.48
120	1.66	1.93	2.08	2.18	2.26	2.32	2.37	2.41	2.45
∞	1.64	1.92	2.06	2.16	2.23	2.29	2.34	2.38	2.42

(Continued)

TABLE A.13 (Continued)

				$d_{0.01}(a-1, f)$ One-Sided Comparisons (continued) $a-1$ = Number of Treatment Means (excluding control)					
f	1	2	3	4	5	6	7	8	9
5	3.37	3.90	4.21	4.43	4.60	4.73	4.85	4.94	5.03
6	3.14	3.61	3.88	4.07	4.21	4.33	4.43	4.51	4.59
7	3.00	3.42	3.66	3.83	3.96	4.07	4.15	4.23	4.30
8	2.90	3.29	3.51	3.67	3.79	3.88	3.96	4.03	4.09
9	2.82	3.19	3.40	3.55	3.66	3.75	3.82	3.89	3.94
10	2.76	3.11	3.31	3.45	3.56	3.64	3.71	3.78	3.83
11	2.72	3.06	3.25	3.38	3.48	3.56	3.63	3.69	3.74
12	2.68	3.01	3.19	3.32	3.42	3.50	3.56	3.62	3.67
13	2.65	2.97	3.15	3.27	3.37	3.44	3.51	3.56	3.61
14	2.62	2.94	3.11	3.23	3.32	3.40	3.46	3.51	3.56
15	2.60	2.91	3.08	3.20	3.29	3.36	3.42	3.47	3.52
16	2.58	2.88	3.05	3.17	3.26	3.33	3.39	3.44	3.48
17	2.57	2.86	3.03	3.14	3.23	3.30	3.36	3.41	3.45
18	2.55	2.84	3.01	3.12	3.21	3.27	3.33	3.38	3.42
19	2.54	2.83	2.99	3.10	3.18	3.25	3.31	3.36	3.40
20	2.53	2.81	2.97	3.08	3.17	3.23	3.29	3.34	3.38
24	2.49	2.77	2.92	3.03	3.11	3.17	3.22	3.27	3.31
30	2.46	2.72	2.87	2.97	3.05	3.11	3.16	3.21	3.24
40	2.42	2.68	2.82	2.92	2.99	3.05	3.10	3.14	3.18
60	2.39	2.64	2.78	2.87	2.94	3.00	3.04	3.08	3.12
120	2.36	2.60	2.73	2.82	2.89	2.94	2.99	3.03	3.06
∞	2.33	2.56	2.68	2.77	2.84	2.89	2.93	2.97	3.00

TABLE A.14   Hartley Distribution
Entry Is $H(1 - \alpha; r, df)$ where $P\{H \leqslant H(1 - \alpha; r, df)\} = 1 - \alpha$

$1-\alpha = 0.95$

r

df	2	3	4	5	6	7	8	9	10	11	12
2	39.0	87.5	142	202	266	333	403	475	550	626	704
3	15.4	27.8	39.2	50.7	62.0	72.9	83.5	93.9	104	114	124
4	9.60	15.5	20.6	25.2	29.5	33.6	37.5	41.1	44.6	48.0	51.4
5	7.15	10.8	13.7	16.3	18.7	20.8	22.9	24.7	26.5	28.2	29.9
6	5.82	8.38	10.4	12.1	13.7	15.0	16.3	17.5	18.6	19.7	20.7
7	4.99	6.94	8.44	9.70	10.8	11.8	12.7	13.5	14.3	15.1	15.8
8	4.43	6.00	7.18	8.12	9.03	9.78	10.5	11.1	11.7	12.2	12.7
9	4.03	5.34	6.31	7.11	7.80	8.41	8.95	9.45	9.91	10.3	10.7
10	3.72	4.85	5.67	6.34	6.92	7.42	7.87	8.28	8.66	9.01	9.34
12	3.28	4.16	4.79	5.30	5.72	6.09	6.42	6.72	7.00	7.25	7.48
15	2.86	3.54	4.01	4.37	4.68	4.95	5.19	5.40	5.59	5.77	5.93
20	2.46	2.95	3.29	3.54	3.76	3.94	4.10	4.24	4.37	4.49	4.59
30	2.07	2.40	2.61	2.78	2.91	3.02	3.12	3.21	3.29	3.36	3.39
60	1.67	1.85	1.96	2.04	2.11	2.17	2.22	2.2	2.30	2.33	2.36
∞	1.00	1.00	1.00	1.00	1.00	1.00	1.00	1.00	1.00	1.00	1.00

$1-\alpha = 0.99$

r

df	2	3	4	5	6	7	8	9	10	11	12
2	199	448	729	1,036	1,362	1,705	2,063	2,432	2,813	3,204	3,605
3	47.5	85	120	151	184	216	249	281	310	337	361
4	23.2	37	49	59	69	79	89	97	106	113	120
5	14.9	22	28	33	38	42	46	50	54	57	60
6	11.1	15.5	19.1	22	25	27	30	32	34	36	37
7	8.89	12.1	14.5	16.5	18.4	20	22	23	24	26	27
8	7.50	9.9	11.7	13.2	14.5	15.8	16.9	17.9	18.9	19.8	21
9	6.54	8.5	9.9	11.1	12.1	13.1	13.9	14.7	15.3	16.0	16.6
10	5.85	7.4	8.6	9.6	10.4	11.1	11.8	12.4	12.9	13.4	13.9
12	4.91	6.1	6.9	7.6	8.2	8.7	9.1	9.5	9.9	10.2	10.6
15	4.07	4.9	5.5	6.0	6.4	6.7	7.1	7.3	7.5	7.8	8.0
20	3.32	3.8	4.3	4.6	4.9	5.1	5.3	5.5	5.6	5.8	5.9
30	2.63	3.0	3.3	3.4	3.6	3.7	3.8	3.9	4.0	4.1	4.2
60	1.96	2.2	2.3	2.4	2.4	2.5	2.5	2.6	2.6	2.7	2.7
∞	1.00	1.0	1.0	1.0	1.0	1.0	1.0	1.0	1.0	1.0	1.0

TABLE A.15 Spearman Test Statistic Table
Critical Values of Spearman Test Statistic
Approximate Upper Tail Critical Values $r \not< s_1$,
Where $P(r_s > r_s) = \alpha, n = 4(1)30$.

n	.001	.005	.010	.025	.050	.100
4	—	—	—	—	.8000	.8000
5	—	—	.9000	.9000	.8000	.7000
6	—	.9429	.8857	.8286	.7714	.6000
7	.9643	.8929	.8571	.7450	.6786	.5357
8	.9286	.8571	.8095	.7143	.6190	.5000
9	.9000	.8167	.7667	.6833	.5833	.4667
10	.8667	.7818	.7333	.6364	.5515	.4424
11	.8364	.7545	.7000	.6091	.5273	.4182
12	.8182	.7273	.6713	.5804	.4965	.3986
13	.7912	.6978	.6429	.5549	.4780	.3791
14	.7670	.6747	.6220	.5341	.4593	.3626
15	.7464	.6536	.6000	.5179	.4429	.3500
16	.7265	.6324	.5824	.5000	.4265	.3382
17	.7083	.6152	.5637	.4853	.4118	.3260
18	.6904	.5975	.5480	.4716	.3994	.3148
19	.6737	.5825	.5333	.4579	.3895	.3070
20	.6586	.5684	.5203	.4451	.3789	.2977
21	.6455	.5545	.5078	.4351	.3688	.2909
22	.6318	.5426	.4963	.4241	.3597	.2829
23	.6186	.5306	.4852	.4150	.3518	.2767
24	.6070	.5200	.4748	.4061	.3435	.2704
25	.5962	.5100	.4654	.3977	.3362	.2646
26	.5856	.5002	.4564	.3894	.3299	.2588
27	.5757	.4915	.4481	.3822	.3236	.2540
28	.5660	.4828	.4401	.3749	.3175	.2490
29	.5567	.4744	.4320	.3685	.3113	.2443
30	.5479	.4665	.4251	.3620	.3059	.2400

Note: The corresponding lower tail critical value for r_s is $-r_s^*$.
Source: Glasser GJ, Winter RF. Values of the coefficient of rank correlation for testing the hypothesis of independence. *Biometrika* 48:444–448. This table incorporates corrections appearing in Conover WJ. Practical Nonparametric Statistics. New York: Wiley, 1971.

TABLE A.16 Fisher Z Transformation Table

$$Values\ of\ \frac{1}{2}log_{10}\frac{1+r}{1-r}\ for\ Given\ Values\ of\ r$$

r	0.000	0.001	0.002	0.003	0.004	0.005	0.006	0.007	0.008	0.009
0.000	0.0000	0.0010	0.0020	0.0030	0.0040	0.0050	0.0060	0.0070	0.0080	0.0090
0.010	0.0100	0.0110	0.0120	0.0130	0.0140	0.0150	0.0160	0.0170	0.0180	0.0190
0.020	0.0200	0.0210	0.0220	0.0230	0.0240	0.0250	0.0260	0.0270	0.0280	0.0290
0.030	0.0300	0.0310	0.0320	0.0330	0.0340	0.0350	0.0360	0.0370	0.0380	0.0390
0.040	0.0400	0.0410	0.0420	0.0430	0.0440	0.0450	0.0460	0.0470	0.0480	0.0490
0.050	0.0501	0.0511	0.0521	0.0531	0.0541	0.0551	0.0561	0.0571	0.0581	0.0591
0.060	0.0601	0.0611	0.0621	0.0631	0.0641	0.0651	0.0661	0.0671	0.0681	0.0691
0.070	0.0701	0.0711	0.0721	0.0731	0.0741	0.0751	0.0761	0.0771	0.0782	0.0792
0.080	0.0802	0.0812	0.0822	0.0832	0.0842	0.0852	0.0862	0.0872	0.0882	0.0892
0.090	0.0902	0.0912	0.0922	0.0933	0.0943	0.0953	0.0963	0.0973	0.0983	0.0993
0.100	0.1003	0.1013	0.1024	0.1034	0.1044	0.1054	0.1064	0.1074	0.1084	0.1094
0.110	0.1105	0.1115	0.1125	0.1135	0.1145	0.1155	0.1165	0.1175	0.1185	0.1195
0.120	0.1206	0.1216	0.1226	0.1236	0.1246	0.1257	0.1267	0.1277	0.1287	0.1297
0.130	0.1308	0.1318	0.1328	0.1338	0.1348	0.1358	0.1368	0.1379	0.1389	0.1399
0.140	0.1409	0.1419	0.1430	0.1440	0.1450	0.1460	0.1470	0.1481	0.1491	0.1501
0.150	0.1511	0.1522	0.1532	0.1542	0.1552	0.1563	0.1573	0.1583	0.1593	0.1604
0.160	0.1614	0.1624	0.1634	0.1644	0.1655	0.1665	0.1676	0.1686	0.1696	0.1706
0.170	0.1717	0.1727	0.1737	0.1748	0.1758	0.1768	0.1779	0.1789	0.1799	0.1810
0.180	0.1820	0.1830	0.1841	0.1851	0.1861	0.1872	0.1882	0.1892	0.1903	0.1913
0.190	0.1923	0.1934	0.1944	0.1954	0.1965	0.1975	0.1986	0.1996	0.2007	0.2017
0.200	0.2027	0.2038	0.2048	0.2059	0.2069	0.2079	0.2090	0.2100	0.2111	0.2121
0.210	0.2132	0.2142	0.2153	0.2163	0.2174	0.2184	0.2194	0.2205	0.2215	0.2226
0.220	0.2237	0.2247	0.2258	0.2268	0.2279	0.2289	0.2300	0.2310	0.2321	0.2331
0.230	0.2342	0.2353	0.2363	0.2374	0.2384	0.2395	0.2405	0.2416	0.2427	0.2437
0.240	0.2448	0.2458	0.2469	0.2480	0.2490	0.2501	0.2511	0.2522	0.2533	0.2543
0.250	0.2554	0.2565	0.2575	0.2586	0.2597	0.2608	0.2618	0.2629	0.2640	0.2650
0.260	0.2661	0.2672	0.2682	0.2693	0.2704	0.2715	0.2726	0.2736	0.2747	0.2758
0.270	0.2769	0.2779	0.2790	0.2801	0.2812	0.2823	0.2833	0.2844	0.2855	0.2866
0.280	0.2877	0.2888	0.2898	0.2909	0.2920	0.2931	0.2942	0.2953	0.2964	0.2975
0.290	0.2986	0.2997	0.3008	0.3019	0.3029	0.3040	0.3051	0.3062	0.3073	0.3084
0.300	0.3095	0.3106	0.3117	0.3128	0.3139	0.3150	0.3161	0.3172	0.3183	0.3195
0.310	0.3206	0.3217	0.3228	0.3239	0.3250	0.3261	0.3272	0.3283	0.3294	0.3305
0.320	0.3317	0.3328	0.3339	0.3350	0.3361	0.3372	0.3384	0.3395	0.3406	0.3417
0.330	0.3428	0.3439	0.3451	0.3462	0.3473	0.3484	0.3496	0.3507	0.3518	0.3530
0.340	0.3541	0.3552	0.3564	0.3575	0.3586	0.3597	0.3609	0.3620	0.3632	0.3643
0.350	0.3654	0.3666	0.3677	0.3689	0.3700	0.3712	0.3723	0.3734	0.3746	0.3757
0.360	0.3769	0.3780	0.3792	0.3803	0.3815	0.3826	0.3838	0.3850	0.3861	0.3873

(Continued)

TABLE A.16 (Continued)

r	0.000	0.001	0.002	0.003	0.004	0.005	0.006	0.007	0.008	0.009
0.370	0.3884	0.3896	0.3907	0.3919	0.3931	0.3942	0.3954	0.3966	0.3977	0.3989
0.380	0.4001	0.4012	0.4024	0.4036	0.4047	0.4059	0.4071	0.4083	0.4094	0.4106
0.390	0.4118	0.4130	0.4142	0.4153	0.4165	0.4177	0.4189	0.4201	0.4213	0.4225
0.400	0.4236	0.4248	0.4260	0.4272	0.4284	0.4296	0.4308	0.4320	0.4332	0.4344
0.410	0.4356	0.4368	0.4380	0.4392	0.4404	0.4416	0.4429	0.4441	0.4453	0.4465
0.420	0.4477	0.4489	0.4501	0.4513	0.4526	0.4538	0.4550	0.4562	0.4574	0.4587
0.430	0.4599	0.4611	0.4623	0.4636	0.4648	0.4660	0.4673	0.4685	0.4697	0.4710
0.440	0.4722	0.4735	0.4747	0.4760	0.4772	0.4784	0.4797	0.4809	0.4822	0.4835
0.450	0.4847	0.4860	0.4872	0.4885	0.4897	0.4910	0.4923	0.4935	0.4948	0.4061
0.460	0.4973	0.4986	0.4999	0.5011	0.5024	0.5037	0.5049	0.5062	0.5075	0.5088
0.470	0.5101	0.5114	0.5126	0.5139	0.5152	0.5165	0.5178	0.5191	0.5204	0.5217
0.480	0.5230	0.5243	0.5256	0.5279	0.5282	0.5295	0.5308	0.5321	0.5334	0.5347
0.490	0.5361	0.5374	0.5387	0.5400	0.5413	0.5427	0.5440	0.5453	0.5466	0.5480
0.500	0.5493	0.5506	0.5520	0.5533	0.5547	0.5560	0.5573	0.5587	0.5600	0.5614
0.510	0.5627	0.5641	0.5654	0.5668	0.5681	0.5695	0.5709	0.5722	0.5736	0.5750
0.520	0.5763	0.5777	0.5791	0.5805	0.5818	0.5832	0.5846	0.5860	0.5874	0.5888
0.530	0.5901	0.5915	0.5929	0.5943	0.5957	0.5971	0.5985	0.5999	0.6013	0.6027
0.540	0.6042	0.6056	0.6070	0.6084	0.6098	0.6112	0.6127	0.6141	0.6155	0.6170
0.550	0.6184	0.6198	0.6213	0.6227	0.6241	0.6256	0.6270	0.6285	0.6299	0.6314
0.560	0.6328	0.6343	0.6358	0.6372	0.6387	0.6401	0.6416	0.6431	0.6446	0.6460
0.570	0.6475	0.6490	0.6505	0.6520	0.6535	0.6550	0.6565	0.6579	0.6594	0.6610
0.580	0.6625	0.6640	0.6655	0.6670	0.6685	0.6700	0.6715	0.6731	0.6746	0.6761
0.590	0.6777	0.6792	0.6807	0.6823	0.6838	0.6854	0.6869	0.6885	0.6900	0.6916
0.600	0.6931	0.6947	0.6963	0.6978	0.6994	0.7010	0.7026	0.7042	0.7057	0.7073
0.610	0.7089	0.7105	0.7121	0.7137	0.7153	0.7169	0.7185	0.7201	0.7218	0.7234
0.620	0.7250	0.7266	0.7283	0.7299	0.7315	0.7332	0.7348	0.7364	0.7381	0.7398
0.630	0.7414	0.7431	0.7447	0.7464	0.7481	0.7497	0.7514	0.7531	0.7548	0.7565
0.640	0.7582	0.7599	0.7616	0.7633	0.7650	0.7667	0.7684	0.7701	0.7718	0.7736
0.650	0.7753	0.7770	0.7788	0.7805	0.7823	0.7840	0.7858	0.7875	0.7893	0.7910
0.660	0.7928	0.7946	0.7964	0.7981	0.7999	0.8017	0.8035	0.8053	0.8071	0.8089
0.670	0.8107	0.8126	0.8144	0.8162	0.8180	0.8199	0.8217	0.8236	0.8254	0.8273
0.680	0.8291	0.8310	0.8328	0.8347	0.8366	0.8385	0.8404	0.8423	0.8442	0.8461
0.690	0.8480	0.8499	0.8518	0.8537	0.8556	0.8576	0.8595	0.8614	0.8634	0.8653
0.700	0.8673	0.8693	0.8712	0.8732	0.8752	0.8772	0.8792	0.8812	0.8832	0.8852
0.710	0.8872	0.8892	0.8912	0.8933	0.8953	0.8973	0.8994	0.9014	0.9035	0.9056
0.720	0.9076	0.9097	0.9118	0.9139	9.9160	0.9181	0.9202	0.9223	0.9245	0.9266
0.730	0.9287	0.9309	0.9330	0.9352	0.9373	0.9395	0.9417	0.9439	0.9461	0.9483
0.740	0.9505	0.9527	0.9549	0.9571	0.9594	0.9616	0.9639	0.9661	0.9684	0.9707
0.750	0.9730	0.9752	0.9775	0.9799	0.9822	0.9845	0.9868	0.9892	0.9915	0.9939
0.760	0.9962	0.9986	1.0010	1.0034	1.0058	1.0082	1.0106	1.0130	1.0154	1.0179

(Continued)

TABLE A.16 (Continued)

r	0.000	0.001	0.002	0.003	0.004	0.005	0.006	0.007	0.008	0.009
0.770	1.0203	1.0228	1.0253	1.0277	1.0302	1.0327	1.0352	1.0378	1.0403	1.0428
0.780	1.0454	1.0479	1.0505	1.0531	1.0557	1.0583	1.0609	1.0635	1.0661	1.0688
0.790	1.0714	1.0741	1.0768	1.0795	1.0822	1.0849	1.0876	1.0903	1.0931	1.0958
0.800	1.0986	1.1014	1.1041	1.1070	1.1098	1.1127	1.1155	1.1184	1.1212	1.1241
0.810	1.1270	1.1299	1.1329	1.1358	1.1388	1.1417	1.1447	1.1477	1.1507	1.1538
0.820	1.1568	1.1599	1.1630	1.1660	1.1692	1.1723	1.1754	1.1786	1.1817	1.1849
0.830	1.1870	1.1913	1.1946	1.1979	1.2011	1.2044	1.2077	1.2111	1.2144	1.2178
0.840	1.2212	1.2246	1.2280	1.2315	1.2349	1.2384	1.2419	1.2454	1.2490	1.2526
0.850	1.2561	1.2598	1.2634	1.2670	1.2708	1.2744	1.2782	1.2819	1.2857	1.2895
0.860	1.2934	1.2972	1.3011	1.3050	1.3089	1.3129	1.3168	1.3209	1.3249	1.3290
0.870	1.3331	1.3372	1.3414	1.3456	1.3498	1.3540	1.3583	1.3626	1.3670	1.3714
0.880	1.3758	1.3802	1.3847	1.3892	1.3938	1.3984	1.4030	1.4077	1.4124	1.4171
0.890	1.4219	1.4268	1.4316	1.4366	1.4415	1.4465	1.4516	1.4566	1.4618	1.4670
0.900	1.4722	1.4775	1.4828	1.4883	1.4937	1.4992	1.5047	1.5103	1.5160	1.5217
0.910	1.5275	1.5334	1.5393	1.5453	1.5513	1.5574	1.5636	1.5698	1.5762	1.5825
0.920	1.5890	1.5956	1.6022	1.6089	1.6157	1.6226	1.6296	1.6366	1.6438	1.6510
0.930	1.6584	1.6659	1.6734	1.6811	1.6888	1.6967	1.7047	1.7129	1.7211	1.7295
0.940	1.7380	1.7467	1.7555	1.7645	1.7736	1.7828	1.7923	1.8019	1.8117	1.8216
0.950	1.8318	1.8421	1.8527	1.8635	1.8745	1.8857	1.8972	1.9090	1.9210	1.9333
0.960	1.9459	1.9588	1.9721	1.9857	1.9996	2.0140	2.0287	2.0439	2.0595	2.0756
0.970	2.0923	2.1095	2.1273	2.1457	2.1649	2.1847	2.2054	2.2269	2.2494	2.2729
0.980	2.2976	2.3223	2.3507	2.3796	2.4101	2.4426	2.4774	2.5147	2.5550	2.5988
0.990	2.6467	2.6996	2.7587	2.8257	2.9031	2.9945	3.1063	3.2504	3.4534	3.8002

r	z
0.9999	4.95172
0.99999	6.10303

Note: To obtain $\frac{1}{2}\log_e\left[(1+r)/(1-r)\right]$ when r is negative, use the negative of the value corresponding to the absolute value of r, e.g., $r = -0.242$, $\frac{1}{2}\log_e\left[(1+0.242)/(1-0.242)\right] = -0.2469$.
Source: Waugh AE. Statistical Tables and Problems. New York: McGraw-Hill, 1952, Table A11, pp 40–41.

TABLE A.17   POWER VALUES FOR TWO-TAIL t TEST

df	1.0	2.0	3.0	4.0	α = 0.01 δ 5.0	6.0	7.0	8.0	9.0
1	.01	.03	.04	.05	.06	.08	.09	.10	.11
2	.02	.05	.09	.16	.23	.31	.39	.48	.56
3	.02	.08	.17	.31	.47	.62	.75	.85	.92
4	.03	.10	.25	.45	.65	.82	.92	.97	.99
5	.03	.12	.31	.55	.77	.91	.97	.99	1.00
6	.04	.14	.36	.63	.84	.95	.99	1.00	1.00
7	.04	.16	.40	.68	.88	.97	1.00	1.00	1.00
8	.04	.17	.43	.72	.91	.98	1.00	1.00	1.00
9	.04	.18	.45	.75	.93	.99	1.00	1.00	1.00
10	.04	.19	.47	.77	.94	.99	1.00	1.00	1.00
11	.04	.19	.49	.79	.95	.99	1.00	1.00	1.00
12	.04	.20	.50	.80	.96	.99	1.00	1.00	1.00
13	.05	.21	.52	.82	.96	1.00	1.00	1.00	1.00
14	.05	.21	.53	.83	.96	1.00	1.00	1.00	1.00
15	.05	.21	.54	.83	.97	1.00	1.00	1.00	1.00
16	.05	.22	.55	.84	.97	1.00	1.00	1.00	1.00
17	.05	.22	.55	.85	.97	1.00	1.00	1.00	1.00
18	.05	.22	.56	.85	.97	1.00	1.00	1.00	1.00
19	.05	.23	.56	.86	.98	1.00	1.00	1.00	1.00
20	.05	.23	.57	.86	.98	1.00	1.00	1.00	1.00
21	.05	.23	.57	.86	.98	1.00	1.00	1.00	1.00
22	.05	.23	.58	.87	.98	1.00	1.00	1.00	1.00
23	.05	.24	.58	.87	.98	1.00	1.00	1.00	1.00
24	.05	.24	.59	.87	.98	1.00	1.00	1.00	1.00
25	.05	.24	.59	.88	.98	1.00	1.00	1.00	1.00
26	.05	.24	.59	.88	.98	1.00	1.00	1.00	1.00
27	.05	.24	.59	.88	.98	1.00	1.00	1.00	1.00
28	.05	.24	.60	.88	.98	1.00	1.00	1.00	1.00
29	.05	.25	.60	.88	.98	1.00	1.00	1.00	1.00
30	.05	.25	.60	.88	.98	1.00	1.00	1.00	1.00
40	.05	.26	.62	.90	.99	1.00	1.00	1.00	1.00
50	.05	.26	.63	.90	.99	1.00	1.00	1.00	1.00
60	.05	.26	.63	.91	.99	1.00	1.00	1.00	1.00
100	.06	.27	.65	.91	.99	1.00	1.00	1.00	1.00
120	.06	.27	.65	.91	.99	1.00	1.00	1.00	1.00
∞	.06	.28	.66	.92	.99	1.00	1.00	1.00	1.00

(Continued)

TABLE A.17 (Continued)

df	1.0	2.0	3.0	4.0	5.0	6.0	7.0	8.0	9.0
					$\alpha = 0.05$ δ				
1	.07	.13	.19	.25	.31	.36	.42	.47	.52
2	.10	.22	.39	.56	.72	.84	.91	.96	.98
3	.11	.29	.53	.75	.90	.97	.99	1.00	1.00
4	.12	.34	.62	.84	.95	.99	1.00	1.00	1.00
5	.13	.37	.67	.89	.98	1.00	1.00	1.00	1.00
6	.14	.39	.71	.91	.98	1.00	1.00	1.00	1.00
7	.14	.41	.73	.93	.99	1.00	1.00	1.00	1.00
8	.14	.42	.75	.94	.99	1.00	1.00	1.00	1.00
9	.15	.43	.76	.94	.99	1.00	1.00	1.00	1.00
10	.15	.44	.77	.95	.99	1.00	1.00	1.00	1.00
11	.15	.45	.78	.95	.99	1.00	1.00	1.00	1.00
12	.15	.45	.79	.96	1.00	1.00	1.00	1.00	1.00
13	.15	.46	.79	.96	1.00	1.00	1.00	1.00	1.00
14	.15	.46	.80	.96	1.00	1.00	1.00	1.00	1.00
15	.16	.46	.80	.96	1.00	1.00	1.00	1.00	1.00
16	.16	.47	.80	.96	1.00	1.00	1.00	1.00	1.00
17	.16	.47	.81	.96	1.00	1.00	1.00	1.00	1.00
18	.16	.47	.81	.97	1.00	1.00	1.00	1.00	1.00
19	.16	.48	.81	.97	1.00	1.00	1.00	1.00	1.00
20	.16	.48	.81	.97	1.00	1.00	1.00	1.00	1.00
21	.16	.48	.82	.97	1.00	1.00	1.00	1.00	1.00
22	.16	.48	.82	.97	1.00	1.00	1.00	1.00	1.00
23	.16	.48	.82	.97	1.00	1.00	1.00	1.00	1.00
24	.16	.48	.82	.97	1.00	1.00	1.00	1.00	1.00
25	.16	.49	.82	.97	1.00	1.00	1.00	1.00	1.00
26	.16	.49	.82	.97	1.00	1.00	1.00	1.00	1.00
27	.16	.49	.82	.97	1.00	1.00	1.00	1.00	1.00
28	.16	.49	.83	.97	1.00	1.00	1.00	1.00	1.00
29	.16	.49	.83	.97	1.00	1.00	1.00	1.00	1.00
30	.16	.49	.83	.97	1.00	1.00	1.00	1.00	1.00
40	.16	.50	.83	.97	1.00	1.00	1.00	1.00	1.00
50	.17	.50	.84	.98	1.00	1.00	1.00	1.00	1.00
60	.17	.50	.84	.98	1.00	1.00	1.00	1.00	1.00
100	.17	.51	.84	.98	1.00	1.00	1.00	1.00	1.00
120	.17	.51	.85	.98	1.00	1.00	1.00	1.00	1.00
∞	.17	.52	.85	.98	1.00	1.00	1.00	1.00	1.00

References

1. DS Paulson. *Topical Antimicrobial Testing and Evaluation*. New York: Marcel Dekker, 1999.
2. WW Daniel. *Biostatistics*. New York: John Wiley & Sons, 1999.
3. CR Hicks, KV Turner, Jr. *Fundamental Concepts in the Design of Experiments*, 5th ed. New York: Oxford Press, 1999.
4. DO Sears, LA Peplau, SE Taylor. *Social Psychology*, 7th ed. New York: McGraw-Hill, 1991.
5. D Polkinghorne. *Methodology for the Human Sciences*. State University of Albany: New York Press, NY, 1983.
6. R Searle. *The Construction of Social Reality*. New York: Free Press, 1995.
7. F Varela, J Shear. *The View from Within*. Lawrence, KS: Imprint Academic Press, 1999.
8. GW Snedecor, WG Cochran. *Statistical Methods*, 6th ed. Ames, IA: Iowa State University Press, 1967.
9. BW Brown, Jr., M Hollander. *Statistics: A Biomedical Introduction*. John Wiley & Sons, New York, 1977.
10. HE Rheinhardt, DO Loftsgaarden. *Elementary Probability and Statistical Reasoning*. Lexington, MA: D C Heath & Company, 1977.
11. LH Koopmans. *An Introduction to Contemporary Statistics*. Boston, MA: Duxbury Press, 1981.
12. RH Green. *Sampling Designs and Statistical Methods for Environmental Biologists*. New York: John Wiley & Sons, 1979.
13. E Peresini. Personal communication. College of Great Falls, Great Falls, MT, 1978.
14. JW Tukey. *Exploratory Data Analysis*. Reading, MA: Addison-Wesley, 1971.

15. F Mosteller, JW Tukey. *Data Analysis and Regression: A Second Course in Statistics*. Reading, MA: Addison-Wesley, 1977.
16. R McGill, JW Tukey, WA Larsen. Varieties of box plots. The American statistician 32:12–16, Washington, DC: American Statistical Association, 1978.
17. DS Paulson. *Topical Antimicrobial Testing and Evaluation*. New York: Marcel Dekker, 1999.
18. PF Velkman, DC Hoaglin. Applications, Basics and Computing of Exploratory Data Analysis. Boston, MA: Duxbury Press, 1981.
19. RGT Steel, JH Torrie, DA Dickey. *Principles and Procedures of Statistics: A Biometrical Approach*, 3rd ed. New York: McGraw-Hill, 1997.
20. WJ Dixon, FJ Massey. *Introduction to Statistical Analysis*, 4th ed. New York: McGraw-Hill, 1983.
21. RE Kirk. *Experimental Design*, 3rd ed. Pacific Grove, CA: Brooks-Cole Publishing, 1995.
22. OJ Dunn, VA Clark. *Applied Statistics*. New York: John Wiley & Sons, 1974.
23. RA Newton, KE Rudstam. *Your Statistical Consultant*. Thousand Oaks, CA: Sage Publishing, 1999.
24. JH Zar. *Biostatistical Analysis*, 4th ed. Upper Saddle River: Prentice-Hall, NJ, 1999.
25. RA Fisher. *Statistical Methods for Research Workers*, 13th ed. Oliver & Boyd: Edinburgh, Scotland, 1958.
26. J Neter, MH Kutner, CJ Nachtsheim & W. Wasserman. *Applied Statistical Models*, 4th ed. New York: McGraw-Hill, 1996.
27. RO Kuehl. *Design of Experiments*, 2nd ed. Pacific Grove, CA: Brooks/Cole, 2000.
28. DC Montgomery. *Design and Analysis of Experiments*, 5th ed. New York: John Wiley & Sons, 2001.
29. GEP Box, WG Hunger, SJ Hunter. *Statistics for Experiments*. New York: John Wiley, 1978.
30. VG Anderson, RA McClean. *Design of Experiments: A Realistic Approach*. New York: Marcel Dekker, 1974.
31. BL Bowerman, RT O'Connell. *Forecasting and Time Series: An Applied Approach*. Belmont, CA: Duxbury Press, 1979.
32. NR Draper, H Smith. *Applied Regression Analysis*, 3rd ed. New York: John Wiley & Sons, 1998.
33. J Neter, W Wasserman, MH Kutner. *Applied Linear Regression Models*. Homewood, IL: Richard Irwin, 1983.
34. AJ Hayter. The maximum family-wise error rate of Fisher's least significant difference test. *Journal of the American Statistical Association*, 81:1000–1004, 1986.
35. DG Kleinbaum, LL Kupper, KE Muller. *Applied Regression Analysis and Other Multivariable Methods*, 2nd ed. Boston, MA: Plus-Kent Publishing, 1988.
36. SJ Pocock. *Clinical Trials*. New York: John Wiley & Sons, 1983.

37. DG Kleinbaum, LL Kupper. *Applied Regression Analysis and Other Multivariable Methods.* Belmont, CA: Duxbury Press, 1978.
38. C Daniel, FS Wood. *Fitting Equations to Data*, 2nd ed. New York: John Wiley & Sons, 1980.
39. TH Wonnacott, RJ Wonnacott. *Regression: A Second Course in Statistics.* New York: John Wiley & Sons, 1980.
40. DC Hoaglin, F Mostellar, JW Tukey. *Exploring Data Tables, Trends, and Shapes.* New York: John Wiley & Sons, 1985.
41. WW Daniel. *Applied Nonparametric Statistics.* Boston, MA: Houghton Mifflin, 1978.
42. WJ Conover. *Practical Nonparametric Statistics*, 2nd ed. New York: John Wiley & Sons, 1980.
43. WJ Conover. *Practical Nonparametric Statistics*, 3rd ed. New York: John Wiley & Sons, 1999.
44. S Siegel, NJ Castellan. *Nonparametric Statistics for the Behavioral Sciences*, 2nd ed. New York: McGraw Hill, 1988.
45. JD Gibbons. *Nonparametric Methods for Quantitative Analysis.* New York: Holt, Rinehart & Winston, 1976.
46. F Mostellar, REK Rourke. *Sturdy Statistics: Nonparametric and Order Statistics.* Reading, MA: Addison-Wesley, 1973.
47. EL Lehmann. *Nonparametrics: Statistical Methods Based on Ranks.* San Francisco: Holden-Day, Inc., 1975.
48. WH Kruskal. A nonparametric test for the several sample problems. *Ann Math Stat* 23:525–540, 1952.
49. M Hollander. A distribution-free test for parallelism. *Journal of American Statistical Association* 65:387–394, 1970.
50. LV Hedges, I Olkin. *Statistical Methods for Meta-analysis.* New York: Academic Press, 1985.
51. H Cooper, LV Hedges. *The Handbook of Research Synthesis.* New York: Sage, 1994.
52. GV Glass, B McGraw, ML Smith. *Meta-analysis in Social Research.* Newbury Park, CA: Sage, 1989.
53. S Piantadosi. *Clinical Trials.* New York: John Wiley & Sons, 1997.

Index

Milton Keynes UK
Ingram Content Group UK Ltd.
UKHW020002071024
449327UK00031B/2627